2/26/68

Gerald E. Swanson, M.D.

1330 St. Paul Ave. St. Paul, Minn.

Principles of HEMATOLOGY

Principles of
HEMATOLOGY

James W. Linman, M.D., F.A.C.P.

Consultant, Section of Clinical Pathology (Hematology), Mayo
Clinic; Associate Professor of Medicine, Mayo Graduate School
of Medicine (University of Minnesota), Rochester. Formerly,
Associate Professor of Medicine, Northwestern University Medical School; Chief, Hematology Section, Veterans Administration Research Hospital, Chicago.

THE MACMILLAN COMPANY, New York
COLLIER-MACMILLAN LIMITED, London

First Printing, 1966

Library of Congress catalog card number: 66–20819

The Macmillan Company, New York

Collier-Macmillan Canada, Ltd., Toronto, Ontario

Printed in the United States of America

*Dedicated to my wife, Fran, and
our children—John, Jean, Jim, and Jeff*

Preface

All phases of medicine have benefited greatly in recent years by the acquisition of a tremendous amount of new information. Hematology has gained much from this "biologic revolution." As a result, the physiology and pathophysiology of hematopoiesis have been clarified, mechanisms of disease have been elucidated, diagnosis has been facilitated, and treatment has been made more effective. Rational explanations are now available or are emerging for many hematologic disorders and responses that formerly were understood poorly, if at all. However, it has become a time-consuming and formidable task to keep abreast of the many diverse research accomplishments in this rapidly growing field. Furthermore, it has become increasingly difficult to evaluate complex techniques, interpret experimental results, and assess the significance of new observations without some background training and experience on which to draw.

For these reasons, the teaching of medicine has been at once made easier and harder. It is easier because logical answers can be supplied for many questions that formerly were unanswerable except by empiric statements; it is harder because of the need to make available to students of clinical medicine (undergraduate and graduate) new information in a form they can use and in a quantity with which they can cope. In the past most textbooks followed the encyclopedic approach; however, the growth of medical knowledge has been such that attempts to encompass all available data are no longer practical. Condensation is essential. On the other hand, brief listings of clinical manifestations are totally inadequate for the student of today.

Principles of Hematology was written especially for medical students, interns, resident physicians, and medical practitioners in specialties other than hematology. Its goal is to provide concise clinical descriptions based on modern physiologic and pathophysiologic concepts. Because an understanding of the pathophysiology of disease is requisite for accurate diagnosis and proper treatment, the discussion of each hematologic disorder is preceded by an account of the pertinent physiology. For example, the chapter dealing with iron deficiency anemia begins with a consideration of normal iron metabolism; the section on hemorrhagic disorders, with a description of the normal coagulation mechanism; the chapter on plasmacytic myeloma, with a discussion of immunoglobulin synthesis; and so on. The diagnostic significance of basic clinical observations (the history, physical examination, and routine hematologic studies) is emphasized, and an attempt is made to place certain newer and more complicated techniques in their proper perspective.

This book is not meant to be all-inclusive. Instead, it was planned as an introduction to clinical hematology and as a source of information on which those who desire more detailed knowledge can build. For the latter purpose the reader is referred to existing books that cover the field in a more comprehensive manner, particularly *Clinical Hematology* by Wintrobe. In addition, a selected bibliography is provided. The purpose and nature of this book militated against an attempt to support all conclusions with appropriate references; neither was it intended to serve as a review of the available literature. Consequently, only a fraction of the articles and books used in its preparation have been included in the bibliography; they were selected because of their scope or the basic importance of the observation. In addition to being listed by chapter, the references have been indexed. The reader who desires more information about a particular subject will find, under the appropriate heading(s) in the index, the number(s) of the references containing this material.

Technical details have been omitted intentionally, and the discussions of laboratory procedures have been restricted to the nature of the information they reveal, its interpretation, and significance. Many excellent laboratory manuals and textbooks of clinical pathology are available and should be consulted for instruction in the actual performance of these tests. To have repeated all this information here would have defeated the book's purpose; the alternative, to have arbitrarily included descriptions of a few techniques, would have accomplished little.

Many persons have assisted with this undertaking. I am first of all indebted to my fellow hematologists, past and present, whose clinical and experimental observations have contributed to the development of this subspecialty. It gives me particular pleasure to acknowledge the counsel and encouragement of Dr. Muriel C. Meyers, who reviewed the entire manuscript. I have also been benefited by the advice of Dr. Thomas L. Grisamore, who contributed to all sections, and Dr. Charles A. Owen, Jr., who reviewed the chapter dealing with the hemorrhagic disorders. I am grateful to Dr. Robert V. Pierre for most of the photomicrographs.

I owe a special debt to Mrs. Ivy W. Cordell, who gave important editorial assistance and typed most of the manuscript. Thanks are also due Mrs. Nancy Ashby for her able secretarial help. Mrs. Margaret Hopkinson, librarian at the Veterans Administration Research Hospital, made available promptly and efficiently the many journals and books consulted during this project.

I am most appreciative of the indulgence and support of my colleagues at the Veterans Administration Research Hospital in Chicago and, more recently, the Mayo Clinic. Last, but by no means least, I wish to thank the medical students and residents at the Northwestern University Medical Center who encouraged me to undertake this task and who, together with Fellows at the Mayo Graduate School of Medicine, offered many valuable suggestions. The preparation of this book has been a richly rewarding experience.

J. W. L.

Rochester, Minnesota
February, 1966

Contents

xi

Principles of HEMATOLOGY

The Blood Cells
(*General Considerations*)

CHAPTER

1

There are three types of cellular elements in the blood: *erythrocytes* (red cells), *leukocytes* (white cells), and *thrombocytes* (platelets). Each has its own functions and differs clearly from the others. Because blood cells have finite life-spans, effete cells are being continuously destroyed and replaced. In health destruction is balanced by production, and the quantity and quality of circulating cells remain remarkably constant. Because of their unique activities, singular constituents, and rapid rates of proliferation, the physiology of the blood cells and of the blood-forming organs is at first glance a subject of awesome complexity. However, recent years have witnessed great strides in our understanding of hematopoiesis and its products. Despite many questions remaining unanswered, it is now possible to approach most hematologic problems from the standpoint of their pathophysiology (in some instances at the molecular level). Basic knowledge of the formation, morphology and ultrastructure, biochemistry, and physiology of the blood cells is the foundation of modern clinical hematology.

EMBRYONIC HEMATOPOIESIS

Mesenchyme, the embryonic connective tissue, constitutes the ontogenetic anlage of the blood cells which are first formed in the numerous blood islands of the yolk sac. These mesoblastic elements differentiate in two directions. The peripheral cells form the endothelial lining of the first blood vessels, whereas those that are more centrally located become the

1

primitive blood cells. This *mesoblastic phase* of hematopoiesis is active throughout the first two months of embryonic development; nucleated erythroblasts or hemoglobin-containing cells predominate. At two months intravascular blood formation is replaced by the *hepatic phase*, which is distinguished by active erythropoiesis in the liver as well as in the spleen and, briefly, in the thymus. Granulocytes and megakaryocytes make their appearance about this time; lymphocytes are detectable by the fourth month and monocytes, by the fifth.

During the fifth month of gestation the final or *myeloid phase* has its onset. Proliferation of mesenchymal cells in bone primordia brings about resorption of cartilage and the formation of islets of active hematopoiesis. Early in the myeloid phase the bone marrow is largely concerned with granulopoiesis. Erythropoiesis continues to take place chiefly in the liver (splenic erythropoiesis terminates near the end of the fifth month); however, the bone marrow gradually takes over. At birth intramedullary blood formation has supplanted that occurring in other sites with the exception of lymphocytes, plasmacytes, and probably monocytes. These cell types continue to be formed in extramedullary tissues; for example, in the spleen, thymus, and lymph nodes.

Consequent to the establishment of hematopoiesis in the bone marrow, the primitive mesenchymal cells are reduced to a minimal reticular stroma. These multipotential cells persist throughout life as part of the reticuloendothelial system in the bone marrow, liver, spleen, lymph nodes, and so forth. In the marrow they continue to undergo active hematopoietic differentiation. Elsewhere they remain hematopoietically quiescent but retain intact all of their embryonic potentialities.

POSTNATAL HEMATOPOIESIS

Normal peripheral blood counts are attained only after birth, but the transition from embryonic to postnatal life is not marked by any sudden changes in hematopoiesis. The processes of proliferation and differentiation previously established continue without interruption. After differentiation into a certain cell lineage, multiplication of blood cell precursors occurs chiefly, if not entirely, by homeoplastic mitosis; that is, one cell gives rise to two like cells at a comparable stage of development. In addition to the proliferation of specific precursor cells, hematopoiesis involves progressive maturation with the evolution of the structural and physiologic attributes of each cell type. This process eventuates in a cell that is no longer capable of undergoing mitotic division. Having lost the ability to replicate itself, such a cell has acquired a finite life-span; although still developing, it is now destined for destruction at a predictable time in the future. Thus continued hematopoiesis is contingent on constant replenishment of each cell compartment by the primitive, multipotential stem cells. Hematopoietic tissue is the most rapidly proliferating cellular system in the body.

Origin and Relationship of the Blood Cells. Knowledge of the multiple physiologic activities culminating in the formation of mature blood cells is incomplete. Numerous experimental models have been devised in an attempt to elucidate the many intricacies of hematopoiesis. Much has been learned, but many questions remain unanswered. One of the most perplexing problems concerns the origin of the blood cells and their relationship to each other.

Despite the attention of many investigators for almost a century, dispute and controversy persist. Monophyletic, dualistic, and polyphyletic theories of hematopoiesis have been advanced, depending on the number of precursor cells envisaged. Some workers have maintained that each cell lineage has its own primitive blast cell; others have proposed one precursor for lymphocytes and another for the rest of the blood cells. The third and most popular theory contends that all hemic cells are derived from a common progenitor; such a scheme is depicted in Figure 1-1. There is little doubt that a primitive, pluripotential reticulum

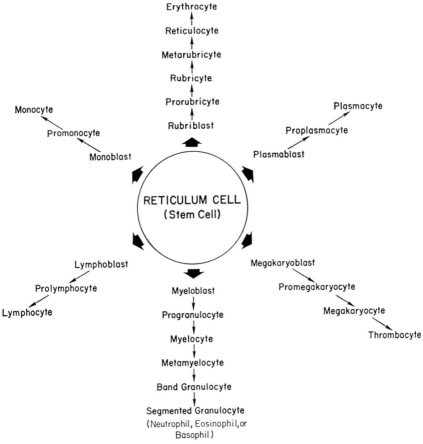

Figure 1-1. Origin of the blood cells.

cell or "stem cell" can undergo differentiation into a specific blood cell compartment. Still problematical are the mechanisms controlling such differentiation, the intermediate steps in this process, and the precise relationship between the lymphoid and myeloid cells. This area of hematologic research is currently an active one, and recent technological advances should contribute importantly to this subject. Pending the revision that may be indicated by future studies, the theory of hematopoiesis shown in Figure 1-1 provides a rational and clinically useful plan.

Although there is persuasive support for the existence of a stem cell compartment, its size cannot be accurately ascertained; neither are the cytologic features of the stem cell well defined. Primitive reticulum cells (Fig. 1-2) make up less than 1 per cent of the nucleated cells

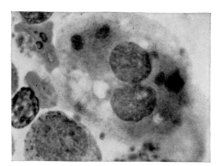 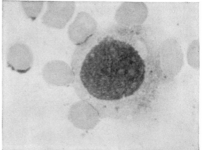

Figure 1-2.   Reticulum cells in a normal marrow aspirate.

in normal bone marrow aspirates. They are more numerous in conditions associated with myeloid hyperplasia; for example, the acute blood loss anemias. In Wright-stained preparations these cells are relatively large (20 to 30 μ in diameter), with abundant, light-blue, opaque cytoplasm occasionally containing a few azurophilic granules. The cell borders are typically irregular. Because reticulum cells are quite fragile, few remain intact in stained films. The nuclei are round to oval, with a finely to coarsely reticulated chromatin pattern which displays sharp contrast between parachromatin and basichromatin; they ordinarily have one to two nucleoli. Marrow reticulum cells are presumably those from which the differentiated blood cell precursors arise. Small numbers of similar cells are demonstrable in Wright-stained imprints of other tissues such as the spleen and lymph nodes. However, it remains conjectural whether marrow reticulum cells and the elusive stem cells are one and the same.

The precursors of each type of blood cell are divisible into several developmental stages based on differences in the cells' activities and morphology. In the past many different names have been given to the developing blood cells, thus leading to confusion and misunderstanding.

A uniform nomenclature is essential. The terminology contained in Figure 1-1 is used throughout this text.

Myelopoiesis. The production of blood cells by the bone marrow is designated *myelopoiesis*. It should be noted that the prefix "myelo-" generally refers to all aspects of bone marrow activity and is not limited to granulocytic elements alone. The only exceptions to this rule are the terms myeloblast, myelocyte, and metamyelocyte, which refer to specific stages in granulocyte maturation (p. 22). Myelopoiesis consists chiefly of erythropoiesis, granulopoiesis, and thrombopoiesis; monocytes also appear to be formed in the marrow as well as elsewhere. Although there are scattered lymphoid follicles in the bone marrow, lymphopoiesis occurs largely in extramedullary sites; for example, the thymus, spleen, and lymph nodes.

Marrow is encased within the medullary cavities of bones and is enclosed by the endosteum. Myelopoiesis takes place extravascularly. Developing and mature blood cells (together with fat cells) lie free in a jellylike substance within a framework made up of scattered reticulum cells and a fibrous network loosely connected to the endosteum and vascular structures. The blood supply is derived from the nutrient arteries, and the arterioles and venules are connected by sinusoids. The sinusoidal walls consist of a single layer of flattened endothelial cells (Fig. 1-3) which make simple contacts with the processes of neigh-

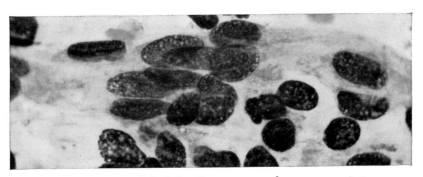

Figure 1-3.   Endothelial cells in a normal marrow aspirate.

boring cells, often leaving visible gaps in the sinusoidal wall. The cells lining the marrow sinusoids have no basement membrane and hardly any stromal support. The sinusoids have a functional flexibility that is absent in most blood vessels. Because of the rigid enclosure surrounding the marrow, the sinusoids cannot all be dilated at the same time. There is no evidence to support the existence of intersinusoidal capillaries. The mechanisms concerned with the release of mature cells from the marrow and their entrance into the circulation are, for the most part, unknown. Because myelopoiesis takes place extravascularly, the cells obviously must traverse the vessel wall. They apparently gain entrance into the sinusoids by diapedesis or, more likely, through gaps or temporary defects in the endothelial wall.

In infants and young children all bones contain red, that is, actively myelopoietic marrow. At four to six years of age fat cells make their appearance. Fat gradually increases and blood cell precursors decrease until the age of 18 to 20 years, when approximately half the marrow is red and the rest is yellow; the yellow marrow consists largely of fat and a few reticulum cells. During the first two decades of life active myelopoiesis recedes centripetally toward the trunk and is confined in adults to the bones of the thorax, vertebrae, skull, pelvis, and proximal portions of the humeri and femora. In the adult the marrow (red and yellow) occupies a volume of about 3000 to 4000 ml and makes up approximately 3.5 to 6 per cent of the body weight; there are about three times as many granulocytes (15×10^9/kg of body weight) as nucleated red cells (5×10^9/ kg).

The precise functions of the large quantity of marrow fat are unknown; 25 to 30 per cent of red bone marrow is fat, and the amount increases with advancing age. This fat, together with that making up the yellow bone marrow, is extremely labile. In situations calling for increased blood cell production, the fat contained in the red marrow is replaced by actively proliferating blood cell precursors. Depending on the persistence and magnitude of the stimulus to myelopoiesis, yellow marrow in other sites such as the shafts of the long bones will eventually be replaced by red marrow. Thus the bone marrow has a substantial functional reserve and can increase its output severalfold (maximum erythrocyte production appears to be six to eight times the normal).

Extramedullary Hematopoiesis. In normal subjects extramedullary hematopoiesis is limited largely to lymphopoiesis. Some lymphocyte production takes place in the bone marrow, but most of the lymphocytes are formed in the thymus, spleen, lymph nodes, and other lymphoid tissues like the Peyer's patches of the intestines and the tonsils. Knowledge of the production of monocytes and plasmacytes is limited, but there is good reason to believe that these blood cells are also formed in extramedullary sites. Erythropoiesis, granulopoiesis, and megakaryocyte production are normally restricted to the bone marrow; the formation of these blood cells in other tissues is an abnormal finding. However, multipotential mesenchymal cells persist throughout life in the spleen, liver, lymph nodes, and other tissues as part of the reticuloendothelial system. The hematopoietic potentialities of these primitive cells, so evident in embryonic development, are intact. They resume active blood cell production in response to a variety of stimuli; for example, severe anemias and leukemia.

MORPHOLOGY, FORMATION, BIOCHEMISTRY, AND PHYSIOLOGY OF THE BLOOD CELLS

The blood cells have much in common, including their sites of formation and apparent derivation from a common stem cell. Under certain circumstances hematopoietic tissue functions as a unit; for example, the increase in erythropoiesis, granulopoiesis, and thrombopoiesis accompanying acute hemorrhage (p. 70). More often, however, each generative compartment functions independently of the others. Furthermore, there are clear-cut differences in the morphology, chemical composition, and physiologic attributes of the different blood cells. Consequently, it is pertinent to consider each type separately.

Erythrocytes

The nonnucleated red cells in the peripheral blood are derived from nucleated precursors in the bone marrow. A number of distinct morphologic and functional stages can be recognized in the development of an erythrocyte and serve as a useful outline of erythropoiesis. As a group, all of the immature and mature erythrocytes in the body are designated the *erythron*. The adjective, *normoblastic*, signifies normal morphology of the nucleated erythrocytic precursors; *megaloblastic* indicates the abnormal morphology of erythrocytic elements characterizing vitamin B_{12} or folic acid deficiency (p. 209). The term *erythroblast* is often used in a generic sense to refer to any or all nucleated red cells. Many names have been used for the developmental stages of an erythrocyte. The following terminology is preferred since accurate definitions are available; a second commonly used set of terms is indicated in parentheses.

MORPHOLOGY

Unless stated otherwise, all morphologic descriptions refer to the appearance of the cells in Wright-stained preparations.

Rubriblast (Proerythroblast). The first recognizable cell of the erythrocytic series is characterized by rather coarsely stippled-to-clumped nuclear chromatin, multiple nucleoli, and scant, hyperchromatic, greenish-blue cytoplasm (Fig. 1-4).

Prorubricyte (Early Normoblast). Nucleoli are still discernible in a prorubricyte, but the nuclear chromatin structure is too coarse to permit its classification as a rubriblast; the nucleus is ordinarily smaller and the basophilic cytoplasm is more abundant than in a more immature cell (Fig. 1-4).

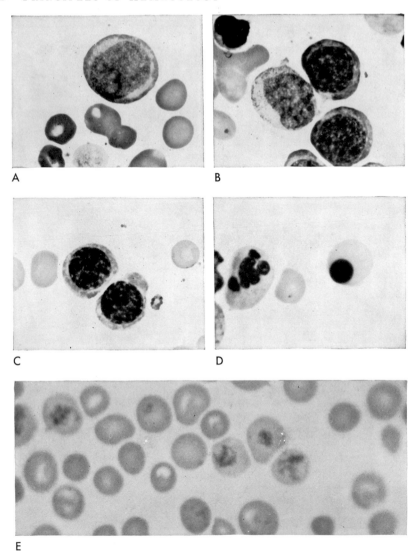

Figure 1-4.   Normal developing erythrocytes. *A.* Rubriblast (proerythroblast). *B.* Prorubricytes (early normoblasts). *C.* Rubricytes (intermediate normoblasts). *D.* Metarubricyte (late normoblast). *E.* Reticulocytes (stained with brilliant cresyl blue and counterstained with Wright's stain).

Rubricyte (Intermediate Normoblast). This erythrocytic precursor possesses a definitive (coarsely clumped) nuclear chromatin structure without nucleoli (Fig. 1-4). These cells may be subdivided into basophilic, polychromatic, or orthochromatic rubricytes based on their complement of hemoglobin.

Metarubricyte (Late Normoblast). A metarubricyte is a nucleated red cell with a pyknotic, fragmented, or partly extruded nucleus consisting of a dense, solid, structureless mass (Fig. 1-4). As a rule, these cells contain nearly normal quantities of hemoglobin, and their cytoplasm is acidophilic or polychromatic.

Reticulocyte. A reticulocyte is a nonnucleated erythrocyte containing, when stained supravitally (usually with brilliant cresyl blue), one or more granules, strands, or a diffuse network of fibrils of precipitated RNA (Fig. 1-4). Most reticulocytes appear polychromatic when stained with Wright's stain (p. 61).

Erythrocyte. All nonnucleated red cells are erythrocytes. The normal erythrocyte is a biconcave disk; details of its structure are considered elsewhere (p. 73).

FORMATION

Erythropoiesis is initiated by differentiation of the multipotential reticulum cell or stem cell into a rubriblast. A phase of cell proliferation and beginning maturation follows. The exact number of cellular divisions that the erythrocytic precursors undergo during their development is not known, but mitotic activity shows a progressive increase with maturation. Consequently, the more mature mitotable cells contribute most of the proliferative activity. The growth rate then declines, and a stage characterized by a pyknotic nucleus is reached. These cells are incapable of further replication and have acquired a finite life-span. The nucleus is extruded, and the cell becomes a reticulocyte. Cytoplasmic maturation, for example, hemoglobin synthesis, continues despite the absence of a nucleus. When the last vestiges of RNA disappear, the cell is no longer able to synthesize hemoglobin, and maturation is complete.

Development from the rubriblast stage to a mature erythrocyte requires approximately four days. About 10 to 15 per cent of the erythrocytic precursors fail to reach maturity and are destroyed at some stage in their generation; a few cells appear to skip mitotic division(s). However, most erythrocytic precursors undergo an orderly maturation that is intimately and inseparably associated with the acquisition of the cells' unique cytoplasmic constituents and enzyme systems. This process takes place at a relatively fixed rate, probably predetermined by the nutritional and hormonal environment; accelerated erythropoiesis appears to reflect the entrance of more stem cells into the erythrocytic compartment rather than a shortening of the maturation time.

The marrow contains a large pool of reticulocytes about equal to the total number of nucleated erythrocytic precursors. Most of these cells remain in the marrow for two to four days before they are released into the circulation; during this time maturation and active hemoglobin synthesis continue. Surprisingly little is known about the mechanisms governing the release of red blood cells from the marrow into the peripheral blood. In response to increased need, such as an acute hypoxic stimulus, reticulocytes are released prematurely and temporarily increase the blood's oxygen-carrying capacity. If all the marrow reticulocytes entered the circulation, the absolute circulating reticulocyte count would be about doubled.

CONTROL OF ERYTHROPOIESIS

The regulatory mechanisms responsible for the normal erythroid steady state and the nature of the stimuli to increased erythropoiesis during periods of need have been the subject of much research. The level of the peripheral erythroid values is determined normally by the rate of erythropoiesis and is not regulated by changes in red cell life-span. It is apparent that the formation, maturation, and release of erythrocytes from the marrow into the circulation are governed by equilibrated forces that maintain a red cell mass commensurate with the tissues' oxygen needs and determine responses to physiologic and pathologic stimuli. Until recently, little was known about the mechanisms that maintain or restore erythrocytic equilibrium. Substances such as iron, vitamin B_{12}, and folic acid are required for the production of erythrocytes and the synthesis of hemoglobin, their major constituent; however, they do not exert a direct influence on the rate of erythropoiesis. These necessary building blocks evoke an increase in red cell production *only* in the presence of their respective deficiencies; they will *not* stimulate erythropoiesis in normal recipients. Hypoxia, humoral factor(s), and the endocrine glands are all capable of affecting erythropoiesis.

Erythropoietic Effects of Hypoxia. The erythropoietic stimulus imparted by hypoxia was first recognized by Bert in 1878. In 1893 Miescher suggested that hypoxia exerted primary control over erythropoiesis. This theory has received abundant clinical and experimental support over the years and *hypoxia* is now generally accepted as the *fundamental erythropoietic stimulus.* However, the original hypothesis that hypoxia of the erythrocytic precursors themselves constituted the stimulus to erythropoiesis has been disproved. Current data indicate that the hypoxic stimulus is mediated to the bone marrow by the humoral erythropoietic regulatory mechanism.

Humoral Control of Erythropoiesis. In 1906 two Frenchmen, Carnot and Deflandre, first described an erythropoietic stimulating factor in the serum of bled rabbits and suggested that it might exert a regulatory effect over erythropoiesis. In the ensuing two decades this intriguing concept was responsible for a number of attempts to confirm the existence of a humoral erythrocytogenic agent; some studies were in accord but most were in disagreement. Because of evident discrepancies in experimental results, the humoral control of erythropoiesis was considered by most to be speculative and lacking in support. Bonsdorff and Jalavisto revived the humoral theory in 1948 and first proposed that the responsible substance be called erythropoietin.

The last 15 years have seen great strides in our understanding of the physiologic and pathophysiologic control of erythropoiesis. The existence of a humoral regulatory mechanism is now indisputable; however, the complete solution to the complex problem of erythropoietic control is not yet at hand. Although the presence of erythrocytogenic stimuli in certain plasmas and urines cannot be denied, the precise nature, site of production, physiologic effect, and pathophysiologic significance of the erythropoietic substance or substances contained in such test materials remain to be elucidated. Nonetheless, it is entirely reasonable to conclude, on the basis of available information, that humoral factors exert homeostatic control over erythropoiesis.

There is compelling support for the current consensus that a humoral factor regulates the quantity of hemoglobin synthesized. This factor is termed *erythropoietin*. Although it has not yet been isolated in pure form, much is known about its structure. Erythropoietin, which is detectable in plasma and urine, appears to be a glycoprotein migrating electrophoretically as an alpha globulin; it has a molecular weight of about 27,000 and is water-soluble, nondialyzable, inactivated by proteolytic enzymes, and relatively thermostable (it withstands heat for short periods but is destroyed by prolonged exposure). There is persuasive evidence that erythropoietin is elaborated, at least for the most part, by the kidneys and that its erythropoietic effect is to bring about stem cell-erythrocytic differentiation.

Limitations in bioassay techniques have retarded observations on the humoral control of erythropoiesis. The concept of a physiologic humoral regulator demands that the responsible substance (or substances) be found in normal blood as well as in certain abnormal situations. Detection of small amounts of erythropoietin has proved to be a problem. Recent studies indicate that erythropoietin is present in normal plasma as well as normal urine, but it has not yet been possible to demonstrate unequivocally less than normal plasma erythropoietin levels. On the other hand, humoral erythropoietic activity can be augmented by a variety of experimental means and is demonstrable in each instance as well as in their clinical counterparts. Every method that will enhance erythropoietin elaboration involves some form of hypoxia. For example, (1) acute hemorrhagic or hemolytic anemia (anemic hypoxia), (2) residence at real or simulated high altitude (hypoxic hypoxia), and (3) the administration of cobalt, which appears to interfere with the utilization of oxygen by the cells (histotoxic hypoxia). Thus it is difficult to avoid the conclusion that hypoxia, irrespective of type, is the chief determinant of erythropoietin activity.

Unfortunately, the problem is not quite so simple as this discussion might tend to imply. Numerous questions, including the likelihood of additional humoral factors, remain unanswered. Another erythropoietic substance that differs clearly from erythropoietin in its chemical, physical, and physiologic effects has been studied. This agent is markedly thermo-stable, ether-soluble, and most likely a lipid; it resists destruction by proteolytic enzymes and is active orally. Further details in regard to its structure and site (or sites) of production are not yet available. When given alone to normal rats, this factor induces a singular type of response characterized by erythrocytosis due to the production of microcytes, reticulocytosis, and myeloid erythrocytic hyperplasia without associated increases in the hemoglobin or hematocrit levels. It has been suggested that this erythrocytosis-stimulating factor determines the number of mitotic divisions that erythrocytic precursors undergo during maturation. Increased activity attributable to this substance is demonstrable in the same experimental and clinical conditions as those that are known to enhance the elaboration of erythropoietin.

The precise significance of the thermostable, ether-soluble plasma erythropoietic factor awaits further study. On the basis of data now at hand, however, it is hypothesized that erythropoiesis is subject to both quantitative and qualitative humoral control. Hemoglobin synthesis and the maturation of erythrocytic precursors are envisaged as proceeding at relatively fixed rates, probably reflecting the inherent growth poten-tial of the rubriblasts to mature into nonnucleated, hemoglobin-containing erythrocytes. Erythropoietin (a glycoprotein that is relatively ther-molabile, soluble in water, inactive orally, and formed in the kidneys) determines the amount of hemoglobin synthesized by regulating the input from the stem cell into the erythrocytic compartment. A second humoral factor, which is markedly thermostable, ether-soluble, active orally, and probably a lipid, appears to affect mitotic proliferation of erythrocytic precursors, thereby controlling the number of erythrocytes formed. In the presence of adequate building blocks and an intact mye-loid reticulum the humoral mechanism would in this manner ensure an oxygen-carrying capacity of the blood commensurate with metabolic needs, together with the production of red cells of optimum size and hemoglobin content for the most efficient completion of their physiologic functions. The amount of hemoglobin synthesized per unit of time is important; so are individual cellular characteristics such as size, shape, and hemoglobin content.

At this time the physiologic and pathophysiologic control of erythro-poiesis cannot be defined precisely. Future studies may require drastic changes in current concepts. The possibility of additional erythropoietic agents cannot be excluded. It also seems likely that erythropoietic in-hibitors and/or humoral factor activators may contribute to the control of erythropoiesis. Therefore, pending clarification of its various components, it is more desirable to refer to the *humoral erythropoietic regulatory mechanism* than to single factors such as erythropoietin.

Although there is little doubt that the fundamental erythropoietic stimulus (hypoxia) is mediated via the humoral erythropoietic regulatory mechanism, it cannot be stated with certainty that this is the sole means by which erythrocytic equilibrium is maintained or restored. Such a unitarian concept of erythropoietic control is obviously desirable, but, in a living organism in which the blood and oxygen supply to various tissues is under continuous flux, the possibility that other regulatory mechanisms might be operating must not be overlooked. However, it appears entirely reasonable to conclude on the basis of existent data that the humoral erythropoietic regulatory mechanism does exert homeo-static control over erythropoiesis and is responsive even to minor disturbances in the dynamic relationship between tissue oxygen tension and metabolic requirements. Such a theory of erythropoietic control is represented schematically in Figure 1-5. Any disorder affecting arterial

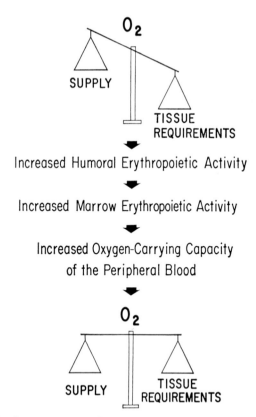

Figure 1-5. Erythropoietic stimulation via the humoral regulatory mechanism.

oxygen saturation (hypoxic hypoxia), the oxygen-carrying capacity of the blood (anemic hypoxia), transport of oxygen to the cells, for example, circulatory insufficiency consequent to congestive heart failure (stagnant hypoxia), or cellular utilization of oxygen (histotoxic hypoxia) will, sequentially, produce tissue hypoxia, enhance humoral factor activity, stimulate the bone marrow, and augment red cell mass. An increase in cellular metabolic requirements would have the same effect.

Conversely, it is logical to surmise that tissue hyperoxia might curtail endogenous erythropoietic factor elaboration which, in turn, would lead to a reduction in the oxygen-carrying capacity of the blood and restoration of the balance between oxygen supply and cellular requirements (Fig. 1-6). Increasing the oxygen tension of inspired air suppresses red cell production, and transfusion-induced polycythemia causes an almost complete cessation of erythropoiesis. The supposition that these suppressive effects are transmitted to the marrow by the humoral mechanism

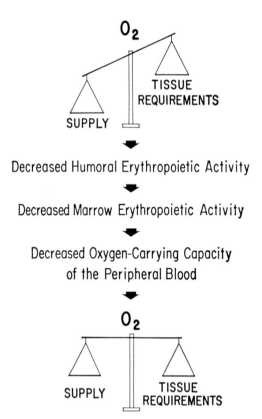

Figure 1-6. Erythropoietic suppression via the humoral regulatory mechanism.

possesses strong indirect and teleological support. However, technical problems concerned with the quantification of less than normal levels of plasma erythropoietic factor activity have, to date, precluded direct documentation. It is noteworthy that decreased cellular requirements would, according to this premise (Fig. 1-6), be expected to have a depressing effect on erythropoiesis similar to that caused by increasing the oxygen content of the blood. Such a mechanism is most likely responsible for the decreased erythropoiesis and peripheral erythroid values accompanying certain hypometabolic states; for example, hypothyroidism.

Erythropoietic Effects of the Endocrine Glands. Abundant evidence, experimental and clinical—both direct and indirect—establishes beyond doubt the ability of the secretions of the pituitary, thyroid, adrenals, and gonads to affect erythropoiesis. Available data indicate that the erythropoietic effects of the endocrine glands are contingent on their roles as determinants of general metabolic activity and cellular oxygen requirements.

THYROID. The thyroid exerts a clear-cut effect on red cell production as evidenced by the decrease in circulating hemoglobin that follows thyroidectomy in experimental animals and human subjects. In addition, most patients with hypothyroidism manifest less than normal peripheral erythroid values (p. 154). In these situations a normal red cell mass is restored consequent to adequate replacement therapy. Since ablation of the thyroid does not abolish the erythropoietic response to hypoxia, it is not possible to assign the thyroid a primary role in the control of erythropoiesis. However, its modifying influence, which appears to reflect alterations in metabolic activity and oxygen consumption and is presumably mediated via the humoral erythropoietic regulatory mechanism (Fig. 1-6), cannot be denied. Hypothyroidism is characterized by a decrease in the metabolic rate, oxygen consumption, and red cell production; thyroid therapy increases the metabolic rate, oxygen consumption, and erythropoiesis.

On the other hand, thyroid hormone is not an effective erythropoietic stimulant in euthyroid recipients. Although thyroxin enhances ^{59}Fe uptake in normal animals, it is not possible to produce a true polycythemia by this means. Neither do patients with hyperthyroidism manifest erythrocytosis. On the premise that erythropoietic activity is dependent on the relationship between oxygen supply and tissue requirements, hyperthyroidism theoretically should be accompanied by erythrocytosis (Fig. 1-5). The failure of the circulating hemoglobin to increase in the face of an increased metabolic rate probably reflects such compensatory measures as tachypnea, tachycardia, and an increased cardiac output which fulfill the cells' increased requirements for oxygen.

GONADS. A slight to moderate decrease in the peripheral erythroid values is evident in castrated male animals and eunuchoid men; treatment with testosterone restores normal levels. Castration in females is followed by an increase in the circulating hemoglobin, which is preventable by the administration of estrogens. Thus androgens stimulate and estrogens inhibit erythropoiesis. The erythropoietic effects of the sex hormones are undoubtedly responsible for the higher peripheral erythroid values in the males of species, including man.

The slight alterations in erythropoiesis consequent to a deficiency of androgens are probably mediated by the humoral erythropoietic regulatory mechanism (Fig. 1-6). They most likely reflect loss of the anabolic effect of testosterone and a decrease in metabolic activity (the curve of the erythropoietic response in eunuchoid men given exogenous testosterone parallels the increase in their basal metabolic rates). Orchidectomy does not prevent the erythropoietic response to hypoxia.

Small doses of testosterone do not significantly affect erythropoiesis in normal persons; however, large amounts given over a long period of time will augment erythropoiesis and total red cell mass. The mechanism(s) by which pharmacologic doses of testosterone enhance erythropoiesis in certain patients with disorders like agnogenic myeloid metaplasia (p. 439) and hypoplastic anemia (p. 235) is not known. Because these anemic patients are already hypoxic and have increased plasma erythropoietic factor activity, large amounts of testosterone obviously do not act through the humoral mechanism (Fig. 1-5). Recent experimental studies suggest that massive doses of testosterone may exert a direct effect on stem cell-erythrocytic differentiation, thus potentiating the action of erythropoietin.

ADRENALS. Adrenalectomy produces a slight anemia in experimental animals and corticosteroids stimulate erythropoiesis in both normal and adrenalectomized recipients. The clinical counterparts of these experimental observations are the decreased peripheral erythroid values in patients with Addison's disease (p. 155) and the erythrocytosis in some persons with Cushing's syndrome (p. 298). However, these changes are slight, and the adrenals are not essential to the maintenance of active erythropoiesis or to the mediation of the hypoxic stimulus. Available data indicate that the erythropoietic effect of the adrenals is due to the ability of the corticosteroids to affect cellular metabolic activities and oxygen consumption and that it is transmitted to the marrow by the humoral erythropoietic regulatory mechanism.

PITUITARY. Hypophysectomy in experimental animals and hypopituitarism in human subjects are regularly accompanied by a decrease in erythropoiesis and red cell mass (p. 156). However, the concept of a discrete pituitary erythropoietic factor is no longer tenable. The erythropoietic suppression consequent to hypoactivity of the anterior pituitary appears to reflect a reduction in metabolic activity and cellular oxygen requirements secondary to adrenal and thyroid deficiencies. This effect is most likely transmitted to the bone marrow by the humoral regulatory mechanism (Fig. 1-6). Combination therapy with thyroxin and corticosteroids enhances oxygen consumption and repairs the anemia in hypophysectomized animals, but marrow hypoplasia persists until growth hormone is added. Thus the erythropoietic alterations due to hypopituitarism are caused by deficiencies of adrenocorticotropic, thyrotropic, and growth-stimulating hormones.

BIOCHEMISTRY

The mature erythrocyte is composed chiefly of water (about 65 per cent) and hemoglobin (about 33 per cent of the wet weight and 95 per cent of the dry weight). The remainder consists of numerous enzymes and coenzymes, other proteins (predominately constituents of the stroma), lipids, carbohydrates, phosphorus, sulfur, zinc, copper, lead, tin, manganese, aluminum, silver, cations (K^+, Na^+, Ca^{++}, Mg^{++}), anions (Cl^-, HCO_3^-, PO_4^{---}, SO_4^{--}), vitamins, and other organic compounds, such as urea, uric acid, creatine, creatinine, adenosine di- and triphosphate, and di- and triphosphopyridine nucleotides. The fully mature, nonnucleated erythrocyte contains no DNA or RNA. It is incapable of replication and cannot synthesize hemoglobin or its components. Nonetheless, an erythrocyte takes part in a number of complex metabolic activities.

Red cell stroma consists primarily of a lipoprotein complex; the erythrocyte has an ordered physicochemical structure and must expend energy to maintain its integrity and discoidal shape (p. 73). The predominate erythrocyte ion is potassium; the maintenance of electrolyte equilibrium is also endergonic (p. 77). Erythrocytes possess all the enzymes needed to catabolize glucose aerobically and anaerobically; red cell energetics are discussed elsewhere (p. 74). Because hemoglobin is the major component of an erythrocyte and is necessary for the cell's prime physiologic function, it is pertinent to consider its structure and synthesis in detail.

Hemoglobin Structure. Hemoglobin consists of *globin*, a colorless protein, and four *heme* radicals (Fig. 1-7) which give hemoglobin its red color. Hemoglobin has a molecular weight of 64,458. Globin is comprised of four polypeptide chains made up of amino acids arranged in a definite sequential and spatial pattern. The globin portion of a molecule of normal adult hemoglobin (Hgb A) contains two α and two β peptide chains; there are 141 amino acids in each α chain and 146

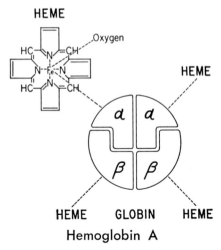

Hemoglobin A

Figure 1-7.   Structure of the hemoglobin molecule.

in the β chains. The compositions of the globin moieties of the other normal hemoglobins (Hgb F and Hgb A₂) and of certain abnormal hemoglobins are described in another chapter (p. 246).

The heme groups of the hemoglobin molecule are metal complexes with an iron atom in the center of a porphyrin structure which consists of four pyrrole rings attached together by methene linkages (Fig. 1-7). Substitutions at the outer corners of the pyrrole rings determine the type of porphyrin. There are three naturally occurring porphyrins (uroporphyrin, coproporphyrin, and protoporphyrin). The porphyrin in heme is protoporphyrin, whose eight side chains include four methyl, two vinyl, and two proprionic acid residues. Because there are three types of substitution, 15 isomeric configurations are possible. The protoporphyrin in heme is the No. 9 isomer. Porphyrins have been synthesized artificially, and four isomeric configurations (etioporphyrins) have been recognized; only types I and III occur naturally. The protoporphyrin 9 in heme is type III. The iron atom contained in the heme radical is hexacovalent. Four of these coordination valences are attached to the four nitrogen atoms of the pyrrole rings, the fifth is bound to a globin polypeptide chain (probably to the imidazole group of a histidine residue), and the sixth bond combines reversibly with oxygen (Fig. 1-7).

Biosynthesis of Hemoglobin.   The porphyrin and globin moieties of hemoglobin are synthesized independently by erythrocytic precursors in the bone marrow. The synthesis of the globin peptide chains and the genetic factors controlling this process are considered in another chapter (p. 246), as are details of iron metabolism (p. 158).

Protoporphyrin synthesis is shown schematically in Figure 1-8. Por-

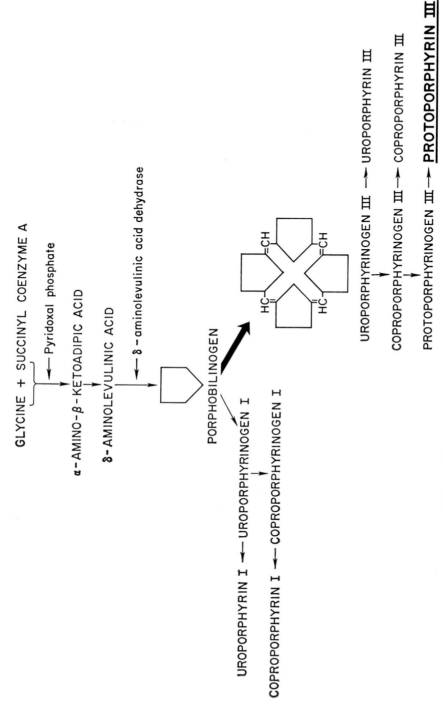

Figure 1-8. Steps in the biosynthesis of protoporphyrin.

phyrins are formed from simple substances, glycine and succinyl-coenzyme A (a four-carbon intermediate of the tricarboxylic acid cycle which operates in nucleated red cells but is inactive in mature erythrocytes). The first step in this synthetic process requires pyridoxal phosphate (vitamin B_6). Although compounds having both type I and III isomeric configurations are formed, type III predominates; it should be noted that type I protoporphyrin has never been found in nature. The "-ogen" compounds are the reduced forms of the porphyrins. Uroporphyrin and coproporphyrin are not intermediate compounds in the direct synthetic pathway (Fig. 1-8); however, they are byproducts of protoporphyrin synthesis, and small quantities are present normally in the feces and urine (coproporphyrin predominates). Normal red cells contain a small amount of free protoporphyrin (20 to 40 µg/100 ml of erythrocytes) and minute quantities of free coproporphyrin.

The final step in the biosynthesis of hemoglobin involves the combination of iron, protoporphyrin, and globin. Precise details of this reaction, which requires one or more enzymes (the heme synthetase system), are not known. It is commonly assumed that iron is inserted into the porphyrin nucleus to form ferroprotoporphyrin 9, type III or heme, which then combines with one of the globin peptide chains. However, the possibilities that protoporphyrin-globin or iron-globin complexes may be formed first cannot be excluded. Although iron uptake and the various other components of this complex synthetic process begin in the most immature erythrocytic precursors, the actual formation of the hemoglobin molecule per se takes place, for the most part, in the more mature precursors, including reticulocytes.

PHYSIOLOGY

The primary function of the red cells is to carry oxygen to the tissues and to assist in the removal of carbon dioxide. Combustion is the essential chemical process of life and requires a constant supply of oxygen. In a normal human subject at rest approximately 250 ml of oxygen are utilized each minute and 200 ml of carbon dioxide are produced. If these respiratory gases were carried in physical solution, man's activity would be only a fraction of his present capabilities. Hemoglobin permits the transport of about 100 times more oxygen than could be handled by the plasma alone. The iron atoms contained in the hemoglobin molecule possess the important attribute of reversible oxygenation; that is, they can bind and release oxygen without changing their valency. When oxygen combines with hemoglobin, its two unpaired electrons are paired with those of iron; as a consequence, oxygen is unable to accept electrons in transfer and cannot act as an oxidizing agent.

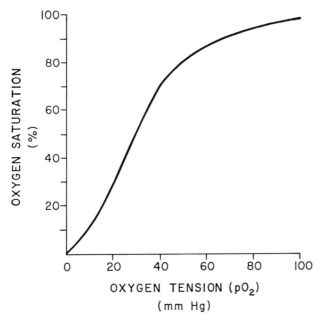

Figure 1-9. Oxyhemoglobin dissociation curve.

The association and dissociation of oxygen and hemoglobin are complex and depend on several factors, including oxygen tension, pH, and temperature. The normal sigmoidal oxyhemoglobin dissociation curve (Fig. 1-9) imparts an important physiologic advantage; at low oxygen tensions minor changes in pO_2 bring about the association with or dissociation from hemoglobin of large quantities of oxygen. At one given time the four atoms of iron in a molecule of hemoglobin may be bound to none, one, two, three, or four molecules of oxygen. When one heme group joins with oxygen, the affinity for oxygen of the other heme moieties is increased. Thus hemoglobin is ideally suited to pick up oxygen in the lungs in which the tension in the alveolar air (about 100 mm Hg) is higher than in the venous blood (about 35 mm Hg) and to give it up to the cells where the oxygen pressure in arterial blood (about 90 mm Hg) greatly exceeds that of the tissues. When fully saturated, 1 gm of hemoglobin can carry 1.34 ml of oxygen.

In addition to its vital role in the transport of oxygen, hemoglobin and the erythrocytes have other functions. These include the transport of carbon dioxide from the tissues to the lungs, where it is given up and eliminated from the body in the expired air. Hemoglobin also contributes to the buffering action of the blood and thereby to the maintenance of normal acid-base balance.

Granulocytes

There are three kinds of granulocytes, *neutrophils, eosinophils,* and *basophils;* the neutrophils predominate (p. 309). Although myeloid is often used as a generic term for these cells, it should be abandoned; the designations *granulocytes* or *the granulocytic series* are much more appropriate. All these cells are distinguished by the acquisition of specific cytoplasmic granules during maturation. Granulocytes are formed in the bone marrow; several distinct developmental stages can be recognized morphologically.

MORPHOLOGY

The following descriptions pertain to the appearance of cells when stained with Wright's stain.

Myeloblast. The most immature granulocyte precursor possesses a relatively large, round-to-oval nucleus with an indistinct nuclear membrane, a finely stippled or "ground-glasslike" chromatin pattern, and two to five nucleoli; the scanty, dark-blue, opaque cytoplasm normally does not contain granules (Fig. 1-10).

Progranulocyte. This hyperchromatic, immature cell has a nuclear chromatin pattern that is coarser and slightly more clumped than that of a myeloblast; nucleoli are still discernible. The major difference between a progranulocyte and a myeloblast is the presence in the former of blue-black or reddish-blue, nonspecific cytoplasmic granules (Fig. 1-10) which overlie and sometimes partly obscure the nucleus. The number of granules ordinarily increases with maturation; however, cells should be classified as progranulocytes as soon as one or more nonspecific granules are evident and as long as specific granules are not seen.

Myelocyte. When a developing granulocyte acquires specific cytoplasmic granules, it should be classified as a myelocyte even though nonspecific granules persist (Fig. 1-10). Specific granules include (1) the small pink-to-lilac granules of a neutrophil, (2) the larger, uniform, orange-red, refractile granules of an eosinophil, and (3) the large, variable-sized, blue-black granules of a basophil. Consequently, myelocytes and all subsequent granulocytic elements must be subdivided into neutrophilic, eosinophilic, or basophilic types. The nucleus of a myelocyte remains round to oval, although the chromatin pattern is more coarsely clumped. Depending on the stage of maturity, that is, an early or late myelocyte, nucleoli may or may not be present. As maturation progresses through this developmental stage, specific granules increase and nonspecific granules disappear.

Metamyelocyte. The next stage in granulocytic maturation is dis-

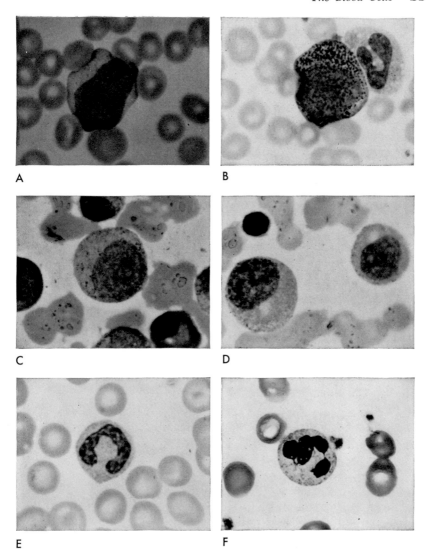

Figure 1-10. Normal developing granulocytes. *A.* Myeloblast. *B.* Progranulocyte. *C.* Myelocyte (neutrophilic). *D.* Metamyelocytes (neutrophilic). *E.* Band neutrophil. *F.* Segmented neutrophil.

tinguished by indentation of the nucleus and progressive clumping and aggregation of the nuclear chromatin (Fig. 1-10). The nucleus is characteristically bean- or kidney-shaped; however, a granulocytic precursor should be classified as a metamyelocyte as long as the diameter of the midportion of the nucleus is greater than that of the ends. Nucleoli are not evident, and metamyelocytes generally contain a nearly full complement of specific granules (a few nonspecific granules may still be present in early metamyelocytes).

Band Granulocyte. These cells have a U-shaped nucleus in which the diameter of the midportion is equal to or less than that of the ends; the nuclear chromatin is present in coarse aggregates, and the cytoplasm appears fully mature (Fig. 1-10).

Segmented Granulocyte. A mature granulocyte is characterized by a nucleus consisting of two or more lobes connected by a filament. It is noteworthy that even marked nuclear constriction does not permit inclusion in this category unless the nuclear lobes are joined by a threadlike structure. However, when doubt exists because one nuclear lobe is overlying another, the cell should be classified as a segmented form, for they are the more differentiated and commonest granulocytes. The nuclear chromatin is coarsely clumped with clear-cut contrast between basichromatin and parachromatin. Segmented granulocytes should be subdivided on the basis of their specific granules into neutrophils, eosinophils, or basophils.

Neutrophils possess a nucleus with two to four lobes; about 50 per cent of these cells have three. The cytoplasm contains a large number of small, evenly distributed acidophilic or pinkish-lilac granules (Fig. 1-10). In a female certain of the segmented neutrophils display a hyperchromatic nuclear "drumstick" consisting of a well-defined, solid appendage about 1.5 μ in diameter attached to one of the nuclear lobes by a single fine chromatin strand (Fig. 1-11). These sex chromatin

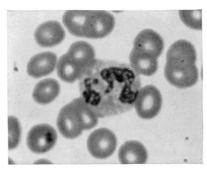

Figure 1-11. Segmented neutrophil from a normal female showing "drumstick" nuclear appendage.

bodies are demonstrable from birth to old age and must be distinguished from "sessile nodules" which are attached to the nucleus by a relatively thick stalk and from "rackets" which differ from drumsticks in having a pale center. The latter two appendages occur in both sexes. There must be typical nuclear drumsticks in at least 6 out of 500 neutrophils to permit the conclusion that the chromosomal sex pattern is female. Less than this number does not imply genetic maleness, for a number of healthy, normal women fall into this category.

Eosinophils and *basophils* are easily identified by their unique cytoplasmic granules (Fig. 1-12). These segmented granulocytes rarely

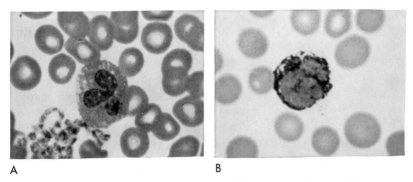

A   B

Figure 1-12. *A.* Mature eosinophil. *B.* Normal basophil.

display nuclei with more than two lobes. The granules overlie and often obscure the nucleus and ordinarily hide the faintly basophilic cytoplasm of an eosinophil and the cobwebby cytoplasm of a basophil.

FORMATION

The kinetics of granulopoiesis have been greatly clarified in recent years, although many problems remain to be solved. Since granulopoiesis is a complex, multicompartmental system, direct measurement of the size and turnover rate of each component has not yet been achieved. Nevertheless, much information has been gained through experimental approaches employing radioisotopic labeling and leukocytopheretic techniques. Granulocytes differ from erythrocytes in several important respects. Red cells normally function within the circulation. In contrast, granulocytes carry out their physiologic activities extravascularly, and those cells in the peripheral blood are merely in transit from the marrow to the tissues. Consequently, the period of time that the granulocytes circulate must not be confused with their actual life-span. The number of granulocytes present in the circulation at any one time represents but a small fraction of the total body granulocyte population.

Granulocytes are produced in the marrow. The first step involves differentiation of a stem cell into a myeloblast and entrance into the granulocytic compartment. All granulocytes are derived from morphologically similar myeloblasts and progranulocytes. When a cell reaches the myelocyte stage and has acquired specific cytoplasmic granules, the nature of the mature product, that is, a neutrophil, eosinophil, or basophil, is evident. The following discussion pertains to neutrophils only.

Marrow granulocytic elements can be appropriately divided into three subcompartments: (1) a primitive or undifferentiated proliferative pool (myeloblasts and progranulocytes), (2) a differentiated, proliferative pool (myelocytes), and (3) a maturing, postmitotable pool (metamyelocytes, band, and segmented neutrophils). The myelocyte subcompartment appears to be self-perpetuating and functions more or less as a stem cell. The more primitive cell population (myeloblasts and progranulocytes) does not contribute an appreciable number of cells to the myelocyte compartment unless an increased demand exists for mature neutrophils. Myelocytes are actively proliferating cells. After mitotic division, one cell can be envisaged as remaining in this compartment to divide again; the other becomes a metamyelocyte and is no longer capable of division. It is now committed to eventual destruction and moves in a sequential pattern through the subsequent stages of maturation into the mature marrow granulocyte pool and then the peripheral blood and thus to the tissues.

Available data indicate that around 11 to 12 days are required for a myelocyte to divide, mature, and appear in the peripheral blood. In this time about two to three days are spent in the myelocyte compartment, approximately four to five days as a metamyelocyte, and about four days as part of the mature (band or segmented forms) marrow granulocyte reserve. There are evident discrepancies in the available figures for the total number of marrow granulocytes. Approximately 15 to 20 $\times$ 10^9/kg of body weight appears to be a reasonable number for a normal adult; about 75 per cent of these cells are in the more mature compartment and are incapable of undergoing cellular division; that is, metamyelocytes, band, and segmented neutrophils.

Mature granulocytes are released from the marrow into the circulation in which they remain for a median of six to seven hours and an average of about 10. Thus the granulocytes in the peripheral blood turn over about 2.5 times each day. Neutrophils are removed from the circulation and enter the tissues in a random fashion. If a neutrophil remains in the circulation, about 24 to 30 hours are required for it to be transformed into a senescent, pyknotic cell. The movement of granulocytes from the marrow to the tissues is unidirectional. There is no evidence that these cells re-enter the circulation or return to the marrow from the tissues. It should be re-emphasized that the short time in which the granulocytes remain in transit in the peripheral blood is *not* synonymous with the cell's life-span; granulocytes do their work in the tissues, not in the circulation.

The marrow granulocyte pool is approximately 20 to 30 times larger than the total blood granulocyte pool. The blood pool can be subdivided into circulating and marginal compartments, in each of which there are approximately equal numbers of cells. The leukocyte count assesses the circulating pool, and the marginal granulocyte pool is composed of cells adherent to the walls of small blood vessels. The two blood granulocyte compartments, which are in a state of dynamic equilibrium, maintain a continuous and rapid exchange of cells. Alterations in the ratio between the circulating and marginal granulocytes are reflected by changes in the leukocyte count, even though the total blood granulocyte pool remains unchanged. The prompt leukocytosis evoked by epinephrine (p. 314) reflects such a shift.

An absolute increase in the granulocytes within the circulation reflects either prolonged survival in the peripheral blood or increased production by the bone marrow. The former mechanism probably has no physiologic significance; however, granulocytes do circulate for significantly longer periods of time in patients with chronic granulocytic leukemia (p. 362) than in normal subjects. Granulocyte output by the marrow can be enhanced in several ways, including (1) release of larger numbers of mature cells from the marrow granulocyte reserve (there are enough cells in this compartment to maintain a normal peripheral blood count for about four days, even if input from the more immature compartments ceased entirely), (2) accelerated proliferative activity in the myelocyte compartment, and (3) increased stem cell-myeloblastic differentiation.

Despite recent advances in our knowledge of granulopoiesis, little is known about the mechanisms that exert normal homeostatic control over this complex process or those that enhance the availability of granulocytes in times of need. Preliminary reports point to the probable existence of several types of humoral factors. It has been suggested that such agents may affect the release of cells from the marrow granulocyte reserve, stimulate mitotic division, and/or enhance input from the stem cell into the granulocyte compartment; however, the preliminary nature of these experimental observations must be stressed. In view of the profound effect exerted by humoral factors on erythropoiesis, it is logical to surmise that other products of the multipotential marrow reticulum cells might be subject to similar regulatory control. Future research along these lines should be informative.

The manner in which granulocytes are destroyed and removed from the body is obscure. It seems likely that significant numbers of senescent cells are released into the oral cavity and gastrointestinal tract. However, the role of these mechanisms in the regulation of the total granulocyte population or in the removal of effete cells is conjectural.

Virtually nothing is known about the mechanisms that govern the formation of eosinophils and basophils. All granulocytic elements participate in certain of the myeloproliferative disorders; for example, polycythemia vera. More often than not an increase in one type of granulocyte is not associated with an increase in another. The eosinophilia that characterizes certain skin diseases or parasitic infestations, for example, is not accompanied by increased neutrophils or basophils in the marrow or peripheral blood. The lack of knowledge about the production of eosinophils and basophils and the factors controlling their levels in the peripheral blood and tissues is not surprising in view of the meager information concerning their normal functions.

BIOCHEMISTRY AND PHYSIOLOGY

Although neutrophils, eosinophils, and basophils have much in common, important quantitative and qualitative differences warrant separate discussions of their chemical constituents and biologic functions.

Neutrophils. Neutrophils are metabolically quite active and are capable of both aerobic and anaerobic glycolysis. They possess glycogen, which increases during maturation and may reflect a storehouse of potential energy. In addition to the enzymes needed to catabolize glucose, neutrophils contain many others, including nucleotidases, proteases, peptidases, oxidases, diastases, lipases, esterases, lysozyme, and cathepsin. Changes in the content of some enzymes, for example, alkaline phosphatase, have diagnostic significance (p. 437).

Neutrophils are motile and move in a characteristic ameboid fashion. These leukocytes constitute the body's first line of defense against invasion by microorganisms. They are actively phagocytic and can engulf a variety of foreign particles, especially small particulate matter such as bacteria. Phagocytosed material apparently is destroyed by enzymatic digestion. The many enzymes in a neutrophil are contained within the cell's granules; thus cytoplasmic degranulation is a reflection of increased cellular activity. It also seems likely that enzymes released from disintegrating granulocytes react with invading bacteria or other microorganisms at sites of infection.

Eosinophils. Despite their unique and characteristic morphology, relatively little is known about the biochemistry or physiology of the eosinophils. Their granules contain proteins, lipids, and a variety of enzymes. Profibrinolysin has been demonstrated recently in eosinophil granules. Although these cells display ameboid motility, they move more slowly than neutrophils. They also possess the ability to phagocytize.

To date, most of the functions of an eosinophil have been inferred from knowledge of the types of disorders associated with eosinophilia or eosinopenia. They appear to participate chiefly in detoxification and defensive processes, especially as a protection against foreign proteins. In addition, there is convincing evidence that eosinophils act to neutralize the effect of histamine. The presence in these cells of profibrinolysin suggests that they may play a role in maintaining the fluidity of the blood. Corticosteroids induce a prompt (within four hours) fall in the circulating eosinophil count, which lasts as long as they are continued. This eosinopenic effect can be utilized to assess the functional capacity of the adrenal cortex to respond to such a stimulus as ACTH.

Basophils. In the past basophils were viewed by most as functionless evolutionary rests, but recent studies have clarified their physiologic significance. Their large metachromatic granules contain heparin, and basophils appear to be a natural source of this substance. Heparin is released for its fat-clearing effect after alimentary lipemia and is reflected by degranulation of basophils. These granulocytes also contain large quantities of histamine, which they apparently synthesize. Thus it seems likely that basophils participate in allergic reactions as well as in fat metabolism. They are motile but quite sluggish.

Basophils appear to be chemically and functionally related to tissue mast cells. Their origin and morphology differ; for example, mast cells have round or oval nuclei and smaller, more uniform granules that do not overlie the nucleus (Fig. 1-13). However, mast cells also contain

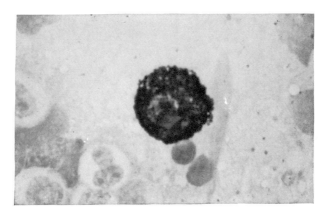

Figure 1-13. Mast cell in a bone marrow aspirate.

heparin and histamine (as well as hyaluronic acid and 5-hydroxytryptamine or serotonin) and participate in many of the same reactions as basophils.

Monocytes

The monocytes in the peripheral blood appear to be the circulating counterparts of tissue macrophages (histiocytes or clasmatocytes). Their origin is speculative and disputable. There are no clear-cut foci of monocyte formation as for granulocytes, erythrocytes, and megakaryocytes (the marrow) and lymphocytes (lymphoid organs such as the spleen and nodes). Monocytes are more closely aligned with the granulocytic than with the lymphocytic series. Current data support their derivation from reticuloendothelial elements in the marrow as well as in extramedullary sites. The mechanisms controlling their formation are obscure.

MORPHOLOGY

Normally it is not possible to follow a developing monocyte through a sequence of stages like those characterizing granulopoiesis or erythropoiesis. However, mature monocytes display distinctive morphologic attributes, and observations in patients with monocytic leukemia point to the existence of specific immature precursors. The following descriptions pertain to the appearance of the cells in Wright-stained preparations.

Monoblast. This primitive cell has a round, oval, or, less often, an irregularly shaped or lobulated nucleus with an indistinct nuclear membrane, one to two nucleoli, and a chromatin pattern distinguished by a fine, lacy architecture (the latter is typical of all cells of the monocytic series). The cytoplasm is opaque and deeply basophilic, and it may contain a few reddish granules. The cell borders are often irregular, with small, pseudopodlike protuberances. However, a monoblast is nonmotile. Some monoblasts are difficult to separate from myeloblasts. Cells with blast morphology associated with promonocytes and monocytes should be classified tentatively as monoblasts (Fig. 8-6, p. 346).

Promonocyte. This cell is intermediate in its morphology between a monoblast and a monocyte. The nucleus is irregularly shaped, and the lacy chromatin pattern is coarser than that of a monoblast. Promonocytes generally possess one or more nucleoli. The opaque, "muddy," blue-gray cytoplasm is abundant and contains granules like those of an adult monocyte. The over-all configuration of a promonocyte is similar to that of a more mature cell (Fig. 8-4, p. 346).

Monocyte. The mature monocyte (Fig. 1-14) is a large cell with abundant, opaque, blue-gray cytoplasm containing numerous small lilac or reddish-blue granules which appear more concentrated at the periphery of the cell. Cytoplasmic vacuoles are common, the cell contour is typically irregular, and there is no perinuclear clear zone. The nucleus is lobulated or convoluted. The nuclear chromatin pattern is fine and lacy with clear-cut points of condensation where strands cross. Nucleoli are not evident.

BIOCHEMISTRY AND PHYSIOLOGY

Relatively little is known about the biochemistry of monocytes. A variety of enzymes has been detected; monocytes are particularly rich

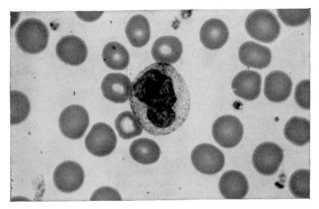

Figure 1-14. Normal, mature monocyte.

in lipases. In contrast to the mature granulocytes, these leukocytes do not contain alkaline phosphatase. Monocytes are actively motile and progress in a sliding movement by putting out pseudopods of variable size and shape. They advance more slowly than neutrophils.

Monocytes are actively phagocytic and can ingest many kinds of substances from molecules to microscopically visible particles such as bacteria, yeast, fungi, and even red cells and other leukocytes. Because of their ability to ingest quite large particulate matter, monocytes are often referred to as macrophages. These leukocytes function chiefly in the tissues, where they assist or more likely merge with and become tissue histiocytes. Monocytes contribute importantly to the body's defense mechanisms. They participate to the greatest extent in chronic infectious processes such as tuberculosis; for example, the epithelioid and giant cells characterizing tuberculosis appear to be derived from monocytic (or histiocytic) elements.

Thrombocytes

Wright pointed out in 1910 that the nonnucleated thrombocytes or platelets are formed by megakaryocytes in the bone marrow. This view has since received absolute documentation—direct and indirect—clinical and experimental. Thus the smallest of the formed elements in the peripheral blood is derived from the largest of the normal marrow cells.

MORPHOLOGY

Three developmental stages can be recognized in the maturation of a megakaryocyte. The following descriptions are based on the cells' appearances in Wright-stained marrow specimens.

Megakaryoblast. This large blast cell has a diameter about twice that of a myeloblast. The nucleus is round, oval, or sometimes slightly irregular with several nucleoli; the nuclear chromatin pattern is non-descript. The scanty, deeply basophilic cytoplasm contains no granules. Megakaryoblasts do not form platelets.

Promegakaryocyte. A promegakaryocyte is intermediate in its morphology between a megakaryoblast and a megakaryocyte. It is usually larger than a megakaryoblast with more abundant, less basophilic cytoplasm with granules. The nucleus is characteristically irregular; nucleoli are still evident.

Megakaryocyte. Adult megakaryocytes (Fig. 1-15) are giant cells (50 to 150 μ in diameter) and are conspicuous in bone marrow prep-

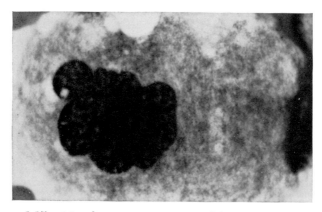

Figure 1-15. Megakaryocyte in a normal bone marrow aspirate.

arations even with the low-power objective. They are by far the largest of all normal marrow cells. The nucleus is typically twisted, lobulated, and quite irregularly shaped. Occasionally there are multiple, separate nuclei; because all of a megakaryocyte's nuclei undergo division synchronously, a normal, multinucleated megakaryocyte contains an even number of nuclei. A megakaryocyte nucleus is pachychromatic without discernible nucleoli. The abundant light-blue cytoplasm is ordinarily packed with numerous small azurophilic granules. Cell borders are often indistinct. Normally, small cytoplasmic particles (thrombocytes or platelets) can be seen breaking away from some of the megakaryocytes.

Thrombocytes. Thrombocytes or platelets are small nonnucleated structures measuring 2 to 4 μ in diameter. Normal platelets are round, oval, or rod-shaped, but bizarre shapes and giant forms are encountered in certain proliferative disorders such as agnogenic myeloid metaplasia (p. 434). When platelets are examined by phase microscopy, or if fixation is delayed, their shape is grossly irregular and numerous filamentous-like pseudopods are present; these dendritic forms reflect contact with a foreign surface. Platelets consist of light blue cytoplasm containing a variable number of azurophilic granules. The granules are characteristically collected in the center (the "granulomere") and are surrounded by a clear "hyalomere."

FORMATION

Megakaryocytes shed or "bud" platelets by forming small cytoplasmic pseudopods followed by progressive thinning of the stalk and eventual shearing of the platelet. Platelet budding is evident in the bone marrow, which is generally presumed to be the site of their formation. However, recent evidence also implicates the lungs in thrombopoiesis. Although megakaryocytes are not detectable in routine peripheral blood films, they can be found with some regularity in buffy coat preparations and are present in relatively large numbers in the pulmonary capillaries. They are also readily demonstrable in blood from the right heart, and many of these cells possess a full complement of cytoplasm. In addition, pulmonary megakaryocytes exhibit histologic evidence of platelet formation. Thus some mature megakaryocytes appear to be carried by the circulation from the bone marrow to the lungs, in which they remain and release platelets. It has been estimated that as many as 25 per cent of the body's platelets may be derived from pulmonary megakaryocytes.

Little information is available about the mechanisms that exert physiologic and pathophysiologic regulatory control over thrombopoiesis and the circulating platelet count. Preliminary data point to the possible existence of a humoral thrombopoietic regulatory mechanism. Platelet production is enhanced by thrombocytopheresis and depressed by platelet transfusions. Thrombocytosis-promoting activity has been demonstrated in normal plasma and urine as well as in plasmas from donors with a variety of disorders involving thrombopoiesis; for example, polycythemia vera (p. 298), primary thrombocythemia (p. 440), acute blood loss anemias—hemorrhagic (p. 70) and hemolytic (p. 89), and thrombocytopenias of various causes. Although these observations support the existence of a humoral thrombopoietic regulator (or regulators), many important questions remain unanswered. For example, how does this hypothetical agent affect platelet production or the circulating platelet count? Alternative possibilities include increased stem cell-megakaryocyte differentiation, augmented proliferation of megakaryocyte precursors, enhanced platelet formation by individual megakaryocytes, vascular redistribution, and even prolonged survival in the circulation. Future developments in this area of hematopoietic control promise to be enlightening.

Knowledge of the kinetics of thrombopoiesis is meager. There is no marrow platelet reserve comparable to the marrow granulocyte reserve. After increased peripheral loss, restoration of a normal platelet count requires three to four days. Based on several techniques the maximum platelet survival time appears to be about 8 to 11 days. Available data point to a finite life-span with a factor such as senescence determining the ultimate destruction of some platelets as well as random loss of others consequent to their utilization. Effete platelets are probably destroyed by reticuloendothelial cells in the spleen and elsewhere.

BIOCHEMISTRY

Platelets are metabolically quite active. They contain a variety of proteins, lipids, carbohydrates, elements (calcium, magnesium, copper, iron, and manganese), and enzymes, which include, among others, esterases, phosphatases, dehydrogenases, oxidases, transaminases, proteases, and carbohydrases. Other platelet constituents are serotonin (5-hydroxytryptamine), epinephrine, norepinephrine, and a variety of coagulation factors (p. 466). Certain of these substances apparently are adsorbed to the platelet's surface or exist in the periplatelet environment. Platelets carry on both anaerobic and aerobic glycolysis and contain relatively large amounts of adenosine triphosphate (ATP). As living cellular particles, they are able to generate energy and perform work.

PHYSIOLOGY

Platelets contribute in several important ways to hemostasis. In addition to their role in the coagulation process, they have several other functions. Because of their adhesiveness, platelets can by themselves occlude breaks in small vessels. They are essential for clot retraction, they liberate serotonin (a vasoconstrictor) at the site of an injury or break in a vessel wall, and they participate in a poorly defined manner in the maintenance of normal capillary integrity. The functions of platelets are discussed in more detail in Chapter 13, which deals with abnormal bleeding (p. 464).

Lymphocytes

Lymphocytes are normally present in relatively large numbers in the peripheral blood (p. 309). Mature lymphocytes possess distinctive features, but their maturation cycle lacks the clearly defined steps that characterize granulopoiesis.

MORPHOLOGY

Four categories of lymphocytes, presumably representing progressive stages of maturity, are recognized. The following morphologic descriptions are based on the cells' appearances in Wright-stained preparations.

Lymphoblast. The most immature lymphocyte precursor is a blast cell with a round nucleus, a distinct nuclear membrane, and one to two prominent nucleoli. The nuclear chromatin pattern is that of a diffusely homogeneous background with scattered small, and seemingly superimposed, more darkly stained clumps or aggregates of basichromatin. This morphologic feature distinguishes all cells of the lymphocytic series, regardless of their stage of maturity or normalcy. The scanty, dark-blue cytoplasm is without granules; a perinuclear clear zone is ordinarily evident. Blast cells associated with prolymphocytes should be tentatively classified as lymphoblasts (Fig. 8-2, p. 345).

Prolymphocyte. A prolymphocyte is a cell of the lymphocytic series with a morphology intermediate between that of a lymphoblast and a mature large lymphocyte. The nuclear chromatin clumps are coarser than those in a lymphoblast; one or occasionally two nucleoli are evident. Classification of a cell in this category more often than not is arbitrary, for prolymphocytes possess attributes of both lymphoblasts and lymphocytes.

Lymphocyte. Large Lymphocyte. A mature large lymphocyte (Fig. 1-16) has a round nucleus with coarse clumps of basichromatin superimposed on a homogeneous, darkly stained background; a nucleolus

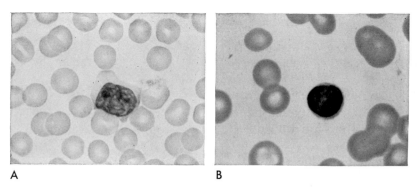

A   B

Figure 1-16. Normal lymphocytes. *A.* Large lymphocyte. *B.* Small lymphocyte.

may be present. The nuclear membrane is dense. The clear, sky-blue cytoplasm is relatively abundant and occasionally contains a few reddish granules. These granules are never numerous; they vary in size and are typically present in a small group. A perinuclear clear zone is often apparent.

Small Lymphocyte. The adult small lymphocyte of the peripheral blood has a nuclear diameter equal to or less than that of a normal erythrocyte (Fig. 1-16). Cytoplasm is scanty (usually just a narrow rim) to almost absent. Small lymphocytes do not have discernible nucleoli.

FORMATION

Lymphocytes are formed in the spleen, lymph nodes, thymus, bone marrow, and lymphoid foci in other tissues, such as Peyer's patches in the intestines. The relative contribution by different organs is not clear, and little is known about the kinetics of lymphopoiesis or its control. The majority of these cells enter the circulation by way of the thoracic duct. In most lymphoid tissues mitotic figures are rare; mature lymphocytes predominate, and lymphoblasts are infrequent in contrast to the prominence of immature erythrocyte and granulocyte precursors in the bone marrow. Large lymphocytes can synthesize DNA and undergo cellular division; small lymphocytes are apparently not capable of mitotic proliferation.

Despite the attention of many investigators, the lymphocyte remains, in large part, an enigma. Recent observations have helped to clarify the situation, but it is problematical whether all the data obtained in experimental animals are applicable to man. Although large numbers of lymphocytes enter the circulation each day, their proliferative capacity is small and their normal life-span appears to be long (about 100 days). These apparent discrepancies are the result of recirculation of lymphocytes through the blood and lymphoid tissues; for example, spleen, nodes, and bone marrow.

It has been generally assumed that the majority of the circulating lymphocytes were formed in the spleen and lymph nodes. It now appears that the thymus is a major source of small lymphocytes. Thymic lymphocytes apparently enter the blood and are carried to the spleen and lymph nodes, where they take up residence and are probably concerned with immune functions. Others such as those in the bone marrow appear to represent a second population of cells derived from alternative source organs and perhaps with different physiologic attributes (function and life-span).

In addition to the role of the thymus as a supplier of lymphocytes, some evidence suggests that this organ may produce a humoral factor that affects lymphocyte production ("lymphocytosis-stimulating factor"). The precise significance of this factor (or factors) must await further study. However, other hormones do exert clear-cut effects on lymphocytes and lymphopoiesis; most notable is the prompt fall in circulating lymphocytes and subsequent involution of lymphoid tissue evoked by corticosteroids. Although corticosteroids cause lymphocytolysis as well as decreased lymphopoiesis, the precise manner by which they affect lymphocytes and their precursors has resisted detection.

BIOCHEMISTRY AND PHYSIOLOGY

Lymphocytes are capable of both aerobic and anaerobic glycolysis, but these metabolic activities are more limited than in granulocytes. Although they possess a variety of enzymes, none is known to be specific for lymphocytes. These leukocytes contain a relatively large amount of RNA and exhibit a high rate of protein turnover. Lymphocytes are actively motile and move in a characteristic fashion without pseudopod formation and with the nucleus in the anterior end of the cell. They possess only limited phagocytic function, which is probably not physiologically significant.

Over the years many physiologic activities have been ascribed to the lymphocytes, most on tenuous and, at best, indirect evidence. A persistent hypothesis envisages the small lymphocyte as a hematologic stem cell capable of differentiating into other cell lineages; for example, a rubriblast or myeloblast. Numerous observations militate against the tenability of this concept. However, the possibility that lymphocytes participate in some way in the production of other blood cells cannot be excluded. There is increasing support that lymphocytes, rather than transforming into primitive precursors of another cell series, contribute DNA, enzymes, or some other vital cellular constituent to the multipotential reticulum cell. After appropriate stem cell differentiation components of lymphocytes would then be incorporated into a new proliferating cell lineage. Such a mechanism would explain many observations that seemingly attest to the totipotentiality of the lymphocyte.

A second proposed function of lymphocytes which deals with the body's defense mechanisms has acquired compelling experimental and clinical support. There is no longer any doubt that lymphocytes are intimately concerned with immune reactions. Plasmacytes synthesize immunoglobulins or humoral antibodies; lymphocytes are primarily concerned with tissue immunity, an essential but still poorly understood component of the body's immunologic defenses. Current evidence indicates that immunologically competent lymphocytes are derived from the thymus, the only lymphoid tissue fully developed and functional at birth.

Details of the relative contributions of plasmacytes (circulating antibody) and lymphocytes (tissue immune reactions) to the body's over-all defense remain to be worked out. It would appear, however, that both are essential, as are the different but nonetheless important functions of granulocytes and monocytes. Differences exist and contribute to varying clinical responses. A decrease in plasmacytes is associated with deficient circulating antibody elaboration and enhanced susceptibility to acute pyogenic infections; lymphopenia (or decreased lymphocytic function) is accompanied by alterations in tissue immunity and a loss of resistance to fungal, viral, and certain chronic bacterial infections. Thus plasmacytic myeloma, which is accompanied by decreased production of normal (or biologically specific) immunoglobulins, is often complicated by acute pyogenic infections; for example, pneumococcal pneumonia (p. 415). On the other hand, lymphomas, which involve lymphoid tissue primarily, are distinguished by little, if any, impairment in humoral antibody production; however, abnormalities in tissue immunity, for example, delayed skin tests and an increased frequency of fungal, viral, and chronic bacterial infections are evident (p. 408).

Plasmacytes

These cells are not normal constituents of the peripheral blood. However, they are present normally in the bone marrow and other blood-forming organs such as the spleen and lymph nodes. Morphologically and functionally they are closely related to the other leukocytes, especially lymphocytes. Therefore plasmacytes may be appropriately classified as blood cells even though they do not circulate. The designation *plasmacyte* is preferred over the frequently used term plasma cell, for it conforms with the nomenclature used for the other hemic cells and their precursors.

MORPHOLOGY

Plasmacytes display a distinctive morphology (Fig. 1-17). When stained with Wright's stain, they possess abundant hyperchromatic (dark

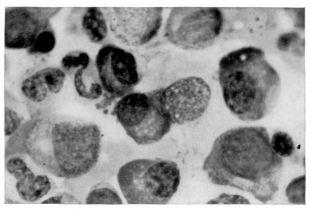

Figure 1-17. Normal, mature plasmacytes in a bone marrow aspirate.

blue) opaque cytoplasm that sometimes contains a few vacuoles or reddish granules. The round or oval nucleus is eccentrically placed with large sharply demarcated clumps of chromatin. Nucleoli are generally absent, although a small nucleolus may be seen in an occasional cell. Normally most plasmacytes are mature. However, a maturation cycle with two developmental stages has been described in patients with plasmacytic myeloma (p. 419). *Plasmablasts* are primitive cells with a fine chromatin structure and one or, rarely, two prominent nucleoli. The nucleus is larger and the basophilic cytoplasm is relatively less abundant than in a mature plasmacyte. A *proplasmacyte* has a morphology intermediate between that of a plasmablast and a plasmacyte. Nucleoli are present, and the nuclear chromatin pattern is coarser than that of a plasmablast and finer than that of a mature cell.

FORMATION

Little is known about the derivation of plasmacytes and the manner by which their production is controlled. They are not demonstrable during embryonic life. It is reasonable to assume that, if one goes back far enough, they are derived from the common multipotential reticulum cell (Fig. 1-1, p. 3). Plasmacytes are closely related to lymphocytes, and it has been suggested, with some support, that they actually arise from primitive lymphocytic elements. Proliferative disorders such as primary macroglobulinemia (p. 442), in which lymphocytoid cells are actively synthesizing proteins similar to those normally produced by plasmacytes, lend credibility to a close plasmacyte-lymphocyte relationship. Plasmacytes are apparently produced for the most part in the marrow and germinal centers of the spleen and lymph nodes. Immature cells are seen rarely in normal persons in whom mature cells predominate. Since nuclear division often occurs without cytoplasmic division, multinucleated forms are frequent. Accurate data pertaining to the lifespan of plasmacytes are not available. Most observations indicate a relatively long survival.

BIOCHEMISTRY AND PHYSIOLOGY

Plasmacytes contain abundant amounts of RNA and are capable of intense protein synthesis. Electron microscopy reveals a well-developed endoplasmic reticulum. It has been demonstrated unequivocally that plasmacytes synthesize immunoglobulins (p. 413).

Examination of the Blood
and Blood-Forming Organs

All phases of diagnostic medicine depend to some extent on laboratory support. However, there are few branches of clinical medicine in which the laboratory figures as importantly as it does in hematology. Modern clinical hematology was born in the laboratory, and its practice demands the availability of a variety of laboratory procedures. Without appropriate laboratory data, few hematologic disorders could be recognized or treated. On the other hand, laboratory studies alone are rarely adequate regardless of their type or quantity. The fundamental importance of a detailed history and a carefully performed physical examination must not be overlooked. Laboratory examinations supplement these indispensable clinical observations; they do not supplant them.

Hematology has been affected profoundly in recent years by rapid and, on occasion, breathtaking advances in technology. The development of an impressive array of ingenious techniques provided a dramatic impetus to research which has revolutionized our concepts of hematopoietic physiology and the pathophysiology of many hematologic diseases. The list of laboratory procedures available to study the blood and blood-forming organs is lengthy and continuing to grow; a description of them all would be a formidable task and far beyond the scope of this book. Furthermore, such a listing would have little clinical usefulness.

Only a few of the recently developed, specialized techniques have become routine; most are investigative tools with, at best, limited clinical applications.

They are considered, when appropriate, in the discussions of individual diseases, for example, ^{51}Cr-tagged red cell life-spans (p. 82) and radioactive cobalt-labeled vitamin B_{12} absorption tests (p. 216). Certain laboratory examinations are routine and comprise an essential part of the work-up of all patients suspected of having a hematologic disorder, primary or secondary. Consequently, it is pertinent to consider them separately and in some detail.

The blood and blood-forming organs possess three attributes that facilitate the laboratory diagnosis of hematologic disease.

1. They can be sampled easily and repeatedly with virtually no untoward side effects and minimal discomfort to the patient.

2. Single-cell systems can be studied.

3. Simple quantitative and qualitative techniques provide accurate and relevant information about complex processes of cell production and destruction as well as biochemical defects and cellular dysfunction.

Basic hematologic studies include quantification of the blood cells in the circulation, study of the peripheral blood film, and examination of the bone marrow and/or other blood-forming organs; for example, lymph nodes. These data provide a readily accessible approach to diagnosis and a means of following responses to therapy. Newer and more directly informative techniques have neither replaced these simpler laboratory examinations nor lessened their value. Recent years have witnessed a tendency to substitute for clinically proved procedures newer, complex, more expensive, and less widely available techniques ostensibly because they yield more accurate information of greater diagnostic import. Therefore a restatement of the role of the routine studies in the present-day diagnosis and treatment of hematologic diseases is of practical and academic interest.

The science of hematology was founded on morphologic observations. Astute clinicians were quick to perceive the clinical implications of these studies, and morphologic techniques were adapted for clinical use and widely adopted as diagnostic aids. Hematology as a biologic discipline grew and flourished in this "morphologic phase" of its development, but, as research began to yield answers at a molecular level to important problems dealing with physiology and pathophysiology, the limitations of this approach became apparent. New techniques were needed to cope with the challenges of molecular biology, and hematology entered the "biochemical phase" of its development.

The dramatic impact of the large amount of recently acquired fundamental information pertaining to the blood in health and in disease has tended to overshadow the contributions that can still be made by morphologic techniques. The belief that the morphologic approach to hematologic problems has outlived its usefulness is, regrettably, being encountered with greater frequency. As a result, some now view the clinical hematologist who continues to rely on hematologic morphology as old-fashioned and out of step with the times. This concept must be dispelled if the patient is to continue to benefit by the advances being made in the research laboratory. Because of the complexity of certain of the techniques used as investigative tools, it has been assumed erroneously that accurate hematologic diagnosis is predicated on such tests. Many of these procedures are available only in a few of the larger medical centers. In addition, they are expensive, often cause the patient discomfort and/or inconvenience, and require the services of highly trained personnel. For these reasons it is necessary to place certain newer and more complicated techniques in their proper perspective. Although they have made invaluable contributions to basic knowledge, most hematologic disorders can be diagnosed with relatively simple laboratory support.

Morphology remains the foundation of clinical hematology. The results of recent hematologic research do not detract from this statement; they attest to its validity. Hematologic morphology rests on a stronger footing now than at any time in the past. It is no longer necessary to interpret morphologic abnormalities on the basis of empiric observations. Instead, rational explanations for many morphologic findings now exist or are emerging, thus contributing to their significance. The morphologic approach to clinical hematologic problems remains the surest, quickest, easiest, and most logical path for the clinician to follow, provided he interprets this information in the light of modern pathophysiologic concepts and supplements it when needed by additional laboratory support. For example, an *accurate* diagnosis of a spherocytic hemolytic anemia based on morphologic criteria is *no less accurate* because the mean red cell life-span is not quantified in days. However, a morphologic diagnosis of a spherocytic hemolytic anemia is not enough, and a precise etiologic diagnosis is contingent on additional laboratory documentation (p. 85).

Thus the modern hematologist continues to rely on the time-proved morphologic techniques of the early workers in this field. However, the many important advantages his predecessors did not have include detailed knowledge of the pathophysiologic mechanisms responsible for many morphologic aberrations and the availability of additional laboratory techniques which, when indicated, provide specific and invaluable information. The study of the morphology of the blood and blood cell precursors remains as important to the present-day student of hematology as it was in the past. Today, however, it has much more meaning.

PERIPHERAL BLOOD

Under normal conditions the cellular composition of the peripheral blood exhibits remarkable quantitative and qualitative stability. Therefore deviations from the norm can be detected with relative ease and serve as valuable indicators of a variety of hematologic and nonhematologic diseases. Routine examination of the peripheral blood includes measurement of the erythroid values, total and differential leukocyte counts, evaluation of blood cell morphology, and a platelet count; in all patients suspected of having a hematologic disorder, a reticulocyte count should be added to the list. Although these simple procedures require a minimum of equipment, they do demand a certain amount of dexterity and skill obtained only by practice. Standardization and uniformity of techniques are requisites for the establishment of normal values and the correct interpretation of results. The ease with which specimens can be procured permits repeat or serial determinations.

Erythroid Values. The peripheral erythroid values include a hematocrit determination, measurement of the hemoglobin content of the blood, and an erythrocyte count. They ordinarily provide comparable information, although some morphologic abnormalities affect certain parameters differently. For example, the presence of a large number of hypochromic microcytes will be reflected by a disproportionately higher erythrocyte count than hemoglobin level, and an anemia distinguished by normochromic macrocytes will be manifested by a greater decrease in the erythrocyte count than in the hemoglobin or hematocrit levels. For reasons discussed elsewhere (p. 59) the erythroid measurements should not be used to classify an anemia morphologically. In most laboratories all three determinations are performed routinely; however, any one will suffice if accurately done. In practice it is desirable to obtain at least two different measurements so that one can be used to check the accuracy of the other. Because of their technical simplicity and the lesser likelihood of error, a hematocrit and hemoglobin level are preferred. The normal ranges for the erythroid values are listed in Chapter 3 (p. 56).

HEMATOCRIT. When properly carried out, the hematocrit or packed red cell volume is the most reliable of all the erythroid measurements. Important ancillary information may be obtained from the appearance of the supernatant plasma; for example, colored in the presence of hyperbilirubinemia and almost colorless in patients with iron deficiency anemia. The height of the white cell column may also be informative. The microhematocrit technique is now widely used and has several distinct advantages which include (1) very small amounts of blood (a venipuncture is not needed), (2) a simple, accurate, reproducible, and fast technique (5 minutes as opposed to 30 minutes for a Wintrobe hematocrit), and (3) easily obtained duplicate determinations which decrease the chances of an erroneous result. The microhematocrit technique does not permit the simultaneous determination of an erythrocyte sedimentation rate.

HEMOGLOBINOMETRY. This relatively simple test can yield accurate results, although it is subject to observational errors and certain other variations. The cyanmethemoglobin method utilizing a photoelectric colorimeter is the preferred technique. Visual colorimetry with a Sahli (acid hematin) type of hemoglobinometer provides acceptable results if a photoelectric cell is not available. Standardization of individual instruments under actual working conditions is imperative, regardless of the method used, and should be rechecked at frequent intervals. If a technique does not permit standardization, it should be avoided. Standards are commercially available for the cyanmethemoglobin technique.

ERYTHROCYTE COUNT. This erythroid measurement is more time-consuming and subject to much greater error than are the hematocrit and hemoglobin determinations. There are three sources of inaccuracies. The error associated with any estimation based on a small random sample and applied to an entire population cannot be eliminated; for hemacytometer counting this amounts to about ±10 per cent. The second error is the result of structural defects in pipettes and counting chambers; it is virtually negligible. The third and most important type of error, introduced by technical imperfections, can be reduced to a minimum only by practice and special attention to all details of the technique. The introduction of electronic cell counters has done much to eliminate errors and to enhance the value of an erythrocyte count.

Leukocyte Counts. A leukocyte count involves the accurate dilution of a representative sample of the peripheral blood in a diluent that destroys the non-nucleated erythrocytes and renders more refractile the leukocytes; the cells contained within a measured volume are then enumerated. In adults the normal leukocyte count ranges between 4000 to 10,000/cu mm; in children the count is slightly higher (p. 308). Leukocytes may be counted by hemacytometer or with an electronic counter; these counts are subject to many of the errors associated with red cell counts. It should be noted that a leukocyte (or white cell) count is actually a total nucleated cell count. Nucleated red cells are included, and the count should be corrected if there are 10 or more/100 leukocytes.

Blood Film. *Microscopic study of a stained peripheral blood film of good quality constitutes the most important part of any hematologic examination.* Frequently, all information needed to determine the cause of a hematologic disorder can be obtained by a trained observer from the inspection of a well-made, well-stained blood film. Since interpretation is based on differences in cell morphology, careful standardization of the preparation and staining of blood films is mandatory.

Peripheral blood films may be made on glass slides or coverslips. Coverslips are preferred because they permit a more uniform distribution of the cellular components of the blood; in some slide smears smaller cells such as lymphocytes congregate in the middle, whereas larger cells such as neutrophils and monocytes accumulate near the edges. In addition, staining of coverslip films can be more easily controlled. Preparation of coverslips is time-consuming (they must be scrupulously clean) and the actual technique of handling them and making the films requires practice. Once familiar with this technique, however, most persons find it to be just as easy and convenient as the slide method. The end product, that is, the stained film, is almost always superior. Blood films should not be made from blood to which an anticoagulant has been added, for all such agents induce unwanted morphologic aberrations—some more than others.

A variety of stains is available; a Romanowsky stain consisting of polychrome methylene blue and eosin is recommended. Wright's stain is widely used and is preferred for its general staining characteristics and simplicity. Briefly, the principle of staining with Wright's stain consists of flooding the film with stain for one minute; this process serves only to fix the film (the stain is dissolved in absolute methyl alcohol), and staining does not take place until water is added to bring about partial dissociation of the compound dye. Staining time varies somewhat with different batches of stain; ordinarily it requires around three minutes. Therefore the entire staining process can be completed in about four minutes. The staining technique must be rigidly monitored or the blood film may appear too light (understained), too dark (overstained), too red (acid), or too blue (alkaline). It may be necessary to double-stain peripheral blood films from patients with very high leukocyte counts.

Interpretation of a peripheral blood film is contingent on the examiner's ability to recognize normal cells and to detect abnormalities in their appearance. Thus some training in hematologic morphology is essential. In this regard there is no short cut to becoming an accomplished morphologist and there is no substitute for time spent at the microscope examining normal and abnormal blood films. For this purpose an experienced teacher who can help in the identification of cells is indispensable. It is extremely difficult to describe verbally the many morphologic attributes that contribute to a cell's appearance. One glance through a microscope is more revealing than pages of detailed descriptions; even photomicrographs have their shortcomings, despite technical perfection. All physicians, regardless of their primary interests, should acquire the training and skill needed to evaluate a normal peripheral blood film and to recognize the more commonly encountered abnormalities. The importance of this examination in all branches of clinical medicine cannot be overemphasized.

Erythrocytes and platelets should be evaluated in addition to a differential leukocyte count. The differential count should include at least 100 (and preferably more) consecutive cells; normal values are given elsewhere (p. 309). The number and type of abnormal cells should be noted. When evaluating red cells, it is helpful for the beginner to have available a well-made, well-stained normal blood film for purposes of comparing size, shape, and chromicity. Although platelets are less likely to be clumped in a supravitally stained preparation, it is possible to obtain a fairly accurate estimate of the platelet count by scanning a Wright-stained blood film. Normally, there should be about three to eight platelets per oil-immersion field.

Many different stains and techniques have been devised for the morphologic study of the blood cells. Some are quite helpful in the identification of abnormal cells, but in most instances a simple Wright-stained film suffices. Study of living cells by phase microscopy is often revealing but requires a certain amount of training and experience which most physicians do not possess. The electron microscope is still a research tool. A variety of stains has been used in an attempt to achieve selective staining of leukocytes, that is, specific staining of one cell type, thus permitting its ready recognition. None has been entirely successful, for no single leukocyte possesses a component that can be so used and is not found in other cell types. Therefore learning how to recognize the different leukocytes in a blood film stained with a Romanowsky stain is much more accurate.

Supravital staining techniques have been widely employed. Again, they require additional training because the cells' morphology differs from that in an ordinary Wright-stained film. Brilliant cresyl blue films are technically simple. A 0.3 per cent solution of brilliant cresyl blue in absolute ethyl alcohol is spread on clean coverslips or slides and allowed to dry. These coverslips or slides can then be stored indefinitely. Just before use they are polished lightly on a piece of hard-finish white paper until their color changes from a blue-gray to a light lavender. Blood films are then made and counterstained with Wright's stain. Advantages of this technique include (1) morphologic changes, for example, nucleoli are made more evident, thereby aiding in the identification of certain abnormalities such as lymphosarcoma cells (p. 376), (2) evenly distributed platelets can be accurately quantified, and (3) reticulocytes are made visible (p. 8); this technique provides a permanent preparation from which an accurate reticulocyte count can be made (the number of reticulocytes encountered per 1000 erythrocytes).

Platelet Counts.   Many different techniques have been devised for platelet enumeration. The most accurate involves phase microscopy; this direct method uses a 1 per cent solution of ammonium oxalate as the diluent and yields normal values of 140,000 to 440,000/cu mm. For routine clinical use the dried film or indirect method is recommended as a simpler procedure which gives quite accurate and reproducible results. In brief, the platelets per 1000 erythrocytes are counted on brilliant cresyl blue blood films which have been counterstained with Wright's stain. The number counted multiplied by the erythrocyte count and divided by 1000 yields the platelets per cubic millimeter. The normal range with this method is 200,000 to 400,000/cu mm. Before counting, the blood film should be scanned; if platelet clumps are present, the preparation is not suitable. With practice it soon becomes possible merely to estimate the platelet count with considerable accuracy.

EXAMINATION OF THE BLOOD-FORMING ORGANS

Bone Marrow. Most of the blood cells are formed in the bone marrow. Consequently, examination of a marrow specimen often provides information of great value in the diagnosis and treatment of hematologic disorders. Sternal marrow aspiration was introduced by Arinkin in 1929 and quickly adopted because of its simplicity, the general excellence of the preparations obtained, and the opportunity to make repeated examinations. With few exceptions aspiration is the technique of choice.

TECHNIQUE FOR PROCURING SPECIMENS. Any bone that contains red marrow and is sufficiently close to the surface of the body is suitable. In the adult the sternum is preferred because of its accessibility, the thinness of the bone and the consequent ease with which the myeloid cavity can be entered, and the cellularity of the marrow in this site. A variety of needles is available. Any short-beveled, wide-bore needle with a stylet will do; for example, a 3- to 4-cm 18-gage lumbar puncture needle. A valuable modification is the addition of an adjustable guard to control the depth the needle can be advanced. The preferred location is the upper part of the body of the sternum at the level of the second intercostal space. In the adult the sternum averages about 1 cm in thickness; the outer plate varies from 0.5 to 5 mm and the myeloid cavity is 5 to 10 mm in depth.

The operator wears sterile gloves, and the area is shaved (if necessary), cleansed, and draped as for any minor surgical procedure. With the patient lying on his back without a pillow (preferably on a hard surface such as an examining table), the skin and periosteum are infiltrated with procaine or some other suitable local anesthetic. The operator then outlines again the lateral borders of the sternum between the second and third ribs, and while standing at the patient's side, introduces the needle and advances it until bone is touched. He then moves to the head of the table and penetrates the myeloid cavity at about a 45° angle with a back and forth rotary or boring motion. During this process the consistency of the bone should be noted. For example, it may be extremely soft in patients with plasmacytic myeloma (p. 424) and excessively hard in others with agnogenic myeloid metaplasia (p. 434).

Ordinarily a "give" is felt when the myeloid cavity is entered; as soon as this happens (or, in the absence of a give, as soon as the needle is firmly fixed in bone), aspiration should be attempted. The stylet is removed and a dry 10- or 20-ml syringe attached to the needle. Maximal suction should be applied as quickly as possible, although care must be taken not to dislodge the needle in the process. The slow application of negative pressure is to be avoided, for this maneuver is more likely to procure sinusoidal blood than it is to dislodge marrow particles. As soon as material appears in the syringe, the plunger should be returned and the needle and syringe removed from the sternum in a single movement. Continued suction in an effort to obtain a larger specimen will only dilute the marrow with sinusoidal blood. The plunger should always be released before the needle is removed from the marrow cavity or the specimen will be splattered over the inside of the syringe.

If the first aspiration does not yield material, the stylet should be reintroduced and the needle rotated about a quarter of a turn without being advanced farther. If subsequent attempts to aspirate marrow are still unsuccessful, the stylet should be returned and the needle advanced slowly with repeated tries to obtain marrow. If there is *any* doubt of the location of the needle in reference to the posterior plate of the sternum, the needle should be removed and reintroduced at another site.

Alternative locations from which marrow can be aspirated are the anterior or posterior iliac crests and the spinous processes of the third or fourth lumbar vertebrae. The most easily accessible site is the anterior iliac crest. With the patient lying on his back on a hard flat surface, the needle is inserted at right angles to the crest just behind the anterior superior iliac spine or perpendicular to the flat surface about 2 cm posterior and 2 cm inferior to the anterior superior spine. When using a spinous process, the patient may sit leaning slightly forward or lie on his side. The spinous process must be easily palpable. The needle is inserted perpendicular to the skin slightly to one side of the midline and about midway between the upper and lower borders. In general, it is technically more difficult to introduce the needle into these sites than it is to enter the sternal myeloid cavity. In addition, iliac crest and spinous process aspirates are likely to be slightly less cellular than sternal marrow. However, sites other than the sternum offer certain important advantages. The anterior iliac crest is the preferred site in children over the age of two because of the thinness of the sternum and the likelihood that they might move during the procedure; under the age of two, marrow is best aspirated from the medial aspect of the upper tibia just below the tibial tuberosity. The iliac crest is also the preferred site for use by untrained operators, since the possibility of serious untoward effects are virtually nil. Rare deaths have occurred consequent to penetration of the posterior plate of the sternum (usually by inexperienced operators) with resultant injury to the heart or great vessels. In selected patients an "aimed" puncture at a site of pain or tenderness may be especially rewarding; for example, it may yield carcinoma cells (p. 243).

A marrow aspiration is the source of little discomfort to the patient and can be likened to such procedures as a lumbar puncture or a pleural tap. Often, patients indicate that a marrow aspiration is less painful than a venipuncture. Most patients experience a peculiar "drawing" pain as marrow is being aspirated. It is transient and disappears as soon as suction is stopped. There is no way to prevent or lessen this discomfort. When it occurs, it indicates with certainty that the needle is in the myeloid cavity. Complications of marrow aspirations are few. Bleeding has been observed, most often in patients with hemophilia or some allied coagulation disorder; bleeding is rare in thrombocytopenic patients, even those with extremely low platelet counts. Collodion seals and/or tight dressings decrease the chances of bleeding. As already mentioned, a few fatalities have been ascribed to sternal punctures. Sternal fractures may occur, especially in persons with plasmacytic myeloma or some comparable disorder of bone. Under these circumstances another site such as the iliac crest should be selected.

If repeated attempts to aspirate marrow are unsuccessful ("dry taps") or produce only a small amount of sinusoidal or peripheral blood, it may be necessary to resort to a marrow biopsy. An open surgical biopsy yields the most suitable material; however, this technique possesses all the disadvantages of a surgical procedure. Closed biopsies can be obtained with Vim-Silverman or Turkel-Bethell needles which also permit another attempt at aspiration in addition to providing a small bone plug. Aspirates are much easier to procure and cytologic detail is ordinarily superior. Therefore a marrow biopsy is indicated only as a last resort.

TECHNIQUE FOR PROCESSING SPECIMENS. Since marrow specimens clot very quickly, they must be processed for study with great speed. Many different techniques have been recommended. In general, the simplest is the best. Wright-stained coverslip or slide smears of freshly aspirated marrow provide excellent morphologic detail and furnish adequate information. Inasmuch as anticoagulants induce certain undesirable changes in morphology, they should be avoided. All marrow aspirates are diluted with variable amounts of sinusoidal blood; in addition, a marrow aspirate is only a small sample and may not be representative of myelopoietic activity at other sites. Consequently, attempts to quantify the cellular and fat content of a marrow specimen serve relatively little purpose.

The most satisfactory preparations are made directly at the patient's side. Immediately on removing the syringe and needle from the bone marrow cavity a small amount of material should be expelled on a cover-slip or slide held by a technologist or assistant. Marrow clumps or particles are ordinarily evident, and it is possible to aspirate excess blood back into the syringe; this blood is then discarded. Using another coverslip or slide, the assistant makes a marrow film in the same way a peripheral blood film is made. This process is repeated, and several films can be made before the specimen clots unless the aspirate is very limited. An alternative method is to expel the entire aspirate on a watch glass or some similar surface. Marrow clumps can then be picked out with a pipette. This method has the advantage of not requiring an assistant. On the other hand, the additional maneuver increases the likelihood that the specimen will clot before the preparations can be made.

Marrow films are stained as peripheral blood films. Wright's or some other Romanowsky stain is preferred; because of the large number of nucleated cells, it is often necessary to double stain. It is noteworthy that gross marrow clumps are not always evident. A single drop of marrow in the lumen of the needle may be diagnostic; therefore, all material should be smeared and stained.

In addition to Wright-stained preparations, some laboratories utilize fixed-tissue sections. Marrow clumps or units are fixed, blocked, sectioned, and stained with hematoxylin and eosin. It has been pointed out that this technique increases the chances of detecting certain focal marrow lesions such as metastatic carcinoma, sarcoidosis, tuberculosis, amyloidosis, and thrombotic thrombocytopenic purpura. Serial sections may also give a truer picture of marrow cellularity. These advantages cannot be denied; however, individual cellular morphology is poor in fixed sections. Furthermore, it is generally possible to make an accurate estimate of cellularity from Wright-stained smears. Therefore the additional information that might be obtained from fixed sections does not warrant the inclusion of this time-consuming process as a routine part of every marrow examination. If it is necessary to resort to a marrow biopsy, imprints should be prepared and stained with Wright's stain in addition to fixed sections of the decalcified bone plug stained with hematoxylin and eosin. The imprints, which are made by gently touching and streaking the specimen to a slide, permit detailed study and easy identification of single cells; the fixed sections reveal over-all cellularity, focal lesions, and myelofibrosis.

INTERPRETATION. Bone marrow interpretation is a complicated, difficult task and requires considerable training and experience. It would be presumptuous to infer otherwise. Only those physicians who have had appropriate subspecialty training in hematology can be expected to evaluate a marrow specimen accurately. On the other hand, all clinicians must be aware of the kind of information obtainable in this manner so that they can properly determine the indications for the procedure.

The types and relative numbers of normal marrow cells are listed in Table 2-1. It must be emphasized that a marrow differential count

Table 2-1. *Approximate Values for Nucleated Cells in Sternal Marrow Aspirates of Adults, Both Sexes*

	MEAN %	RANGE %
Myeloblasts	1.5	0.25–3.0
Progranulocytes	6.0	1.0–8.0
Neutrophilic myelocytes	12.0	7.0–20.0
Neutrophilic metamyelocytes	20.0	10.0–30.0
Neutrophils—band and segmented	24.0	15.0–35.0
Eosinophils—all stages	1.5	0.5–3.0
Basophils—all stages	0.3	0.0–1.0
Lymphocytes	7.0	2.0–12.0
Monocytes	2.0	0.5–5.0
Reticulum cells	0.2	0.2–1.0
Plasmacytes	0.5	0.0–2.0
Megakaryocytes	(less than 0.01)	
Rubriblasts (proerythroblasts) / Prorubricytes (early normoblasts)	4.0	2.0–6.0
Rubricytes (intermediate normoblasts)	14.0	12.0–20.0
Metarubricytes (late normoblasts)	7.0	6.0–10.0
Erythroid:granulocyte (E:G) ratio	1:3	1:1.5–1:8

is at best an approximation, regardless of how many cells are counted (100 cell counts are valueless). Because myeloid cells proliferate *in situ* by homeoplastic mitosis, the marrow is composed of scattered clumps of similar cells; it is not a mixture of different cell types uniformly dispersed.

A bone marrow aspirate is a small sample of a large organ and may not be representative of myelopoiesis at other sites. Therefore marrow specimens must *always* be interpreted in the light of other clinical and hematologic findings. Abnormalities in myeloid activity are commonly reflected by appropriate changes in the peripheral blood. Consequently, the marrow findings can usually be predicted with accuracy by study of the peripheral blood, especially the blood film.

The following types of information can be obtained from a bone marrow examination (more detailed descriptions of marrow pictures are to be found in the discussions of specific disorders): (1) over-all cellularity, including fat content and the presence or absence of clumps of cells, (2) relationship between erythropoiesis and granulopoiesis (the erythroid:granulocyte or E:G ratio), (3) quantitative assessment (both relative and absolute) of all aspects of myelopoiesis, (4) changes in the morphology of blood cell precursors (e.g., the megaloblastic morphology of the nucleated erythrocytes in the anemias caused by deficiencies of vitamin B_{12} or folic acid [p. 209]), (5) status of maturation within a cell compartment (e.g., the disorderly maturation characterizing leukemia [p. 337]) as well as asynchronism between nuclear and cytoplasmic maturation, (6) cellular function (e.g., are the more mature nucleated red cells being properly hemoglobinized?), (7) appraisal of iron stores, (8) presence or absence of abnormal cells (e.g., carcinoma cells or certain microorganisms), and (9) with the use of special techniques, chromosomal abnormalities like the Ph^1 chromosome in chronic granulocytic leukemia (p. 365).

INDICATIONS. A bone marrow examination contributes importantly to the diagnosis of certain hematologic disorders and in the assessment of responses to treatment. However, it does not always provide specific or even relevant information, and the presence of a hematologic abnormality, for example, an anemia, or the suspicion of a hematologic disorder is not always an indication to study the bone marrow. The decision to employ this procedure must be made for each patient on the basis of the history, physical findings, and examination of the peripheral blood (with or without other laboratory tests). For example, a bone marrow adds little to the work-up of a patient with a microcytic, hypochromic anemia caused by documented bleeding; on the other hand, the demonstration of normal or increased iron stores may be of great value in the work-up of a patient with a microcytic, hypochromic anemia caused by thalassemia (p. 268). A list of the disorders in which a marrow examination may or may not be of value is of little practical use. Instead, knowledge of marrow pathophysiology in the disorder believed to be present provides a much more rational basis for the decision to procure a marrow specimen. Consequently, the precise indications for marrow examinations are more appropriately considered in those sections that deal with specific hematologic disorders.

Bone marrow examination is invaluable to the hematologist; it should not be inferred otherwise. The point that deserves emphasis is the frequent misuse of this procedure because of the physician's failure to delineate the conditions in which it will or will not be of value. Although the source of little discomfort to the patient and virtually innocuous in trained hands, complications have occurred, especially with sternal punctures. In addition, the preparation, staining, and interpretation of bone marrow specimens are time-consuming tasks that require experienced personnel. Therefore clear-cut indications for a marrow aspiration must exist.

Lymph Nodes. Although marrow aspirations have been widely adopted as a clinical and research tool of great value, lymph node aspirations are rarely used. Yet there are a number of situations in which a lymph node aspirate may be helpful. Most often an involved node is biopsied and fixed sections are examined. This technique provides important information regarding over-all changes in node architecture; however, individual cellular morphology is poorly maintained. A node biopsy is a surgical procedure with all the attendant disadvantages; a node aspiration is a simple, painless office or bedside procedure. Furthermore, it permits detailed morphologic study of individual cells.

The skin overlying the palpable node selected to be aspirated is shaved (if necessary) and cleansed as for a marrow aspiration. There is no need for a local anesthetic because the procedure causes the patient no more discomfort than a venipuncture. The operator grasps and immobilizes the node with the thumb and forefinger of one hand and introduces in a single movement directly into the substance of the node an 18- or 20-gage needle attached to a 10- or 20-ml syringe. Moderate suction should be applied quickly. If no material appears in the syringe (a common occurrence), the plunger may be released and two or three more attempts made. The plunger should always be returned to its original position before the syringe and needle are removed from the node or the small aspirate (frequently just a drop in the lumen of the needle) may be irretrievably drawn up into the syringe. The aspirate is blown out on a coverslip or slide and films are made and stained with Wright's stain.

A normal lymph node aspirate consists of about 90 per cent small mature lymphocytes; the rest are large lymphocytes (most of which are mature) with rare plasmacytes and reticulum cells. In patients with lymph node pathology distinguished by morphologically specific cells (e.g., Reed-Sternberg cells [p. 383], lymphosarcoma cells [p. 377], or carcinoma cells), a node aspirate may establish the diagnosis. It should be emphasized that a node aspirate will not reveal distortion in node architecture by morphologically normal cells; neither will a normal aspirate exclude diagnoses like lymphoma or metastatic carcinoma. However, it is such a simple procedure that it is worthwhile in almost every patient with enlarged nodes in whom a malignant disorder is suspected. Even when a node is surgically removed, in addition to fixed sections, imprints should be prepared and stained with Wright's stain. Imprints permit detailed cytologic study unobtainable with the fixed-section technique.

Spleen. Splenic aspiration has been advised in the diagnosis of certain disorders; for example, agnogenic myeloid metaplasia (p. 435) or lymphoma associated with specific cells (i.e., Hodgkin's disease [Reed-Sternberg cells] or lymphosarcoma). However, a splenic aspiration is not without hazard. Lacerations are fairly common and bleeding may require an emergency splenectomy. In view of the limited information obtainable with this technique, there are few indications for its use. The decision to aspirate the spleen requires seasoned clinical judgment, and the procedure should be carried out only if adequate facilities and personnel are available to perform, if necessary, an emergency splenectomy.

Anemia
(General Considerations
and Classification)

Anemia is a decrease in hemoglobin per unit volume of blood below the level previously established as normal with respect to age and sex. This definition is not necessarily synonymous with a decrease in total body hemoglobin or red cell mass. However, the relationship between venous and body hematocrits is quite constant and total blood volume is relatively stable under a variety of conditions. Following acute hemorrhage, a normal blood volume is rapidly restored by appropriate changes in plasma volume. Even in chronic anemias an increased plasma volume maintains a near normal blood volume. Hypervolemia due to an expanded plasma volume causes a fall in the peripheral erythroid values even in the presence of a normal red cell mass, but, with the exception of the physiologic "anemia" of pregnancy and acute (but rarely chronic) congestive heart failure, such situations are not often encountered. Furthermore, the hemoglobin contained in a given quantity of blood accurately reflects the functional competency of the blood to supply oxygen to the tissues. Therefore the definition is valid and clinically useful.

NORMAL VALUES

The peripheral erythroid values depend on age, sex, elevation above sea level, and, to a certain extent, the techniques employed. Ideally, the normal range should be determined for each individual laboratory, but this is not always practical. Based on the cyanmethemoglobin method, the microhematocrit technique, and hemacytometer erythrocyte counts, the ranges of normal values for an altitude comparable to that of Chicago (about 600 ft above sea level) are listed in Table 3-1. In the newborn the hemo-

Table 3-1. *Normal Range of Peripheral Erythroid Values*

Determination	Adults		Children— Both Sexes (3 mo.–13 yr.)
	Males	Females	
Hemoglobin (gm/100 ml)	13.5–17.5	12.0–15.5	10.0–14.5
Hematocrit (%)	42–53	38–46	31–43
Erythrocytes (millions/cu mm)	4.6–6.2	4.2–5.4	3.8–5.2

globin varies between 18 and 22 gm/100 ml of blood; by the second week of life it has decreased about 4 gm/100 ml, and by the second to third month normal childhood levels are reached. During the first two years of life the average hemoglobin is about 11 gm/100 ml; the erythroid values then increase slowly throughout childhood and reach adult levels at about the age of 14.

ETIOLOGIC CLASSIFICATION

An anemia is a manifestation of some underlying disorder and is not a disease *sui generis*. Its exact nature must be sought by careful study of all phases of red cell production and destruction and by elucidation of their disturbances. Inasmuch as the causes of anemia are multiple and diverse, a simple and workable etiologic classification is needed. Although all anemias are the result of inadequate blood formation (production failing to keep pace with peripheral need), they can be divided into two broad groups on the basis of the *fundamental* pathogenic mechanism responsible for the lowered erythroid values. These two categories and their subgroups with representative examples of specific diseases are shown in Table 3-2. It is not unusual for an anemia to reflect both blood loss and impaired production.

Table 3-2. *Etiologic Classification of Anemia*

I. *Blood Loss*
   A. Hemorrhage
   B. Hemolysis

II. *Impaired Erythropoiesis*
   A. Deficiencies   Vitamin B_{12}, folic acid, and iron
   B. Destruction   Hypoplastic anemia
   C. Diversion of growth potential   Granulocytic leukemia
   D. Displacement   Lymphocytic leukemia and metastatic carcinoma
   E. Defective   Hereditary hemoglobinopathies
   F. "Depression" (etiology unknown)   Anemia of chronic infection and liver disease

PATHOPHYSIOLOGY

A reduction in the oxygen-carrying capacity of the blood produces tissue hypoxia and activates a number of corrective mechanisms which attempt to compensate for the interference with oxygen transport. The clinical manifestations of anemia reflect these physiologic adjustments as well as cellular hypoxia. The physiologic adjustments include tachycardia, an augmented cardiac output, accelerated velocity of blood flow (caused by a decrease in blood viscosity and peripheral resistance), and increased pulmonary ventilation. In addition, a shift to the right in the oxyhemoglobin dissociation curve (Fig. 1-9, p. 21), together with a reduction in tissue oxygen tension, decreases the affinity of hemoglobin for oxygen and permits better extraction of oxygen in the peripheral vascular beds.

The response to a reduction in circulating hemoglobin is dependent on the rate at which the anemia develops, the competency of the physiologic corrective mechanisms, the degree of activity (or oxygen requirements), and, of course, the level of the erythroid values. Acute hemorrhage with rapid loss of about one third (or even less) of the blood volume will evoke a profound reaction (i.e., shock). If anemia develops gradually, however, an otherwise normal person may tolerate as much as a 50 per cent reduction in hemoglobin without conspicuous untoward effects. A long-standing anemia with a hemoglobin of 9 to 11 gm/100 ml of blood is not associated with significant symptoms (fatigability) or findings other than minimal pallor and slight tachycardia. In an individual without underlying cardiac or pulmonary disease exertional dyspnea has its onset at a hemoglobin of about 7.5, dyspnea at rest at approximately 3, and congestive heart failure at 2 to 2.5 gm/100 ml. Hemoglobin levels below 2.0 gm/100 ml are ordinarily incompatible with life. Weakness is not marked until the hemoglobin falls to 6 gm/100 ml or less. Other manifestations of anemia include headache (often severe), low-grade fever (usually associated with a hemoglobin of 4 gm/100 ml or less), cardiac murmurs (typically apical or pulmonic systolic murmurs), and electrocardiographic abnormalities (most often nonspecific T-wave changes). The effects of anemia are often obscured or complicated by other manifestations of the primary disease. Furthermore, inadequate physiologic adjustment will drastically alter the individual's ability to tolerate low erythroid values. Thus children and young adults compensate amazingly well and often deny all symptoms even with marked anemia. On the other hand, a moderate anemia may precipitate congestive failure or contribute to myocardial ischemia in patients with underlying cardiac disease or coronary insufficiency. In general, one need not be seriously concerned about the deleterious effects of the anemia per se if the hemoglobin is above 7.0 to 7.5 gm/100 ml of blood.

EVALUATION OF THE ANEMIC PATIENT

Recently developed radioisotopic, electrophoretic, immunologic, cyto-chemical, and other techniques have been responsible for a dramatic increase in the tempo of hematologic research. These methods have contributed greatly to our basic knowledge of the physiology and pathophysiology of erythropoiesis and have clarified the patho-genesis of a number of heretofore poorly understood anemias. In addition to their use as investigative tools, most of the newer techniques have undergone rapid clinical adaptation and are now widely employed as diagnostic aids. As a result, evaluation of the anemic patient, basi-cally a simple task, is now viewed by many as a specialized procedure that can be accomplished only in a well-equipped laboratory staffed with a variety of highly trained personnel. Such is *not* the case. A diagnosis of a hemolytic anemia is not dependent on ^{51}Cr red cell sur-vival data (p. 107), nor is the diagnosis of pernicious anemia predi-cated on the failure to excrete in the urine a certain percentage of orally administered radioactive vitamin B_{12} (p. 216). Furthermore, the complexity, cost, and limited availability of such methods are impor-tant disadvantages. It is pertinent, therefore, to place recent techno-logic advances in their proper perspective and to reassess diagnostic approaches in the light of information obtainable by these means.

The clinician's observations which rely heavily on hematologic mor-phology have *not* become obsolete parameters of little use in the work-up of an anemic patient. Newer and more sophisticated techniques sup-plement such clinical studies but do not replace them. A history, physi-cal examination, some measure of the erythroid values (hemoglobin, hematocrit, and/or erythrocyte count—a single determination will suffice if correctly done), a leukocyte count, and examination of the periph-eral blood film are the basic studies required to evaluate an anemic patient. More often than not these data permit a precise etiologic di-agnosis. The importance of a detailed history and careful physical ex-amination must not be overlooked. This information is indispensable to the clinical hematologist; without it a rational approach to the problem of the anemic patient is precluded, irrespective of the type or quantity of laboratory observations available. With these clinical data exami-nation of the peripheral blood then affords relevant information. When there is knowledge of normal values and the results, in duplicate, of the peripheral erythroid measurements are provided, an anemia can usually be detected with ease. It should be recognized that a small number of otherwise normal subjects will have erythroid values slightly below the lower limits of normal; however, all possible abnormal causes must be excluded before such values can be considered normal for that particular individual.

Morphologic Classification. After the establishment of the existence of an anemia, the next step is to classify the process morphologically. Depending on the size of the erythrocytes, an anemia is categorized as *normocytic, microcytic,* or *macrocytic.* The chromicity of a red cell refers to its hemoglobin concentration or to the ratio of hemoglobin to total red cell mass; it is not a measure of the quantity of hemoglobin contained in the cell. Hemoglobin normally accounts for 30 to 36 per cent of the wet weight of a human erythrocyte. If the red cells have a normal concentration of hemoglobin, they are described as normochromic, regardless of their size. If the concentration of hemoglobin falls below normal, the cells are termed hypochromic. Since a mammalian erythrocyte cannot become supersaturated with hemoglobin, there is no place in hematologic nomenclature for the term hyperchromic. Thus an anemia may be characterized as *hypochromic* or *normochromic* but never as hyperchromic. Theoretically, several morphologic diagnoses are possible. Actually, most anemias are *normocytic-normochromic, microcytic-hypochromic,* or *macrocytic-normochromic.*

Cell measurements derived from the hemoglobin, hematocrit, and erythrocyte count have been widely used as indicators of the size, hemoglobin concentration, and hemoglobin content of the average erythrocyte (Table 3-3). Inasmuch as the MCH reflects both the size and

Table 3-3. *Normal Mean Erythrocytic Measurements in the Adult*

Mean corpuscular volume [1]	82–96 μ^3
Mean corpuscular hemoglobin concentration [2]	30–36 %
Mean corpuscular hemoglobin [3]	26–32 $\mu\mu g$

$$^1 MCV = \frac{\text{hematocrit }(\%)}{\text{RBC (millions/cu mm)}} \times 10$$

$$^2 MCHC = \frac{\text{hemoglobin (gm/100 ml)}}{\text{Hematocrit }(\%)} \times 100$$

$$^3 MCH = \frac{\text{hemoglobin (gm/100 ml)}}{\text{RBC (millions/cu mm)}} \times 10$$

hemoglobin concentration, it is without clinical significance. Knowledge of the other morphologic characteristics is extremely significant; for example, a microcytic, hypochromic anemia in an adult male implies iron deficiency caused by chronic bleeding until proved otherwise. Mean cell measurements, however, are not infallible; all too often they are actually misleading. The erythroid values from which they are derived are subject to error. Although accurate determinations can be made by strict observance of all technical details by well-trained and experienced personnel, errors inherent in the methods alone may lead to erroneous conclusions. For example, a hemoglobin of 7.5 gm/100 ml and a hematocrit of 24 per cent would yield a MCHC of 31 per cent;

a hemoglobin of 7.0 and a hematocrit of 25 (variations within an acceptable range for laboratory error) would indicate hypochromia (MCHC = 28 per cent). It must also be borne in mind that these cell measurements are averages and reflect the presence of all cells, regardless of their size or hemoglobin content. Macrocytes may be counteracted by microcytes, with the net result a normal MCV. For these reasons the morphologic classification cannot be accurately established on the basis of the peripheral erythroid values and mean red cell measurements. Calculation of these measurements serves no useful purpose, and an anemia should be classified morphologically from information derived from the peripheral blood film, irrespective of the calculated red cell indexes. Whereas each of the peripheral erythroid determinations is subject to error, a well-made, well-stained blood film is not. Microcytes cannot be transformed artifactually into macrocytes, and hypochromic cells cannot be hidden from the examiner's eye.

Erythrocyte Morphology. Detailed study of the peripheral blood film yields data of tremendous diagnostic import and is a fundamental observation in the evaluation of all anemic patients. Therefore adequately prepared and standardized films *must* be available. For this purpose coverslip films are greatly preferred (p. 44). Both Wright's stained coverslip films and brilliant cresyl blue films counterstained with Wright's stain should be used; the latter permit a reticulocyte count and an estimate of the numerical status of the platelets as well as recognition of certain erythrocytic and leukocytic abnormalities.

Normal erythrocytes are described as *normocytic* and *normochromic*. Morphologic abnormalities in red cells include alterations in size, shape, and staining characteristics, together with a variety of inclusion bodies. Slight differences in size and shape are normal; major deviations are designated, respectively, *anisocytosis* and *poikilocytosis*.

Microcytes are small cells with diameters less than 6 μ (Fig. 5-1, p. 174); they are present in a number of anemias, such as iron deficiency and pernicious anemias and the thalassemia syndromes, and are not diagnostically specific. Cells with diameters of more than 8.5 μ are called *macrocytes*. They are most characteristic of anemia caused by vitamin B_{12} or folic acid deficiency (Fig. 5-3, p. 206) but are also found in patients with liver disease or reticulocytosis (Fig. 5-8, p. 213).

A decreased cellular concentration of hemoglobin is manifested morphologically by accentuation of the normal central pale area and is termed *hypochromia* (Fig. 5-1, p. 174). In most cases hypochromia is due to iron deficiency, but abnormalities in the utilization of iron or in the synthesis of porphyrin or globin will evoke similar changes. Large or excessively thick cells that stain more darkly than normal are described as being *hyperchromatic* or as displaying *hyperchromasia*. The term hyperchromia should be avoided, for it might tend to infer that the cells were supersaturated with hemoglobin, that is, the opposite of hypochromia. Although the hemoglobin content of a macrocyte may be increased by virtue of its size, the concentration of hemoglobin does not exceed 36 per cent.

A young erythrocyte retains sufficient basophilic material (chiefly RNA) to be evident in a Wright-stained film by the light blue-gray color of the entire cell (*diffuse basophilia*) or by a punctate or mottled blue-gray appearance (*polychromasia*). When these cells are exposed to a supravital stain, such as brilliant cresyl blue, the basophilic material is precipitated into strands, granules, or a reticular arrangement; the cells are then termed *reticulocytes* (Fig. 1-4, p. 8). There is good but not exact correlation between the degree of polychromasia or diffuse basophilia in a Wright-stained film and the reticulocyte count (all of the former cells will be reticulocytes when stained supravitally, but the converse is not true). Slight polychromasia is normal (a normal reticulocyte count is 0.5 to 2.5 per cent). For the most part increased polychromasia and reticulocytosis reflect increased erythropoietic activity regardless of cause (e.g., acute blood loss anemia or response to specific therapy such as vitamin B_{12} in a patient with pernicious anemia). Occasionally basophilic material, called *punctate basophilia*, may be clumped or present in small aggregates in a Wright-stained film (Fig. 3-1). These cells are especially frequent in patients

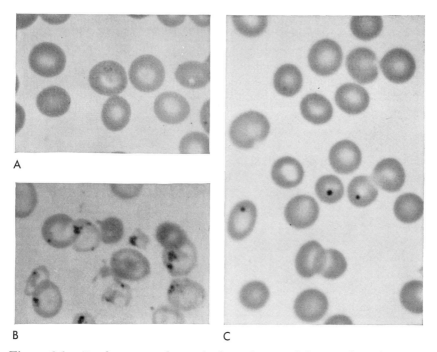

A

B   C

Figure 3-1. Erythrocyte inclusion bodies. *A.* Basophilic stippling (punctate basophilia). *B.* Pappenheimer bodies. *C.* Howell-Jolly bodies.

with lead poisoning or thalassemia but can also be found in other situations accompanied by accelerated red cell production.

Spherocytes are rounded red cells which have lost their normal biconcave configurations because of damage to their surface membranes or because of some interference with the normal metabolic processes needed to supply the energy that must be expended by these cells to maintain their normal biconcavity. Spherocytes are thicker than normal; consequently they lack central pallor and appear smaller and darker than normal cells (Fig. 4-4, p. 92). These cells are often called microspherocytes because of their decreased diameters; however, their volumes remain near normal because of increased thickness. Spherocytes have impaired viability and display increased osmotic and mechanical fragility; their presence in vivo usually indicates an active hemolytic process (either intrinsic or extrinsic). It should be noted that transfused cells often assume a spheroidal shape and do not necessarily indicate significant hemolysis. A rare spheroidal cell can be found in normal blood films and probably reflects decreased glycolytic activity as a result of normal aging of the cell.

Leptocytes are abnormally thin cells. *Target cells* are leptocytes with a dark staining center (probably caused by apposition of surface membranes). The central "bull's eye" is surrounded by an achromic ring, and the well-stained periphery creates the appearance of a target (Fig. 5-16, p. 263). Leptocytes and target cells are demonstrable after splenectomy and in patients with certain hemoglobinopathies (e.g., hemoglobin C disease or one of the thalassemia syndromes), or liver disease of varied etiology with or without jaundice.

Oval red cells (*ovalocytes* or *elliptocytes*) are characteristic of the megaloblastic, macrocytic anemias (Fig. 5-3, p. 206). They are inherited rarely as a simple mendelian dominant (Fig. 4-6, p. 95); in most cases this anomaly is without clinical significance but occasional patients manifest hemolysis.

Sickle cells (*depranocytes*) are bizarre, sickle- or crescent-shaped cells with tailed, filamentous, and spinelike processes (Fig. 5-15, p. 254). They are misshapen because of the presence in the cell of Hgb S.

Burr cells are peculiar poikilocytes with one or more spiny projections along their peripheries (Fig. 3-2); they are most often associated with uremia. The pathogenesis of these cells is obscure; their nucleated precursors exhibit similar morphologic abnormalities.

Acanthocytes are erythrocytes with numerous, large, thornlike projections of variable size and length (Fig. 3-2). "Thorny" red cells occur in a rare inborn disorder of lipid or lipoprotein metabolism associated with several other defects, including steatorrhea, atypical retinitis pigmentosa, and progressive neurologic abnormalities. Burr cells and acanthocytes must be distinguished from crenated cells which are

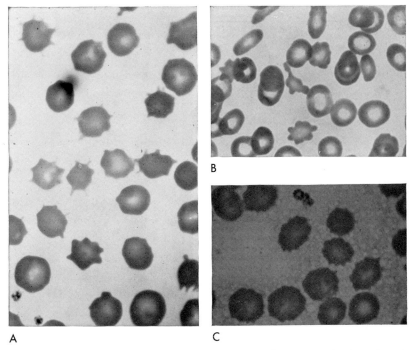

Figure 3-2. Abnormalities in the shape of erythrocytes. *A.* Acanthocytes. *B.* Burr cells. *C.* Crenated red cells.

covered with fairly uniform blunt, knoblike projections (Fig. 3-2). Crenation is artifactual and represents exposure in vitro to a hypertonic medium.

Schistocytes, which are irregular cell fragments (Fig. 13-3, p. 502), reflect erythrocyte damage and breakdown.

Howell-Jolly bodies are round, dense inclusion bodies (1 μ or less in diameter) situated near the periphery of an erythrocyte (Fig. 3-1). They occur singly (rarely doubly), are visible in the living cell with phase microscopy, stain a dark blue-black with the Romanowsky stains, are Feulgen positive for DNA, and do not contain iron. Howell-Jolly bodies appear to be nuclear remnants and are seen in a variety of severe anemias, especially hemolytic disorders. They are characteristic of hyposplenism and are invariably present after removal of the spleen.

Siderocytes are red cells that contain one or more hemosiderin granules; these inclusion bodies vary in size and are usually demonstrable only with special stains, such as Prussian blue. Occasionally they are associated with sufficient basophilic material to be evident with Romanowsky stains and are then referred to as *Pappenheimer bodies* (Fig. 3-1). The majority of the nucleated red cells in the marrow contain hemosiderin granules. After cells with inclusion bodies enter the peripheral blood the granules are rapidly and efficiently removed from the erythrocytes by the spleen. Therefore siderocytes are not normally evident in the circulating blood. Because of the loss of the spleen's normal "pitting function," siderocytes are most numerous after splenectomy; with the exception of iron deficiency, they also accompany a variety of anemias (especially hemolytic processes).

Cabot rings are filamentous or threadlike structures that often assume bizarre configurations; they are purple in Wright-stained films and not visible in unstained preparations. Their nature is obscure and they may be artifactual. These inclusion bodies are associated with marked disturbances in erythropoiesis (e.g., severe pernicious anemia) and lack specificity.

Heinz bodies are single or multiple refractile granules of precipitated hemoglobin (Fig. 4-5, p. 94). These erythrocyte inclusion bodies are detectable in wet preparations and with supravital staining techniques, but not with the usual Romanowsky stains. They reflect erythrocyte injury and are prominent in a variety of hemolytic disorders.

Bone Marrow. The failure to include a bone marrow examination in the list of basic observations needed in the work-up of an anemic patient deserves comment. The peripheral blood reflects abnormalities in marrow activity; therefore marrow findings can usually be predicted with accuracy by study of the peripheral blood, especially the blood film. An anemia is not necessarily a valid indication to examine the marrow, because the changes associated with many anemic states are nonspecific; for example, the erythrocytic hyperplasia accompanying acute hemorrhage is identical in appearance with that caused by hemolysis. Even when an anemia is associated with relatively specific marrow abnormalities, such as the megaloblastic morphology of the erythrocytic precursors in a patient with pernicious anemia, the characteristic findings in the peripheral blood and the other clinical and laboratory observations often preclude the need for marrow studies. Furthermore, the demonstration of a megaloblastic marrow, although diagnostic of vitamin B_{12} or folic acid deficiency, does not elucidate the pathogenesis of the deficiency state. An examination of the bone marrow is invaluable to the hematologist; no other inference is intended or possible. The point deserving emphasis is the frequent misuse of this procedure because of the physician's failure to delineate the conditions in which it may or may not be of diagnostic value. Although it is the source of little discomfort to the patient and virtually innocuous in trained hands, fatalities have been ascribed to sternal punctures. In addition, the preparation, staining, and interpretation of bone marrow films are time-consuming tasks that require experienced personnel. Consequently, the marrow should be examined only in the presence of a clear-cut indication.

The following examples point out the ease with which most problems can be solved; each type of anemia is discussed in more detail elsewhere.

Acute Blood Loss (p. 67). Polychromasia, reticulocytosis, and nucleated red cells in the peripheral blood are manifestations of accelerated erythropoiesis brought about by acute blood loss, that is, acute hemorrhage or hemolysis. The normocytic, normochromic anemia of acute hemorrhage rarely presents a diagnostic problem and can usually be confirmed by the history and physical examination. If spherocytes are present, a diagnosis of a spherocytic hemolytic anemia can be made. In nonspherocytic hemolytic anemias a palpable spleen and jaundice ordinarily suggest hemolysis and the other studies needed to clarify the problem (e.g., a Coombs' or bromelin test, pigment studies, and fragility measurements). Hemolytic activity sufficient to produce an anemia is always reflected by changes in these readily assessable parameters. ^{51}Chromium red cell survival data are rarely needed clinically.

Deficiency States. The microcytic, hypochromic anemia of iron deficiency is easily recognized in the peripheral blood (p. 174). The magnitude of the morphologic abnormalities varies directly with the severity of the deficiency; however, it is difficult to envisage a deficit sufficient to produce an anemia without morphologic evidence of its presence. Poorly prepared or stained blood films will, of course, preclude the recognition of minimal deficiencies. Vitamin B_{12} or folic acid deficiencies are also manifested by pathognomonic changes in the peripheral blood, that is, macrocytic ovalocytes, microcytes, large hypersegmented neutrophils, leukopenia, and thrombocytopenia (p. 206). These and other routine clinical observations will generally suffice. The demonstration of a megaloblastic marrow or an abnormal Schilling test is rarely needed to make the diagnosis in an anemic patient.

Marrow Destruction or Hypocellularity (p. 222). In addition to an anemia (usually normocytic and normochromic), a hypoplastic or "aplastic" anemia is typically accompanied by leukopenia and thrombocytopenia. The absence of splenomegaly, enlarged lymph nodes, or immature cells in the peripheral blood completes the clinical picture; a hypocellular marrow confirms the diagnosis.

Diversion of Growth Potential (p. 338). Immature leukocytes in the peripheral blood, abnormalities in the leukocyte count, thrombocytopenia, symptoms, and physical findings will usually suggest that a normocytic, normochromic anemia is the result of granulocytic or myelomonocytic leukemia. Marrow examination will establish the diagnosis.

Displacement of Normal Marrow Elements (p. 240). A combination of abnormalities in the peripheral blood which is hard to explain on the basis of any known primary hematologic disorder should point to a myelophthisic process. This diagnosis can often be confirmed by the demonstration of abnormal cells such as carcinoma or Gaucher cells in the bone marrow.

Defective Hemoglobin Synthesis. Sickle and target cells, polychromasia, and reticulocytosis, especially in a Negro, clearly indicate the need for other studies, most notably hemoglobin electrophoresis, to rule in or out a hereditary qualitative hemoglobinopathy (p. 248). Hypochromia, polychromasia, target cells, reticulocytosis, and splenomegaly suggest a thalassemia syndrome (p. 268).

Depressed Erythropoiesis (p. 283). A normocytic, normochromic anemia without any other hematologic abnormalities excludes the well-established causes of anemia and eliminates the need for more detailed hematologic studies. Under these circumstances the diagnosis of the basic disease is dependent on nonhematologic data (e.g., renal or liver function studies and the demonstration of a chronic infection).

Thus the evaluation of most anemic patients is a relatively simple task based on knowledge of the physiology and pathophysiology of erythropoiesis, symptoms, physical abnormalities, and peripheral blood findings. Because treatment of an anemia cannot be intelligently selected until the cause is known and because clarification of the type of secondary anemia may serve as an important clue to the primary diagnosis, the precise cause of all anemias must be ascertained. An anemia, even though slight, should never be ignored; neither should it be treated with "shotgun" therapy. Indications for such antianemic agents *do not exist*. Although a therapeutic trial is often the easiest path to follow, it is an irrational and unscientific approach which can never be justified and is often hazardous; for example, progression of neurologic damage in the face of a return to hematologic normalcy in a patient with pernicious anemia treated with folic acid (p. 196) or correction of an iron deficiency anemia due to chronic blood loss from a colonic carcinoma, thereby obscuring the primary disease until it reaches an inoperable stage (p. 180). For these reasons and because of the frequency with which anemia is encountered it behooves every physician, regardless of specialty or primary interests, to possess a clear understanding of the pathogenesis and significance of all types of anemia.

Anemia Caused by Blood Loss

CHAPTER

4

The blood-loss anemias are caused by the removal of erythrocytes from the circulation before the end of their finite life-span. The resulting fall in the red cell mass activates the humoral erythropoietic regulatory mechanism, which in turn serves to increase erythropoiesis. Thus the blood loss anemias are characterized by evidence of *augmented erythrocyte production* (erythrocytic hyperplasia in the marrow and increased polychromasia, reticulocytosis, and nucleated red cells in the peripheral blood). There are only two routes by which erythrocytes can be lost. One is hemorrhage, the other is premature destruction (hemolysis). The hematologic manifestations of both types of blood loss anemia are similar; however, other important differences in clinical pictures permit their separation. Because of the relatively long survival times of normal erythrocytes, a sudden decrement in the peripheral erythroid values always indicates acute blood loss, whether by hemorrhage or hemolysis.

Acute Hemorrhagic Anemia

The clinical manifestations of acute hemorrhage are variable and depend on the amount of blood lost, the rapidity of the bleeding, the status of the patient before the sudden lowering of the blood volume, and the nature of the underlying disease or trauma responsible for the hemorrhage. An otherwise normal person may tolerate as much as a 40 per cent reduction in blood volume without serious untoward

67

effects, provided the blood loss occurs slowly (e.g., over a period of 24 hours). On the other hand, a smaller hemorrhage over a shorter period of time or in a patient with pre-existent anemia or other abnormalities that alter or prevent the normal physiologic compensatory responses may result in profound shock and death.

PATHOPHYSIOLOGY

The initial and immediate effect of acute hemorrhage is a decrease in blood volume caused by equivalent reductions in red cell mass and plasma volume. Since comparable amounts of cells and plasma are lost, an anemia (less than a normal amount of hemoglobin per unit volume of blood) does not become evident until extravascular fluid begins to enter the intravascular compartment to correct the hypovolemic state (Fig. 4-1). Hence the early manifestations of acute hemorrhage are attributable to hypovolemia rather than to a decrease in the oxygen-carrying capacity of the blood. A number of cardiac, pulmonary, and

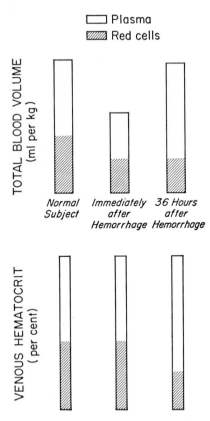

Figure 4-1. Effects of acute hemorrhage on the plasma volume, total red cell mass, and venous hematocrit.

vascular (splanchnic and cutaneous vasoconstriction) adjustments are immediately brought into play in an attempt to prevent circulatory collapse and to maintain the oxygen supply to vital organs such as the brain. These corrective mechanisms are reflected by tachycardia, hyperpnea, cold extremities, and so forth. If the cardiovascular-pulmonary responses are unable to cope with the hypovolemia, cardiac output decreases, the pulse becomes weak and thready, the patient exhibits air hunger, diaphoresis, and hypothermia, the blood pressure falls, and shock ensues.

A normal total blood volume is usually restored within 12 to 36 hours after acute bleeding stops. The speed with which tissue fluids enter the intravascular compartment is controlled by the rate that new proteins are added to the circulation. Protein replenishment begins shortly after an acute hemorrhage and occurs more rapidly than hemoglobin regeneration. In an individual whose nutritional status is satisfactory plasma protein content is generally normal within 24 to 48 hours after acute hemorrhage has ceased.

Consequent to expansion of the contracted plasma volume, the already reduced red cell mass is diluted (Fig. 4-1). As a result, the peripheral erythroid values (hemoglobin, hematocrit, and erythrocyte count) fall, and a normocytic, normochromic anemia develops. It is accompanied by the typical manifestations of a reduction in circulating hemoglobin, irrespective of cause (e.g., weakness, exertional tachycardia and dyspnea, and pallor). The anemia imparts a potent stimulus to the marrow, presumably mediated by the humoral erythropoietic regulatory mechanism (p. 10). In the presence of an intact marrow reticulum increased numbers of stem cells undergo erythrocytic differentiation and enter the red cell compartment. Proliferation and maturation proceed in a normal and orderly fashion, provided the nutritional and hormonal environment is adequate. The normal ratio of immature to mature nucleated red cells is maintained, and the erythrocyte generation time is not significantly altered. Total red bone marrow mass increases and is reflected by increased cellularity of marrow aspirates, erythrocytic hyperplasia, and a reversal of the E:G ratio.

Evidence of active red cell regeneration (increased polychromasia, reticulocytosis, and circulating nucleated red cells) appears in the peripheral blood within 24 to 48 hours after an episode of bleeding. The magnitude of these findings depends on the severity of the acute hemorrhagic anemia. The reticulocyte count is ordinarily between 5 and 10 per cent and rarely exceeds 15 per cent; it reaches a peak between the fifth and seventh day after the hemorrhage and returns to normal between the tenth and fourteenth day. As a rule, the circulating nucleated red cells range from 0 to 5/100 leukocytes. If all requirements for erythropoiesis are met, if no other disorder that impairs red cell production exists, and hemorrhage does not recur, peripheral erythroid values will be normal within three to six weeks.

In addition to an enhancing effect on erythropoiesis, acute hemorrhage also affects the circulating leukocyte and platelet counts. Leukocytosis (a relative and absolute neutrophilia) and thrombocytosis develop within a few hours and persist for several days after bleeding ceases. The magnitude of these changes reflects the severity of the hemorrhage. The leukocyte count usually ranges between 10,000 to 20,-000/cu mm; it is occasionally higher but seldom exceeds 35,000/cu mm. It is common to observe a few immature granulocytes in the peripheral blood, which are most often neutrophilic metamyelocytes and band neutrophils. The platelet count generally varies from 500,000 to 1,000,-000/cu mm.

The pathogenesis of the leukocytosis and thrombocytosis accompanying acute blood loss is obscure. The rapidity with which these cellular increases occur indicates an initial release of cells from the marrow or other storage sites. A severe hemorrhage will eventually enhance marrow granulopoiesis and thrombopoiesis. There is an absolute increase in the number of granulocytic precursors and megakaryocytes in the marrow, although erythrocytic hyperplasia is always more marked and dominates the picture. Preliminary observations suggest that the leukocytosis and thrombocytosis induced by acute blood loss may reflect enhanced activity of a humoral factor or factors affecting these aspects of hemopoiesis (p. 89); further studies along these lines are needed.

DIAGNOSIS

The diagnosis of acute hemorrhage seldom presents a problem, for overt bleeding is usually apparent. Bleeding into the gastrointestinal tract, body cavities, or tissues may cause some confusion, especially if the patient is unable to provide a history. Early, the peripheral erythroid values may be normal. However, the manifestations of hypovolemia are fairly specific, and acute hemorrhage must always be considered in any patient in shock. Later, after the blood volume has returned to normal, the chief manifestations may be attributable to anemia. By this time there is generally some indication of bleeding; for example, black, tarry stools or an elevated blood urea nitrogen if the bleeding has been into the gastrointestinal tract. Furthermore, evidence of active red cell regeneration associated with rapidly increasing peripheral erythroid values provides useful information. Consequently, an acute hemorrhagic anemia rarely masquerades as any other type of anemia.

It is noteworthy that only an acute, self-limited hemorrhage or intermittent episodes of acute bleeding will produce a normocytic, normochromic anemia. Chronic bleeding will eventually deplete iron stores and cause a chronic microcytic, hypochromic (iron deficiency) anemia. However, in the face of adequate amounts of iron the effects of chronic hemorrhage will be compensated by increased marrow production and will *not* result in a chronic normocytic, normochromic anemia. The functional reserve of the bone marrow is such that it can, under optimal conditions, increase production six to eight times. Therefore it is theoretically possible for an adult to lose 250 to 350 ml of blood a day without the level of the circulating hemoglobin being affected (reticulocytosis and marrow erythrocytic hyperplasia would, of course, be evident). Persistent hemorrhage of this magnitude obviously would not be occult. Furthermore, 125 to 175 mg of elemental iron would be lost daily. Even therapeutic doses of inorganic iron would be unable to prevent negative iron balance (p. 181). Under these circumstances iron stores would be quickly exhausted and a profound microcytic, hypochromic anemia would ensue. In addition, depletion of plasma proteins and other blood constituents would soon cause serious and life-threatening problems. For these reasons hemorrhage cannot bring about a chronic normocytic, normochromic anemia, that is, peripheral erythroid values that remain relatively stable for two to three weeks or longer. It should be emphasized, however, that fortuitously spaced acute hemorrhages might appear to cause such an anemia; for example, an acute hemorrhagic anemia followed by an increase in the erythroid values with a subsequent fall due to a second hemorrhagic episode. Because the erythropoietic response to hemolysis is not limited by the availability of iron, a chronic hemolytic anemia is characterized by a chronic normocytic, normochromic anemia (p. 86). Therefore time alone will distinguish between the two types of acute blood-loss anemias.

TREATMENT AND COURSE

Because of the many factors that influence the body's response to acute hemorrhage, treatment must be individualized; the obvious exception in all cases is the necessity for the prompt institution of appropriate measures to control the bleeding. Therapy of an acute hemorrhagic anemia is divided into that of the acute phase and the recovery phase.

Acute Phase. If the hemorrhage has ceased and the physiologic compensatory mechanisms are able to maintain the integrity of the circulatory system, further emergency treatment is not required; but if bleeding is expected to recur, surgical intervention appears imminent, or the classic manifestations of shock and/or acute anemic hypoxia are present, the depleted blood volume and oxygen-carrying capacity of the blood must be augmented immediately by the transfusion of whole blood. Plasma, dextran, glucose solutions, or normal saline may be given intravenously in the interim until whole blood is available. However, these materials will not substitute for blood because they fail to correct the deficit in the red cell mass. Once bleeding has ceased and the symptoms and findings of shock and/or acute anemic hypoxia have abated, further transfusions in an attempt to replace all of the blood are neither necessary nor advisable.

Although the hemoglobin, hematocrit, and erythrocyte counts are useful indicators of the amount of blood lost and the persistence of active bleeding, it must be emphasized that these measurements may be misleading (Fig. 4-1). The initial determinations will be falsely high, for red cell and plasma volumes are reduced by equivalent amounts. Immediately following an acute hemorrhage the peripheral erythroid values, which reflect the relative amount of hemoglobin or number of erythrocytes contained in a unit volume of whole blood, will not change, despite a marked reduction in whole body red cell mass. As tissue fluid begins to enter the intravascular compartment, the peripheral erythroid values will fall (even though all bleeding has ceased) and will continue to fall for several hours until the blood volume is restored to normal. Inasmuch as these changes in the peripheral values suggest further blood loss, serial blood-volume determinations by a technique such as that employing radioactive iodine-labeled human serum albumin serve as a more useful guide to therapy during the acute phase of a hemorrhagic anemia (Fig. 4-1). As long as the blood volume is reduced, whole blood transfusions are indicated. As soon as the blood volume is replenished, packed red cells constitute the treatment of choice, provided additional replacement is still deemed necessary by the likelihood of recurrent bleeding or in preparation for surgery. Otherwise the hypervolemia induced by the continued administration of whole blood may precipitate serious complications, especially in patients with an impaired cardiac reserve.

Recovery Phase. In the presence of a normal bone marrow and sufficient metabolic building blocks, prompt re-establishment of erythrocytic equilibrium is ensured after acute hemorrhage through the homeostatic erythropoietic regulatory mechanism (p. 13). No additional treatment is required. However, the administration of iron is advisable, for it has been shown to hasten recovery and will replenish iron stores (p. 182). Ferrous sulfate in oral doses of 0.3 gm three times daily after meals is preferred. Iron therapy should be continued for at least 8 to 12 weeks or longer if hypochromia, which indicates prior blood loss, is present (p. 172).

Hemolytic Anemias

Under physiologic conditions normal red cells circulate for about 120 days after they leave the bone marrow. During this time the erythrocytes are subjected to severe mechanical buffeting and metabolic stresses and must expend a considerable amount of energy to maintain their physical and functional integrity. An erythrocyte is not a physiologically inert, passive carrier of oxygen. Although incapable of reproduction, non-nucleated erythrocytes are very much alive and carry on a variety of complex metabolic processes, some of which are essential for their survival.

Any abnormality that shortens red cell life-span will interfere with the normal erythroid steady state. A compensatory augmentation in erythropoiesis follows via the humoral erythropoietic regulatory mechanism (p. 13). A normal marrow can increase red cell production approximately six to eight times. Therefore slight impairment in red cell viability will not be manifested by changes in the peripheral erythroid values and is appropriately designated a *compensated hemolytic disorder*. When erythrocyte survival times are shortened to less than 15 to 20 days (one eighth to one sixth of normal), the rate of peripheral destruction exceeds maximum production capacity. As a consequence, normal peripheral erythroid values can no longer be maintained and a *hemolytic anemia* results. Because of the large functional reserve of the marrow, impaired erythrocytogenesis contributes importantly to the development of an overt hemolytic anemia. An inhibited marrow may be unable to compensate for a decrease in erythrocyte life-span which, in the presence of a normal marrow, would not cause a detectable lowering of the circulating hemoglobin. Many hemolytic anemias reflect an element of relative bone marrow failure in addition to increased peripheral destruction, although the latter ordinarily predominates.

The causes of hemolysis are many and varied. However, the hematologic manifestations are similar, irrespective of the nature of the primary disease or erythrocytic defect. As a result, differential diagnosis may be difficult, even though hemolytic activity is readily apparent.

NORMAL ERYTHROCYTE STRUCTURE, METABOLISM, AGING, AND DESTRUCTION

Knowledge of the physical characteristics of a normal red cell, its metabolic activities, the changes that accompany aging, and the mechanisms by which it is destroyed is requisite for a rational classification and for an understanding of the pathophysiology of the hemolytic disorders.

Structure. The mammalian erythrocyte is ideally structured for the successful completion of its physiologic functions. The normal biconcave erythrocyte is an appropriate container for hemoglobin with a large surface area for gaseous exchange (the sum total of which is about 1500 times that of the body) and a configuration that permits diffusion of gases into and out of the cell with maximal ease. If hemoglobin existed free in the plasma, it would exert an osmotic pressure approximately five times that of the normal plasma proteins. Furthermore, the life-span of free plasma hemoglobin is only a few hours at best, whereas intra-erythrocytic hemoglobin remains functional for about 120 days. In addition, the erythrocyte ultrastructure provides a convenient enclosure in which the metabolic processes required to maintain hemoglobin in a chemically functional state can take place.

Red cell stroma consists primarily of a lipoprotein complex. Since the surface area of an erythrocyte is larger than that required merely to enclose hemoglobin and other cell constituents, it follows that an ordered molecular structure exists. An erythrocyte ghost (a cell from which almost all hemoglobin has been removed) can be made to assume a normal biconcave discoidal shape. Consequently, the stroma, rather than the hemoglobin, is the major contributor to the cells' architecture. Maintenance of this desired shape requires an expenditure of energy, and there is evidence that this goal is achieved through an adenosine triphosphate (ATP)–dependent contractile protein. The normal erythrocyte is quite pliable (an important attribute facilitating navigation through small capillaries), and its over-all configuration can be altered by external pressures or internal changes (e.g., ingress of water). Minor deviations from normal are reversible. However, the relatively inelastic surface membrane will not permit large increases in cell volume or drastic changes in shape without irreparable harm to the cell.

The precise molecular architecture of an erythrocyte is not known. Electron microscopic studies indicate that the surface consists of a series of plaquelike structures; the interstices between these plaques may act as pores or openings for the ingress and egress of water and electrolytes. Under the outermost plaques is a fibrillary protein latticework, which runs parallel to the surface; individual elements may be linked together by lipids. The major ABO and CDE (Rh) blood group factors are associated with this fraction of the erythrocyte stroma. Progressing toward the interior of the cell, structural order decreases as the concentration of hemoglobin increases. However, there is some pattern to the positioning of the hemoglobin molecules, even in the center of the cell. There is no clear-cut dividing line between hemoglobin and stroma, and small amounts of hemoglobin appear to be an essential but not inseparable component of the stroma.

Maintenance of the complex, ordered, ultrastructure of a red cell is an active process that is dependent on a variety of factors, both extrinsic and intrinsic, and requires the expenditure of energy. The mammalian erythrocyte does not possess its characteristic morphology as the result of chance. Instead, the biconcave discoidal shape contributes to the efficiency and physiologic competency of this intricate, highly specialized cell.

Metabolism.   In addition to proteins, lipids, and carbohydrates, normal erythrocytes contain an impressive array of enzymes, anions, and cations. Nucleated erythrocytes possess all the necessary building blocks and enzymes for the synthesis of numerous substances, most notably the hemoglobin molecule. To supply its energy requirements, the immature erythrocytic precursor has available for the catabolism of glucose the tricarboxylic acid cycle as well as the Embden-Meyerhof and pentose phosphate pathways. The tricarboxylic acid cycle is no longer operative in the nonnucleated, nonreticulated erythrocyte, even though certain of its enzymes remain; the other two pathways account for all the glucose metabolized by adult erythrocytes.

Mature red cells are rather deficient in stored energy and continuously depend on glycolysis via the anaerobic Embden-Meyerhof and the oxidative pentose phosphate pathways. These glycolytic activities supply the compounds of high potential energy and reductive capacity that keep the cell functioning and alive. Glucose metabolism in a normal mature erythrocyte is depicted schematically in Figure 4-2.

Anaerobic catabolism of glucose to lactate through the Embden-

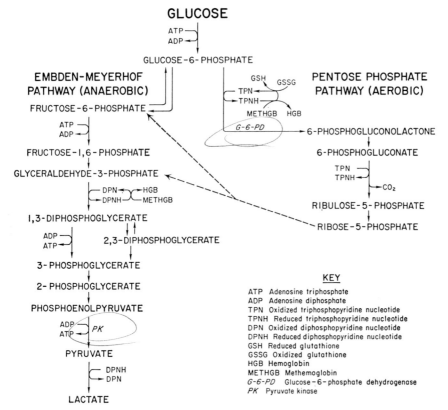

Figure 4-2. Schematic representation of erythrocytic glycolysis.

Meyerhof pathway accounts for about 90 per cent of the glucose utilized and supplies, largely in the form of the high-energy phosphate bonds in ATP, approximately 75 per cent of the cell's energy. This glycolytic process results in a net gain of two moles of ATP for each mole of glucose that is catabolized and is the sole source of ATP. During the initial steps in the degradation of glucose to lactate, ATP is utilized (ATP → ADP) in a series of phosphorylative reactions; ATP is reformed (ADP → ATP) during the dephosphorylation involved in the conversion of the intermediate metabolites to pyruvate and lactate (Fig. 4-2). In addition to its vital role in the transfer of energy, ATP acts as a coenzyme in a number of essential metabolic reactions, serves as a precursor of other coenzymes, and primes or initiates glycolysis.

The Embden-Meyerhof glycolytic pathway also provides the cell with DPNH (Fig. 4-2), which acts as the preferred coenzyme for the physiologic reduction of methemoglobin and participates in the production of lactate from pyruvate. Although DPNH constitutes another source of potential energy for the erythrocyte, anaerobic glycolysis does not result in a net gain of DPNH (the concentration of DPN in a normal erythrocyte is several times that of DPNH). Therefore it would appear that the Embden-Meyerhof pathway normally provides just enough DPNH to reduce physiologic amounts of methemoglobin and to complete the last step in this metabolic process, the transformation of pyruvate to lactate.

Approximately 10 per cent of the glucose metabolized by an erythrocyte is diverted into the pentose phosphate pathway (also known as the hexose monophosphate pathway or "shunt"). This oxidative process (Fig. 4-2) provides approximately 25 per cent of the cell's potential energy in the form of TPNH, an essential cofactor in many reductive activities. For each mole of glucose catabolized through this aerobic pathway, two moles of TPN are reduced to TPNH. Glucose metabolism via the pentose phosphate pathway is the sole source of TPNH and accounts for all the oxygen consumed and carbon dioxide produced by mature erythrocytes. Both glycolytic pathways require priming with ATP and the formation of glucose-6-phosphate. The first step in the pentose phosphate pathway depends on the enzyme, glucose-6-phosphate dehydrogenase (Fig. 4-2). In addition to carbon dioxide, aerobic glycolysis culminates in the formation of a hexose monophosphate (fructose-6-phosphate) and a triose phosphate (glyceraldehyde-3-phosphate). Thus the pentose phosphate pathway is linked to the Embden-Meyerhof pathway (Fig. 4-2). The fate of these intermediate metabolites is not known. They may be catabolized anaerobically to lactate, thereby contributing to the potential energy capacity of the cell. A possible alternative is conversion to glucose-6-phosphate by reverse glycolysis and recycling through the hexose monophosphate shunt.

There are many voids in our knowledge of erythrocyte metabolism.

The physiologic significance of some steps in the glycolytic pathways and the role of certain intermediary metabolites range from conjecture to enigma. For example, catabolism of 1,3-diphosphoglycerate directly to 3-phosphoglycerate results in a gain of potential energy (ADP → ATP); conversion of 1,3-diphosphoglycerate to 3-phosphoglycerate through the intermediary metabolite, 2,3-diphosphoglycerate, does not (Fig. 4-2). Therefore the formation of 2,3-diphosphoglycerate would appear to waste energy, a reaction at odds with other highly efficient erythrocytic activities. Even so, the adult erythrocyte contains abundant amounts of 2,3-diphosphoglycerate. It is possible that this compound may serve a regulatory function in the ATP ⇌ ADP equilibrium in the form of a reserve store of phosphate which is available for the rephosphorylation of ADP, should the cell be deprived of glucose. Thus 2,3-diphosphoglycerate may serve a function analogous to that of glycogen in other cells (red cells do not contain significant quantities of this carbohydrate).

Other unanswered questions appear to be even more pertinent than elucidation of all the intricacies of red cell glycolysis. For example, there is much to be learned about the purposes for which the erythrocyte needs and utilizes the energy that is available to it. Transport of oxygen and carbon dioxide are passive functions that do not require the expenditure of energy. However, energy is required for several processes that are essential to maintain an erythrocyte in a physiologically functional state and to preserve its physical and chemical integrity.

MAINTENANCE OF ELECTROLYTE EQUILIBRIUM. The principal constituent of an erythrocyte is an almost saturated solution of hemoglobin. Control of ion transport into and out of the cell is essential to counteract the excess osmotic pressure caused by the hemoglobin; otherwise, movement of water into the erythrocyte would cause the cell to swell and lyse. The erythrocytic membrane is freely permeable to Cl^- and HCO_3^- anions as well as to water. Cationic equilibrium is maintained by active transport mechanisms involving exergonic chemical reactions. The intracellular concentration of K^+ greatly exceeds that of the plasma; for Na^+ the reverse is true. As a result, total cation concentrations of plasma and cell are approximately equal. Influx of K^+ and efflux of Na^+ involve work. These two active processes are linked and interdependent. Both of these cations are in a constant state of flux. To prevent an unlimited ingress of K^+ and egress of Na^+, the active cationic transport mechanisms are counterbalanced by relatively slow passive diffusion of Na^+ into and K^+ out of the cell. The end result is an electrolyte steady state. Formation of the ATP needed to run the "cation pump" requires about 10 per cent of the potential energy output of the Embden-Meyerhof glycolytic pathway.

REDUCTION OF METHEMOGLOBIN. Since erythrocytes transport large quantities of molecular oxygen, hemoglobin is constantly in danger of being oxidized to methemoglobin. The iron in methemoglobin is in the ferric form, and oxygen linked thereto is not dissociable by physiologic changes in oxygen tension. Consequently, methemoglobin does not function as a carrier of oxygen. If the iron in methemoglobin is reduced to the ferrous form, the hemoglobin again becomes functional. Small amounts of methemoglobin are being formed continuously; however, they are also being reduced constantly and methemoglobin is normally present in a concentration of only 1 to 2 per cent. Methemoglobin reduction is accomplished by DPNH and TPNH acting as hydrogen donors with the assistance of their respective and specific enzymes, both termed methemoglobin reductase (Fig. 4-2). DPNH appears to be the preferred coenzyme for the reduction of physiologic amounts of methemoglobin. In the presence of certain oxidant drugs, the TPNH-dependent methemoglobin reductase system is of major importance. Therefore methemoglobin reduction depends on both anaerobic and aerobic glycolysis.

PROTECTION FROM OXIDATION. Because of the abundant amounts of molecular oxygen within erythrocytes, reducing agents must be continuously generated to prevent spontaneous oxidation of hemoglobin, enzymes, coenzymes, and other cell components. In the absence of such reducing systems, attempts to establish redox equilibrium would result in a flow of electrons from red cell constituents to oxygen. TPNH is the most important reducing substance in an erythrocyte; the sole mechanism for its formation is the aerobic catabolism of glucose via the pentose phosphate pathway (Fig. 4-2). TPNH acts as the hydrogen donor for many reductive processes, but its major role is in the maintenance of the proper equilibrium between reduced and oxidized glutathione (TPNH is the preferred coenzyme for glutathione reduction). Reduced glutathione (GSH) in turn participates as a hydrogen donor in a number of vital metabolic activities and protects the sulfhydryl groups of many proteins (hemoglobin, enzymes, and coenzymes) against oxidative destruction. In addition, GSH is bound to at least one enzyme and is the cofactor of another. TPNH also contributes to other cell activities such as the reduction of methemoglobin in the presence of redox compounds and the degradation of certain drugs that facilitate the transfer of electrons from various cellular components to oxygen. Thus the functional and physical integrity of mature erythrocytes is contingent on adequate amounts of TPNH and GSH (GSH being dependent on TPNH).

LIPID TURNOVER AND SYNTHESIS. Most of the lipids in an erythrocyte are contained in the lipoproteins of the cell membrane. Red cell lipids are in continuous flux and energy is apparently required for this purpose. Lipid turnover appears to be essential for the maintenance of the proper molecular configuration and electrical and chemical conditions of the red cell membrane. Evidence also exists that TPNH plays an important role in the synthesis of lipids by developing erythrocytes. It is not known whether lipids are being synthesized by mature erythrocytes; if they are, energy would be required.

MISCELLANEOUS USES OF GLYCOLYTIC ENERGY. Other red cell functions or activities known to involve the expenditure of energy include the synthesis of TPN and DPN as well as the probable synthesis of other nucleotides. In addition, ATP is needed to initiate both aerobic and anaerobic glycolysis (Fig. 4-2). Despite the recent clarification of many aspects of erythrocyte energetics, the uses of a considerable amount of available energy remain to be elucidated by future studies. Even so, it is quite apparent that glycolysis contributes to the integrity of the mature erythrocyte and that interference with the production and/or utilization of energy will seriously affect cell function and viability.

Aging. Following the release of an erythrocyte from the bone marrow, a series of changes occurs which culminates in the cell's destruction about 120 days later. Young cells are larger, contain more water, possess a lower density, and display greater resistance to osmotic lysis than do older cells. In addition, erythrocytes that have recently lost their nuclei contain RNA and other cytoplasmic constituents detectable as polychromasia in Wright-stained films and as precipitated strands or granules (reticulocytes) in supravitally stained preparations. These cells retain the ability to synthesize hemoglobin, but after a few days in the circulation, they lose this property (concomitantly with disappearance of RNA) and acquire the morphologic, physical, and chemical characteristics of a fully mature erythrocyte (p. 9). Throughout the life-span of an erythrocyte, alterations are detectable in structure and composition; presumably they are responsible for (or reflect other still unrecognized changes) the removal of the cell from the circulation and its subsequent destruction. The effects of aging include, among others, (1) a decrease in the concentrations of a variety of enzymes concerned with glucose metabolism, for example, glucose-6-phosphate dehydrogenase, (2) a decrease in ATP and an increase in ADP, (3) a decrease in lipid content, (4) a decrease in the cell's capacity to reduce methemoglobin, degrade certain oxidant drugs or dyes, and prevent oxidation of other cell constituents (all manifestations of declining glycolytic activity), and (5) a decrease in intracellular potassium and an increase in intracellular sodium and water. Electron microscopy has shown that the granular membrane of a young erythrocyte is replaced in an old cell by a smooth membrane. With light microscopy, erythrocytes do not display morphologic evidence of aging. However, it should be noted that an occasional spheroidal cell is detectable in all normal blood films. Although proof is lacking, it seems reasonable to assume that these cells reflect the structural changes brought about by aging.

Destruction. Normally, red cells survive for about 110 to 130 days after they leave the bone marrow (120 days is the figure customarily used for the normal erythrocyte life-span). At the end of this time, the erythrocyte is destroyed. Despite the careful attention of investigators for many years and the fact that about 250 billion erythrocytes are destroyed each day in a normal adult, the actual site of cell destruction and the mechanism (or mechanisms) by which the cells are destroyed remain obscure. The spleen sequesters and eliminates certain damaged or abnormal cells (p. 451) and probably plays a role in the removal of normal aged cells; however, this organ is obviously not essential, for splenectomy does not significantly alter red cell survival times. The reticuloendothelial system is intimately concerned with erythrocyte destruction and hemoglobin catabolism. An attractive but unproved and largely conjectural hypothesis is that of destruction by progressive erythrocyte cytoclasis. Consequent to a "wearing out" of the complex enzyme systems needed to ensure adequate energy to maintain the cell's physiologic, physical, oncotic, and chemical integrity, the erythrocyte may no longer be able to resist the detrimental effects of mechanical trauma and metabolic stresses. Following cytoclasis, small erythrocyte fragments might be removed by phagocytic reticuloendothelial cells.

It is possible to study erythrocyte destruction in vitro under a variety of unphysiologic conditions, such as lysis by osmosis (suspension of cells in hypotonic media) and destruction by antibodies, physical agents, or surface active chemicals. Contrary to a once widely held view, hemolysis induced by these means does not involve a tear or break in the erythrocyte membrane with release of the hemoglobin molecules. Instead, the restraining forces holding the hemoglobin molecules in place appear to be overcome, and hemoglobin escapes from the cell by generalized oozing. For example, extrinsic injury to the surface membrane affects permeability and permits alterations in ionic equilibrium leading to the ingress of water, swelling, assumption of the spheroidal shape, distention of surface "pores," and the egress of hemoglobin. However, erythrocyte destruction is not always preceded by sphering, and many facets of in vitro red cell lysis remain to be elucidated. In addition, the relationship between hemolysis induced in vitro and that occurring in vivo is speculative and the subject of much dispute.

Even if in vivo hemolysis reflects mechanisms similar to those that cause hemolysis in vitro, the physiologic destruction of normal red cells which have reached the end of their life-spans may be accomplished in quite a different manner. Two kinds of in vivo hemolysis are recognized. Intravascular cell disruption with release of hemoglobin into the circulating plasma is uncommon even in active hemolytic disorders. Therefore it seems quite unlikely that effete erythrocytes are normally destroyed within the circulation. Extravascular hemolysis (especially in organs with large numbers of reticuloendothelial cells such as the spleen, liver, and bone marrow) is the commonest type of accelerated erythrocyte destruction and is probably the way normal aged red cells are eliminated from the body.

Although the changes that accompany erythrocyte aging can be followed up to the time of cell destruction, the actual mechanism by which the cell is removed continues to elude detection. Even so, it is possible to measure red cell survival times and to follow the catabolism of hemoglobin after the erythrocyte has been destroyed. Because red cell survival times and the manifestations of hemoglobin degradation are parameters that reflect increased hemolytic activity, they are considered in detail.

ERYTHROCYTE SURVIVAL TIMES. Reproducible and meaningful red cell survival data can be obtained by several techniques, even though precise measurements are difficult at best and often impossible. It is necessary to be able to recognize and separate the cells present at the start of the study from those that are formed at a later date; otherwise it would not be possible to determine the rate of disappearance of the erythrocytes from the circulation. Therefore the aliquot of cells being studied must differ clearly from the rest of the erythrocytes. Transfusion with donor cells of a different but compatible blood type (the Ashby technique) permits this separation. For example, type O erythrocytes are serologically separable from type A or B red cells, yet they are compatible and will survive normally in a recipient whose blood type is A or B (p. 528). In specimens consisting of mixtures of types O and A or B cells it is possible to remove the A or B cells by potent anti-A or anti-B sera, leaving the donor type O cells, which can then be enumerated and their rate of removal ascertained. When the number of donor erythrocytes remaining is plotted against time, the curve is linear, provided the cells are being removed as they reach a certain age. If the cells are being destroyed randomly, regardless of age, the curve will be exponential.

The differential agglutination or Ashby technique does not permit observations on the survival of erythrocytes in their natural surroundings. Other disadvantages include its time-consuming nature, the need to rely on red cell counts with their inherent errors, the limitations imposed by the requirement that donor erythrocytes be compatible with but serologically distinguishable from the recipient's cells, and the necessity to transfuse large quantities of test cells (500 to 1000 ml). For these reasons it is more desirable to tag the subject's own cells and then measure the rate at which they are removed.

By using cells that have been labeled at random, it is possible to determine life-span rather quickly by extrapolation from data obtained during the first 20 to 30 days. However, accurate determinations are predicated on the maintenance of a steady state consisting of erythrocytes of all ages. If, at the time of labeling, the predominant cells are young, the survival time will be abnormally long; if most of the tagged cells are old, it will be abnormally short. During the period of observation a constant relationship must be maintained between erythrocyte production and destruction, and no significant change in red cell mass should occur. If the red cell mass is increased by transfusions, enhanced production, or decreased destruction, labeled cells will be diluted; if the red cell mass is decreased by bleeding, tagged cells will be lost. Either event will result in an apparent (but not real) shortening of the survival time. An ideal red cell tag would label erythrocytes of all ages promptly and irreversibly, would not in itself affect the cell's viability, and would be detectable in small quantities of blood. In addition, the label should not be reused to tag new cells when the originally tagged cell is destroyed.

Radioactive chromium in the form of Na_2 $^{51}CrO_4$ is the label currently used most often for the measurement of red cell survival times; it has virtually supplanted the Ashby technique. Although all of these requirements are rarely met, the radiochromium method generally provides valuable information. When an aliquot of red cells is incubated in vitro with radioactive sodium chromate, the chromium is firmly bound to the β globin chains of the hemoglobin molecule. Chromium released subsequent to the destruction of tagged cells (or that which is eluted—about 1 per cent per day) is promptly excreted by the kidneys and does not relabel other cells. This isotope is also detectable with routine equipment in small samples of blood. The chief disadvantage of the technique is random elution of the ^{51}Cr regardless of cell age. Even in normal subjects elution is responsible for an exponential rather than a linear survival curve. There is no accurate and acceptable means to correct for elution because of variable and unpredictable differences in the rate that the label is lost. When survival times are markedly shortened, differences in the correction factors lack significance, for they do not alter the results by more than a day or so. With longer life-spans, however, the correction factor used can seriously affect the results, which may vary as much as 20 days or more. Thus a normal survival time may appear to be abnormally short and vice versa. In general, chromium elution is ignored and correction factors are not used.

It is customary to report the uncorrected radiochromium survival time as the half-life ($T/2$) of the tagged cells, that is, the time required for half of the labeled cells to be removed. Normally, the $T/2$ of ^{51}Cr tagged erythrocytes is about 25 to 35 days. It is noteworthy that these values differ from the normal half-life of about 60 days obtained with the Ashby technique. This difference is the result of the elution of the chromium tag. If accurately corrected, the results would be comparable. In other words, the half-life of normal erythrocytes is actually 60 days and not 30 days, as suggested by the chromium method. Practically, however, it makes little difference as long as the normal range for the radiochromium technique is known and we are aware that such data do not indicate the true life-span of the erythrocytes in days.

Random labeling of erythrocytes with radioactive phosphorus-labeled diisopropylfluorophosophate (DF ^{32}P) appears to offer certain advantages. DFP irreversibly inhibits the activity of red cell esterases. Isotopically labeled DFP is an excellent erythrocyte label which does not in itself interfere with red cell viability. To date DF ^{32}P has not been widely adopted, but it seems likely that further experience will show it to be superior to the radiochromium method. Several other techniques are available. For example, it is possible to label a cohort of cells by giving some substance that is incorporated into newly formed erythrocytes, such as glycine ^{14}C, glycine ^{15}N, or ^{59}Fe. Under these circumstances, all labeled cells are of a comparable age, and the survival curve differs clearly from that obtained with random labeling. The necessity to collect data until all labeled cells have been destroyed (more than 120 days in a normal person) detracts from the usefulness of cohort labeling as a diagnostic tool.

HEMOGLOBIN CATABOLISM. Hemoglobin is degraded by reticulo-endothelial cells in the liver, bone marrow, spleen, and elsewhere. This process is depicted schematically in Figure 4-3. Iron is conserved and reutilized; globin is broken down, and the component amino acids are returned to the general amino acid pool; the porphyrin moiety is catabolized to bilirubin and excreted. The first step in the degradation of the hemoglobin molecule has not been clearly elucidated. Globin may be separated from the iron-protoporphyrin complex to yield the hydroxide of ferric protoporphyrin or hematin. A second possibility consists in opening the porphyrin ring to a straight-chain bilirubin-iron-globin complex (choleglobin). By either route iron and globin are eventually split off, leaving biliverdin (a green pigment). Biliverdin is rapidly reduced to free or unconjugated bilirubin, which is carried by the plasma in the form of protein complexes (especially with albumin) to the liver. Plasma bilirubin has a normal life-span of about 90 minutes. Unconjugated bilirubin is not water-soluble and is not excreted by the kidneys. It has often been called the indirect bilirubin fraction because it will not participate in the color reaction with Ehrlich's diazo reagent until it is solubilized by the addition of alcohol. In the liver unconjugated bilirubin enters the parenchymal cells and, in the region of the microsomes, is conjugated enzymatically with glucuronic acid. Conjugated bilirubin or bilirubin glucuronide is water-soluble and will give an immediate color reaction with Ehrlich's reagent; for this reason it has often been designated the direct bilirubin fraction. A small amount of bilirubin glucuronide escapes back into the plasma; although conjugated

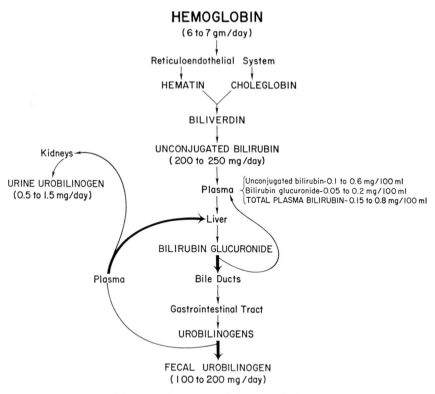

Figure 4-3.   Hemoglobin catabolism.

bilirubin is excretable by the kidneys (presumably because of its water-solubility), it is not detectable in the urine under normal circumstances.

Most of the bilirubin glucuronide formed by the liver is excreted into the intestinal tract, in which it is reduced by bacterial action to uro-bilinogen (reduced forms) and urobilin (oxidized forms) compounds. These protoporphyrin catabolites are referred to collectively as uro-bilinogens. The majority of these substances are excreted in the feces, but some are absorbed from the gastrointestinal tract and re-excreted by the liver. The urobilinogens are also excretable by the kidneys. How-ever, most of the pigments that enter the "enterohepatic circulation" are cleared promptly and efficiently by the liver. Therefore only small amounts of urobilinogen are present normally in the urine.

Based on a mean survival time of 120 days, about 6 to 7 gm of hemo-globin (0.83 per cent of the red cell mass) are degraded in a normal adult each day and replaced by newly formed erythrocytes. Since 1 gm of hemoglobin yields 35 mg of bilirubin (or urobilinogen), daily pig-ment production should amount to about 200 to 250 mg. However, it is not possible to quantify precisely the rate of red cell destruction or the amount of hemoglobin catabolized from urobilinogen excretion data. Technical problems exist; for example, fecal urobilinogen measurements are contingent on accurate stool collections continued over a period of several days, and only 50 per cent or so of the pigment produced is recoverable in the feces. More important is the knowledge that total bilirubin production exceeds by a significant amount that derived from the breakdown of effete red cells. Approximately 10 to 20 per cent of the daily bilirubin production appears to originate from ineffective erythropoiesis, that is, nucleated red cells that never reach maturity or erythrocytes destroyed before or immediately after release into the circulation. Various other heme-containing compounds (e.g., myoglobin, catalase, cytochromes, and peroxidase) also contribute to total bilirubin production. For these reasons only 75 per cent or so of the urobilinogen excretion reflects destruction of mature circulating red cells.

When hemoglobin is released directly into the plasma, it attaches promptly to haptoglobin, an α_2 globulin capable of binding two molecules of hemoglobin. The haptoglobin-hemoglobin complex is cleared by the reticuloendothelial system at a rate of about 15 mg/hour and the protoporphyrin is degraded as already described. Because of its molecular weight, the haptoglobin-hemoglobin complex is not excreted by the kidneys. Normal haptoglobin levels are capable of binding approximately 100 mg hemoglobin/100 ml plasma. Several genetically determined haptoglobin variants have been described; each transports hemoglobin equally well. Haptoglobin plays its greatest role in those hemolytic disorders characterized by intravascular hemolysis; for example, hemolytic transfusion reactions (p. 532). The precise contribution of haptoglobin to normal hemoglobin catabolism is not known. This globulin probably does not participate to any great extent. However, a certain amount of hemoglobin derived from extravascular erythrocyte destruction does diffuse into the plasma, in which it is bound to haptoglobin. Therefore it is logical to assume that haptoglobin contributes, at least minimally, to the degradation of hemoglobin in a normal person.

PATHOPHYSIOLOGY OF THE HEMOLYTIC DISORDERS

The pathophysiologic effects of impaired red cell viability are the same, regardless of the nature of the abnormality in the erythrocytes or their environment. The premature destruction of circulating red cells imparts a potent stimulus to marrow erythrocyte production. The predominant manifestations of the hemolytic anemias are divisible into those reflecting increased erythrocyte destruction and those attributable to increased erythropoiesis. Because all hemolytic syndromes are characterized by a mixture of findings falling into these two categories, their clinical pictures have much in common.

Manifestations of Increased Erythrocyte Destruction. Decreased red cell viability, which is demonstrable by techniques that quantify erythrocyte survival times, alters the finely balanced equilibrium between erythrocyte production and destruction. Current data are in accord with the thesis that the decrease in circulating hemoglobin affects the dynamic relationship between tissue oxygen tension and cellular requirements; enhanced humoral erythropoietic factor elaboration ensues and is, in turn, responsible for augmented marrow erythropoiesis (p. 13). If the balance between erythrocyte production and destruction can be restored by increasing marrow output, the peripheral erythroid values will remain normal and the hemolytic disorder is compensated. If production fails to keep pace with peripheral destruction (either because the functional reserve of the marrow is exceeded or because a superimposed abnormality prevents a maximal response), anemia develops; the hemolytic disorder is now uncompensated and is appropriately designated a hemolytic anemia.

A hemolytic anemia may vary from mild to profound and may develop slowly or with great speed. Because of the relatively long red cell lifespan, a rapid onset is characteristic of blood loss anemia, indicating either acute hemorrhage or hemolysis. In patients with chronic uncompensated hemolysis, the symptoms caused by the anemia are nonspecific (e.g., weakness, tachycardia, and exertional dyspnea). On the other hand, acute hemolysis may be manifested by severe pain in the back, abdomen, or extremeties, chills, fever, prostration, hypotension, and even shock followed by renal failure. The explanations for most of these findings are obscure. In some patients shock may be the result of acute hypovolemia, secondary to a rapid decrease in red cell mass.

The other clinical manifestations of increased erythrocyte destruction directly reflect the catabolism of increased amounts of hemoglobin. The typical pigment changes of hemolytic jaundice are (1) hyperbilirubinemia due to free or unconjugated bilirubin, (2) increased fecal urobilinogen (500 to 4000 mg/24 hours), and (3) increased urine urobilinogen (usually 5 to 30 but occasionally as high as 200 mg/24 hours). However, several variables significantly influence these findings. The concentration of bilirubin in the blood is dependent on the rate and severity of the hemolytic process as well as on the functional status of the liver. The normal liver is capable of handling large quantities of bilirubin without permitting the plasma concentration to increase. For example, in a normal-sized adult with hemolysis and a sixfold increase in erythropoiesis, bilirubin production would be six times normal, or 1200 to 1500 mg daily; however, such a person would not, as a rule, be jaundiced. In addition, the size of the red cell mass limits the availability of cells to be destroyed, and hemolysis superimposed on some other type of anemia may play an essential role in the pathogenesis of a severe anemia without providing enough bilirubin to produce hyper-bilirubinemia. Liver dysfunction also contributes to the actual concentration of bilirubin in the blood. Thus neither chemical nor clinical jaundice is requisite for the diagnosis of a hemolytic anemia, even though they are common findings (the total serum bilirubin may be normal, slightly increased, or reach concentrations of 10 mg [or more]/100 ml). Theoretically, blood bilirubin glucuronide levels should not be increased by hemolysis (Fig. 4-3). However, a slight increase in direct-reacting bilirubin is usual in patients with hemolytic jaundice because of the solubilizing effect of certain plasma constituents which permit a small amount of unconjugated bilirubin to participate in an immediate color reaction with Ehrlich's reagent. Significant elevations in bilirubin glucuronide concentration in the blood ordinarily reflect such complications as biliary tract obstruction or superimposed hepatic parenchymal disease. Consequently, persons with uncomplicated hemolytic jaundice have no bile in their urine. For this reason it has been designated *acholuric jaundice*.

In general, most hemolytic disorders (compensated and uncompensated) are accompanied by increased fecal and urine urobilinogen levels. Fecal urobilinogen content depends on several factors, such as bacterial flora (broad-spectrum antibiotics will curtail urobilinogen formation) and the size of the red cell mass (in the presence of anemia there are fewer cells to contribute to bilirubin production). Therefore it is difficult to quantify hemolytic activity on this basis, even using a correction device such as the hemolytic index, which takes red cell mass into consideration. Furthermore, the need to collect all feces over a period of several days, together with the unpleasant nature of the technique, detracts considerably from the clinical usefulness of fecal urobilinogen determinations. Although an increase in fecal urobilinogen confirms the presence of hemolytic disease, its absence by no means excludes the diagnosis. Urine urobilinogen concentrations are even less reliable because the liver can clear large amounts of pigment from the plasma with relative ease. As a result, clear-cut hemolytic activity may be associated with only minimal increases in urine urobilinogen. Despite the failure of these pigment measurements to correlate well with the peripheral erythroid values or rate of hemolysis, they constitute important tools for the clinical and investigative study of the hemolytic anemias and often provide valuable information.

Accelerated hemoglobin catabolism also affects the extracorpuscular hemoglobin transport mechanism, or haptoglobin. Normally, haptoglobin is able to bind about 100 mg of hemoglobin/100 ml plasma. Following acute intravascular hemolysis, all available haptoglobin may be bound to hemoglobin; even in chronic hemolytic disorders, in which extravascular hemolysis predominates, haptoglobin is ordinarily metabolized at a faster rate than it can be synthesized. Therefore most of the hemolytic anemias are characterized by markedly decreased to undetectable plasma haptoglobin levels. If there is not enough haptoglobin to bind all the extracorpuscular hemoglobin, free hemoglobin can be detected in the plasma (the plasma appears pink when the hemoglobin concentration exceeds 20 and red when it reaches 100 mg/100 ml). A small amount of free plasma hemoglobin may be broken down and the heme moiety oxidized to hematin, which then combines with albumin to form methemalbumin. Because this compound is cleared rapidly from the plasma, its presence is always indicative of recent intravascular hemolysis.

When the free plasma hemoglobin reaches 25 mg/100 ml, the resorptive capacity of the renal tubules is exceeded and hemoglobinuria ensues. Hemosiderinuria is another manifestation of hemolytic disease; however, in contrast to hemoglobinuria, which reflects recent acute intravascular hemolysis, hemosiderinuria is the result of chronic hemolytic activity. Free hemoglobin filtered by the glomeruli is absorbed by the tubular cells, in which it is broken down and the iron is converted to hemosiderin and ferritin. Although some of this iron appears to be transported elsewhere and reused, a significant amount is lost in the urine, chiefly that contained in desquamated cells.

Increased bilirubin production is also responsible for a greatly increased incidence of cholelithiasis (pigment stones). Indeed, few patients with chronic hemolysis escape the development of gallstones, and cholelithiasis in a young person (especially under the age of 30) demands the exclusion of a hemolytic disorder.

Splenomegaly comes very close to being a *sine qua non* of hemolysis. It may reflect multiple and varied causes such as extramedullary hematopoiesis or the basic disease (e.g., lymphoma). However, splenic enlargement is often the result, at least in part, of "work hypertrophy," that is, the need to remove increased numbers of defective or damaged cells. Under these circumstances splenomegaly is a manifestation of increased erythrocyte destruction. In some instances it is possible to define more clearly the role of the spleen in this condition. For example, ^{51}Cr-tagged red cells can be detected in the spleen by external counting techniques; a disproportionately greater number of counts over the spleen than over other sites such as the liver and precordium is indicative of excessive splenic red cell sequestration. Following the injection of ^{51}Cr-labeled red cells, an initial high uptake over the spleen and a relatively slow drop over the subsequent hour suggests a "big spleen" syndrome and slow mixing of the tagged cells with the circulating cells because of an expanded splenic stasis compartment.

Decreased red cell viability also contributes to the development of tissue hemosiderosis, a common finding in long-standing hemolytic disorders. The presence of anemia, together with increased erythropoietic activity, serves to enhance the absorption of iron from the gastrointestinal tract (p. 161). As a result, body iron stores are augmented. With the exception of a very few patients who lose excessive amounts of iron in their urine, for example, those with paroxysmal nocturnal hemoglobinuria (p. 150), hemolysis is not accompanied by increased iron loss. Instead, iron is carefully conserved and iron stores are progressively expanded. For this reason, the administration of therapeutic amounts of inorganic iron to a patient with a chronic hemolytic anemia is contraindicated unless superimposed iron deficiency and negative iron balance are unequivocally present.

Manifestations of Accelerated Erythropoiesis. A decrease in erythrocyte life-span imparts a potent stimulus to the marrow; accelerated erythropoiesis ensues. This stimulus appears to be mediated by the humoral erythropoietic regulatory mechanism, and increased plasma erythropoietic activity is demonstrable in most hemolytic disorders. In fact, an acute phenylhydrazine-induced hemolytic anemia is an effective and commonly used means to enhance humoral erythropoietic factor elaboration in experimental animals. The consequence of this increased humoral stimulus is myeloid erythrocytic hyperplasia. Erythropoiesis is augmented by increasing input from the stem cell into the erythrocytic compartment.

The increased erythropoietic tissue is accommodated in bones that are normally concerned with myelopoiesis (ribs, vertebrae, pelvis, and skull), as well as in others that do not otherwise participate in blood cell production (e.g., femurs and humeri). Augmented erythropoiesis is manifested in routine marrow specimens by decreased fat and hypercellularity; the latter is due predominantly to erythrocytic hyperplasia, and there may be two or three times as many developing erythrocytic as granulocytic elements. If all other requirements are met, erythropoiesis is normoblastic and orderly and the normal ratio between immature and mature nucleated red cells is maintained. Because of the erythrocytic hyperplasia, there is a relative decrease in granulopoiesis and the number of megakaryocytes. However, there is no absolute decrease in these aspects of myelopoiesis, and, in certain types of hemolytic anemias, they are actually increased. These quantitative changes in granulopoiesis and thrombopoiesis have not been clearly defined; some preliminary experimental data suggest that they may reflect enhanced activity of humoral factors, but clarification of these findings must await further study.

Increased marrow activity is responsible for bone pain in some patients with acute and severe hemolysis and may cause certain bony changes such as widening of medullary cavities, cortical atrophy, and "tower" skulls. The stimulus (presumably humoral) that evokes the increase in marrow erythropoiesis also affects pluripotential reticulum cells elsewhere; these cells resume their embryonic myelopoietic tasks, and foci of extramedullary hematopoiesis appear in the spleen, liver, and other tissues. Even posterior mediastinal masses consisting of developing blood cells have been observed in a few patients with such chronic hemolytic anemias as hereditary spherocytosis and the hereditary hemoglobinopathies.

If increased marrow production cannot keep pace with peripheral destruction, anemia develops. Other peripheral blood manifestations of accelerated erythropoiesis are attributable to the release from the marrow of increased numbers of immature cells. Increased polychromasia, an absolute reticulocytosis, and circulating nucleated red cells are the hallmark of increased erythropoiesis, irrespective of cause. The magnitude of these findings varies with the severity of the hemolytic process. The degree of polychromasia parallels the reticulocyte count, since all polychromatophilic cells in a Wright-stained film are reticulocytes when stained supravitally with brilliant cresyl blue. The reticulocyte count may range from slightly elevated (3 to 5 per cent) to 50 per cent or higher; in most patients it is between 5 to 20 per cent. Typically, there are one to five nucleated red cells per 100 leukocytes. Because young erythrocytes are larger than older cells, reticulocytosis is reflected by increased numbers of round macrocytes (p. 213). Occasionally, Howell-Jolly bodies (p. 63) and siderocytes (p. 63) may be observed.

Since hemolytic disorders are often associated with marrow granulocytic and megakaryocytic hyperplasia as well as increased numbers of developing erythrocytes, it is not surprising that leukocytosis and thrombocytosis should accompany these findings. The exceptions are few and appear to consist of certain of the autoimmune hemolytic anemias and the rare entity, paroxsymal nocturnal hemoglobinuria. In the autoimmune hemolytic anemias the lack of leukocytosis and/or thrombocytosis (or more likely the presence of leukopenia and/or thrombocytopenia) probably reflects abnormal immunoglobulins or autoantibodies directed against these blood cells (p. 135). The leukopenia and thrombocytopenia in paroxysmal nocturnal hemoglobinuria may be due to marrow hypoplasia (p. 151). Patients with other hemolytic anemias can be expected to have normal or increased leukocyte and platelet counts. In most cases the increases are modest (a leukocyte count of 10,000 to 20,000 and a platelet count of 400,000 to 600,000/ cu mm). However, some patients manifest more striking leukemoid reactions (p. 333), and leukocyte counts of 100,000/cu mm have been observed. A few immature granulocytes are common in the peripheral blood of an actively hemolyzing patient; they probably reflect premature release from the marrow, but remarkably little is known about the mechanisms governing this process.

Additional pathophysiologic manifestations of increased erythropoiesis are a decreased plasma iron turnover time and an increased rate of incorporation of radioiron into newly formed erythrocytes. It should be noted that these findings lack specificity and are similar to those caused by acute hemorrhage. The increased rate of erythropoiesis also contributes, along with the anemia, to the absorption of increased amounts of dietary iron and the eventual enlargement of body iron stores.

The hemolytic disorders are ordinarily associated with increased erythropoiesis and hypercellular bone marrows; however, *aplastic* or, more appropriately, *hypoplastic crises* have been observed in all types of hemolytic anemias, hereditary and acquired. The explanations for these occurrences, which are fortunately quite rare, are conjectural. In some patients folate deficiency appears to play a role; these individuals respond to appropriate replacement therapy. Such a deficiency is probably the result of increased folic acid requirements consequent to the accelerated erythropoiesis in the face of suboptimal intake (p. 201). However, patients with hypoplastic crises usually have hypocellular marrows. Although profound folate deficiency might produce a decrease in the number of erythrocytic precursors in the marrow, it is characteristically manifested by a cellular marrow with megaloblastic morphology (p. 209). Thus other ill-defined pathogenic mechanisms must exist. Infections, hypersensitivity phenomena, adverse reactions to drugs, and an abnormality in the humoral erythropoietic regulatory mechanism have been suggested as possible causes, but proof is lacking. Since this rare complication of a hemolytic anemia has occurred in more than one member of a family with a hereditary hemolytic disorder, genetic factors may also contribute.

The clinical manifestations of a hypoplastic crisis develop with dramatic suddenness. Because the rate of hemolysis ordinarily does not change, the curtailed red cell production causes an abrupt fall in the peripheral erythroid values. The reticulocyte count decreases to near zero, and, since there are fewer cells to be lysed, bilirubin production declines; jaundice may subside and fecal and urine urobilinogen levels decrease. As a rule, the bone marrow reveals striking erythrocytic hypoplasia. Some patients have hypoplasia of all marrow elements, and leukopenia and thrombocytopenia accompany the rapidly increasing anemia. The cause of the crisis, for example, decreased production or folic acid deficiency, will influence the marrow picture as will the stage of the crisis (normoblastic hyperplasia may be a manifestation of beginning recovery). When and if bone marrow function is restored, it is reflected by a striking reticulocytosis and the re-establishment of the peripheral blood values that characterized the patient's hemolytic disorder before the development of this complication.

Manifestations of Specific Causes. Certain varieties of hemolytic disease are associated with specific (or at least relatively specific) findings reflecting their underlying pathogenesis. Even though some of these manifestations are common to several hemolytic syndromes, they are not found in all hemolytic disorders. Therefore it seems appropriate to consider them separately.

ERYTHROCYTE MORPHOLOGY. A variety of abnormalities in red cell morphology distinguish certain of the hemolytic disorders. Among them, *spherocytes* (Fig. 4-4) are most specific, most commonly encountered,

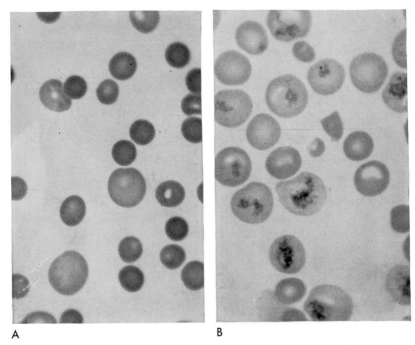

A   B

Figure 4-4. Spherocytes. A. Wright-stained peripheral blood film. B. Blood film stained supravitally with brilliant cresyl blue and counterstained with Wright's stain (reticulocytes are seldom spherocytic).

and most significant. A great deal has been written about the pathophysiologic importance of these cells, which have been the subject of much study. Basically, a spherocyte is an erythrocyte that has lost its normal biconcave configuration and assumed a spherical form. Since these cells represent the greatest volume that can be maintained within their surface areas, their diameter is less and their thickness greater than similar measurements of the biconcave discs from which they are derived. Therefore spherocytes lack a central pale area and appear smaller and more hyperchromatic than normal erythrocytes.

In vitro, a normal red cell behaves as a near perfect osmometer.

When suspended in a hypotonic medium, water enters the cell and causes it to assume a spheroidal shape. When the maximal volume permitted by the nonelastic surface membrane is reached, the cell undergoes lysis. Erythrocytes can be transformed in vitro into spherocytes by means other than disturbances in osmotic equilibrium. Injury to the red cell consequent to physical factors such as heat, contact with erythrocyte antibodies, or exposure to surface-active substances such as saponin, ionic detergents, or lysolecithin will produce spherocytes; deprivation of glucose in vitro results in similar morphologic changes. In each of these instances the assumption of the spheroidal configuration reflects some injury or change that immediately precedes in vitro lysis or seriously affects the cells' viability when returned to the donors.

In vivo, spherocytes distinguish a variety of hemolytic disorders, including hereditary spherocytosis, autoimmune hemolytic anemias (primary and secondary), certain isoimmune hemolytic anemias (e.g., erythroblastosis fetalis due to ABO blood group incompatibility), Zieve's syndrome (hyperlipemic hemolysis), and "big spleen" syndromes such as agnogenic myeloid metaplasia and Gaucher's disease. Careful study of a well-made, well-stained blood film will ordinarily reveal a rare spherocyte in a normal person; similar cells may be found in recipients of recent blood transfusions and probably represent red cells soon to be destroyed. Otherwise spherocytosis indicates a hemolytic process and therefore is a finding of considerable diagnostic significance. Spherocytes, together with the peripheral blood manifestations of increased erythropoiesis—polychromasia, reticulocytosis, and nucleated red cells—are pathognomonic of a spherocytic hemolytic anemia. Although many hemolytic disorders are characterized by the presence of spherocytes, it is noteworthy that some are not; consequently, their absence does not exclude the diagnosis of a hemolytic anemia.

The precise relationship between spherocytosis and in vivo erythrocyte destruction has not been clearly defined. There is convincing support for the theory that spherocytes represent the last morphologic stage preceding cell destruction. Therefore spheroidal erythrocytes, which are particularly susceptible to sequestration in the spleen and equally attractive to reticuloendothelial cells elsewhere, may be viewed as red cells destined for early death. However, all spherocytes are not irreversibly damaged. Furthermore, the actual shape of a spherocyte is not necessarily the factor responsible for its destruction. It is quite possible that the spheroidal configuration is merely a reflection of some serious derangement in the cells' metabolic activities, osmotic equilibrium, or surface membranes and that these abnormalities rather than the peculiar shape determine their fate. In any event, spherocytic morphology remains an invaluable clinical sign of some abnormality

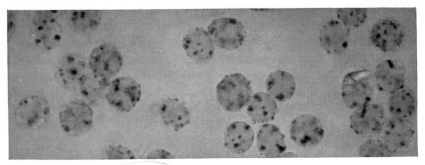

Figure 4-5. Heinz bodies in erythrocytes from a patient with glucose-6-phosphate dehydrogenase deficiency. Red cells were incubated with acetylphenylhydrazine and the wet preparation was stained with crystal violet (the majority of these cells contain more than five inclusion bodies).

(either intra- or extracorpuscular) that prevents survival for a normal period of time.

Heinz bodies (Fig. 4-5) are multiple coccoid granules of denatured hemoglobin formed as the result of exposure to an oxidant compound such as acetylphenylhydrazine. These intraerythrocytic inclusion bodies are not demonstrable with ordinary polychrome stains and require special supravital techniques with dyes such as brilliant cresyl blue or crystal violet. Heinz bodies reflect an insufficient complement of the glycolytic enzymes needed to generate sufficient reducing capacity (chiefly in the form of TPNH) to prevent spontaneous oxidation of glutathione and hemoglobin (Fig. 4-2). As a result, hemoglobin is eventually denatured and precipitated as Heinz bodies. Since normal aging is accompanied by a wearing out of the erythrocytes' vital enzyme systems, occasional Heinz bodies can be seen in normal erythrocytes. However, the presence of large numbers of cells containing multiple cytoplasmic inclusions (five or more Heinz bodies in 40 per cent or more of the cells) usually indicates a genetically determined hemolytic disorder such as that caused by glucose-6-phosphate dehydrogenase deficiency.

Other morphologic abnormalities of red cells are often more specific, but in most the mechanism of their formation is obscure. These misshapen erythrocytes include the ovalocytes (or elliptocytes) of hereditary elliptocytosis (Fig. 4-6) and the target cells of hemoglobin C disease (p. 263). On the other hand, the pathogenesis of the peculiar sickle cells (or depranocytes) that characterize hemoglobin S disease is well known and the structural changes are, in turn, directly responsible for the cell's decreased survival time (p. 254). Additional erythrocytic changes associated with hemolytic disorders include the microcytes, target cells, and hypochromia of the thalassemia syndromes.

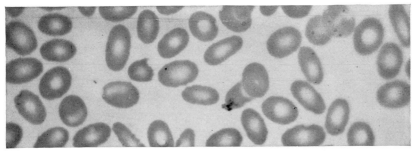

Figure 4-6. Peripheral blood film from a patient with hereditary elliptocytosis.

Although these findings appear to reflect a genetically determined quantitative defect in hemoglobin synthesis, their role in or relationship to the hemolytic component of these hemoglobinopathies is unknown (p. 272).

ERYTHROCYTE OSMOTIC AND MECHANICAL FRAGILITY. Evaluation of the ability of erythrocytes to tolerate osmotic stress in vitro has provided important information in the study of the hemolytic disorders. There are few in vivo counterparts other than hemolysis due to the injection of large amounts of water or some other hypotonic solution. However, the behavior of red cells in hypotonic salt solutions in vitro is often a reflection of their survival times in vivo. Normal osmotic behavior does not exclude impaired red cell viability. On the other hand, the correlation between decreased osmotic resistance and a shortened life-span possesses compelling experimental and clinical support. Although the demonstration of decreased red cell survival in vivo is not strictly analogous to the finding of increased osmotic fragility in vitro, these techniques provide information of comparable clinical importance.

Erythrocyte osmotic fragility is dependent on ionic equilibrium. Any change in this equilibrium will interfere with the cells' behavior in hypotonic media. Since spherocytes already possess the maximum volume permitted by their surface area, they are much less resistant to hypotonic stress than are normal cells. In other words, a spherocyte has already progressed to the point of lysis, whereas a normal cell can accommodate a certain amount of water and is, as a result, protected by being able to assume the spheroidal configuration. Therefore spherocytes always display abnormal osmotic behavior and undergo lysis in solutions of graded hypotonicity before normal cells. Hence, on the basis of the demonstration of spherocytes in a peripheral blood film, it can be predicted that erythrocyte osmotic fragility measurements will be abnormal. However, abnormal osmotic behavior can exist in the absence of spherocytes (some cells may be able to maintain a normal shape in plasma but have an inadequate reserve to resist even minor changes in ionic flux).

Slight abnormalities in osmotic fragility may be made more evident by incubation in vitro. If normal erythrocytes are deprived of glucose (the source of the energy needed to maintain their electrolyte pump and replenish redox systems), they will, after a period of time, be unable to resist osmotic stress. Consequently, osmotic resistance varies inversely with the duration of in vitro incubation. The latter will then "magnify" minor erythrocyte abnormalities affecting their osmotic behavior and in vivo survival.

A modification of the effect of incubation on osmotic behavior is the assessment of *autohemolysis*. After incubation for 48 hours, about 5 per cent of normal erythrocytes will undergo lysis; if glucose is added, autohemolysis can be reduced to about 1 per cent. In many hemolytic disorders the erythrocytes are less able to withstand glucose deprivation, and more than 20 per cent of the cells will be destroyed after the 48-hour incubation period. In some instances this greatly increased rate of autohemolysis can be corrected by the addition of glucose.

Resistance of red cells to graded degrees of mechanical trauma occasioned by shaking with glass beads (mechanical fragility) has also been used to detect cellular changes interfering with survival. In general, abnormalities in mechanical fragility parallel changes in osmotic resistance. Sickle cells are a notable exception; despite their normal osmotic behavior, these cells have markedly increased mechanical fragility (p. 258).

ERYTHROCYTE ANTIBODIES. Hemolytic disorders caused by erythrocyte antibodies are associated with complex serologic manifestations of the immune process. With the exception of hemolytic transfusion reactions caused by ABO blood group incompatibility (p. 532), these serum factors are, for the most part, immunoglobulins with sedimentation constants of 7S and molecular weights of about 160,000; the majority are *warm agglutinins*, that is, they are most active at 37°C and produce agglutination rather than hemolysis. Naturally occurring erythrocyte antibodies, for example, anti-A and anti-B (p. 520), are most active in the cold (4 to 20°C) and are complete (or polyvalent), attaching to more than one erythrocyte at a time. As a result, visible clumping occurs in saline. In contrast, virtually all immune erythrocyte antibodies (isoimmune and autoimmune) are incomplete (or univalent) and attach to only one cell at a time. Therefore incomplete immunoglobulins act as blocking antibodies; red cells to which these substances are adsorbed will not agglutinate in saline. However, they will conglutinate or stick together when suspended in a medium of high molecular weight such as 20 to 30 per cent bovine albumin. Such erythrocytes can also be made to clump in saline if the antibody-coated surfaces of the cells are treated with a proteolytic enzyme such as trypsin, papain, or bromelin. A third means to detect incomplete erythrocyte antibodies is clinically the most useful and is designated the *Coombs'* or *antiglobulin* test.

Incomplete erythrocyte antibodies are immunoglobulins. Cells coated with these substances will be agglutinated by antihuman globulin antibodies (Coombs' sera) which are obtained from rabbits that have been injected with human immunoglobulins. A positive *direct Coombs' test* consists of the agglutination of washed erythrocytes suspended in Coombs' reagent. With few exceptions, it indicates the presence of an abnormal protein (usually an incomplete antibody) adsorbed to the surface of the cell. Most autoimmune and isoimmune erythrocyte antibodies attach to erythrocytes at body temperature; therefore a positive direct Coombs' test is the most consistent serologic finding in patients with acquired isoimmune and autoimmune hemolytic disorders, both primary (or idiopathic) and secondary. The direct Coombs' test is fairly specific, but false positives and false negatives do occur. Although most of the false negatives reflect technical defects (weak Coombs' sera or improper dilutions), it is unlikely that this technique will detect all serum factors (presumably antibodies) capable of producing hemolysis. False positive direct Coombs' tests create more clinical confusion.

Originally, Coombs' sera were prepared by immunizing rabbits against whole human serum. Such rabbit sera are capable of reacting with any of the plasma proteins. As a result, they will cause agglutination of reticulocytes which are coated with transferrin, a normal β_1 globulin. Because reticulocytosis is a feature of almost all hemolytic anemias, clumping of young red cells by broad spectrum Coombs' sera may be mistaken for the presence on the cells of an abnormal protein factor, that is, an incomplete erythrocyte antibody. This effect can be inhibited if the Coombs' serum is incubated with transferrin before its use. The specificity of Coombs' sera can also be enhanced by injecting the donor rabbits with "pure" human immunoglobulins.

Incomplete cold agglutinins are often present in low titers in normal persons and storage of blood specimens in the refrigerator may permit their attachment to erythrocytes; when these cells are suspended in Coombs' serum, the result is a false positive direct antiglobulin test. This type of false positive reaction can be avoided by keeping the specimen warm and can be inhibited to a large degree by anticoagulating the blood. False positive direct Coombs' tests have been reported in various disorders associated with hyperglobulinemia such as sarcoidosis, systemic lupus erythematosus, and rheumatoid arthritis. It is becoming more and more evident, however, that most of these disorders are accompanied by an element of decreased red cell survival due to an extracorpuscular factor. Therefore the designation in such a disorder of a positive direct Coombs' test as a "false positive" may be an invalid assumption.

The *indirect Coombs' test* detects the presence of a circulating incomplete erythrocyte antibody. Normal cells are incubated in the plasma being tested. If the plasma contains erythrocyte autoantibodies, they will be fixed to normal cells regardless of blood type; these "sensitized" erythrocytes will now give a positive direct Coombs' test. Incomplete warm reacting erythrocyte autoagglutinins are rarely present in high titers in plasma because they are continuously being adsorbed to the erythrocytes. Consequently, the indirect Coombs' test is not always positive in the acquired autoimmune hemolytic disorders.

Circulating immune isoantibodies in infants with erythroblastosis fetalis or in adults who have been sensitized by the administration of mismatched transfusions or by blood group incompatible pregnancies are blood type specific. These antibodies can be detected by the indirect Coombs' test only if appropriate red cells are used. For example, anti-D (anti-Rh_o) antibodies will be adsorbed to D(Rh_o) positive cells but not to those that are D(Rh_o) negative (p. 523). The direct Coombs' test is also positive in infants with erythroblastosis fetalis, for the antibodies are derived from the mother and are directed against the infants' own erythrocytes; the direct Coombs' test is negative in the other situations.

Isoimmune erythrocyte antibodies are occasionally complete or saline agglutinating. However, it is very rare to find a complete autoimmune erythrocyte antibody. In the few patients in whom they do occur, such antibodies are almost always most active in the cold (usually at 4°C). Cold agglutinins may be demonstrable in titers up to 1:16 in normal persons. In rare patients with acquired autoimmune hemolytic disorders, cold agglutinins may reach titers of 1:1,000,000 or higher. These cold antibodies display little or no lytic activity, affect erythrocytes regardless of blood type, and can be quantified in the cold by using normal type O erythrocytes or preferably the patient's own red cells. The possible existence of an incomplete cold agglutinin is conjectural. Patients with high titers of cold agglutinins ordinarily have positive direct Coombs' tests; such findings probably reflect attachment of the antibody to the erythrocytes consequent to cooling in peripheral vascular beds or in vitro. Some cold agglutinins are macroglobulins with sedimentation constants of 19 to 20S and molecular weights of about 1,000,000.

Most acquired erythrocyte antibodies are agglutinins and do not possess lytic properties. *Warm hemolysins* are extremely rare; however, *cold hemolysins* are responsible for an uncommon type of acquired hemolytic anemia. This antibody, which has only minimal agglutinating properties, is often termed the Donath-Landsteiner antibody. In brief, it requires two steps to produce hemolysis. The first consists of chilling, during which time the antibody attaches, in the presence of complement, to the erythrocytes. The cells must then be warmed before hemolysis will take place.

MISCELLANEOUS FINDINGS. Other pathophysiological manifestations of the hemolytic syndromes reflect their individual causes rather than increased erythrocyte destruction per se. Consequently, they possess greater diagnostic significance and are discussed in the sections devoted to specific types of hemolytic disorders.

CLASSIFICATION OF THE HEMOLYTIC DISORDERS

A clinical classification of the hemolytic disorders is given in Table 4-1. In general, the hemolytic anemias have been divided into (1) those that are inherited or inborn and those that are acquired or (2) those that reflect an intrinsic or intracorpuscular abnormality (red cells that are defective when they leave the bone marrow) and those that are

Table 4-1. Classification of the Hemolytic Disorders

I. *Hereditary*
  A. Hereditary spherocytosis
  B. Hereditary hemoglobinopathies
  C. Hereditary glycolytic enzyme deficiencies
    1. Pentose phosphate pathway
      a. Glucose-6-phosphate dehydrogenase
        (1) "Primaquine-sensitive" anemias
        (2) Favism
      b. Others
    2. Embden-Meyerhof pathway
      a. Pyruvate kinase
      b. Others
  D. Hereditary elliptocytosis
  E. Erythropoietic porphyria
II. *Acquired*
  A. Isoimmune
    1. Hemolytic transfusion reactions
    2. Erythroblastosis fetalis
  B. Autoimmune
    1. Primary (idiopathic)
    2. Secondary (lymphoma, chronic lymphocytic leukemia, nonhematologic neoplasms, collagen diseases)
  C. Chemical and physical factors
  D. Infections
  E. Splenomegaly ("big spleen" syndrome)
  F. Vitamin B_{12} or folic acid deficiency
  G. Paroxysmal nocturnal hemoglobinuria

the result of extrinsic or extracorpuscular abnormalities (red cells that are injured after their release from the bone marrow). It seems less artificial to separate the hemolytic anemias into hereditary and acquired types. Furthermore, all hereditary hemolytic disorders reflect an intrinsic cellular defect, whereas almost all acquired hemolytic anemias are due to extrinsic or extracorpuscular factors (the only exceptions are paroxysmal nocturnal hemoglobinuria and vitamin B_{12} or folic acid deficiency).

The hereditary hemolytic disorders are distinguished by erythrocytes that have decreased survival times in the patient as well as in normal recipients and by normal survival of normal donor cells in the patient. Therefore the defect resides in the cell rather than in the cell's environment. Erythrocyte survival curves are linear because each cell has a similar, albeit shortened, finite life-span.

Most of the acquired hemolytic disorders are characterized by erythrocytes that have decreased survival times in the patient; however, these cells will survive normally in a normal recipient, provided they have not been irreparably damaged. On the other hand, normal cells will be destroyed prematurely when transfused into the patient. Consequently, the defect lies in the cell's environment rather than in the cell itself. Erythrocyte survival curves are exponential, for cells are destroyed at random irrespective of age.

Despite the many similarities in the clinical manifestations of the hemolytic disorders, there are important differences that make it desirable to discuss them separately. As a rule a hemolytic anemia can be recognized with ease; however, a precise etiologic diagnosis requires detailed knowledge of the many facets of each of the hemolytic disorders.

Hereditary Spherocytosis

Hereditary spherocytosis is a genetically determined hemolytic disorder due to a poorly defined intrinsic erythrocyte defect. When fully developed, it is characterized by a spherocytic hemolytic anemia, splenomegaly, and jaundice. Two widely used synonyms are congenital hemolytic jaundice and congenital hemolytic anemia. Because there are other types of congenital hemolytic jaundice as well as other congenital hemolytic anemias, hereditary spherocytosis is preferred. Furthermore, it stresses the constant presence of spherocytes.

HISTORY

Vanlair and Masius published the first clinical description of hereditary spherocytosis in 1871 and with remarkable perspicacity pointed out most of the features of the disease, including the jaundice, splenomegaly, small hyperchromatic erythrocytes, and familial nature. Min-kowski, with others, focused attention on this disorder near the turn of the century. Chauffard described the erythrocyte osmotic fragility abnormalities in 1907. Shortly thereafter the term spherocyte came into common usage. Kahn reported a favorable response to splenectomy in 1913, and within a decade removal of the spleen was being described as "curative." Recent contributions have dealt with the nature of the erythrocytic abnormality.

PATHOGENESIS

Hereditary spherocytosis reflects a mutant gene that appears to be-have as a nonsex-linked simple mendelian dominant. Although it af-fects both sexes with equal frequency, most genetic studies raise certain objections to this mode of inheritance. Approximately half the offspring of persons with hereditary spherocytosis manifest the disease, but there are too many instances of failure to detect disease in a patient's siblings or his parents. Possible explanations include, among others, spontaneous mutation and incomplete penetrance. Since few patients with hereditary spherocytosis succumb before they reach the reproductive age, a spon-taneous mutation rate high enough to explain the fairly large number of patients without demonstrable disease in their families should cause a sharp increase in incidence. Such is not the case. Current data favor variable expressivity or penetrance so low that the disorder resists de-tection by available techniques. In view of widely differing degrees of severity, hereditary spherocytosis is probably not genetically homoge-neous. A disease remarkably similar to hereditary spherocytosis in man has been observed in the deer mouse; however, the murine disorder is due to a recessive gene and thus differs from that in man.

The nature of the red cell abnormality remains enigmatic. Although spherocytosis is a reflection of the cellular defect, the spheroidal con-figuration is not in itself the primary reason for the cell's premature destruction. Erythrocytes are ordinarily not spherocytes when they leave the bone marrow but become so soon after they reach the circulation. Thus sphering appears to depend on aging and/or exposure to some spherocyte conditioning factor; both mechanisms probably operate.

The spleen plays an essential role in hereditary spherocytosis as it does in the pathogenesis of most other hemolytic disorders. However, splenic histology is nonspecific and there is no demonstrable abnormal-ity in the spleen, which apparently behaves in an essentially normal manner toward a group of abnormal red cells (p. 451). Erythrocytes from donors with hereditary spherocytosis survive poorly in normal subjects whose spleens are intact; on the other hand, they survive normally if the recipient has been splenectomized. Normal erythrocytes exhibit normal survival times in recipients with hereditary spherocytosis.

Therefore the abnormality is within the cells and not in their environment or in the functions of the spleen.

Despite scattered reports to the contrary, there is no convincing evidence that erythrocytic glycolysis is quantitatively impaired or qualitatively abnormal. No enzymatic deficiencies have been detected. Instead, these erythrocytes appear to utilize greater than normal amounts of glucose. There is persuasive evidence pointing to the cell membrane as the site of the defect in hereditary spherocytosis. Abnormalities in lipid synthesis and/or turnover have been described, but they lack confirmation and may be nonspecific manifestations of a generalized breakdown in cellular energetics and integrity before the cell's destruction. Increased permeability of the membrane to sodium appears to be more important.

The erythrocytes in persons with hereditary spherocytosis display a decrease in intracellular potassium and water; as a result, the cellular concentration of hemoglobin increases. Although sodium content is normal, there is a significant increase in sodium turnover. An enhanced influx of sodium (a process that is accomplished by passive diffusion) is balanced by augmented efflux, an active process that requires the expenditure of energy in the form of ATP (Fig. 4-2). Thus increased amounts of glucose must be catabolized to maintain ionic equilibrium, and the erythrocytes of hereditary spherocytosis are abnormally susceptible to glucose deprivation, including that which occurs normally during temporary sequestration in the spleen (p. 452). Although normal erythrocytes are able to resist the metabolic stresses occasioned by the short periods of splenic stasis, hereditary spherocytosis cells accumulate abnormal quantities of sodium. Further changes in membrane permeability follow such disturbances in ionic equilibrium with eventual sphering and cellular destruction. In addition, a vicious circle would be expected because spherocytes are more susceptible to splenic stasis (p. 451). The constant need for greater than normal glucose catabolism can be envisaged as depleting prematurely the cells' complements of glycolytic enzymes. Because the finite life-span of an erythrocyte appears to be determined largely by the time required for these essential enzyme systems to "wear out," increased glycolytic activity should hasten the aging process and contribute to shortened red cell survival times.

The foregoing explanation is in part speculative and still lacks proof. However, it is compatible with existent data and provides a rational explanation for the pathogenesis of hereditary spherocytosis. Many voids in our knowledge of this disorder remain to be filled. Pending further studies, it is entirely reasonable to consider hereditary spherocytosis as an inborn defect in the red cell membrane which makes it abnormally permeable to sodium. As a result the erythrocytes are particularly susceptible to glucose deprivation, the deleterious effects of normal splenic stasis, and sphering that leads to a shortened life-span. Because splenectomy restores red cell survival times to normal without eliminating the spherocytes (or presumably without altering the basic cellular defect), the spleen obviously plays an essential role in determining whether this erythrocytic abnormality causes clinically recognizable disease. The manifestations of hereditary spherocytosis are attributable to increased erythrocyte destruction, accelerated erythropoiesis, and the findings peculiar to the presence of spherocytes.

CLINICAL MANIFESTATIONS

Hereditary spherocytosis is generally described as a rare disorder; however, it is probably much more common than most series indicate because of the high incidence of compensated, asymptomatic disease which often goes undetected. Because it is inheritable, the frequency varies somewhat in different locales. It is particularly common in persons of north European origin, but hereditary spherocytosis occurs in all races and all parts of the world. It affects both sexes equally. The age at diagnosis is variable and contingent on the severity of the process. In some patients it can be recognized within a few hours after birth or within the first year of life; in others the hemolytic disorder may remain hidden until the eighth or ninth decades of life. Most often hereditary spherocytosis becomes clinically apparent or is diagnosed as an unexpected coincidental finding in childhood, adolescence, or early adult life.

Symptoms. Some persons with hereditary spherocytosis are entirely asymptomatic; most admit to mild symptoms, whereas others are severely and acutely ill. Typical complaints are jaundice, dark urine, pallor, and the nonspecific manifestations of anemia (weakness, tachycardia, and exertional dyspnea). Since the age at diagnosis is dependent on the severity of the hemolytic process, the severer forms of the disease are diagnosed earlier. Consequently, children are generally more symptomatic than adults. Some patients give a history of intermittent jaundice, dark urine, and weakness often triggered by some infection and frequently accompanied by fever, headache, and pain in the abdomen, back, and/or extremities. In between such episodes symptoms may be so slight as to pass unnoticed. Jaundice often fluctuates in intensity, presumably a reflection of varying rates of hemolysis. In those rare patients who develop a hypoplastic crisis the symptoms are those of rapidly developing anemia in the face of lessening jaundice. Complaints attributable to cholelithiasis (abdominal pain and obstructive jaundice) are common, for 80 to 90 per cent of adults have gallstones. The older the patient, the more likely he is to have developed cholelithiasis.

Physical Findings. Splenomegaly is a constant occurrence, ranging from slight to occasionally marked; in most patients the spleen is readily palpable. Jaundice is the second most common physical abnormality; it varies greatly in degree and is often detectable only in the scleral conjunctivae. The liver is usually enlarged, especially in patients with marked or long-standing hemolysis. Depending on the severity of the anemia, there are varying degrees of pallor and tachycardia. Fever indicates substantial hemolytic activity or a superimposed infection. Severe disease early in life may be responsible for enlargement of the skull (tower skull), impaired growth, or infantilism; however, few patients manifest developmental or other congenital abnormalities. Chronic leg ulcers are most unusual.

Laboratory Findings. PERIPHERAL BLOOD. In patients with compensated disease the peripheral erythroid values are normal. When production is unable to keep pace with destruction, a mild to profound anemia develops. *Spherocytes* are constant findings (Fig. 4-4). These erythrocytes are hyperchromatic; they lack a central pale area and have a decreased diameter and increased thickness. The spherocytes in hereditary spherocytosis are true microspherocytes and are ordinarily smaller than the spherocytes in the acquired autoimmune hemolytic disorders. The number of spherocytes varies from a few to many; however, in well-made, well-stained blood films they are apparent even in persons with mild compensated disease. Erythrocyte osmotic and mechanical fragility are increased, often markedly so. Autohemolysis is abnormal (20 per cent or more of the cells are destroyed after incubation for 48 hours); the addition of glucose reduces autohemolysis to near normal.

Other erythrocytic abnormalities reflect accelerated erythropoiesis and consist of increased polychromasia, reticulocytosis, and circulating nucleated cells. In individuals with compensated hereditary spherocytosis, the reticulocyte count is only slightly increased (3 to 5 per cent); in the majority of anemic patients the reticulocyte count ranges between 5 and 20 per cent; in rare instances 80 to 90 per cent of the erythrocytes may be reticulocytes. The degree of polychromasia parallels the reticulocyte count. Since reticulocytes are rarely spherocytes, reticulocytosis is reflected in Wright-stained films by the presence of round (and usually polychromatophilic) macrocytes. Ordinarily there are only one or two circulating nucleated red cells per 100 leukocytes, but severe hemolysis will evoke a much higher count.

The leukocyte and platelet counts may be normal. However, patients with active hemolysis often have leukocytosis (generally between 10,-000 and 15,000/cu mm) and slight to moderate thrombocytosis. It is common to find an occasional metamyelocyte, myelocyte, or even a more immature granulocyte in the peripheral blood.

BONE MARROW. The marrow is typically hypercellular because of a relative and absolute increase in erythrocytic precursors. The E:G ratio usually varies between 1:1 and 3:1. Erythropoiesis is orderly and normoblastic (Fig. 4-7). Marrow iron is ordinarily increased. There

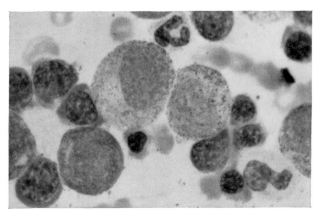

Figure 4-7. Normoblastic, erythrocytic hyperplasia in the bone marrow aspirate of a patient with hereditary spherocytosis.

is often an absolute increase in granulopoiesis and thrombopoiesis, but these marrow compartments are always quantitatively less hyperactive than the erythrocytic. Therefore the marrow in patients with hereditary spherocytosis customarily reveals a relative decrease in granulopoiesis and thrombopoiesis, which remains orderly without evidence of maturation defects.

OTHER LABORATORY FINDINGS. The characteristic biochemical abnormalities reflect increased hemoglobin catabolism. As in each of the other clinical manifestations of hereditary spherocytosis, these changes may be absent, slight, moderate, or marked. Most patients exhibit *hyperbilirubinemia* caused by free or unconjugated bilirubin; significant increases in serum bilirubin glucuronide concentrations point to some complication such as obstruction of the biliary tree consequent to a strategically positioned gallstone. *Fecal urobilinogen* content is generally increased, as is *urine urobilinogen;* however, it must be borne in mind that the size of the red cell mass, administration of oral broad-spectrum antibiotics, and the functional reserve of the liver (p. 86) all influence these determinations. Acholic or clay-colored stools and/or bile in the urine point to some kind of jaundice other than hemolytic, usually obstructive due to cholelithiasis. *Plasma haptoglobin* levels are ordinarily markedly reduced and frequently undetectable. *Direct and indirect Coombs' tests* are negative. In some patients the *serum uric acid* may be slightly to moderately increased. *Erythrocyte survival times* are decreased and external counting techniques reveal *sequestration of* ^{51}Cr-*tagged erythrocytes in the spleen. Radioiron turnover time* is decreased and *erythrocyte* ^{59}Fe *uptake* is increased. *Plasma iron* is normal or slightly increased. *Bone x-rays* may reveal decreased mineralization and widening of the medullary cavities. *Cholecystography* demonstrates a high incidence of nonradiopaque (pigment) stones. Other findings lack specificity and reflect long-standing and/or severe hemolysis; for example, laboratory evidence of hepatic dysfunction, cardiomegaly consequent to severe anemia, and electrocardiographic abnormalities attributable to anemia.

DIAGNOSIS

The diagnosis of hereditary spherocytosis is based on the finding of a spherocytic hemolytic disorder in a person without evidence of any other cause for a spherocytic hemolytic anemia. An absolute diagnosis demands that a similar disorder be demonstrated in some member of the patient's family; however, confirmation is often unobtainable. Therefore a presumptive diagnosis is permitted in the absence of genetic corroboration, provided all other hemolytic disorders have been excluded.

The first step to the diagnosis of hereditary spherocytosis is the demonstration of spherocytes (the hallmark of this hemolytic disorder) and a decreased red cell life-span. The spherocytes are responsible for such findings as abnormal osmotic behavior and increased autohemolysis, but their presence can be established with certainty only by morphologic study. Consequently, well-made, well-stained peripheral blood films are mandatory. Rare spheroidal cells are detectable in normal blood films and can be found in persons who have recently been transfused. In addition, improper technique may create confusion (cells that are poorly pulled out lack the normal central pale area). However, artifactual "spherocytes" are not hyperchromatic, for they are not really spheres; furthermore, other technical imperfections point to the likelihood of artifact. If an anemia is the result of spherocytic hemolysis, it is difficult to hide the presence of spherocytes, regardless of how poor the blood film may be. On the other hand, a few spherocytes in a person with compensated disease may be easily missed. As a rule, spherocytosis is probably not a pertinent finding if a trained examiner, given an adequate blood film, encounters difficulty in ascertaining the significance of a few spheroidal cells.

The *sine qua non* of any hemolytic disorder is the direct demonstration of a decrease in the erythrocyte life-span. There are methods available to measure in days the average red cell survival time. Among the existent techniques isotopically labeled cells (^{51}Cr or DF^{32}P) are preferred. However, there are cogent reasons why red cell survival data are rarely needed or indicated in the clinical evaluation of patients suspected of having a hemolytic disorder. Disadvantages of these techniques that limit their routine use include (1) the need for special laboratory equipment and trained personnel to handle radioisotopes, (2) the inability to obtain meaningful figures for two to three weeks, (3) the potential hazards to the patient and/or his progeny associated with exposure to radioactive materials, (4) the rarity with which hemolyzing patients can maintain a steady relationship between production and destruction (a requisite for accurate survival measurements, p. 81), and (5) technical defects that influence the results; for example, the problem of chromium elution (p. 82).

With few exceptions, simpler parameters afford comparable information. Thus increased polychromasia, reticulocytosis, circulating nucleated red cells, and myeloid erythrocytic hyperplasia point clearly to an acute blood-loss anemia (hemorrhage or hemolysis). When these hematologic abnormalities occur in an anemic patient without evidence of bleeding and, especially when coupled with splenomegaly, the appropriate pigment changes of hemolysis, or cholelithiasis, there is room for little if any question of the existence of impaired erythrocyte viability. When these peripheral blood and marrow findings coexist with spherocytes, abnormal osmotic behavior, and increased autohemolysis corrected by glucose, a diagnosis of a spherocytic hemolytic disorder has been established.

For these reasons it is possible to predict with accuracy the decreases in red cell viability capable of causing clinical disease without actually measuring red cell survival times. The shorter the life-span, the more marked the evidences of increased erythrocyte destruction. Therefore an overt hemolytic anemia can be easily recognized without red cell survival data. In fact, the significance of the former manifestations of hemolysis is such that in their presence a normal ^{51}Cr survival time would have to be viewed as a laboratory error and repetition would be indicated. In slightly anemic patients or those with compensated disease the diagnosis is more apt to present difficulties. These are the situations in which precise measurements of red cell life-span would provide the greatest diagnostic assistance. Unfortunately, they are also the ones in which the techniques are least likely to provide accurate data (p. 82). Therefore the clinician must rely on other manifestations of the hemolytic disorder. It is noteworthy that evidence of increased red cell destruction can be found when sought, even in nonanemic individuals with occult hemolysis. Thus measurement of erythrocyte life-span is rarely essential for clinical diagnosis; it has proved most valuable as a research tool.

The second step to the diagnosis of hereditary spherocytosis is the exclusion of other causes of a spherocytic hemolytic disorder. Acquired autoimmune hemolytic disorders (primary or secondary) are most likely to be confused with hereditary spherocytosis. Positive Coombs' tests, leukopenia and/or thrombocytopenia, and, if the hemolytic disorder is secondary, other manifestations of the primary disease (e.g., lymphoma and chronic lymphocytic leukemia) characterize the acquired type. Hereditary spherocytosis in the newborn may simulate erythroblastosis fetalis due to ABO incompatibility, but these two kinds of hemolytic jaundice of the newborn are separable on the basis of the serologic manifestations of erythroblastosis fetalis (p. 123). Certain hemolytic anemias attributable to chemical (Zieve's syndrome) and physical (burns) factors are associated with spherocytosis as are some of the "big spleen" syndromes; for example, agnogenic myeloid metaplasia (p. 452). However, other manifestations of these disorders prevent confusion. Other hemolytic processes are not characterized by spherocytes.

Some aspects of hereditary spherocytosis resemble those of a variety of nonhemolytic hematologic disorders as well as other diseases that are associated with jaundice. However, careful evaluation of the entire clinical picture eliminates these possibilities with relative ease. For example, anemia, reticulocytosis, circulating nucleated red cells, leukocytosis with immature granulocytes, splenomegaly, and bone pain are manifestations of leukemia as well as hereditary spherocytosis; jaundice, the presence of spherocytes, and a bone marrow that reveals orderly, controlled myelopoiesis quickly eliminate the likelihood of leukemia. Spherocytes and evidence of hemolysis delineate between the jaundice of hereditary spherocytosis and the nonhemolytic, acholuric jaundice that characterizes constitutional hepatic dysfunction or Gilbert's disease. Gilbert's disease reflects a hepatic enzyme deficiency that interferes with the conjugation of free bilirubin and glucuronic acid; as a result, there is hyperbilirubinemia caused by unconjugated bilirubin, but erythrocyte survival is normal.

The third and final step to the diagnosis of hereditary spherocytosis is proof of the heritable nature of the hemolytic disorder. Although this information is often difficult to procure or is actually unobtainable, an effort to find a similar abnormality in some member of the patient's family is *always* indicated. A detailed family history is important, especially knowledge of anemia, splenomegaly, or jaundice. Another point that is commonly overlooked is cholelithiasis (or a history of gallbladder disease of some type) occurring at an early age. Cholelithiasis developing before the age of 30 in some member of the patient's family is strong indirect support for the existence in that person of a hereditary hemolytic disorder.

If they are alive and available, it is much more rewarding to examine other members of the patient's family. Since the gene causing hereditary spherocytosis behaves as a nonsex-linked mendelian dominant, there is no reason to select specific relatives (e.g., paternal as opposed to maternal). The incidence of demonstrable disease is significantly higher in the offspring of an individual with hereditary spherocytosis than in his siblings or parents. Therefore, if a patient suspected of having this hemolytic disorder has children, they offer the best chance of obtaining genetic confirmation of the diagnosis. Even if the diagnosis has been established, a patient's children should be studied because of the likelihood that they also have hereditary spherocytosis.

Inasmuch as it is often necessary to examine asymptomatic family members, some mention should be made of the number and types of studies that are most likely to be productive. A complete history and physical examination, with detailed hematologic evaluation and determination of the concentration of bilirubin in the blood and of urobilinogen in the feces and urine, would permit easy detection of disease. However, such an approach is obviously impractical. With few exceptions, the following will suffice to confirm or to exclude the diagnosis of hereditary spherocytosis, provided a spherocytic hemolytic disorder has already been found in some other member of the family:

1. Assessment of the peripheral erythroid values, for example, a hemoglobin or hematocrit determination.
2. Evaluation of the peripheral blood film for spherocytes.
3. A reticulocyte count.
4. Examination of the abdomen for splenic enlargement.

TREATMENT AND COURSE

Although the course of hereditary spherocytosis varies greatly, it is generally characterized by relative benignity. It is likely that a significant number of persons die of other causes without ever having had the diagnosis made and without ever having been seriously affected by the disease. Some of these individuals obviously survive until old age, because the diagnosis of hereditary spherocytosis is frequently made in the elderly. In others with severer disease, varying degrees of anemia, jaundice, or symptomatic cholelithiasis occur at some time during their lives.

In most cases clinical manifestations persist once they become sufficiently developed to call attention to the disease. For example, a patient with an overt hemolytic anemia and/or jaundice can be expected to remain anemic and/or jaundiced unless the course is altered by appropriate therapy. Because completely effective treatment has been available since shortly after hereditary spherocytosis was delineated as a specific entity, information is not available on the course and subsequent outcome in the untreated patient with overt disease. It is reasonable to predict that they would become progressively more incapacitated by an increasingly severe hemolytic anemia and would eventually develop such complications as cholelithiasis with biliary obstruction and hepatic dysfunction, a hypoplastic crisis, tissue hemosiderosis, and cardiac failure. There is little doubt that persistent hemolytic activity would increase morbidity and adversely affect longevity. Therefore all but the most exceptional patients should be treated.

The treatment for hereditary spherocytosis is splenectomy. The primary defect is intracorpuscular and is unaffected by the presence or absence of the spleen, but the spleen is requisite for the shortening of the finite life-span of these defective erythrocytes. Following splenectomy, spherocytes persist, as do abnormalities in osmotic and mechanical fragility and in autohemolysis; however, the red cells no longer have decreased survival times, and all the manifestations of increased erythrocyte destruction and accelerated erythropoiesis disappear. Hence the peripheral erythroid values, reticulocyte count, and marrow cellularity return to normal, as do the parameters reflecting increased hemoglobin catabolism. Spherocytes remain, but they are now without pathophysiologic significance. In other words, the patient has been "cured," even though the genetically controlled red cell abnormality persists unchanged.

Splenectomy is completely effective; that is, hemolysis ceases, in virtually 100 per cent of the patients with hereditary spherocytosis, a therapeutic response that can be equaled in few other disorders. In fact, the results of splenectomy are so uniform that hemolysis persisting after the spleen has been removed strongly suggests another diagnosis or an accessory spleen (or spleens) that may have been missed at the time of surgery (p. 463). If the patient has cholelithiasis, it is often desirable to defer cholecystectomy until a later date.

Failure to splenectomize a person with an overt hemolytic anemia due to hereditary spherocytosis cannot be condoned unless the patient has some complication or other disease that greatly increases operative risk or could logically be expected to cause his death before he encounters serious trouble consequent to the hemolytic process. Cholelithiasis is another clear-cut indication for splenectomy. In children it is wise to postpone splenectomy until the age of four or five years, provided satisfactory peripheral erythroid values can be maintained without transfusions. If not, splenectomy should be performed at once, even during the first year of life. It has been suggested that young children may be more susceptible to infections after splenectomy, possibly because of altered immunologic responses. However, there is no proof that splenectomy has a deleterious effect on the body's immunologic mechanisms. Pending further study, the possibility of infection is an inadequate reason to defer splenectomy until adolescence or adulthood. Although the relationship between splenectomy and susceptibility to infection is conjectural, certain of the effects of chronic hemolysis are well established; for example, a child with hereditary spherocytosis has an excellent chance of developing cholelithiasis if his spleen is not removed before the second decade of life.

Hereditary spherocytosis rarely causes severe hemolysis in the immediate neonatal period. However, it is sometimes responsible for hemolytic jaundice of the newborn and must then be handled somewhat differently. If hyperbilirubinemia becomes sufficiently marked, exchange transfusions are indicated to prevent kernicterus (p. 130). In most cases conservative therapy is adequate and splenectomy can ordinarily be deferred until the child is older.

The role of splenectomy in the asymptomatic patient with compensated hereditary spherocytosis is somewhat disputable. The knowledge that a number of these patients reach an advanced age without serious untoward effects has been cited as a reason to withhold splenectomy. However, the advantages to be gained by removing the spleen outweigh the possible risks of surgery. It is the consensus of most hematologists that the diagnosis of hereditary spherocytosis in a person without another disease or contraindication to surgery is in itself a clear-cut indication for elective splenectomy regardless of the absence of symptoms, anemia, or jaundice; I concur with this view.

With the exception of patients who develop hypoplastic crises or sudden severe increases in hemolytic activity and a rapid fall in their peripheral erythroid values, there is little need for blood transfusions in the management of patients with hereditary spherocytosis. Barring these circumstances in which transfusions may be life-saving, anemia of such severity that transfusions are needed is an indication for splenectomy rather than for maintenance of a satisfactory red cell mass by transfusions.

The rare patient who develops superimposed folate deficiency should, of course, be treated with folic acid. In view of the potential seriousness of hypoplastic crises, it is appropriate to give all patients who manifest this complication the benefit of supplemental folic acid, even in the absence of definite proof of a deficiency state. No other therapeutic agent (e.g., iron, vitamin B_{12}, pyridoxine, cobalt, or testosterone) is indicated in patients with uncomplicated hereditary spherocytosis. Iron, in particular, is contraindicated. These patients absorb greater than normal amounts of iron from the gastrointestinal tract. In chronically hemolyzing patients the prolonged administration of therapeutic doses of inorganic iron may be responsible for the development of hemosiderosis with serious sequelae.

Hereditary Hemoglobinopathies

The hereditary hemoglobinopathies (qualitative and quantitative) reflect impaired or abnormal globin synthesis as well as hemolysis. They are discussed in detail in Chapter 5 (p. 246).

Hereditary Glycolytic Enzyme Deficiencies

The chemical, functional, and physical integrity of an erythrocyte is contingent on glycolysis, which in turn is dependent on a number of enzymes and coenzymes. Interference with glucose metabolism will shorten a red cell's life-span. Genetically determined glycolytic enzyme deficiencies occur and are manifested clinically by hemolytic anemias. These disorders were originally classified together as the congenital nonspherocytic hemolytic anemias in order to separate them from hereditary spherocytosis. When it became evident that they were a heterogeneous group, attempts were made to subdivide them into types I and II, based on the autohemolytic behavior of the erythrocytes. All these terms have outlived their usefulness and should be discarded for their continued use serves only to confuse. These hereditary hemolytic anemias are caused by deficiencies of enzymes participating in the Embden-Meyerhof glycolytic pathway as well as the pentose phosphate pathway (Fig. 4-2). Most of those falling in the former category have involved pyruvate kinase (PK) and in the latter, glucose-6-phosphate dehydrogenase (G-6-PD). Therefore it is much more appropriate to use such designations as hereditary G-6-PD deficiency and hereditary PK deficiency.

GLUCOSE-6-PHOSPHATE DEHYDROGENASE (G-6-PD) DEFICIENCY

History. The development of knowledge about the hemolytic anemias caused by G-6-PD deficiency is a modern addition to medical history. Although it was first pointed out in 1926 that certain antimalarial drugs were potentially hemolytic, it was not until 1954 that the susceptibility to hemolysis induced by such compounds was shown to reflect an intrinsic abnormality of the erythrocyte. Shortly thereafter numerous important contributions clarified the mode of inheritance and biochemical definition of this inborn error in erythrocyte glucose metabolism. As a result, many drug- and plant-induced hemolytic anemias, previously thought to reflect diverse etiologies, have been shown to have a common pathogenesis. The pioneer observations and subsequent studies of Alving and Beutler and their associates provided invaluable data and stimulated intensive investigation in many laboratories in all parts of the world.

Research in this area remains active and the final chapter has yet to be written.

Pathogenesis. G-6-PD deficiency is transmitted by a mutant gene of partial dominance located on the X chromosome. Affected hemizygous males manifest full expression, for the abnormal gene is unopposed by a normal allele. Full expression also occurs in homozygous females, that is, those with two mutant genes. Heterozygous females exhibit partial expression of the metabolic defect. The mutant gene for G-6-PD deficiency is widely distributed throughout the world, but the incidence is highest in the more darkly pigmented racial and ethnic groups. G-6-PD deficiency is particularly common in certain parts of Africa, the countries surrounding the Mediterranean Sea, and in persons whose ancestors originated in these areas. About 10 to 15 per cent of American Negro males are hemizygous and about 20 per cent of American Negro females are heterozygous for the abnormal gene (female homozygosity is rare because such an individual must acquire a mutant gene from each parent). In certain populations the incidence of G-6-PD deficiency is as high as 50 per cent; for example, Kurdish and Sephardic Jews (it is rare in the Ashkenazim), Sardinians, Greeks, and Turks. The high frequency of G-6-PD deficiency in tropical and semitropical locales parallels the distribution of falciparum malaria. This observation, together with the demonstration that these parasites require reduced glutathione and aerobic glycolysis for optimal growth, suggests that G-6-PD deficiency (like hemoglobin S disease and the thalassemia syndromes) may offer a protective advantage against malaria. The concept of balanced polymorphism is appealing but still lacks proof.

Glucose-6-phosphate dehydrogenase catalyzes the initial step in the pentose phosphate or aerobic glycolytic pathway (Fig. 4-2). Therefore deficient G-6-PD activity is characterized by a decrease in glucose utilization and a fall in oxygen consumption. The oxidative catabolism of glucose is the sole mechanism by which an erythrocyte can reduce TPN to TPNH, which is an important source of red cell reducing power. The first step in reductive detoxification is the formation of increased TPNH, and, in normal erythrocytes, the rate-limiting factor in the pentose phosphate pathway appears to be the availability of TPN. Since G-6-PD deficiency interferes with TPNH regeneration, the G-6-PD-deficient red cell lacks this protective capacity; its ability to resist oxidative damage is contingent on G-6-PD content.

Because TPNH is the preferred hydrogen donor for the reduction of glutathione, the glutathione of G-6-PD-deficient erythrocytes is particularly susceptible to oxidation. The resultant deficiency of reduced glutathione permits the oxidative destruction of certain erythrocytic components. The sulfhydryl groups of the globin chains and the cell membrane are especially vulnerable. Oxidation of hemoglobin culminates in the formation of sulfhemoglobinlike compounds and the precipitation of irreversibly denatured hemoglobin (these degradation products of hemoglobin are demonstrable as Heinz bodies by special staining techniques; see Fig. 4-5). Oxidation of the sulfhydryl groups of the membrane proteins appears to be the decisive event affecting red cell survival.

Normally, G-6-PD activity is highest in the most immature red cells and decreases progressively throughout their finite life-span. Therefore young erythrocytes in G-6-PD-deficient persons behave in an essentially normal manner. However, the supply of this vital enzyme will be exhausted sooner when the initial complement is subnormal. As a result, erythrocyte aging, which appears to reflect enzymatic depletion, occurs prematurely. In the hemizygous American Negro male or homozygous female, with full expression of this inborn error in red cell metabolism, erythrocyte G-6-PD activity is reduced to about 10 to 15 per cent of normal. Despite this significant decrement in enzymatic content, there is only a 25 per cent reduction in red cell life-span. Under otherwise normal conditions the bone marrow compensates easily for this slight impairment in erythrocyte survival times and these individuals have normal peripheral erythroid values. However, such persons are unable to withstand more than normal oxidative stress without serious consequences.

Erythrocytic components are normally protected from the high oxidation potential of molecular oxygen by a metabolic block or hiatus that permits only a minimal essential flow of electrons. Certain drugs and dyes (e.g., primaquine and methylene blue) are potent oxidation-reduction mediators. These compounds are capable of bridging the relative obstruction to the flow of electrons from cell constituents to molecular oxygen. As a result, electron transfer is facilitated and the oxidation of cellular components is accelerated. The cell's defenses against the intrusion of such electron carriers are the important reducing systems generated by the aerobic catabolism of glucose (Fig. 4-2). In the face of G-6-PD deficiency the capacity of a red cell to counteract the deleterious electron flow caused by oxidant drugs and chemicals is limited.

All erythrocytes are potentially susceptible to the oxidative effect of redox compounds. The final result is predicated on the dose of the drug as well as the G-6-PD content of the red cells. Some chemicals, such as phenylhydrazine, readily produce hemolysis in normal persons. Others must be given in very large or suprapharmacologic amounts to affect normal red cells; however, ordinary or pharmacologic doses cause irreversible damage to erythrocytes with less than normal quantities of G-6-PD. Thus the reactions in individuals with hereditary G-6-PD deficiency differ from those of normal subjects only in degree; that is, doses that fail to cause appreciable hemolysis in normal persons produce overt hemolysis in those with G-6-PD deficiency.

The sequence of events in G-6-PD-deficient red cells challenged by a redox compound is as follows:

1. The drug or chemical accelerates the flow of electrons from hemoglobin and other cellular constituents to molecular oxygen.

2. Glucose catabolism via the pentose phosphate pathway is stimulated. However, G-6-PD deficiency prevents the generation of adequate reducing power in the form of TPNH.

3. Insufficient TPNH permits a continued flow of electrons (an unchecked attempt to establish redox equilibrium) with the oxidation of hemoglobin to methemoglobin, the oxidative destruction of the iron-containing enzyme, catalase, and a shift in the $GSSG \rightleftharpoons GSH$ equilibrium to the left.

4. The resultant decrease in reduced glutathione renders the sulfhydryl groups in globin, certain enzymes, and the erythrocytic membrane highly vulnerable to oxidation. As a consequence, hemoglobin is progressively degraded, denatured, and eventually precipitated as hemoglobin-glutathione complexes and sulfhemoglobinlike compounds. In a like manner sulfhydryl-containing enzymes are inactivated and the integrity of the cell membrane, which is dependent on sulfhydryl activity, is compromised.

Depending on the magnitude and reversibility of the oxidative damage caused by a redox drug or chemical, an erythrocyte either undergoes immediate intravascular lysis, is sequestered and destroyed in the liver, is sequestered and destroyed in the spleen, or is earmarked for later but premature destruction. Varying degrees of hemolytic activity ensue. Because current evidence indicates that the normal erythrocyte life-span is determined by the time required for its essential glycolytic enzyme systems to wear out, oxidant compounds may be viewed as accelerating erythrocyte senescence.

The list of agents potentially hemolytic in G-6-PD-deficient persons is lengthy and continuing to grow. The more commonly incriminated compounds include *antimalarials* such as primaquine, pamaquine, and quinine; *sulfonamides* such as sulfanilamide, sulfisoxazole (Gantrisin), salicylazo-sulfapyridine (Azulfidine), and sulfamethoxypyridazine (Kynex); *nitrofurans* [e.g., nitrofurantoin (Furadantin)]; *analgesics* and *antipyretics* such as aspirin and acetophenetidin (phenacetin); *sulfones* [e.g., sulfoxone (Diasone)]; *vitamin K; naphthalene* (moth balls); *trinitrotoluene;* and certain *plants* (most notably the fava bean).

The hemolytic effect of these oxidant compounds is dependent on dose and level of erythrocyte G-6-PD activity. Additional factors influencing the severity of hemolysis induced by these agents in G-6-PD-deficient subjects include the following:

CELL AGE. Since younger cells contain more G-6-PD than older cells, they are less susceptible to oxidative destruction. For example, a standard dose of primaquine (30 mg of the base daily) does not destroy cells that are less than 60 days old. Consequently, the severity of such a hemolytic process will be mitigated by any condition that causes a preponderance of young cells (e.g., hemolysis or recovery from acute bleeding). It is for this reason that prolonged administration of 30 mg of primaquine per day is not associated with a persistent anemia. The first doses destroy all the older cells, leaving only young cells that are able to resist this amount of drug. Although continued exposure to primaquine shortens the average red cell survival time to less than half of normal, increased erythropoiesis is able to compensate for this decrease in life-span; the circulating hemoglobin returns to normal. It should be noted that the resistance of younger G-6-PD-deficient cells is not absolute; progressive increments in drug dose cause destruction of younger and younger cells.

ASSOCIATED DISEASES. A number of other disorders affect the severity of this kind of drug-induced hemolysis. For example, *gastrointestinal disease* may impair absorption and *hepatic* or *renal disease* may interfere with metabolism or excretion of the redox compound. Gastrointestinal disease will lead to a lower blood concentration and less hemolysis, whereas hepatic or renal disease will augment blood levels and enhance cell destruction. A variety of *infections* (bacterial and viral) and *metabolic derangements*, for example, *diabetic acidosis* and *physiologic hypoglycemia of the newborn*, render G-6-PD-deficient erythrocytes more sensitive to oxidative destruction. Under these circumstances contact with some drug such as aspirin in a dose that would otherwise be innocuous may evoke acute hemolysis.

GENETIC VARIATIONS. Less than normal activity of an enzyme may reflect decreased rates of synthesis, formation of abnormal molecules, a deficiency of enzyme activators, or the presence of inhibitor substances. A number of genetic variants express themselves clinically as G-6-PD deficiency. Several different genotypes and phenotypes have been observed, and it is likely that more will be uncovered. Thus the clinical pictures accompanying G-6-PD deficiency in different ethnic and racial groups are somewhat varied. There is also a variety of structurally different enzymes. For example, the enzyme molecule in most G-6-PD-deficient American Negroes differs from the enzyme in deficient Caucasians. In addition, the enzymatic deficiency in the Negro is demonstrable only in nonnucleated cells (erythrocytes, thrombocytes, and the ocular lens); in most affected Caucasians G-6-PD deficiency is readily demonstrable in other tissues. These two groups react somewhat differently to different redox compounds and obviously do not reflect a common genetic defect.

Other less commonly observed variations include a few persons with a complete (or almost complete) absence of G-6-PD; these individuals manifest a chronic hemolytic anemia and differ clearly from the hemizygous Negro male who exhibits overt hemolysis only after contact with some compound such as primaquine. Still other factors have been observed to affect the clinical manifestations of G-6-PD deficiency. In some newborn the development of severe jaundice and even kernicterus appears to require G-6-PD deficiency plus another still poorly defined factor or factors. It is apparent therefore that the in vitro demonstration of decreased erythrocyte G-6-PD activity reflects varied and complex genetic abnormalities.

OTHER EXTRAERYTHROCYTIC FACTORS (FAVISM). Acute hemolysis following exposure to the broad bean (*Vicia fava*) deserves separate consideration. G-6-PD deficiency is a requisite for this hemolytic syndrome; however, an additional factor(s) is required, and all G-6-PD-deficient persons are not sensitive to the fava bean. Favism is most common in Caucasians originating from the northern and eastern portions of the Mediterranean basin (e.g., Sardinians and Greeks). Although these individuals are sensitive to redox compounds that produce hemolysis in other G-6-PD-deficient persons, they also manifest sudden (within a few hours) and generally severe hemolysis following exposure to fava beans. This contact may consist of ingestion of the beans or inhalation of the pollen from the fava-bean plant. These persons do not manifest favism from birth. There is convincing evidence that an acquired immune factor, together with genetically controlled G-6-PD deficiency, determines the sensitivity to fava beans.

Clinical Manifestations. Because hereditary G-6-PD deficiency does not, as a rule, impair longevity, hemolysis affects all age groups. Racial and ethnic group predilections have been discussed. Full expression of this enzymatic deficiency is about ten times commoner in males than in females. Because of the genetic variants and other factors that influence the severity of the process (e.g., type and dose of drug), variable clinical pictures are observed, ranging from mild hemolytic activity to a profound hemolytic anemia. The hemolytic episode created in the hemizygous American Negro male treated with 30 mg of primaquine daily is predictable and reproducible; it will be used as the prototype of hemolytic anemia resulting from G-6-PD deficiency because it emphasizes the manifestations unique to this hemolytic disorder. The clinical course is divisible into acute hemolytic, recovery, and equilibrium phases.

ACUTE HEMOLYTIC PHASE. Hemolysis begins 24 to 48 hours after primaquine is started and increases in intensity over the ensuing four to six days with the destruction of 30 to 50 per cent of the circulating red cell mass. *Symptoms* lack specificity and are those of any hemolytic anemia; their severity is related to the degree of anemia and the rapidity with which it develops. *Physical findings* are likewise nonspecific; jaundice and pallor predominate. The spleen may or may not be palpably enlarged. Because hemolysis is self-limited and short-lasting, splenomegaly is not a typical finding. *Laboratory findings* are chiefly those of any hemolytic anemia (a normocytic, normochromic anemia, increased polychromasia, reticulocytosis, circulating nucleated red cells, marrow erythrocytic hyperplasia, hyperbilirubinemia due to free or unconjugated bilirubin, and increased urobilinogen in the feces and urine). Although a few spherocytes are usually evident, overt spherocytosis does not occur. Osmotic fragility is ordinarily normal to slightly increased. Autohemolysis is normal and is not affected by glucose. Mean red cell survival times are shortened. Coombs' tests are negative. Heinz bodies are numerous, and methemoglobinemia is present early in the acute hemolytic phase; later on methemoglobinemia subsides, and cells containing Heinz bodies disappear (the oldest cells, which form the most methemoglobin and Heinz bodies, are the first to be destroyed). Erythrocyte G-6-PD activity is decreased, and methemoglobin reduction is much slower than normal. Other manifestations include decreases in erythrocyte TPNH, catalase, reduced glutathione, and total lipids.

RECOVERY PHASE. If primaquine is discontinued during the acute hemolytic phase, red cell destruction ceases within 48 to 72 hours. Even if the drug is continued, hemolysis is self-limited, for only the older erythrocytes are sensitive to this dose of primaquine. In the face of continued drug administration, recovery begins as soon as the older, more susceptible cells have been destroyed (about the tenth day). Overt hemolysis ceases, reticulocytosis subsides, and the peripheral erythroid values gradually increase, reaching normal pretreatment levels in four to six weeks.

EQUILIBRIUM PHASE. During this phase mild hemolytic activity persists, and erythrocytes are destroyed as soon as they reach the critical age of about 60 days; however, the marrow is able to compensate for this reduction in erythrocyte life-span, and the hemolytic process can be detected only by red cell survival studies and a slight increase in the reticulocyte count. Since the mean erythrocyte age is less than normal, certain red cell constituents are increased as a reflection of the younger cells; for example, G-6-PD activity will be greater than it was before the administration of primaquine. If the drug is discontinued, a second hemolytic episode of comparable severity cannot be reproduced for four to six months (the time required to restore the pretreatment age distribution). If the dose of primaquine is increased during the equilibrium phase, overt hemolysis recurs (younger cells are susceptible to oxidative destruction by larger daily doses of primaquine).

Diagnosis. The diagnosis of hereditary G-6-PD deficiency is contingent on the exclusion of other hemolytic disorders and on the demonstration of reduced erythrocyte G-6-PD activity or of one of the consequences of a reduction in this enzyme. G-6-PD deficiency must be considered and excluded in all patients with an acute hemolytic anemia, especially those in whom spherocytosis is not a prominent finding. History of exposure to some drug, chemical, or plant known to cause hemolysis in G-6-PD-deficient persons is helpful, as is a detailed family history.

Several laboratory procedures have been devised to detect G-6-PD deficiency. Actual measurement of enzyme activity is the most direct, but the method is technically difficult and is useful chiefly as a research tool. Measurement of reduced glutathione content is likewise difficult. The Heinz body test is relatively simple (more than 40 per cent of the erythrocytes exhibit five or more Heinz bodies in individuals with full expression of the genetic defect); however, it is rather nonspecific because of its considerable overlap and has been largely replaced by other procedures. The methemoglobin reduction test is simple and accurate and has been widely adopted. It is based on the inability of G-6-PD-deficient erythrocytes to reduce methemoglobin in the presence of methylene blue, a potent oxidation-reduction mediator. This technique will pick up all hemizygous males and homozygous females in addition to about 80 per cent of the heterozygous females. A spot test based on the failure of G-6-PD-deficient erythrocytes to reduce a tetrazolium dye because of their decreased TPNH content is commercially available. This technique has a visual end point and will detect all individuals who are susceptible to clinically significant hemolysis. It is noteworthy that evidence of G-6-PD deficiency may be hidden (at least partly) in persons in the recovery or equilibrium phase because of a shift toward a younger mean cell age with a greater enzyme content.

Treatment and Course. The course of hemolysis in G-6-PD-deficient subjects has already been detailed. In general, it occurs in self-limited episodes unresponsive to any therapeutic measures other than discontinuance of exposure to the responsible redox compound. Transfusions are rarely, if ever, needed, and there is no place for corticosteroids or splenectomy in the management of these patients. Corticosteroids are ineffective even in those few persons manifesting a chronic hemolytic anemia. In infants with severe jaundice, the indications for exchange transfusions to prevent kernicterus are the same as those applying to infants with erythroblastosis fetalis (p. 130).

HEREDITARY PYRUVATE KINASE (PK) DEFICIENCY

Pyruvate kinase catalyzes an essential step in the Embden-Meyerhof pathway (Fig. 4-2). Because erythrocytes continuously depend on anaerobic glycolysis for the ATP needed to maintain their integrity, a deficiency of PK is a serious metabolic error that significantly shortens red cell life-span, causing a severe hemolytic anemia. Hereditary PK deficiency is a rare hemolytic disorder with an autosomal recessive mode of inheritance. It has been observed most often in individuals of north European ancestry. Patients with active hemolysis are homozygous and have markedly decreased erythrocyte PK activity. Red cell PK activity is about 50 per cent of normal in heterozygotes, but these persons are clinically normal. Hemolytic anemia resulting from hereditary PK deficiency usually has its onset in infancy or early childhood and is generally severe.

The predominant clinical manifestations are those of any hemolytic process. Splenomegaly has been a common but not a consistent finding. The hematologic abnormalities include anemia, increased polychromasia, reticulocytosis, circulating nucleated red cells, and myeloid erythrocytic hyperplasia. Spherocytes are absent or present in only small numbers, and increased numbers of reticulocytes are reflected in Wright-stained films by macrocytosis. Some patients manifest striking poikilocytosis. Osmotic fragility is near normal. Autohemolysis is increased; it is not corrected by glucose but is decreased by the addition of ATP. Coombs' tests are negative. Assessment of bilirubin metabolism reveals the changes of hemolysis. Erythrocyte survival times are markedly shortened, and erythrocyte PK activity is decreased. Red cell G-6-PD activity is increased (probably a reflection of a younger cell population); reduced glutathione is normal.

The diagnosis of hereditary PK deficiency is dependent on the demonstration of decreased erythrocyte PK activity. The absence of spherocytes and abnormal osmotic behavior serves to distinguish this hemolytic disorder from hereditary spherocytosis. G-6-PD deficiency is readily excluded, for all tests pertaining to the pentose phosphate glycolytic pathway are normal. The only available treatment is transfusions as needed to maintain satisfactory peripheral erythroid values. In those few patients who have been splenectomized, no significant improvement accrued. The prognosis is guarded and reflects the severity of the hemolytic process. Cholelithiasis can be anticipated. In view of the seriousness of this metabolic defect, decreased longevity is to be expected. In those patients who are dependent on transfusions, hemosiderosis and serum hepatitis constitute serious complications.

OTHER HEREDITARY GLYCOLYTIC ENZYME DEFICIENCIES

Until recently all hereditary hemolytic anemias other than hereditary spherocytosis and hereditary elliptocytosis were classified together as the congenital nonspherocytic hemolytic anemias. Rational chemical explanations for certain of these syndromes have now emerged (e.g., G-6-PD and PK deficiencies). Thus some semblance of order is beginning to evolve in what was once a heterogeneous group of disorders. To date inadequacies of glutathione reductase, diphosphoglycerate mutase, and triosephosphate isomerase have been implicated in the causation of hemolytic anemias in a few patients. It seems certain that future studies will uncover additional genetically determined enzyme deficiencies as well as other genetic variants that may have similar clinical expressions.

Hereditary Elliptocytosis

Hereditary elliptocytosis is a genetically determined erythrocyte defect characterized by the presence of elliptical or oval-shaped red cells and sometimes by a hemolytic anemia. The mutant gene behaves as an autosomal dominant. The nature of the red cell abnormality is unknown. Since nucleated red cells and reticulocytes are not elliptocytes, the morphology of the erythrocytes is probably a manifestation of some underlying metabolic error rather than the primary defect, but no biochemical lesion has yet been defined.

Hereditary elliptocytosis is rare; its frequency has been estimated to be about one fiftieth that of hereditary spherocytosis or about four per million population. Only three examples of homozygosity have been observed. About 90 per cent of those affected are asymptomatic and have no clinical manifestations other than the presence of variable numbers of elliptical erythrocytes (Fig. 4-6). The remaining display a hemolytic component characterized by many of the features of hereditary spherocytosis. Normal erythrocytes survive normally in these patients. Elliptocytes have shortened life-spans when transfused into normal recipients unless the recipients have been splenectomized; they then display normal viability. Osmotic fragility and autohemolysis determinations usually resemble those of hereditary spherocytosis. Splenectomy has been almost uniformly effective in alleviating the hemolytic component.

The reasons for the differences in the clinical expression of this mutant gene are not known. They probably reflect genetic variants, with hemolysis occurring in some families and being completely absent in others. Spherocytes are evident in a few families; however, there is no proof that double heterozygosity is the cause of hemolysis (i.e., the gene for hereditary elliptocytosis coexisting with another potentially "anemic" gene such as that which causes hereditary spherocytosis). Morphologically, elliptocytes with decreased viability are indistinguishable from those with normal survival times. Thus only the general features of hemolytic disease set those patients with hemolysis apart from those in whom hereditary elliptocytosis exists as a completely benign condition devoid of clinical significance. In those persons with active hemolysis, the characteristic morphology of the red cells readily permits the diagnosis of hereditary elliptocytosis and the exclusion of other hemolytic disorders. If there are significant numbers of spherocytes, some confusion may exist between hereditary elliptocytosis with hemolysis and hereditary spherocytosis. Because the treatment is the same (i.e., splenectomy), precise differentiation is of little clinical import.

Erythropoietic Porphyria

This rare (only about 50 cases have been reported) congenital disorder is characterized by the overproduction of type I porphyrins by nucleated red cells (Fig. 1-8, p. 19). Available evidence suggests that it is caused by an autosomal recessive gene. Clinically, erythropoietic porphyria is manifested by skin photosensitivity and the formation of bullae and vesicles on exposure to natural light, erythrodontia, red staining of bones, the excretion of red urine, increased amounts of uroporphyrin I and coproporphyrin I in the urine and stools (the former predominates in the urine and the latter in the feces), and overt hemolysis with splenomegaly and the other features of a hemolytic disorder. The cause of the decrease in erythrocyte life-span is not known, although it presumably reflects an intrinsic or intraerythrocytic defect. In some (but not all) patients, the hemolytic component has responded to splenectomy.

Acquired Isoimmune Hemolytic Anemias

A number of genetically determined erythrocytic antigens give red cells their serologic identity and possess the ability to evoke antibody production. In addition to *immune erythrocyte antibodies* produced in response to a specific antigenic stimulus (a mismatched transfusion or a blood-type incompatible pregnancy), there exist *naturally occurring isoantibodies* to several of the erythrocyte antigens. These antibodies are normally present and cannot be attributed to a known antigenic stimulus. Red cell antigens and antibodies are discussed in detail elsewhere (p. 519). Both immune and naturally occurring antibodies are capable of reacting with and causing the destruction of erythrocytes that possess the appropriate antigens. The result is an isoimmune hemolytic anemia. In vivo, naturally occurring antibodies generally cause prompt intravascular lysis. Most immune antibodies injure or condition the red cells, which are then prematurely destroyed by reticuloendothelial cells, especially in the spleen and the liver.

HEMOLYTIC TRANSFUSION REACTIONS

Hemolysis consequent to the administration of incompatible blood is discussed in Chapter 14 (p. 532).

ERYTHROBLASTOSIS FETALIS

Erythroblastosis fetalis is a hemolytic disorder of the fetus and of the newborn caused by blood-group incompatibility between the infant and the mother. Immune erythrocyte isoantibodies formed in the mother readily cross the placental barrier and produce hemolysis in the fetus. The name *erythroblastosis fetalis* has been criticized because it ignores the fact that maternal antibodies are responsible for disease in the fetus. Although this point is well taken, widespread usage dictates retention of the term. It should be modified with respect to the fetal erythrocyte antigen or to the maternal erythrocyte antibody that is at fault [e.g., erythroblastosis fetalis due to anti-D(Rh$_0$)].

History. Knowledge of erythroblastosis fetalis developed in three separate phases, each pertaining to one of the major manifestations of the disorder: (1) edema (hydrops fetalis), (2) jaundice (icterus gravis neonatorum), and (3) certain types of anemia of the newborn. The term erythroblastosis was introduced by Rautmann in 1912, but it was not until 1932 that Diamond and his associates recognized that the seemingly diverse manifestations actually reflected a common pathogenesis. In 1938 Darrow concluded that the disorder was due to a maternal antibody against some component of fetal blood. In 1940 Landsteiner and Wiener identified the Rh blood group system, and in the following year Levine and associates pointed out the importance of fetal-maternal Rh blood factor incompatibility in the causation of erythroblastosis fetalis. Subsequent observations clarified the role of the ABO system and of other erythrocyte antigens in the pathogenesis of this isoimmune hemolytic disorder. The introduction of the Coombs' or antiglobulin test in 1945 provided an invaluable research and diagnostic tool.

Pathogenesis. Erythroblastosis fetalis is the result of maternal erythrocyte antibodies gaining entrance via the placental circulation into the fetus in whom they cause red cell destruction. Naturally occurring antibodies (those that are present normally without known antigenic exposure) are, as a rule, complete antibodies with molecular weights of about 1,000,000. Because these antibodies do not cross the placental barrier or do so to a limited extent, they do not cause erythroblastosis fetalis. In contrast, immune erythrocyte antibodies (those formed in response to a specific antigen) are, for the most part, incomplete and have molecular weights of about 160,000; these antibodies traverse the placenta with ease and can cause hemolysis in the fetus. Therefore an isoimmune hemolytic anemia in the fetus requires prior sensitization of the mother. Maternal sensitization may result from an incompatible transfusion or transplacental immunization. Small numbers of fetal cells consistently find their way into the maternal circulation during every normal pregnancy, and significant placental hemorrhage accompanies certain obstetrical complications. As little as 1.0 ml of blood or less (perhaps as little as 0.1 ml) may effectively sensitize an individual. In the case of the ABO blood group system, the elaboration of anti-A or anti-B antibodies may follow such nonspecific stimuli as the injection of tetanus toxoid.

The clinical significance of the various erythrocyte antigens in the causation of erythroblastosis fetalis depends on several factors, most notably their frequency and antigenicity. Inasmuch as the complete antigenic makeup of an erythrocyte appears to be unique for each individual, every pregnancy and blood transfusion is a potential mechanism for maternal sensitization. Practically, however, all but about 2 per cent of the cases of erythroblastosis fetalis are due to ABO or Rh blood group incompatibility (the other blood group factors either occur with very low frequency or are weakly antigenic). Approximately two thirds are caused by anti-A or anti-B antibodies, predominantly the former; the remaining one third reflect anti-D(Rh$_o$). Although ABO incompatibility is a more common cause of erythroblastosis fetalis, it characteristically produces mild disease. Most of the cases requiring treatment are due to anti-D(Rh$_o$), that is, the fetus is Rh or D(Rh$_o$) positive and the mother is Rh or D(Rh$_o$) negative.

There are several reasons for the mildness of erythroblastosis fetalis that results from ABO incompatibility. Anti-A and anti-B antibodies differ from one another as well as from Rh antibodies. Anti-A antibodies are more potent than anti-B, and those occurring in persons who are type O are much more likely to cause overt hemolysis in the child than are the anti-A antibodies in type B individuals. Thus most instances of overt ABO hemolytic disease involve type A infants and type O mothers. There are also marked differences between maternal and fetal anti-A or anti-B titers in contrast to anti-D(Rh$_o$), which is usually as abundant in the fetus as in the mother. Although maternal titers of anti-D(Rh$_o$) of 1:64 or higher are associated with severe disease in the fetus, anti-A titers are characteristically 1:1000 or higher in mothers giving birth to infants with overt hemolysis. Therefore it would seem that anti-A (or anti-B) antibodies do not cross the placental barrier as easily as anti-D(Rh$_o$). A contributing factor may be the presence of A (or B) antigen in other tissues as well as in the secretions of most persons possessing these antigens in their red cells (p. 521). In contrast to anti-D(Rh$_o$), which has mainly erythrocyte D(Rh$_o$) antigen with which to react, the fetal titer of anti-A (or anti-

B) may be kept down because of the additional extraerythrocytic sources of A (or B) antigen.

Factors other than frequency and antigenicity of erythrocyte antigens obviously contribute to the incidence and severity of clinically recognizable erythroblastosis fetalis. Less than 5 per cent of the children who have an ABO blood type that is incompatible with their mothers are affected, and less than 10 per cent of $D(Rh_o)$ negative women with $D(Rh_o)$ positive husbands will become sensitized. These factors include the following:

1. The presence or absence of naturally occurring antibodies in the mother against the fetal cells; for example, $D(Rh_o)$ positive, type A fetal cells will be destroyed so promptly in a $D(Rh_o)$ negative type O or B mother that they will not have an opportunity to sensitize.

2. The genotype of a father whose phenotype is $D(Rh_o)$ positive [all the offspring of a homozygote will be $D(Rh_o)$ positive; however, 50 per cent of the children of a heterozygote will be $D(Rh_o)$ negative].

3. The type of sensitizing stimulus (an incompatible blood transfusion is much more likely to sensitize than is an incompatible pregnancy).

4. The frequency of exposure to the foreign erythrocyte antigen.

Anti-$D(Rh_o)$ antibodies are seldom detectable during a first pregnancy, and first-born infants are normal. As a rule, anti-$D(Rh_o)$ titers rise progressively with each succeeding pregnancy, thereby increasing the likelihood that the child will have erythroblastosis fetalis. In addition, a mother who has given birth to an infant with anti-$D(Rh_o)$ erythroblastosis fetalis can usually, but not always, expect more serious disease in subsequent offspring. Although the antibody titer ordinarily falls when a pregnancy is terminated and the antigenic stimulus is removed, production continues and increases markedly in response to repeat antigenic exposure like another incompatible pregnancy.

In contrast to anti-$D(Rh_o)$ antibodies, the elaboration of immune anti-A and anti-B antibodies usually reflects heterogenic stimuli such as exposure to bacterial antitoxins or A or B antigens from plant or animal sources. Consequently, primiparae often give birth to children with ABO erythroblastosis fetalis. Furthermore, maternal antibody titers do not show significant increments with subsequent pregnancies, and the likelihood of severe ABO hemolytic disease is no greater in the children of multiparous than primiparous women.

There is no evidence that maternal antibodies directly affect any fetal tissues other than erythrocytes and their precursors. Because most of the antibodies causing erythroblastosis fetalis are incomplete or "blocking" antibodies (p. 96), they may interfere with typing of an infant's cells. For example, $D(Rh_o)$ positive fetal erythrocytes coated with anti-$D(Rh_o)$ will not react with additional anti-$D(Rh_o)$ sera. The absence of agglutination may be falsely interpreted as indicating that the child is $D(Rh_o)$ negative. The presence of maternal antibodies adsorbed on to fetal red cells is detectable by a direct Coombs' test.

The diverse clinical manifestations of isoimmune hemolytic disease of the newborn reflect increased red cell destruction as well as augmented erythrocyte production. They vary from no clinical abnormality (even in some children of sensitized mothers) to a compensated hemolytic disorder to severe anemia of the newborn to death *in utero*. Intense fetal erythropoietic activity is manifested by reticulocytosis, large numbers of nucleated red cells in the peripheral blood, and extensive extramedullary hematopoiesis, which is responsible for such characteristic physical abnormalities as splenomegaly. Massive edema (hydrops fetalis) is the result of congestive heart failure consequent to profound anemia. The degree of edema is more marked than that which is associated with heart failure in postnatal life because a fetus is not dependent on the lungs for his oxygen supply (after birth pulmonary edema causes death before cardiac decompensation can produce such marked edema).

Before birth the catabolism of large amounts of hemoglobin is of no pathophysiologic significance. Despite markedly increased rates of erythrocyte destruction, infants with erythroblastosis fetalis are not jaundiced at birth. There are at least two reasons for this seemingly paradoxical occurrence. First, large amounts of bilirubin are excreted *in utero*, apparently via the placenta and the mother. Second, newborn infants do not appear to be clinically icteric until the serum bilirubin reaches 4 to 6 mg/100 ml; the explanation for this observation is obscure and may reflect differences in capillary permeability or affinity of the skin for bilirubin. Normally, the serum bilirubin of a newborn infant is less than 3 mg/100 ml. Physiologic jaundice is never manifested before 36 hours, and the maximum serum bilirubin concentration (10 to 13 mg/100 ml) is usually reached at about 48 hours, after which it falls to normal over the ensuing 24 to 48 hours. In the premature infant serum bilirubin levels are higher (occasionally more than 20 mg/100 ml) and rise more slowly; maximal values may not be reached until the third or fourth day, and normal values may not be restored until as late as the tenth day of life. As a rule, the newborn with erythroblastosis fetalis has a serum bilirubin at birth that is only slightly above normal (about 3.5 mg/100 ml). More important is the dramatic and prompt neonatal rise with the serum bilirubin occasionally increasing as rapidly as 1.0 mg/100 ml per hour. Clinical jaundice becomes apparent within a short time (jaundice appearing within the first 24 hours of life is always pathologic and most often indicates erythroblastosis fetalis). In an erythroblastotic infant the blood bilirubin progressively increases over the ensuing 10 to 14 days.

At birth certain hepatic enzymes, most notably glucuronyl transferase, are not fully developed. As a result, the ability of a newborn infant to conjugate free bilirubin with glucuronic acid is impaired. Therefore unconjugated bilirubin accumulates more rapidly in an infant with erythroblastosis fetalis than in an older person with a comparable degree of hemolysis. This type of bilirubin is toxic to the central nervous system. The mechanism by which free bilirubin injures nervous tissue is largely conjectural, but it probably interferes with the oxygen uptake of brain cells. Normally, the blood-brain barrier prevents neurologic damage in persons with hyperbilirubinemia. However, the blood-brain barrier in the newborn is not intact for several days. Consequently, a newborn with erythroblastosis fetalis is not equipped to resist the damaging effect of high blood unconjugated bilirubin levels; the result is a bilirubin encephalopathy or *kernicterus.*

The frequency of kernicterus is directly related to the degree of hyperbilirubinemia. As long as the serum bilirubin is less than 20 mg/100 ml, kernicterus will not occur; as soon as it exceeds 20 mg/100 ml, kernicterus can be expected. Therefore this complication of hemolysis is preventable and can be obviated by exchange transfusions. Kernicterus is most often due to erythroblastosis fetalis, but any disorder that causes a sufficient degree of hyperbilirubinemia during the first two weeks of life will produce a similar bilirubin encephalopathy.

A neurologic picture identical with kernicterus occurs in a strain of jaundiced rats deficient in the conjugating enzyme, glucuronyl transferase. In severely jaundiced infants the entire brain may be stained; however, the staining is more marked in the basal ganglia and other nuclei in the medulla and brain stem. Degeneration of ganglion cells is a prominent histologic feature of kernicterus. Although relatively few patients (about 10 per cent) with erythroblastosis fetalis develop kernicterus, the prognosis in those who do is very poor. About 70 per cent of newborn infants with kernicterus die within the few first days; most of the remaining 30 per cent develop severe neurologic sequelae at a later date. It is noteworthy that kernicterus is responsible for about 10 per cent of the cases of cerebral palsy.

Clinical Manifestations. Approximately 1.5 per cent of all newborn infants have an acquired isoimmune hemolytic disorder. In about 1 per cent erythroblastosis fetalis is due to ABO incompatibility; in 0.5 per cent anti-D(Rh_o) is at fault. Virtually every other erythrocyte antigen has been implicated in at least one case, but the incidence is so low that it lacks clinical significance. Erythroblastosis fetalis affects both sexes and occurs in all parts of the world. For obvious reasons the incidence in different racial and ethnic groups reflects differences in the frequency of such important erythrocyte antigens as $D(Rh_o)$.

The physical findings in an infant with erythroblastosis fetalis depend on the severity of the hemolytic disorder. Consequently, the appearance of an affected child may vary from that of a normal infant to one with massive generalized edema (hydrops fetalis). Minimal to marked pallor, jaundice (absent at birth but appearing within the first 24 to 36 hours of life), and hepatosplenomegaly characterize those infants who fall between these two extremes.

Laboratory findings are equally variable. Anemia may be absent, slight, moderate, marked, or profound. The anemia is accompanied by the typical changes of hemolysis (increased polychromasia, reticulocytosis, circulating nucleated red cells, marrow erythrocytic hyperplasia, and hyperbilirubinemia due to free or unconjugated bilirubin). The circulating nucleated red cell and reticulocyte counts may reach very high values. Although a few nucleated red cells (less than 10/100 leukocytes) can be found in the peripheral blood of a normal newborn during the first two days of life, the peripheral nucleated red cell count in an infant with erythroblastosis fetalis may be five to ten times greater than the leukocyte count. As a result of reticulocyte counts of 10 to 70 per cent, macrocytosis is a prominent feature in the peripheral blood. Spherocytosis is a common manifestation of erythroblastosis fetalis due to anti-A or anti-B but does not accompany disease caused by anti-$D(Rh_o)$.

In infants with active hemolysis, leukocytosis (up to 30,000/cu mm) resulting from a neutrophilia is usual (the leukocyte count must be corrected for the high nucleated red cell count). A few immature granulocytes are commonplace. Erythrophagocytosis (monocytes containing erythrocytes) may be prominent. The platelet count may be normal or, in patients with severe disease, thrombocytopenia may be present and sufficiently marked to cause abnormal bleeding.

The other laboratory manifestations of erythroblastosis fetalis deal directly with the serologic abnormalities. In patients with erythroblastosis fetalis due to anti-$D(Rh_o)$, the direct Coombs' test is consistently positive. It is also positive in disease caused by other erythrocyte antigens; the exception is found among infants with ABO incompatibility in whom the direct Coombs' test is, as a rule, weakly positive or even negative. The indirect Coombs' test is generally positive in patients with a positive direct Coombs' test; however, the titer of circulating antibody in the infant bears little relationship to the severity of the hemolytic process.

Diagnosis. The diagnosis of erythroblastosis fetalis is often suggested by a history of abortions or stillbirths or by the knowledge that the mother has already given birth to a child with an acquired isoimmune hemolytic disorder. Jaundice appearing during the first 36 hours of life demands the exclusion of erythroblastosis fetalis, as does the presence of a hemolytic anemia in a newborn. A positive direct Coombs' test in the baby establishes the diagnosis of erythroblastosis fetalis. In most cases it will be due to anti-D, which can be confirmed by demonstrating a maternal-fetal Rh-type incompatibility and by detecting the appropriate antibody in the mother. If the direct Coombs' test in the infant is positive and there is no demonstrable Rh or ABO blood group incompatibility between the mother and the child, the presence of an antibody against one of the rarer and more weakly antigenic blood-group factors must be sought (e.g., anti-c, anti-E, and anti-Kell). If the child's direct Coombs' test is negative or weakly positive and his ABO blood type is incompatible with that of the mother, a hemolytic disorder is most likely due to anti-A or, less often, anti-B (in some cases the responsible antibody can be demonstrated in the infant's serum). If the direct Coombs' test in the child is negative and there is no ABO incompatibility between the infant and the mother and no maternal erythrocyte antibodies other than anti-A and/or anti-B are present, the possibility of erythroblastosis fetalis can be dismissed. The differential diagnosis includes all causes of anemia, jaundice, and hemolysis in the newborn. However, the unique serologic manifestations of erythroblastosis fetalis eliminate most other hemolytic disorders with relative ease.

Treatment and Course. Treatment of the infant with erythroblastosis fetalis has three goals: (1) the birth of a viable infant, (2) the control of anemia and its serious aftermath—congestive heart failure, and (3) the control of hyperbilirubinemia and the prevention of kernicterus. Preparedness is an essential aspect of successful treatment. In this regard, all pregnant women should be tested routinely for Rh and ABO incompatibility. If the mother is type O and the father is type A, B, or AB, the possibility of ABO hemolytic disease exists. There are no other prenatal tests to assess the likelihood of such an occurrence and the history of a prior birth of an infant with erythroblastosis fetalis is of little help. Knowledge of the father's genotype is helpful, for half of his offspring will be type O if he is heterozygous. If the mother is $D(Rh_o)$ negative and the father is $D(Rh_o)$ positive, the stage is set for the development in the fetus of an isoimmune hemolytic disorder. Under these circumstances the mother should be tested for antibodies at the beginning of the pregnancy, at about 28 to 30 weeks, and just before delivery. If the antibodies are absent during the first trimester, it may be concluded that the mother has not been sensitized and that her child will not be affected, at least not seriously. If the maternal anti-$D(Rh_o)$ titer rises during pregnancy, it may be assumed that maternal-fetal incompatibility exists. In general, the higher the maternal antibody, the severer the disease in the infant. Other factors influencing the likelihood of erythroblastosis fetalis include knowledge of the father's genotype [only 50 per cent of a heterozygote's children will be $D(Rh_o)$ positive], as well as the history of stillbirths or of the birth of a child with anemia, jaundice, hydrops fetalis, or a known diagnosis of erythroblastosis fetalis. Thus the physician should be aware of the possibility of an isoimmune hemolytic disorder and should have some idea of its statistical likelihood before delivery.

Although the exact frequency of stillbirths caused by acquired isoimmune hemolytic disease is not known, erythroblastosis fetalis is an important cause of death *in utero*. Because death is caused by profound anemia and congestive heart failure usually after the thirty-seventh week of gestation, the induction of labor at about this time (or delivery by section) has been advised. However, prematurity adds so greatly to postnatal mortality that this approach can be recommended only if the mother has given birth previously to a dead fetus, the father is a $D(Rh_o)$ positive homozygote, and the maternal antibody titer is high (1:64 or more) and rising. In addition, there must be a team of experts available for an immediate exchange transfusion. Recently, techniques for transfusing an affected fetus *in utero* have been described, but their role in the over-all management of erythroblastosis fetalis must await evaluation in more cases.

Treatment after birth consists of blood transfusions, usually exchange transfusions, and is highly effective. The mortality from erythroblastosis fetalis can be reduced to about 5 per cent (or even less) with prompt treatment given by skilled and experienced personnel. The major cause of death during the first 24 hours is cardiac failure; after 48 hours death is ordinarily due to kernicterus. If a child is born alive with marked anemia and severe congestive heart failure, he is likely to die within a few hours. Few such infants can be saved even with judicious and rapid treatment. On the other hand, *kernicterus is preventable by exchange transfusions.* If the major problem is anemia, small infusions of blood are as effective as exchange transfusions; however, to prevent kernicterus, the fetal cells that are being destroyed by the maternal antibody must be removed and replaced by cells that will not be affected by such antibodies. For example, the transfused cells must be those that will survive normally in the mother; therefore a $D(Rh_o)$ positive infant should be given $D(Rh_o)$ negative, ABO type compatible erythrocytes.

The precise indications for exchange transfusions and the details of the technique are complex and beyond the scope of this book. In brief, the goal is to maintain an adequate oxygen-carrying capacity of the blood and to prevent the serum unconjugated bilirubin from exceeding 20 mg/100 ml. As a general rule, an exchange transfusion is indicated if there is overt disease at birth (anemia, splenomegaly, cardiac failure, or hyperbilirubinemia), a maternal anti-D(Rh$_o$) titer of 1:64 or higher, or a history of a stillbirth or kernicterus due to erythroblastosis fetalis in an earlier child. If an exchange transfusion is not done immediately after birth, the infant must be observed closely. Jaundice appearing in less than six hours and rapidly increasing serum bilirubin levels (e.g., 1 mg/100 ml per hour) point to the need for an immediate exchange transfusion. A second transfusion may be required in 12 to 24 hours, but a third is rarely needed, provided that the first exchange transfusion was carried out within a few hours after birth.

Most isoimmune hemolytic disorders of sufficient severity to warrant exchange transfusions are due to Rh incompatibility [i.e., anti-D(Rh$_o$)]. However, all other types of erythroblastosis fetalis requiring treatment are managed in an identical fashion. ABO hemolytic disease deserves special comment, for hyperbilirubinemia and kernicterus may develop in an infant who shows little or no evidence of the disorder at birth. Exchange transfusions are not limited to the treatment of infants with erythroblastosis fetalis. They are equally effective in preventing kernicterus in all other types of hemolysis in the newborn that may cause marked hyperbilirubinemia.

Acquired Autoimmune Hemolytic Anemias

This category of acquired hemolytic disease is characterized by impaired erythrocyte viability consequent to random red cell destruction by extrinsic or extracorpuscular plasma factors. Although these plasma factors display heterogeneity in different patients, they are proteins with the attributes of immunoglobulins; presumably, they are antibodies. However, these globulins differ from erythrocyte isoantibodies in two important respects:

1. They are ordinarily active against all red cells irrespective of their type or antigenic makeup.
2. They are not elaborated in response to a specific antigen.

Since their presence cannot be attributed to a known antigenic exposure, these proteins are termed *autoantibodies*.

HISTORY

Near the close of the nineteenth century and during the first decade of the twentieth, Hayem, Widal, and others pointed out the acquired hemolytic disorders and stressed their differences from congenital hemolytic anemia (hereditary spherocytosis). Autoagglutination of erythrocytes was observed in some of these patients, and Donath and Landsteiner (1904) and Chauffard (1908) demonstrated the presence of autohemolysins in the blood of certain patients with hemolytic anemia. However, little attention was paid to the possibility of immune hemolysis and few accepted the concept of an acquired hemolytic anemia. In 1925 Lederer's report of several patients with acute hemolytic anemias cured by blood transfusions was viewed by most as a new entity. It was not until 1940 that Dameshek and Schwartz established unequivocally the presence of abnormal hemolysins in the blood of patients with acute hemolytic anemia and elucidated experimentally the role of such erythrocyte antibodies in the causation of hemolysis. The subsequent development of serologic techniques (most notably the introduction of the Coombs' or antiglobulin tests in 1945) contributed significantly to our present knowledge of the autoimmune hemolytic anemias.

CLASSIFICATION

The acquired autoimmune hemolytic disorders are divisible into two groups, primary (or idiopathic) and secondary (Table 4-1). At the time of diagnosis, about half of the patients fall into the idiopathic category; that is, there is no evidence of any other disease. After completion of the initial work-up and a short period of observation, 70 to 80 per cent of the patients are found to have some other underlying disease. Continued observation decreases even further the number of primary or idiopathic cases; if these patients live long enough, few will remain in this category. There is increasing support for the concept that an acquired autoimmune hemolytic anemia almost always reflects some other primary disease, although this disease may remain "hidden," sometimes for many months or years.

The causes of a secondary autoimmune hemolytic anemia are seemingly diverse and include (1) hematologic neoplasms (lymphoma, chronic lymphocytic leukemia, plasmacytic myeloma, and primary macroglobulinemia), (2) collagen diseases (systemic lupus erythematosus, polyarteritis, and scleroderma), (3) nonhematologic neoplasms (ovarian cysts, dermoid cysts, renal carcinomas, and, less often, other malignant tumors), (4) infections (infectious mononucleosis, primary atypical pneumonia, infectious hepatitis, syphilis, and a variety of chronic pyogenic infections), and (5) miscellaneous disorders (e.g., ulcerative colitis and thrombotic thrombocytopenic purpura).

The clinical manifestations of the primary and secondary autoimmune hemolytic anemias differ only insofar as the underlying basic disease contributes to the clinical pictures of the secondary forms. The hemolytic mechanisms are the same regardless of the source of the abnormal globulin (or antibody) or of the nature of the stimulus evoking its formation. Furthermore, the diagnosis of a primary autoimmune hemolytic anemia is predicated on the exclusion of all secondary types.

Therefore it is appropriate to discuss together the pathogenesis, clinical manifestations, diagnosis, treatment, and course of all the autoimmune hemolytic anemias.

In addition to the partition of the autoimmune hemolytic anemias into primary and secondary categories, it has been customary to consider separately those anemias due to "warm" antibodies from those caused by antibodies most active in the cold. However, such an arbitrary separation serves no useful purpose. Although certain of the characteristics of "warm" and "cold" antibodies differ and, as a result, influence the clinical manifestations of the hemolytic disorder they cause, their presence reflects similar pathogenic mechanisms. For example, patients with cold hemolysins (often associated with syphilis) are usually classified under the heading of paroxysmal cold hemoglobinuria. However, hemoglobinuria is nonspecific (it accompanies acute intravascular hemolysis of any cause), and these patients ordinarily have a chronic hemolytic anemia that is exacerbated by exposure to cold. The basic difference between these patients and others who have warm antibodies appears to reflect variable molecular structure (and therefore pathophysiologic effects) of the abnormal globulins. The serologic complexity of the autoimmune hemolytic anemias suggests individual patient specificity analogous to that of the myeloma proteins (p. 414). In response to a similar or closely related pathogenic stimulus, one patient produces a warm agglutinin; for reasons still unknown another person elaborates a cold hemolysin.

Current data dictate that all acquired autoimmune hemolytic anemias be so designated and then qualified by such descriptive terms as secondary to lymphosarcoma or primary. Because most of these hemolytic disorders are due to antibodies that are active at 37°C, this attribute of the abnormal protein is inferred. If hemolysis is caused by a cold antibody, it should be so stated (e.g., acquired autoimmune hemolytic anemia, primary, due to a cold agglutinin).

PATHOGENESIS

The acquired autoimmune hemolytic anemias are caused by abnormal globulins that damage erythrocytes, thereby shortening their lifespans. With few exceptions these proteins are 7S globulins with molecular weights of about 160,000; most behave as incomplete or univalent antibodies and are warm agglutinins; that is, they agglutinate rather than lyse, are most active at 37°C, and are adsorbed onto the erythrocytes, thereby requiring special techniques such as the direct Coombs' or antiglobulin test for their detection. Erythrocyte autoantibodies are rarely active in the cold; some of these proteins are macroglobulins with molecular weights around 1,000,000. Because cold antibodies attach to red cells only at low temperatures, the direct

Coombs' test may be negative unless the blood is chilled. Circulating cold antibodies can be accurately quantified (titers of 1:8 to 1:16 are present in many normal persons). Cold hemolysins are particularly apt to be found in patients with syphilis.

There are cogent reasons to implicate normal lymphocytes and plasmacytes as the cells that synthesize immunoglobulins in response to specific antigenic stimuli. There is convincing evidence that these cells (or closely related cells) elaborate the abnormal globulins that cause the autoimmune hemolytic anemias. However, in striking contrast to the production of other antibodies, the antigenic stimulus or stimuli responsible for erythrocyte autoantibody elaboration has not been identified. There are at least two explanations. A popular and widely accepted theory invokes autoimmunity and contends that immune tolerance to one's own tissues is lost. As a result of some ill-defined cellular change consequent to any of several possible endogenous or exogenous factors, red cells may no longer be recognized by the body's immunologically competent cells, which respond by synthesizing an antibody directed against erythrocytes. Another means by which an autoimmune reaction might take place is the emergence of clones of antibody-producing cells that have either not acquired or have lost their immunologic tolerance to erythrocytes. There are convincing arguments both for and against the role of autoimmunity in the pathogenesis of these acquired hemolytic disorders. The over-all importance of autoimmune mechanisms in the production of disease is becoming more and more apparent; however, another equally plausible explanation exists for the production of the "autoimmune" hemolytic anemias.

The protein factors responsible for the destruction of red cells may not be antibodies in the true sense of the word; that is, structurally specific immunoglobulins produced in response to a certain antigenic stimulus. Instead, they may be abnormal globulins possessing by chance a physical makeup that gives them a peculiar affinity for erythrocytes. The end result, that is, a hemolytic anemia, would be the same. Such abnormal proteins could be formed in response to a specific stimulus, or, since they are without known biologic usefulness, they might reflect a byproduct of benign or malignant hyperplasia of cells capable of active protein synthesis. The autoimmune hemolytic anemias might then be envisaged as manifestations of lymphoproliferative disorders and could be likened to plasmacytic myeloma in which the abnormal plasmacytes or myeloma cells retain their ability to synthesize globulins; the myeloma globulins formed by these cells are, in turn, responsible for many of the pathophysiologic manifestations of this malignant plasmacytic neoplasm (p. 415). In line with this possibility is the knowledge that the seemingly diverse causes of a secondary "autoimmune" hemolytic anemia have in common either easily demonstrable lymphocytic or plasmacytic hyperplasia or plasma protein abnormalities (e.g., the hypergammaglobulinemia of the collagen diseases and malignant disorders).

The leukocytic and thrombocytic manifestations of the autoimmune hemolytic anemias also tend to support the concept of a chance affinity of the abnormal globulins for blood cells. Acute blood loss (hemorrhage or hemolysis) typically evokes leukocytosis and thrombocytosis, and the hereditary hemolytic anemias are customarily accompanied by an increase in the leukocyte and platelet counts. In contrast, the autoimmune hemolytic anemias are frequently distinguished by leukopenia and/or thrombocytopenia. These peripheral blood cytopenias also appear to reflect increased destruction by autoantibodies. In those patients with an autoimmune hemolytic anemia and neutropenia or thrombocytopenia, the marrow findings are those of hypersplenic neutropenia and thrombocytopenia (p. 456). In addition, leukocyte and/or platelet agglutinins are often demonstrable. These observations suggest that a variety of immune hypersplenic syndromes (primary and secondary autoimmune hemolytic anemias, primary and secondary immunothrombocytopenias, and primary and secondary immunoneutropenias) may have a common pathogenesis. Minor differences in host response and protein structure may determine whether the major manifestation is a hemolytic anemia, thrombocytopenia, neutropenia, or some combination.

Precise elucidation of the pathogenic mechanisms underlying the autoimmune hemolytic anemias must await further studies. It is possible that both theories are valid in different situations. Pending resolution of the role of autoimmunity, it has been suggested that the designation autoimmune hemolytic anemia may be inappropriate. However, it has been widely adopted and there is no good reason to discard it. Even if the globulins are not classical antibodies formed in response to a particular antigen, they possess the properties of and behave as antibodies. Therefore the mode of erythrocyte destruction is *immune* and the prefix *auto* applies, regardless of the specificity of the affinity of these protein factors for erythrocytes. Irrespective of the nature of the stimulus that is responsible for the production of erythrocyte autoantibodies, it is reasonable to conclude that they are formed by lymphocytes and plasmacytes, either normal or abnormal.

The consequences of erythrocyte destruction by autoantibodies are the same as those of any other hemolytic disorder (anemia, increased polychromasia, reticulocytosis, nucleated red cells in the peripheral blood, marrow erythrocytic hyperplasia, hyperbilirubinemia, and so forth). Erythrocyte destruction is random and affects cells of all ages. Normal donor erythrocytes survive poorly in a patient with an autoimmune hemolytic anemia, whereas the patient's cells display relatively normal life-spans in a normal recipient. The exact manner by which autoantibodies bring about red cell destruction is not known. They apparently injure the surface membrane in such a way that they interfere seriously with the cell's ability to preserve its cation gradients and normal metabolic functions. Spherocytosis is a frequent, but not a consistent, finding in the autoimmune hemolytic anemias. When spherocytes are prominent, osmotic and mechanical fragilities are increased. Autoagglutination (presumably a direct reflection of the autoantibody) is rather common and often precludes an accurate erythrocyte count. Erythrophagocytosis may be a prominent feature. Differing manifestations (e.g., the presence or absence of spherocytes) appear to reflect differences (gross or subtle) in the abnormal globulins. Erythrocyte antibodies differ strikingly among patients. Indeed, it would seem that few, if any, of these protein factors are identical, even in patients with comparable clinical pictures.

CLINICAL MANIFESTATIONS

The exact incidence of the autoimmune hemolytic anemias is not known. Following the introduction of the Coombs' or antiglobulin test and the development of techniques to measure red cell life-span accurately, it soon became evident that hemolysis due to erythrocyte autoantibodies is quite common. Few patients with the diseases known to cause a secondary autoimmune hemolytic anemia (Table 4-1) fail to exhibit at least an occult or compensated hemolytic disorder; many manifest overt hemolysis. In addition, primary (idiopathic) autoimmune hemolytic anemia is by no means a rare occurrence. Because of their varied etiologies, the autoimmune hemolytic anemias affect both sexes of all ages and races. Most reported series suggest a predominance of older males in the secondary and of younger females in the primary autoimmune hemolytic disorders. However, such data have little relevance. The former probably reflect the higher incidence of hematologic neoplasms in older males, whereas the latter may be a reflection of the frequency with which such disorders as systemic lupus erythematosus affect young females. Furthermore, long-term follow-up progressively depletes the category of patients with primary disease. Consequently, the age and sex distribution becomes that of the underlying disease.

Symptoms. An acquired autoimmune hemolytic anemia may start insidiously or develop with dramatic suddenness, bringing about the destruction of as much as 50 per cent of the red cell mass in a period of 24 hours. The symptoms are those of any hemolytic process; their severity depends on the rate of hemolysis and the degree of the anemia. Thus some patients are asymptomatic; others complain of weakness, tachycardia, exertional dyspnea, jaundice, dark urine, and so forth; those with acute hemolysis may manifest fever, pain in the abdomen, back, and extremities, and rapidly developing pallor with or without jaundice. It should be re-emphasized that the presence of jaundice is contingent on the functional capacity of the liver and is not requisite for the diagnosis of a hemolytic anemia. In the primary autoimmune hemolytic anemias the symptoms are solely those attributable to hemolysis. The basic disease significantly affects the clinical pictures of the secondary hemolytic disorders. For example, a patient with Hodgkin's disease and superimposed hemolysis may complain of fever, weight loss, and pruritus instead of symptoms characteristic of hemolysis. For this reason the symptomatology of the secondary autoimmune hemolytic anemias is extremely variable and fails to reveal any consistent pattern over and above those complaints resulting from anemia or increased hemoglobin catabolism. Those rare patients with erythrocyte antibodies that are most active in the cold will complain of cold sensitivity; for example, dark urine, pallor, weakness, jaundice, or dermal manifestations (urticaria, Raynaud's phenomenon, and even superficial gangrene) developing after exposure to cold.

Physical Findings. Splenomegaly, pallor, and jaundice are the characteristic physical manifestations of the autoimmune hemolytic anemias, as they are of any other hemolytic disorder. Their magnitude depends on the severity of the hemolytic process, the degree of anemia, and the functional capacity of the liver. Splenomegaly is quite a constant finding; in general, the larger the spleen, the greater the hemolytic activity. It is noteworthy that variations in the rate of hemolysis are ordinarily reflected by prompt changes in the size of the spleen. Hepatomegaly is a frequent but by no means a universal finding. In addition, patients with a secondary autoimmune hemolytic anemia manifest the physical abnormalities that distinguish their basic disease (e.g., lymphadenopathy and hepatosplenomegaly in persons with lymphoma).

Laboratory Findings. Peripheral Blood. The peripheral erythroid values vary from normal to extremely low levels. Spherocytes are ordinarily prominent and often appear larger than those in hereditary spherocytosis; however, spheroidal cells are not demonstrable in every patient with an autoimmune hemolytic anemia. Macrocytosis parallels the reticulocyte count. The erythrocytes are normochromic and, as a rule, show little variation in shape. Autoagglutination is often present and may interfere with or even preclude an accurate erythrocyte count; if caused by a cold agglutinin, clumping in vitro can be prevented by warming the specimen. Other manifestations of accelerated erythropoiesis include increased polychromasia, reticulocytosis, and circulating nucleated red cells. These findings vary with the rate of hemolysis and, in the secondary autoimmune hemolytic anemias, are also influenced by other factors affecting the ability of the marrow to respond. In the hereditary hemolytic anemias it is possible to correlate fairly well the magnitude of the hemolytic process with the degree of anemia and reticulocytosis (the greater the hemolysis, the lower the peripheral erythroid values and the higher the reticulocyte count). However, in the secondary autoimmune hemolytic anemias there may be other causes for an anemia, for example, marrow depression or infiltration with foreign cells. As a result, marked anemia may actually reflect a minimal hemolytic component; conversely, severe hemolysis may evoke slight evidence of accelerated marrow activity. Thus the reticulocyte count may be normal, slightly elevated, or reach levels of 80 to 90 per cent. In the presence of a significant number of spherocytes, osmotic and mechanical fragilities will be increased. Autohemolysis is variable but usually accelerated and little altered by the addition of glucose.

The leukocyte and platelet counts are normal or quite often decreased (leukocytosis and/or thrombocytosis are distinctly unusual except in patients with leukemia and Hodgkin's disease). It is common to find a few immature granulocytes in the peripheral blood. Erythrophagocytosis is demonstrable in some patients (p. 311).

BONE MARROW.   In those patients without other abnormalities affecting myeloid activity, the marrow is hypercellular, consequent to orderly, normoblastic, erythrocytic hyperplasia. Normal to increased numbers of megakaryocytes with sharply demarcated cytoplasmic borders and little or no evidence of platelet budding are found in patients with immunologic thrombocytopenia (p. 493); immunoneutropenia is associated with normal or increased numbers of granulocytic precursors, often with evidence of a "maturation arrest" (p. 332). The marrow picture will obviously be influenced by other diseases associated with specific marrow defects; for example, chronic lymphocytic leukemia with a secondary autoimmune hemolytic anemia. In these situations the hemolytic process may be at least partly obscured. Marrow iron is generally increased. In those rare patients who develop a hypoplastic crisis the bone marrow usually reveals a paucity of nucleated red cells. Superimposed folic acid deficiency is ordinarily manifested by characteristic megaloblastic morphology (p. 209).

OTHER LABORATORY FINDINGS.   With few exceptions serologic evidence of the abnormal globulin can be elicited in patients with an autoimmune hemolytic anemia (both primary and secondary). A positive *direct Coombs' or antiglobulin test* is the most consistent finding, although it is not found in all patients. When the direct Coombs' test is negative, it may be necessary to utilize one of the many other techniques devised to detect the presence of an incomplete erythrocyte antibody (e.g., treating the erythrocytes with a proteolytic enzyme such as trypsin or bromelin). The *indirect Coombs' test* is positive less often.

An erythrocyte autoantibody is rarely type specific and will agglutinate only those cells that possess a specific Rh antigen. In those hemolytic disorders consequent to autoantibodies that are most active at low temperatures, cold agglutinin titers reach high levels (occasionally 1:1,-000,000 or more). Cold hemolysins require a special technique, the *Donath-Landsteiner test* (an initial cold phase permits the antibody to become fixed to the cell; hemolysis then takes place in the presence of complement upon warming). The other laboratory manifestations of the autoimmune hemolytic anemias lack specificity and include *hyperbilirubinemia* due to unconjugated bilirubin, increased *fecal and urine urobilinogen,* decreased to absent *plasma haptoglobin,* and decreased *erythrocyte survival times* with exponential curves. Following the administration of ^{51}Cr-tagged red cells, external counting often reveals increased sequestration in the spleen; however, the role of the spleen is less important than in patients with hereditary spherocytosis, and the liver also participates actively in cell destruction. *Plasma iron* is normal or slightly increased. Unless some associated disease has impaired marrow activity, *plasma iron turnover* and ^{59}Fe *incorporation in hemoglobin* are increased. *Plasma protein electrophoresis* is sometimes abnormal because of the large amounts of abnormal globulin. *Cholecystography* reveals a high incidence of cholelithiasis in patients with long-standing hemolysis. Other findings are attributable to the anemia or reflect whatever underlying disease might be present; for example, LE cells in systemic lupus erythematosus (p. 313) and plasma protein electrophoretic abnormalities in plasmacytic myeloma (p. 422).

DIAGNOSIS

The clinical manifestations attributable to increased erythrocyte destruction (anemia, spherocytes, and splenomegaly), increased hemoglobin catabolism (acholuric jaundice), and increased erythropoiesis (polychromasia, reticulocytosis, and nucleated red cells in the peripheral blood) ordinarily point to a hemolytic disorder during the initial routine work-up. Special techniques are rarely, if ever, needed for the diagnosis of an overt hemolytic anemia. Procedures such as erythrocyte survival times should never be substituted for simpler clinical parameters (history, physical examination, and routine study of the peripheral blood and urine); erythrocyte survival procedures supplement the clinical parameters but do not replace them. If red cell viability is so slightly impaired that it can be detected only by measuring erythrocyte life-span, it is not in itself an adequate explanation for an anemia.

Following the recognition of a hemolytic anemia, special techniques are needed to establish the exact cause. In the autoimmune hemolytic anemias the direct Coombs' or antiglobulin test produces the most valuable information, although the limitations of this technique must be borne in mind (p. 97). With the exception of the autoimmune hemolytic disorders and erythroblastosis fetalis, the direct Coombs' test is rather consistently negative in the other types of hemolytic anemias. If an autoimmune hemolytic anemia seems likely and the direct Coombs' test is negative, it may be necessary to demonstrate the presence of the incomplete erythrocyte autoantibody in other ways. In a few patients the responsible factor (or autoantibody) will elude detection by available techniques. If all other findings favor an autoimmune process, such a diagnosis is still justified even though an abnormal protein cannot be found.

The presence of leukopenia or thrombocytopenia (most other hemolytic processes evoke leukocytosis and thrombocytosis) or of some disease that is known to be accompanied by an autoimmune hemolytic anemia is often helpful; for example, hemolysis in a patient with lymphoma is probably due to a secondary autoimmune hemolytic anemia even though evidence of erythrocyte antibodies is unobtainable. However, an absolute diagnosis of an autoimmune hemolytic anemia demands the exclusion of all other hemolytic disorders and is always on a more solid basis when the direct Coombs' or some comparable test is positive.

TREATMENT AND COURSE

Meaningful data pertaining to the course, prognosis, and therapeutic responses of the autoimmune hemolytic anemias as a group are not available. These anemias reflect diverse primary diseases which determine the ultimate outcome (a patient with an autoimmune hemolytic anemia secondary to infectious mononucleosis can be expected to recover; a patient with lymphoma will die from his basic disease). Even an attempt to assess course and prognosis in a group of patients with primary or idiopathic autoimmune hemolytic anemia is fraught with hazards. A variety of diseases with different prognoses have an autoimmune hemolytic anemia as their initial manifestation, and the number of patients retaining this diagnosis varies inversely with the period of observation. Therefore average or median survival times serve little, if any, purpose.

The prognosis in a patient with a secondary autoimmune hemolytic anemia is basically that of the underlying disease; however, an autoimmune hemolytic disorder is a serious complication that significantly increases morbidity and mortality. Thus a patient with Hodgkin's disease and an autoimmune hemolytic anemia has a much poorer outlook than a similar patient without superimposed hemolysis. It is virtually impossible to predict the subsequent course of a primary autoimmune hemolytic anemia accurately. During the first 12 to 18 months after the onset of overt hemolysis, about half of these patients will manifest evidence of some underlying disease (e.g., lymphoma). Since this disease is likely to be a progressive one, the ultimate outcome leaves much to be desired. Available data suggest that about 40 to 50 per cent of the remaining patients will die during the first one to two years, despite appropriate therapy. Hence the diagnosis of idiopathic autoimmune hemolytic anemia carries with it a poor prognosis, and only 25 to 30 per cent of the patients so diagnosed initially will be alive without evidence of some other disease one to two years later. Among them less than half (10 to 15 per cent of the original patients) can be expected to recover; the rest will continue to hemolyze. Some run a protracted course characterized by remissions and relapses. Even after periods of several years, the possibility remains of recurrence or the development of overt signs of some disorder like a collagen disease.

The mainstays of treatment are the *corticosteroids* and *splenectomy*. Therapy of the two categories of autoimmune hemolytic disorders is fundamentally the same. However, the secondary type does differ insofar as treatment of the basic disease contributes to control of the hemolytic anemia or to the indications for splenectomy. Therefore detailed treatment programs are considered separately.

Primary (Idiopathic) Autoimmune Hemolytic Anemias. CORTICO-STEROIDS. In general, the diagnosis is an indication for treatment with one of the corticosteroids. The usual starting dose is 15 mg of prednisone (or an equivalent amount of a comparable compound) every six hours. Most patients with warm incomplete erythrocyte autoantibodies will respond; the majority will show substantial or even complete subsidence of hemolytic activity. The anemia is corrected in as many as 80 to 90 per cent of the patients who receive 60 mg of prednisone daily. Improvement, often dramatic, is marked by a prompt fall in the reticulocyte count, a decrease in the size of the spleen, and a rapid increase in the peripheral erythroid values. Despite careful observations, the mode of action of the corticosteroids remains obscure. Among patients with comparable clinical improvement, the erythrocyte autoantibody titer may decrease, stay the same, or rise.

An adequate trial of corticosteroids appears to be about 21 to 28 days; if the hemolysis has not lessened by the end of three to four weeks, it is unlikely that more prolonged treatment will be effective. Under these circumstances a trial of massive corticosteroid therapy, for example, 400 mg of prednisone daily for five to seven days, is justified, although the results ordinarily leave much to be desired. There have been a few reports of patients failing to respond to corticosteroids who subsequently improved when given ACTH; the explanation for such occurrences is not apparent.

In those patients in whom the anemia is corrected and the reticulocytosis subsides, the corticosteroids should be gradually withdrawn. In a few individuals remission will persist even though the prednisone is stopped. These patients require no further treatment but should be followed closely. Rare persons will remain normal, whereas others will begin to hemolyze again at some time in the future. Retreatment with corticosteroids is then indicated. If hemolysis recurs as the prednisone is being tapered or after it has been stopped, the patient is a potential candidate for splenectomy. It is unlikely that a partial response to full doses of corticosteroids will be maintained without continuous therapy. Under these circumstances, therefore, the prednisone dose should be progressively decreased as soon as maximal improvement is attained to the smallest amount that will maintain a satisfactory circulating hemoglobin level. These patients are also potential candidates for splenectomy.

Patients with a primary autoimmune hemolytic anemia caused by cold autoantibodies do not respond so well to corticosteroids as do those with warm antibodies. Avoidance of exposure to cold is often more effective. However, some patients deserve a trial of corticosteroids and a few will improve.

SPLENECTOMY. Splenectomy is much less effective in the acquired autoimmune hemolytic anemias than it is in hereditary spherocytosis (p. 110). After removal of the spleen, hemolysis will cease in about one third of the patients; in another third hemolysis will continue, but at a slower rate; in the remaining third splenectomy fails to affect the hemolytic process. Therefore the role of and indications for splenectomy in the management of patients with autoimmune hemolytic disorders are unclear and disputable. In acutely ill patients who fail to respond to corticosteroids and must be transfused in order to maintain satisfactory peripheral erythroid values, there is little choice, despite the relatively high operative risk and the poor chances for improvement. Patients who require large doses of corticosteroids (60 mg of prednisone or more a day) to maintain an adequate hemoglobin level fall into the same category. However, the decision to operate is much harder to reach in those patients who can be adequately controlled with small doses of corticosteroids (e.g., 10 to 15 mg of prednisone a day). These situations call for astute clinical judgment. The deleterious side effects of long-term corticosteriod therapy (susceptibility to infections, osteoporosis, peptic ulceration, and so forth) must be balanced against the hazards of splenectomy. The factors that influence this decision include the age of the patient, associated diseases, the presence of thrombocytopenia and/or neutropenia, and the likelihood of beneficial effects of splenectomy on the hemolytic process.

Splenectomy offers two theoretical advantages: (1) elimination of the organ that contributes to the destruction of damaged erythrocytes and (2) removal of a large collection of antibody-producing cells (p. 453). However, the relatively poor results are not difficult to explain; many other tissues contain cells capable of synthesizing globulins, and extrasplenic reticuloendothelial cells contribute importantly to red cell destruction. In fact, the liver often plays a greater role in the removal of abnormal erythrocytes than does the spleen (cells severely damaged by erythrocyte antibodies are preferentially sequestered and destroyed in the liver). Some assessment of the spleen's contribution to the hemolytic process can be obtained after the administration of ^{51}Cr-tagged red cells (p. 88). Unless the technique reveals increased splenic sequestration, the chances that splenectomy will be of any real value are poor. The type of antibody also affects the response. For example, hemolysis resulting from a cold hemolysin predominantly reflects intravascular erythrocyte destruction and would not be expected to respond to splenectomy. Disease consequent to cold agglutinins is also less likely to be affected by splenectomy than hemolysis caused by antibodies that are most active at 37°C.

Every patient who does not respond well to corticosteroids or who requires continuous treatment should not be splenectomized. On the other hand, splenectomy exerts a beneficial effect in a significant number of patients and in some all evidence of hemolysis ceases. Therefore splenectomy should not be advised just as a last ditch measure or only after a one- to two-year trial of corticosteroids (the latter is a commonly encountered recommendation). In certain patients the risks of immediate splenectomy, that is, within the first four to six weeks after onset of hemolysis, appear to be considerably less than the untoward effects of long-term corticosteroid therapy.

Each case must be considered separately, and every patient presents a unique problem. Factors favoring early splenectomy include the following:

1. A patient who appears to be a good operative risk, (e.g., a young person without other disease).

2. The presence of significant thrombocytopenia and/or neutropenia (immunothrombocytopenias generally respond well to splenectomy—p. 495).

3. Severe hemolysis requiring relatively large amounts of corticosteroids (e.g., 30 mg of prednisone or more daily).

4. The presence of relative contraindications to prolonged corticosteroid therapy such as pulmonary tuberculosis, diabetes mellitus, congestive heart failure, psychiatric disorders, and peptic ulcer.

5. Manifestations of significant corticosteroid toxicity during the initial treatment (excessive fluid retention, increased susceptibility to infections, emotional problems, peptic ulceration, osteoporosis, hypertension, hyperglycemia).

6. A high index of suspicion of some underlying disease like lymphoma (histologic study of the spleen or other tissue obtained at surgery may establish the diagnosis).

7. The availability of a skilled surgeon and adequate facilities for pre- and postoperative care.

8. Evidence of significant splenic red cell sequestration.

Factors militating against early splenectomy include the following:

1. A patient who is a poor risk, that is, one with some other disease that would increase operative mortality.

2. Mild hemolytic activity requiring only low doses of corticosteroids.

3. Absence of thrombocytopenia and/or neutropenia.

4. Absence of significant contraindications to or ill effects from corticosteroids.

5. Lack of adequate facilities for surgery.

6. The inability to demonstrate selective red cell sequestration in the spleen with the ^{51}Cr technique.

Hemolysis should be under optimum corticosteroid control before splenectomy. In this way transfusions can often be avoided, and the operative risks will be lessened. Therefore patients who exhibit recurrent or increased hemolytic activity as the corticosteroids are being tapered or after the drug has been discontinued should have the dose increased to the level that will bring about maximum improvement, preferably normal or near normal peripheral erythroid values. Splenectomy should be deferred, if possible, until that goal is achieved. After splenectomy, prednisone dosage should be tapered as soon as possible by daily decrements of 10 to 15 mg. If the splenectomy has been successful, prednisone can be stopped within four to seven days; if partly effective, the hemolytic disorder may be controllable by lower doses than were needed before surgery; in those patients who continue to hemolyze actively, the only alternatives are the continued administration of large doses of prednisone and/or one of the other forms of therapy discussed next.

BLOOD TRANSFUSIONS.   Transfusions figure importantly in the treatment of some patients with an autoimmune hemolytic anemia. However, they are only palliative, rarely very effective, and not without risk. Since most erythrocyte autoantibodies affect all red cells, irrespective of their antigenic makeup, it is unlikely that donor cells will survive in the recipient any longer than his own. In fact, the average life-span of transfused erythrocytes is often less because of larger numbers of older and less resistant cells (in patients who are actively hemolyzing, a greater proportion of the cells is young). The end result of a transfusion is all too often enhanced hemolysis (more cells are available to be destroyed) and little or no improvement in the oxygen-carrying capacity of the blood. At best, any benefit that may be obtained is transient and lasts only a few days.

Despite these drawbacks, transfusions are needed in critically anemic patients (especially those with hypoplastic crises) and in others being prepared for surgery. Insofar as possible, corticosteroids should always be started before a patient is transfused; in acutely ill patients, in whom an immediate transfusion is deemed necessary to sustain life, corticosteroids should be given (preferably intravenously) at the time the blood is started. Serious problems are often encountered in typing and cross matching and may be the source of considerable anxiety. Because of incomplete antibody adsorbed onto the patient's erythrocytes, agglutination by type-specific antisera may be blocked; consequently, it may be necessary to elute the incomplete antibody before the cells can be typed. When autoagglutination is present, it will also interfere with typing. A compatible cross match may be difficult to achieve or actually unobtainable as the result of circulating autoantibodies in the patient. Under such circumstances the only recourse is to test as many specimens as possible and administer the one that reacts the least. In those rare patients with Rh type specific autoantibodies, it is possible to select blood that will not react with the autoantibodies. However, such cells would be incompatible with those of the patient; isoimmunization would then be likely and could lead to additional problems in the future.

Patients with hemolytic anemias are not hypovolemic unless massive hemolysis has occurred over a very short period of time. Therefore packed erythrocytes are preferred over whole blood. In addition, the first few milliliters should be given quite slowly under close observation. The possibility of a transfusion reaction is a real threat, even in the face of a seemingly compatible cross match.

OTHER FORMS OF TREATMENT. In a few patients control of an autoimmune hemolytic anemia can be achieved with a *cytotoxic agent* that suppresses the proliferation of the cells synthesizing the abnormal globulin. Several drugs have been shown to be variably effective, including 6-mercaptopurine (p. 356), cyclophosphamide (p. 405), and chlorambucil (p. 373). Treatment must be continued for weeks to months before improvement occurs, and toxicity, most notably bone marrow depression, is an ever-present threat. In general, cytotoxic drugs should be given in daily doses about half the size of those used to treat leukemia or lymphoma; even so, these patients must be followed closely in order to prevent serious marrow depression. Further study is needed before these drugs can be assigned their proper places in the treatment of the autoimmune hemolytic anemias. At the present time their use should be restricted to those patients who do not respond to corticosteroids or splenectomy or to those in whom either or both of these forms of therapy are deemed inadvisable.

Many other therapeutic approaches have been tried without consistent or significant success (e.g., heparin and radioactive gold). Heparin supposedly inhibits antigen-antibody reactions, and the gold is taken up by the reticuloendothelial system where it theoretically suppresses antibody elaboration. If a patient with an autoimmune hemolytic anemia develops a superimposed folic acid deficiency, supplemental folic acid should be given (5 mg/day is many times more than enough—p. 222). Otherwise, there is no indication for the administration of an antianemic agent. In particular, iron is contraindicated. Patients with hemolytic anemias are already overloaded with iron and are absorbing increased amounts from the gastrointestinal tract. Chronic iron therapy may culminate in tissue hemosiderosis with serious consequences.

Secondary Autoimmune Hemolytic Anemias. These hemolytic disorders are treated in much the same way as the primary (idiopathic) type. However, certain differences deserve emphasis. The secondary autoimmune hemolytic anemias ordinarily do not respond so well to corticosteroids. Although the majority of the patients show a lessening of hemolytic activity, normal peripheral erythroid values are rarely restored largely because of the limitations imposed by the underlying disease. Even so, the diagnosis is generally an indication for treatment with corticosteroids. When the peripheral erythroid values have stabilized, the basic disease should be treated, provided treatment is available and indicated. For example, a patient with active lymphoma and a secondary autoimmune hemolytic anemia should receive appropriate suppressive therapy (such as x-radiation or an alkylating agent—p. 399). It is important that such treatment be given while the hemolytic process is under maximum corticosteroid control, for the erythropoietic suppression induced by the cytotoxic therapy will aggravate the anemia. A sudden decrease in erythropoiesis will be reflected by a rapid drop in the peripheral erythroid values, even though red cell life-span remains unchanged.

Control of the primary disease is often accompanied by decreased hemolytic activity. However, some patients actually manifest enhanced hemolysis after treatment of their lymphoma or chronic lymphocytic leukemia; such occurrences may reflect destruction of leukemic or lymphoma cells containing large quantities of preformed globulins (or autoantibodies). When increased erythrocyte destruction follows specific treatment, it is usually transient and recedes in a few weeks to pretreatment levels of hemolytic activity or, hopefully, less.

As soon as maximum hematologic improvement has been achieved and the marrow has recovered from any suppressive therapy that may have been given, the corticosteroid dose should be gradually reduced to the smallest amount that will maintain the desired effect (preferably around 15 mg of prednisone a day or an equivalent amount of a comparable compound). It is unusual to obtain such complete control of a secondary autoimmune hemolytic anemia that corticosteroids can be stopped, and long-term maintenance therapy is required (frequently throughout the rest of the patient's life). In patients with a collagen disorder and an acquired autoimmune hemolytic anemia, corticosteroids are also indicated for the basic disease.

Because most of the diseases associated with a secondary autoimmune hemolytic anemia have a poor prognosis, splenectomy is generally avoided if possible. Many of these patients are relatively poor risks, and the immediate hazards of surgery ordinarily outweigh those of maintenance corticosteroid therapy. Therefore splenectomy is customarily reserved for those patients with life-threatening hemolysis who cannot be adequately controlled with prednisone or by some other means. Despite the increased risks associated with surgery in patients with lymphoma or some other malignancy, selected individuals should still be considered for splenectomy, especially those with thrombocytopenia and/or neutropenia accompanying the hemolytic anemia. The response is sometimes dramatic and quite gratifying. Blood transfusions play an important role in the over-all management of patients with a secondary autoimmune hemolytic anemia.

Patients with cold antibodies deserve special mention. Avoidance of exposure to low temperatures is of value for obvious reasons. In those persons with cold hemolysins and syphilis, the syphilis should, of course, be treated. Patients with primary atypical pneumonia and cold agglutinins rarely require any specific treatment directed at the hemolytic component. Patients with such disorders as lymphoma or chronic lymphocytic leukemia and hemolysis characterized by cold agglutinins are managed in a manner similar to persons with warm agglutinins.

Acquired Hemolytic Anemias Caused by Chemical and Physical Factors

Many chemicals are capable of causing hemolysis, and there are few drugs that have not been implicated in the pathogenesis of a hemolytic disorder. Most of these agents are oxidant compounds that act by interfering with glycolysis (p. 115). Some, such as phenylhydrazine, cause lysis of normal erythrocytes; others, such as primaquine, require a genetically determined deficiency of glucose-6-phosphate dehydrogenase. A few drugs, which act as haptenes, cause hemolysis by evoking antibody production; for example, stibophen (Fuadin), penicillin, quinidine, methylethyl-hydantoin (Mesantoin), and acetophenetidin or phenacetin. Certain heavy metals are also capable of injuring erythrocytes and decreasing their life-span. Among them, hemolysis consequent to acute lead poisoning is best known; arsine (arsenuretted hydrogen) is another common cause of a hemolytic anemia.

Some snake venoms are potent hemolytic agents because of their content of lecithinase. Lecithinase converts lecithin into lysolecithin, which has strong hemolytic properties. Saponin (a glycoside) and sodium taurocholate are other examples of substances possessing a direct lytic effect. *Zieve's syndrome* or *hyperlipemic hemolysis* is of particular interest in this regard. An acute hemolytic anemia is a relatively common finding in chronic alcoholics with minimal hepatic dysfunction but with significant fatty infiltration of their livers. The anemia typically becomes evident shortly after hospitalization and coincides with an improved dietary intake and decreased alcohol consumption. Hemolysis is usually accompanied by hypercholesterolemia; hyperlipemia is common, but the blood may appear milky for only a day or so. Hemolytic activity is generally of minimal to moderate severity; as a rule, spherocytes are demonstrable. The anemia is ordinarily self-limited and disappears as the patient's liver status improves. This hemolytic disorder is presumably caused by some still unidentified lipid (or lipids) with hemolytic properties.

Erythrocytes subjected to heat in vitro become spherocytic and have decreased survival times when returned to the donor. Acute hemolysis in persons who have been badly burned undoubtedly reflects red cell damage consequent to the excessive temperatures.

Following the entrance of large amounts of distilled water (600 ml or more) into the circulation, acute hemolysis occurs, probably consequent to simple osmotic swelling and lysis. This type of hemolysis has complicated transurethral resections and is evident in persons who survive drowning in fresh water.

Mechanical trauma in vitro will bring about erythrocyte destruction. Several types of in vivo trauma also appear to cause premature removal of red cells from the circulation. A number of patients have been observed to develop an acute hemolytic anemia after cardiac surgery (implantation of valve prostheses and repair of septal defects). Available data indicate that the accelerated red cell destruction is the result of physical trauma caused by altered blood velocity, increased turbulence, or actual collision of red cells with some foreign object (e.g., a prosthesis or artificial septum). The presence in such patients of marked poikilocytosis supports erythrocytic fragmentation as the basic mechanism responsible for the decrease in red cell viability. Some of these patients will eventually compensate for the shortened erythrocyte lifespan by increasing red cell production.

Although proof is lacking, it seems likely that those few patients who have been observed to develop acute hemolysis following physical exertion ("march hemoglobinuria") reflect a similar pathogenesis, that is, increased physical trauma. It has also been suggested that the hemolytic anemia characterizing thrombotic thrombocytopenic purpura may be due to trauma to the circulating erythrocytes by vascular lesions; it is noteworthy that bizarre poikilocytes or red cell fragments are evident in this disorder (Fig. 13-3, p. 502).

Acquired Hemolytic Anemias
Caused by Infections

Certain acute infections are consistently associated with overt hemolysis. Malaria and Oroya fever (*Bartonella bacilliformis*) are prominent examples in which the microorganisms directly invade red cells and cause their destruction. A hemolytic anemia is also fairly common in patients with gas gangrene (*Clostridium welchii*) and cholera (*Vibrio comma*). The frequency with which hemolysis accompanies other acute infections has not been clearly elucidated.

Hemolytic anemias have been observed in a variety of infectious diseases, including, among others, primary atypical pneumonia, infectious mononucleosis, infectious hepatitis, typhoid fever, septicemia (pneumococcal, streptococcal, or staphylococcal), psittacosis, miliary tuberculosis, and subacute bacterial endocarditis. However, overt hemolysis is not a common complication of acute infections, despite the fact that such occurrences might be anticipated. For example, primary atypical pneumonia is often associated with demonstrable cold agglutinins, many infections evoke clear-cut plasma protein changes as well as stimulating the reticuloendothelial system, and some bacterial toxins possess hemolytic properties. Although it is generally believed that most acute infections cause hemolytic anemias, such is not the case. In some instances, for example, subacute bacterial endocarditis, only a few such patients have been observed. The relationship between acute infections and hemolysis obviously requires further study. Since an acute infection may make an occult hemolytic disorder clinically apparent, it is possible that some underlying abnormality such as G-6-PD deficiency or hereditary spherocytosis may be responsible for some cases of hemolysis seemingly caused by acute infections.

Chronic infections are frequently accompanied by an anemia. These anemias are in large part due to depressed erythropoiesis and are discussed elsewhere (pp. 178, 289). Overt hemolysis is rarely associated with a chronic infection; however, erythrocyte life-spans are slightly decreased in most of these patients as the result of a poorly defined extrinsic or extracorpuscular factor. It seems likely that this decrease in red cell survival time reflects the presence of an abnormal globulin, that is, a mechanism similar to that operating in the secondary autoimmune hemolytic anemias (p. 133).

Acquired Hemolytic Anemias Caused by Splenomegaly

There is convincing evidence that the expanded vascular bed and stasis compartment of greatly enlarged spleens can cause the premature destruction of red cells and an overt hemolytic anemia. This type of hypersplenism is considered in Chapter 12, page 448. Examples include agnogenic myeloid metaplasia (p. 430), Banti's syndrome (p. 457), and Gaucher's disease (p. 458).

Acquired Hemolytic Anemia Caused by Vitamin B$_{12}$ or Folic Acid Deficiency

Erythrocytes produced in the face of inadequate amounts of vitamin B$_{12}$ or folic acid have decreased survival times. In addition, many erythrocytic precursors are destroyed in the marrow before they reach maturity. The contributions of the hemolytic component to the clinical manifestations of the megaloblastic macrocytic anemias are discussed elsewhere (p. 192).

Paroxysmal Nocturnal Hemoglobinuria

Paroxysmal nocturnal hemoglobinuria is a rare, acquired hemolytic disorder of unknown cause characterized by hemoglobinuria occurring during sleep superimposed on a chronic hemolytic anemia, leukopenia, thrombocytopenia, recurrent infections, and venous thromboses. Its frequency has been estimated to be about one per million population. The disorder usually has its onset in the third or fourth decade of life and shows no sex, race, or geographic predilections. The severity of the hemolytic process varies considerably among different patients and from time to time in a single patient. In some the disorder is benign and of little clinical significance; in others it is life threatening.

The cause of paroxysmal nocturnal hemoglobinuria (PNH) is not known. PNH cells have decreased survival times in normal recipients, whereas normal donor cells survive normally in patients with PNH. Patients with PNH appear to have two populations of cells; one is normal and the other has impaired viability. The number in the second category correlates well with clinical severity. The nature of the intrinsic red cell defect is obscure. PNH erythrocytes are destroyed in vitro when incubated in acidified plasma or serum; cell destruction is also enhanced by the addition of thrombin. Spherocytes are absent. Erythrocyte acetylcholinesterase content is decreased; however, this enzymatic deficiency does not affect erythrocyte survival and cannot be implicated in the pathogenesis of hemolysis. PNH red cells are often lysed by antibodies that ordinarily agglutinate normal cells.

In addition to the poorly defined intracorpuscular abnormality, several extracorpuscular factors participate, including magnesium cations, properdin, components of complement, and possibly other still unidentified plasma constituents. Because maximal hemolysis in vitro occurs at a less than normal physiologic pH and because hemolysis in vivo increases during sleep, a popular thesis has been that of decreased sensitivity of the respiratory center during sleep with increased carbon dioxide retention and a fall in plasma pH. Against this possibility is the demonstration that hemolytic activity increases during sleep even though normal respirations are maintained by mechanical means.

There is no adequate explanation for the frequent findings of leukopenia and thrombocytopenia. Both decreased rates of production and increased peripheral destruction have been proposed. An interesting but unexplained observation is the finding of decreased alkaline phosphatase in the granulocytes.

The clinical manifestations of PNH are basically those of any hemolytic disorder plus nocturnal hemoglobinuria (passage of dark urine after sleep). Slight splenomegaly is usual. Spherocytes and erythrophagocytosis are not present. Prominent hemosiderinuria results in the loss of significant amounts of iron that may in time be responsible for a superimposed microcytic, hypochromic (iron deficiency) anemia. The diagnosis of PNH can be confirmed by the acid hemolysis or Ham test (lysis of PNH cells when incubated in acidified serum).

There is no effective form of treatment. Splenectomy and corticosteroids are without value. In severely anemic patients transfusions may be needed (packed cells should be used, for whole blood may aggravate hemolysis, presumably because of the plasma factors it contains). Dextran has been observed to lessen hemolysis temporarily, perhaps by binding properdin. Although heparin may accelerate hemolysis, dicoumarin has been effective in some patients (thromboembolism causes about half the deaths attributable to PNH). In some patients PNH does not affect longevity, and in others apparent clinical recovery occurs. Therefore the outlook is not always poor.

Anemias Caused by Impaired Production

Erythrocytes have a finite life-span of about 120 days. In a normal adult some 250 billion effete erythrocytes containing approximately 7 gm of hemoglobin are destroyed each day and replaced by new red cells. Normally, erythrocyte production exactly balances peripheral destruction and the oxygen-carrying capacity of the blood remains remarkably uniform. Any abnormality that interferes with erythropoiesis will disrupt the normal steady state. If the marrow is unable to replace aged red cells as they are destroyed, the peripheral erythroid values will decline. Although a decrease in red cell mass ordinarily imparts a stimulus to erythropoiesis (presumably via the humoral erythropoietic regulatory mechanism), an abnormal marrow cannot respond. Because erythrocytes remain viable and continue to circulate for about four months, anemias caused by defective erythrocytogenesis characteristically progress slowly. If erythropoiesis ceased completely and red cell survival times remained normal, the peripheral erythroid values would undergo only a 10 per cent decrement every 12 days. Actually, many of these anemias develop more rapidly because they also reflect a decrease in red cell viability.

The causes of the anemias consequent to impaired erythrocyte production are listed in Table 3-2, page 56. Their diverse etiologies, variable pathophysiologic manifestations, and distinctive clinical pictures warrant separate discussions of these disorders.

Deficiency Anemias

Erythropoiesis is dependent on a complex nutritional and hormonal environment (p. 15). Inadequacy of a variety of hormones and nutrients theoretically would be expected to impair erythrocytogenesis; failure of production to keep pace with peripheral destruction should bring about an anemia. Such is the case in experimental animals. In man, however, there are only a few deficiency states associated with anemia; these involve the secretions of certain of the endocrine glands, iron, vitamin B_{12}, and folic acid.

HORMONES

The humoral erythropoietic regulatory mechanism plays a fundamental role in the homeostatic control of erythropoiesis (p. 13). Therefore it is reasonable to theorize that humoral factor deficiency would be manifested by decreased erythropoiesis and anemia. Although available experimental data are incomplete, most, if not all, well-defined anemias are accompanied by increased plasma erythropoietic factor activity. The only apparent exception is the anemia of chronic renal disease. Preliminary observations point to decreased activity attributable to erythropoietin (the glycoprotein erythropoietic factor that enhances hemoglobin synthesis) in patients with the anemia of uremia. Although these findings are in accord with those that implicate the kidneys in the elaboration of erythropoietin (p. 11), the complex problem of the pathogenesis of the anemia of chronic renal insufficiency has not been solved. Erythropoietin deficiency undoubtedly plays a role, but other factors also appear to operate (e.g., decreased cell survival). Consequently, it is not yet possible to classify the anemia of uremia as a straightforward deficiency anemia; it is discussed in detail in another section (p. 284).

The erythropoietic effects of the thyroid, adrenals, pituitary, and gonads (androgens) have been subjected to extensive investigative study. The hormones elaborated by these endocrine glands exert a modifying or conditioning influence on erythropoiesis based largely on their role as regulators of general metabolic activity and oxygen requirements (p. 15). In this way they serve to determine the level at which erythrocytic equilibrium is to be maintained. This effect appears to be mediated by the humoral erythropoietic regulatory mechanism and, with the possible exception of testosterone, the secretions of the orthodox endocrine glands do not affect the marrow directly. Thus the "anemias" characterizing hormonal deficiencies actually represent "normal" values because of the less than normal metabolic activity. Since the consumption of oxygen is decreased as a result of endocrine insufficiency (e.g., a hypofunctioning thyroid), a normal oxygen-carrying capacity of the blood results in tissue hyperoxia. This hyperoxic effect, which is analogous to transfusion polycythemia or increasing the oxygen tension of the inspired air, serves through the humoral mechanism to depress erythropoiesis. In the face of a hormonal deficiency, therefore, erythrocytic equilibrium is re-established at a new level, which, although lower than normal, is entirely adequate to supply enough oxygen to fulfill the tissues' decreased needs. Consequently, the anemia that accompanies hormonal inadequacy is not really an abnormal finding; instead, the decreased circulating hemoglobin reflects a normal physiologic compensatory mechanism comparable to the erythrocytosis caused by arterial hypoxemia (p. 295).

In laboratory animals hormonal deficiency subsequent to ablation of the thyroid, pituitary, adrenals, or testes is characterized by reduced metabolic activity and oxygen consumption and by less than normal peripheral erythroid values which are correctable by specific replacement therapy. Each of these experimentally induced deficiency states, with the exception of hypogonadism, has a clinical counterpart. Although orchidectomized males tend to have lower peripheral values than normal males, the decrease in red cell mass is so minimal that it does not constitute a clinical problem and usually goes undetected.

Hypothyroidism.   Most patients with decreased thyroid function have a slight to moderate normocytic, normochromic "anemia." The decrease in circulating hemoglobin is unrelated to the cause of the hypothyroidism, that is, surgical removal, idiopathic myxedema, and so forth. In the absence of any other cause for anemia, the hemoglobin rarely falls below 9 to 10 gm/100 ml of blood even in totally thyroidectomized subjects. The actual level of the peripheral erythroid values depends on several factors, such as the degree of hypometabolism and associated pulmonary or cardiac dysfunction. Consequently, every patient with clinical hypothyroidism does not manifest low erythroid values. The erythrocytes are morphologically normal and physiologically competent with normal survival times. There are no consistent or significant changes in the leukocyte or platelet counts. The bone marrow is normoblastic but hypocellular (a reflection of the quantitative decrease in erythropoiesis occasioned by the decreased metabolic activity). There are no demonstrable qualitative defects in erythropoiesis or hemoglobin synthesis, and these patients respond in the usual manner to such stimuli as acute hemorrhage; however, their erythroid values return only to the level previously determined by the decreased oxygen requirements, not to normal. In contrast to other anemic states, cardiac output is not increased (another reflection of the "normalcy" of the reduced hemoglobin content of the blood for the hypothyroid patient).

Symptoms, physical findings, and other laboratory abnormalities are those of hypothyroidism and cannot be attributed to the reduced oxygen-carrying capacity of the blood. This secondary hematologic manifestation of hypothyroidism responds *only* to thyroid replacement therapy. The anemia will not be affected by any other therapeutic agents. In the absence of some complication (e.g., acute hemorrhage), transfusions are *never* indicated. Transfusing a patient with hypothyroidism would be equivalent to transfusing a normal subject; as a result, erythropoiesis would be depressed because of relative tissue hyperoxia. The institution of thyroid therapy is not followed by a reticulocytosis or a rapid increase in the peripheral erythroid values. Instead, increases in red cell mass and marrow cellularity occur slowly and parallel the increase in oxygen consumption. Normal peripheral erythroid values may not be restored for several months.

Two other types of deficiency anemia deserve mention, for they occur with greater frequency in patients with hypothyroidism than in euthyroid subjects. The incidence of addisonian pernicious anemia is many times higher in patients with hypothyroidism than in the rest of the population. In addition, dietary inadequacy consequent to the hypothyroidism (e.g., decreased activity and lack of interest) predisposes to the development of nutritional folic acid deficiency. Thus a deficiency of vitamin B_{12} or folic acid often complicates hypothyroidism and produces the characteristic clinical and hematologic manifestations of a megaloblastic, macrocytic anemia (p. 203). Such occurrences were apparently responsible for the once widely held view that the anemia of hypothyroidism was characteristically macrocytic. Hypothyroid patients with a superimposed megaloblastic anemia respond to appropriate replacement therapy (i.e., vitamin B_{12} or folic acid), but unless the patient is simultaneously treated with thyroid, the peripheral erythroid values will increase only to that level needed to maintain adequate tissue oxygenation in the hypometabolic state. Iron deficiency also occurs with increased frequency in hypothyroid patients. Menorrhagia and metrorrhagia are quite common and contribute importantly to negative iron balance. The diagnosis and treatment of iron deficiency anemia are discussed elsewhere (p. 180).

Addison's Disease (Hypoadrenocorticosteroidism). Patients with Addison's disease typically manifest a slight to moderate normocytic, normochromic anemia which appears to reflect diminished production consequent to hypometabolism and decreased oxygen requirements. Red cell mass is disproportionately more reduced than are the peripheral erythroid values consequent to the contracted plasma volume that characterizes adrenocortical insufficiency. Because of the effects of the corticosteroids on other hemic cells (p. 314), hypoadrenocorticosteroidism is also accompanied by a leukopenia with neutropenia, eosinophilia, and a relative lymphocytosis. Normal hematologic values are restored slowly after the institution of adequate replacement therapy.

Hypopituitarism. Hypofunction of the anterior lobe of the pituitary is accompanied by a slight-to-moderate normocytic, normochromic anemia. Abundant experimental evidence indicates that the decrease in red cell mass is the result of deficiencies of thyrotropic and adrenocorticotropic hormones (the concept of a specific pituitary erythropoietic factor is no longer tenable). Thus the hematologic manifestations of hypopituitarism reflect the combined effects of hypothyroidism and hypoadrenocorticosteroidism and include the leukocyte changes of the latter. The hematologic abnormalities are corrected by thyroid and corticosteroid therapy.

NUTRIENTS

A variety of substances is known to be essential in animals for the maintenance of the normal erythroid steady state. Deficiencies of such nutrients as amino acids, ascorbic acid, riboflavin, nicotinic acid, pyridoxine, tryptophan, pantothenic acid, copper, and cobalt will, in certain species, cause an anemia that is correctable by specific replacement therapy. However, there is no proof that a deficiency of any of these substances is responsible for anemia in man. Thus there are no clinical counterparts for the cobalt deficiency anemia of herbivorous ruminants (cattle and sheep) in such geographic locales as Australia or Florida, the hypochromic anemia of copper-deficient rats, the anemia of hypoproteinemic dogs or rats, and the hypochromic anemia of pyridoxine-deficient swine. A few patients have been observed with pyridoxine-responsive anemias, but these persons are not pyridoxine deficient (p. 178). Vitamin C plays a role in erythropoiesis, and patients with scurvy are commonly anemic; however, the anemia is usually the result of superimposed folic acid deficiency (p. 197), or it reflects chronic bleeding and iron deficiency (p. 171).

Three other nutrients (iron, vitamin B_{12}, and folic acid) are absolutely essential for normal human erythropoietic activity. Deficiencies of these factors are invariably characterized by anemia. Iron deficiency produces a microcytic, hypochromic anemia, and vitamin B_{12} and/or folic acid deficiencies are manifested by a megaloblastic, macrocytic anemia. These deficiency states account for the majority of the anemias encountered in clinical medicine and are considered in detail.

Iron Deficiency Anemia

Iron is an integral part (0.347 per cent) of the hemoglobin molecule. To maintain the erythroid steady state a normal adult requires about 20 to 25 mg of elemental iron each day to replace the hemoglobin lost consequent to normal red cell attrition. When body iron is so depleted that this requirement cannot be met, the amount of hemoglobin synthesized by each developing erythrocyte is quantitatively curtailed; total marrow output of hemoglobin falls, and a microcytic, hypochromic anemia ensues. Iron deficiency is one of the most frequently encountered disorders in clinical medicine and the commonest cause of a microcytic, hypochromic anemia. Although most hypochromic anemias are caused by iron lack, this morphologic diagnosis is *not* synonymous with the designation of iron deficiency anemia or depleted iron stores. Any defect in the ability of a red cell to fabricate the hemoglobin molecule will produce similar morphologic changes. Thus deficient globin formation (e.g., the thalassemia syndromes, p. 268) or porphyrin synthesis (e.g., pyridoxine-responsive anemia, p. 178) decrease corpuscular hemoglobin concentration; morphologically, these cells also appear hypochromic. Practically, however, a microcytic, hypochromic anemia implies iron deficiency until disproved because of the relative rarity of the other causes of this type of anemia. Since most of the body's iron is contained in hemoglobin and because this metal is tenaciously conserved, iron deficiency anemias generally reflect chronic blood loss.

HISTORY

Medicinal attributes were ascribed to iron in ancient civilizations; however, the indications governing its use were largely symbolic and based on certain divine and mystical qualities attributed to the metal (e.g., those of strength). Sydenham introduced iron into clinical medicine in the seventeenth century as a remedy for chlorosis (a malady first described clearly by Lange in 1554 and subsequently shown to be iron deficiency anemia). In 1713 Lemery and Geoffy provided a scientific basis for such therapy when they demonstrated iron in the ash of blood. Menghini showed, in 1746, that iron-rich diets would enhance the iron content of the blood. In 1832 Fodisch pointed out the deficiency of iron in the blood of patients with chlorosis, but even before this discovery Pierre Blaud demonstrated unequivocally the value of large oral doses of ferrous sulfate in the treatment of this disorder. The remarkable efficacy of the "veritable pills of Dr. Blaud" received immediate and widespread confirmation, and the principles of iron therapy laid down by him stand basically intact today. In 1845 Popp noted pallor of the individual red cells in patients with chlorosis. Duncan accurately described hypochromia in 1867 and recognized that the major defect was impaired hemoglobin synthesis.

Toward the close of the nineteenth century, the use of inorganic iron as a therapeutic agent fell into disrepute, despite the incontrovertible evidence of its effectiveness by numerous clinicians, including such astute observers as Osler. The "credit" for this backward step in medical progress goes largely to Bunge, a prestigious person, who concluded, on the basis of inadequate experimental data, that inorganic iron could not be utilized by the human body for the synthesis of hemoglobin. About the same time Quincke and van Noorden advocated the use of very small and ineffectual doses of iron instead of the larger amounts previously employed. These teachings profoundly affected medical practice, and the importance of iron deficiency anemia as a clinical problem increased dramatically. As recently as 1925, it was being stated emphatically that inorganic iron had no therapeutic value in anemia, despite the fact that Lichtenstein reintroduced large doses of inorganic iron and verified their value in 1918. Lindberg (1922) and Meulengracht (1923) published corroborative studies. Shortly thereafter the remarkable results of earlier clinicians were widely reaffirmed, and it was demonstrated conclusively by Heath and co-workers in 1932 that inorganic iron was incorporated into hemoglobin. Thus a completely efficacious treatment was once again available for the patient with iron deficiency anemia.

During the last 25 years, the features of normal iron metabolism have been worked out largely by isotopic tracer techniques. As a result, the pathogenesis and pathophysiology of iron deficiency have been greatly clarified.

IRON METABOLISM

Iron is required for the sustenance of life. This widely distributed metal has several vital functions. It readily undergoes oxidation and reduction and is incorporated into a number of enzymes concerned with electron transport (e.g., cytochromes, catalase, peroxidase, and succinic dehydrogenase). Certain iron-porphyrin-protein complexes have the ability to combine reversibly with oxygen and are used for its transport (hemoglobin) and storage (myoglobin). The body conserves and reuses iron in a miserly fashion. Consequently, knowledge of normal iron metabolism is a prerequisite for a discussion of the causes and pathophysiology of iron deficiency.

Requirements. The approximate distribution of the iron contained in a normal-sized adult is depicted in Table 5-1. At any one time the majority (about two thirds) of the body iron is incorporated in the hemoglobin molecule. Therefore requirements are, for the most part, determined by the amount of hemoglobin needed to replace that lost by normal red cell catabolism. About 20 to 25 mg of elemental iron are required daily for this purpose; however, an equivalent amount is made available by the destruction of effete erythrocytes and can be reutilized for the synthesis of hemoglobin. Consequently, exogenous iron requirements reflect the amount lost from the body. Because the retentive capacity is great (there is no normal effective excretory mechanism to

Table 5-1. *Average Distribution of Iron in a Normal-Sized Adult*

	PER CENT	MILLIGRAMS
Hemoglobin	65	2600
Storage iron		
(ferritin and hemosiderin)	29	1160
Myoglobin	3.5	140
Iron in transit		
(iron-transferrin complex)	0.1	4
Labile iron pool	2.2	88
Enzyme iron	0.2	8
Total	100.0	4000

rid the body of iron), these needs are small; nonetheless, they are quite real and physiologically important.

Average daily exogenous iron requirements are shown in Table 5-2.

Table 5-2. *Normal Daily Iron Requirements*

Adult males and nonmenstruating females	0.5 to 1.5 mg
Menstruating females	1.0 to 2.5 mg
Pregnant females	2.0 to 3.5 mg
Children	0.5 to 1.0 mg

The adult male with a normal complement of iron "excretes" about 0.5 to 1.5 mg/day. There are very small amounts of iron in the urine, and the feces contain about 0.5 mg derived from bile and gastrointestinal mucosal cells (all body cells contain enzymatic iron). The remainder of the daily obligatory loss is dermal (desquamated cells, hair, nails, and sweat). Requirements of the postmenopausal or nonmenstruating female are similar to those of the adult male.

During the childbearing period menses augment the female's needs. "Normal" menstrual bleeding is quite variable and can range from less than 10 to more than 150 ml. Average blood loss per period amounts to 35 to 70 ml and contains about 17.5 to 35 mg of iron (there are approximately 50 mg of iron in each 100 ml of whole blood). Thus most menstruating females require an additional 0.5 to 1.0 mg of elemental iron per day to maintain positive iron balance. Pregnancy constitutes another physiologic drain of about 500 mg of iron; however, conservation of iron consequent to amenorrhea reduces the requirements during pregnancy to only 1.0 mg (or less) per day more than those of a nonpregnant menstruating female. Lactation imposes an additional burden of about 1 mg of iron per day, but the accompanying amenorrhea negates a substantial part of this demand.

At birth the average full-term infant possesses about 250 mg of iron.

Normal growth necessitates the acquisition of an additional 200 to 300 mg during the first year of life (about 0.8 mg/day). Thereafter 0.5 to 1.0 mg/day will maintain positive iron balance and provide for the creation of normal adult stores. During adolescence active growth temporarily increases the need for iron. When adult stature is reached, requirements revert to those of the normal adult.

Absorption.   The iron required to maintain positive iron balance is derived from dietary sources. The average diet in the United States contains about 10 to 20 mg of elemental iron. Of this quantity, 10 per cent or less is absorbed by the normal individual. In persons with increased need, up to 30 per cent of food iron may be absorbed, but this amount appears to be the maximum that can be extracted from a normal diet even in the face of depleted iron stores. Inorganic iron salts are assimilated much more efficiently than organic or food iron. A normal person can absorb as much as 20 per cent of a physiologic amount of inorganic iron, and an iron-deficient subject may retain as much as 60 per cent. Iron is absorbed chiefly, if not entirely, in the bivalent (ferrous) form. Because most of the iron in food occurs as ferric hydroxide complexes or exists as trivalent iron bound to amino acids, proteins, or other organic radicals, it must be split off and chemically reduced before absorption. Contrary to a once widely held view, hydrochloric acid plays no apparent role in the absorption of iron, and an acid medium does not enhance this physiologic process.

The availability of iron in different foodstuffs varies; for example, hemoglobin iron is absorbed more readily than is that contained in vegetables or eggs. Large doses of ascorbic acid facilitate absorption (probably through its reducing capacity); phosphates and phytates retard absorption (probably by forming insoluble compounds). Bile exerts no demonstrable effect on iron absorption, but some experimental data suggest that normal gastric secretions may contain a substance that prevents the precipitation of relatively insoluble iron hydroxide in the alkaline medium of the small intestine. There is also some indirect evidence that pancreatic secretions may retard iron absorption (increased iron stores have been observed in association with pancreatic insufficiency and following pancreatic duct ligation).

A small amount of iron appears to be absorbed in the stomach, but most of it is assimilated in the proximal duodenum, with absorption decreasing progressively in the more distal segments of the small intestine. Iron enters the blood directly and is not absorbed through the lymphatics. Absorption begins promptly and is virtually complete within one to two hours. Little is known about the actual mechanism by which iron enters into and is transported across the mucosal cell. It appears to be an active transport system contingent on an energy-producing metabolic reaction. Numerous theories have been proposed on the basis of rather scant experimental and/or clinical evidence. The most popular hypothesis has envisaged ferritin as playing a fundamental role in the transport of iron across the mucosal cell; however, there is little support for this contention. The ferritin contained in the gastrointestinal mucosa probably reflects a nontoxic form of storage iron, as it does in other tissues. In view of the great avidity of ionic iron for a variety of organic radicals, it most likely traverses the mucosal cell in a chelated or bound form, perhaps as an iron-amino acid complex. More precise definition must await further study.

Inasmuch as there is no effective excretory mechanism for iron, some type of absorptive regulatory control must exist to prevent overload. Despite intensive effort on the part of many investigators, the actual mechanisms governing the absorption of iron are poorly understood and continue to be the subject of much speculation and dispute. Factors known to enhance absorption include (1) depleted iron stores, (2) an increased rate of erythropoiesis, (3) anemia, and (4) hypoxia. It is evident that no single factor exerts primary control to the exclusion of the others. Although their effects may, to a certain extent, be additive, they are capable of affecting iron absorption independently. The manner by which these stimuli are transmitted to the gastrointestinal mucosa is unknown. Attempts to demonstrate a humoral agent or agents have failed. Erythropoietin is not a common mediator; although it enhances iron absorption, it does so by increasing erythropoietic activity. If the normal marrow response is prevented by some myelosuppressive agent, erythropoietin will not affect iron absorption. Furthermore, decreased iron stores augment iron absorption in the absence of anemia or increased erythropoietin levels.

Much has been written about the regulatory effect of ferritin on the absorption of iron and the "mucosal block." According to this theory, apoferritin in the gastrointestinal mucosal cell acts as the acceptor for iron, and, when saturated, no more iron can be absorbed. This concept has now been largely disproved, and such a "mucosal block" appears to be an artificial and unphysiologic phenomenon. Although large quantities of inorganic iron will adversely affect absorption of subsequent doses for a period of four to six hours, it is doubtful that physiologic amounts can activate this mechanism. Moreover, there is a relatively constant relationship between a dose of iron regardless of its size and the amount absorbed; increasing the dose is always associated with the absorption of a greater quantity. Furthermore, assimilation remains high in the face of a stimulus, such as increased erythropoiesis, despite the presence of augmented tissue iron stores. Thus ferritin cannot exert primary control over iron absorption.

It seems likely, however, that the ferritin apparatus may contribute to the maintenance of the iron balance by acting as an excretory mechanism of limited capacity. Since the mucosal lining of the gastrointestinal tract is entirely replaced every three days, ferritin iron is lost when these deciduous cells are shed. Therefore complexing in the mucosal cell of apoferritin and iron (either iron that has just entered the cell from the lumen of the gastrointestinal tract or previously absorbed iron that has been carried to the cell by the normal plasma transport mechanism) may be a means of preventing the entrance into or ridding the body of some (but certainly not all) unwanted iron.

Transport. Iron enters the plasma in the bivalent form, where it is promptly oxidized and tightly bound to transferrin (also known as siderophilin or iron-binding protein). This β_1 globulin is a true iron carrier, and each molecule of transferrin can bind two atoms of trivalent iron. The resulting iron-transferrin complex is extremely stable at a physiologic pH. A number of genetically determined variants of transferrin have been observed; each is equally capable of binding and transporting iron. The half-life of transferrin is about 10 days, whereas the half-life of plasma iron is only one to two hours. Thus the iron-binding protein releases iron to the tissues and becomes free to carry additional iron. Normally the plasma (or serum) iron-binding capacity is around 300 μg/100 ml (range—250 to 400) and is about one third saturated. The mechanisms controlling the blood transferrin level are unknown. The iron-binding capacity is increased in iron deficiency anemia, acute hepatitis, and the last trimester of pregnancy; it is normal or decreased in most other kinds of anemia. Iron-binding capacity is decreased in the presence of acute or chronic infections and in patients with certain types of hypoproteinemia (e.g., those with nephrosis). Rare patients with congenital atransferrinemia have been described.

In the average adult approximately 4 mg of elemental iron are in transit. The normal plasma iron is about 100 μg/100 ml (range—50 to 200) and is firmly chelated with transferrin. Free or ionic iron can be found in the plasma only in persons with acute iron poisoning or following parenteral iron therapy. Plasma iron reflects iron being transported from the gastrointestinal tract and sites of red cell breakdown to or from the marrow or extramedullary storage sites. Daily plasma iron turnover amounts to about 40 mg in the average adult male. Normally, plasma iron levels are characterized by a rather striking diurnal variation (as much as 100 μg/100 ml) with the highest values being observed in the morning and the lowest in the late afternoon or evening. Plasma iron is decreased in iron-deficient subjects as well as in those with infections or hypotransferrinemia. Hyperferremia accompanies iron overload (idiopathic hemochromatosis or transfusion hemosiderosis), acute hepatitis, hemolytic anemias, and anemias due to impaired erythrocytogenesis of varied causes (e.g., megaloblastic and hypoplastic anemia).

Storage. Iron stores in the normal adult amount to about 1.0 to 1.5 gm. Most of this iron is in the liver, spleen, and bone marrow and is about equally divided between two forms—ferritin and hemosiderin. Ferritin is approximately 20 per cent iron and consists of a protein, apoferritin, and scattered micelles of a ferric hydroxide-phosphate complex with an approximate composition of $(FeOOH)_8 FeOPO_3H_2$. This iron compound is water-soluble and is in a unique magnetic state because of the presence of three unpaired electrons in each iron atom. Molecules of ferritin are too small to be visualized with an ordinary microscope but can be demonstrated by electron microscopy. The formation of ferritin appears to depend on energy-producing oxidative metabolic reactions, although the precise details remain to be worked out. Oxidizing agents enhance the complexing of iron and apoferritin. Reducing substances and hypoxia favor release of iron from the ferritin molecules; there is some evidence that xanthine oxidase also participates in this process. In addition to its importance as a readily available, nontoxic form of iron, ferritin may have other physiologic functions. Vasodepressor and antidiuretic effects have been ascribed to ferritin, although proof of such biologic activities is lacking.

The exact nature of hemosiderin is unknown. It contains ferritin, and certain data indicate that hemosiderin is made up of clusters or aggregates of ferritin molecules. However, other observations point to clear-cut differences. Nearly 40 per cent of the dry weight of hemosiderin is iron, and it contains porphyrin and other substances not present in ferritin. Furthermore, hemosiderin does not appear to be a physicochemically homogeneous compound. Hemosiderin is insoluble in water and is visible by ordinary microscopy as golden-yellow refractile granules; it stains readily with Prussian blue.

Although there are evident differences between ferritin and hemosiderin, these substances are closely related insofar as function is concerned. Iron first enters the storage compartment as ferritin. As ferritin stores accumulate hemosiderin begins to appear. In cases of iron overload, hemosiderin predominates. Stored iron is released slowly on demand, and both ferritin and hemosiderin are available and can be used as needed for the synthesis of hemoglobin and to supply the other needs of the body for iron; however, ferritin is more immediately available than hemosiderin. There is no direct continuity between the storage compartment and circulating iron. The latter does not mix uniformly with storage iron; dispersion of a tracer dose of radioactive iron into the total miscible iron pool may require a year or longer. Radioisotopic studies also indicate that a certain proportion of the iron stores is relatively inert, probably the larger hemosiderin granules. Such iron is miscible with the rest of the body iron only with difficulty and over a long period of time.

Labile Iron Pool. The existence of this iron compartment is based on radioisotopic data. Although its chemical nature and anatomic localization are not known, its size has been estimated to be about 85 mg in the normal adult. This labile iron pool might best be envisaged as intermediate between plasma and hemoglobin iron. It is freely mixable with the plasma iron (but not with storage iron) and is available for immediate use. It has been suggested (but not proved) that this iron is reversibly bound to the membrane of marrow erythrocytic precursors. From this location it may enter the cell and be incorporated into the hemoglobin molecule, or it may be transported via transferrin to some other site.

Utilization. Almost 100 per cent of a physiologic amount of iron absorbed from the gastrointestinal tract or injected directly into the blood is destined for the marrow. Half is cleared from the plasma in about 90 minutes; approximately 10 days later about 80 per cent of this iron is contained in hemoglobin of circulating erythrocytes. The mechanisms that prevent plasma iron from mixing freely with stored iron are not well understood. Newly acquired iron does not enter the storage compartment directly but instead becomes a part of the labile pool which is used preferentially for hemoglobin synthesis. Transferrin appears to play a major role in this process. Iron not bound to transferrin (e.g., parenterally administered iron) is cleared rapidly from the plasma and deposited in reticuloendothelial cells in the liver, spleen, and elsewhere. On the other hand, the iron-transferrin complex has a great affinity for developing erythrocytes and resists giving up its iron to other cells or tissues. Maximal transfer of iron to erythrocytic precursors occurs when the plasma iron-binding capacity is 20 to 60 per cent saturated. When the saturation exceeds 60 per cent, nonspecific unloading takes place and iron is "shunted" to storage sites. Observations on patients with atransferrinemia support this mechanism; these persons have a hypochromic, microcytic anemia despite increased iron stores.

Although delivery of iron to the developing erythrocytes by transferrin plays a major role in iron utilization, it may not be the only mechanism. Direct transfer of ferritin molecules from marrow reticulum cells to nucleated erythrocytes has been demonstrated by electron microscopy. This process, which can be likened to pinocytosis, has been termed rhopheocytosis. Transfer of ferritin molecules in this manner cannot be denied; however, its precise physiologic significance has been questioned by some who have suggested that the direction of movement may actually be from the erythrocytic precursor to the reticulum cell. Both mechanisms may operate, but the transfer of iron to erythrocytic precursors by way of transferrin appears to be the more important. This type of iron transfer is related to an energy-producing metabolic reaction. Once within the cell, iron becomes associated with particulate matter, that is, mitochondria and microsomes, and is subsequently incorporated into the hemoglobin molecule (p. 20).

PATHOPHYSIOLOGY OF IRON DEFICIENCY

The clinical manifestations attributable to iron deficiency are the same, regardless of the cause of the negative iron balance. Iron stores are affected first and gradually give up their iron to supply the body's needs and replace that which is lost. The storage compartment must be exhausted before altered physiology occurs; however, there is a small portion that is relatively inert and miscible with the rest of the body iron only after a long period of time. Consequently, some storage iron may be demonstrable (e.g., a few large hemosiderin granules in the bone marrow), even though the readily available iron stores have been exhausted. When reserves are depleted, deficiency exists even though normal function can be maintained because of the body's ability to reutilize iron. As negative iron balance continues, other effects of the deficiency state become evident. Plasma iron falls below 50 µg/100 ml, and plasma iron-binding capacity (the transferrin level) increases. Absorption of food iron undergoes as much as a threefold increase. If this mechanism supplies enough iron (it rarely can), other abnormalities may be prevented, although the storage compartment will remain empty. It is extremely difficult, if not impossible, to replenish iron stores from normal dietary sources alone. In most cases negative iron balance continues and the clinical manifestations of iron deficiency appear. Because most of the body's iron is contained in hemoglobin, it is not surprising that hematologic abnormalities (i.e., an iron deficiency anemia) dominate the clinical picture.

Hematologic Effects. The iron content of hemoglobin is fixed; it is impossible to synthesize a hemoglobin molecule with less than four atoms of iron. Each milliliter of normal erythrocytes contains about 1 mg of iron. When body iron is less than the amount needed to maintain a normal hemoglobin level, anemia is inevitable. Iron deficiency curtails the quantity of hemoglobin produced. Other aspects of erythropoiesis are not affected. For example, porphyrin synthesis is not depressed and free protoporphyrin is increased in the erythrocytes of iron-deficient subjects. As the circulating hemoglobin levels decrease, plasma erythropoietic factor activity increases, and marrow erythrocytic hyperplasia ensues. The normal ratio between immature and mature nucleated red cells is maintained, thus indicating that mitotic proliferation and cell maturation proceed in an essentially normal fashion. Since the erythrocytic precursors are unable to synthesize a normal complement of hemoglobin, the more mature nucleated red cells exhibit impaired hemoglobinization. The concentration and content of hemoglobin in mature erythrocytes decrease and are manifested morphologically by hypochromia and small cells. In other words, hemoglobin synthesis fails to keep pace with cell proliferation and the hemoglobin and hematocrit levels are disproportionately lower than the red cell count. Therefore a microcytic, hypochromic anemia is the hematologic manifestation of iron deficiency.

It is often stated that an iron deficiency anemia is initially normocytic and normochromic. This contention is without proof and is teleologically untenable. If iron lack could produce a normocytic, normochromic anemia, it would be necessary to postulate some mechanism such as decreased input from the stem cell compartment or decreased proliferation of nucleated red cells. Since marked iron deficiency is *always* manifested by a microcytic, hypochromic anemia and a hypercellular marrow, it is difficult to envisage minimal iron deficiency as decreasing stem cell-erythrocytic differentiation or mitotic activity of precursor cells. Provided with well-stained, well-made peripheral blood films, a trained observer can always discern hypochromia and microcytes even in patients whose erythroid values are only slightly below the lower limits of normal. It should be noted that the magnitude of these changes varies directly with the degree of iron depletion. Early, these morphologic findings are slight and can be easily missed in poor preparations; furthermore, derived cell indexes are normal at this stage in the development of an iron deficiency anemia. However, the failure to perceive minimal morphologic abnormalities or to detect the presence of a few abnormal cells by decreases in mean corpuscular volume or hemoglobin concentration (at best an inaccurate means of categorizing an anemia morphologically, p. 59) does not justify the classification of an iron deficiency anemia as normocytic or normochromic.

The symptoms and physical findings of an iron deficiency anemia are basically those attributable to a reduction in the oxygen-carrying capacity of the blood, regardless of cause. Other aspects of hematopoiesis fail to exhibit clear-cut or consistent abnormalities. Splenomegaly occurs in about 10 per cent of patients (usually those with more marked depletion of body iron); its cause is obscure, but extramedullary hematopoiesis may be at least partly responsible for this finding.

Tissue Iron Deficiency. Iron performs functions in addition to its role in the transport of oxygen. Therefore restricted hemoglobin synthesis should not be the only manifestation of iron deficiency. Until recently, it was generally conceded that iron-containing enzymes were inviolable even in the face of profound iron deficiency. It is now known that certain of these enzymes are decreased in iron-depleted subjects, as are myoglobin and the iron content of epithelial and mucosal cells; however, the pathophysiologic significance of such inadequacies has not yet been established. There is no proof that deficiencies of iron-containing enzymes limit normal metabolic processes. Tissue oxygen consumption is normal in the presence of exhausted iron stores and is not influenced by iron repletion.

Attempts to attribute symptoms in nonanemic patients to enzyme deficiencies have not been convincing. In view of the essential function of the iron-containing oxidative enzymes, it is unlikely that their activities would be curtailed before hemoglobin synthesis was affected. On the other hand, as negative iron balance progresses, it seems reasonable that dysfunction would occur as the result of tissue iron deficiency. Tongue changes (atrophy of the filiform papillae and a decrease in keratohyalin granules) are rather commonly associated with marked iron depletion and may be a reflection of inadequate iron in the epithelial cells. Cheilitis, glossitis, stomatitis, esophageal webbing and dysphagia, gastritis, gastric atrophy, and achlorhydria probably reflect a similar pathogenic mechanism. Occasionally, severe deficiency states are associated with changes in other mucous membranes (e.g., vaginitis and proctitis). Koilonychia (flattening or concavity of the nails together with brittleness and irregularities) accompanies iron deficiency anemia with sufficient regularity to suggest a causal relationship. These nail changes may be explicable, at least in part, on the basis of decreased tissue iron.

ETIOLOGY

Iron deficiency may result from inadequate intake, impaired absorption, increased requirements, or excessive loss. An iron deficiency anemia is not a disease *sui generis* but is always secondary to some other primary abnormality. Because of the size of the storage compartment and the efficiency with which iron is reused, most iron deficiency anemias are caused by augmented loss. Since there is no effective excretory mechanism and the majority of the body iron is contained in the hemoglobin molecule, increased iron loss is contingent on abnormal bleeding. For practical purposes, therefore, an iron deficiency anemia indicates blood loss until proved otherwise. In some cases multiple factors act conjointly; for example, dietary inadequacy in a pregnant woman with increased requirements and depleted iron stores consequent to prior menorrhagia.

Inadequate Intake. The normal diet contains approximately 10 to 20 mg of iron; normally, about 10 per cent is absorbed. Because dietary iron barely meets the minimal daily requirements (Table 5-2), decreased intake would theoretically appear to play an important role in the pathogenesis of iron deficiency. Actually, it is almost never the *sole* cause of an iron deficiency anemia. As iron stores fall, daily loss decreases and a greater proportion of food iron is absorbed (up to 30 per cent). Almost every type of food contains some naturally occurring iron; in addition, many foods such as bread are fortified with iron. Consequently, it is almost impossible to subsist on an iron-free diet. Furthermore, several years would be needed to exhaust body stores even if the diet were devoid of iron and daily loss remained at the upper limits of normal. For these reasons nutritional inadequacy alone is *not* an acceptable explanation for an iron deficiency anemia in an otherwise normal adult.

However, inadequate dietary intake may contribute significantly to the development of an iron deficiency anemia during periods of increased need (e.g., infancy, puberty, and pregnancy). Even under prime socioeconomic conditions, an infant's diet rarely provides more than 4 to 6 mg of iron per day during the first four to five months of life (all types of milk are uniquely low in iron). Between the age of 6 to 12 months the minimal daily dietary requirement is about 8 mg (approximately 10 per cent is absorbed). Few diets supply more than this amount. Because an infant's iron stores are quite meager, he is dependent on dietary sources to meet his rapidly increasing needs. Therefore iron balance is in a precarious state in all infants, and a less than optimal intake can readily produce an iron deficiency anemia. Because of their increased needs, even a normal diet fails to supply premature infants with enough iron, and supplementation with inorganic iron is essential to prevent anemia. Suboptimal dietary intake throughout childhood may preclude the acquisition of normal adult stores, thereby contributing to the development of iron deficiency during periods of rapid adolescent growth. Decreased intake of food iron may also potentiate negative iron balance in pregnant women as well as in patients with impaired absorption or chronic blood loss.

Impaired Absorption. Gastrointestinal abnormalities that interfere with the absorption of iron contribute importantly to the development of iron deficiency, especially in conjunction with bleeding or increased iron requirements. Negative iron balance is more marked in the presence of absorptive defects than that which would result from the loss of dietary iron alone because of the quantity of iron (normally about 1 mg/day) contained in bile. Under normal circumstances most of this biliary iron is promptly reabsorbed, but in patients with impaired absorption, it is lost, thus contributing to the depletion of iron stores. Although decreased gastric acidity was once believed to be an important factor in the production of an iron deficiency anemia, it is now clear that achlorhydric patients absorb iron well and maintain iron balance without difficulty. Several gastrointestinal disorders affect iron absorption adversely.

GASTRECTOMY AND GASTROENTEROSTOMY. A significant number of patients develop an iron deficiency anemia during the first 6 to 12 months after gastric resection. These patients absorb inorganic iron salts normally. Although they can also absorb physiologic amounts of food iron without much difficulty, they are unable to increase absorption of dietary iron in response to increased need (e.g., depleted iron stores). Consequently, the gastrectomized patient cannot replenish storage iron from dietary sources alone, a difficult task at best. A requisite for the development of an iron deficiency anemia following gastrectomy appears to be exhausted iron stores secondary to blood loss from the lesion for which the gastrectomy was performed (e.g., a peptic ulcer). These patients are usually transfused before and during surgery so that their peripheral erythroid values are normal at the time of discharge from the hospital. Unless they are treated with inorganic iron, however, their storage compartments remain depleted and even minor defects in absorption are soon manifested by an iron deficiency anemia. Therefore it is not necessary to demonstrate persistent bleeding to explain an iron deficiency anemia developing after gastrectomy. It is unlikely that gastric resection will be followed by iron deficiency if the patient has normal iron stores at the time of surgery, provided, of course, that bleeding does not occur postoperatively.

Inasmuch as iron is assimilated mainly in the duodenum and proximal jejunum, absorption will be affected adversely by a bypass around these sites (e.g., a gastroenterostomy) or by intestinal hurry. Such a mechanism is rarely, if ever, the sole cause of an iron deficiency anemia; however, it is often an important factor in preventing a normal therapeutic response. In some patients iron tablets may not dissolve until after they have passed the absorptive areas (these individuals respond satisfactorily to inorganic iron in liquid form).

MALABSORPTION SYNDROMES. Through loss of absorptive surface, diseases of the upper small intestine, such as celiac disease, idiopathic steatorrhea, and tropical sprue, interfere with the absorption of a variety of nutrients, including iron. As a result, certain of these individuals develop an iron deficiency anemia (a megaloblastic anemia caused by defective absorption of vitamin B_{12} or folic acid may also accompany these disorders, p. 200). Most patients with an iron deficiency anemia secondary to a malabsorption syndrome respond satisfactorily to oral treatment, and it is seldom necessary to resort to parenteral therapy. Therefore the absorptive block must be a relative one. In some cases the defect in absorption acts in a cumulative fashion with other factors such as blood loss to deplete iron stores. Impaired iron absorption may also contribute to the causation of anemia in other diseases of the small intestine (e.g., regional enteritis), but chronic blood loss would appear to be of greater pathogenic importance in most of these situations.

IDIOPATHIC IRON DEFICIENCY ANEMIA. Rare patients appear to have an isolated defect in iron absorption, the nature of which is obscure.

These individuals are usually middle-aged females with achlorhydria and a long history of a microcytic, hypochromic anemia that has been unresponsive to oral iron therapy. They exhibit none of the other manifestations of a malabsorption syndrome (e.g., steatorrhea). Although oral iron is ineffective, response to parenteral iron is prompt and complete. Such individuals must not be confused with those who are iron deficient because of occult bleeding, increased requirements, and so forth. The latter do not exhibit abnormalities in iron absorption and respond optimally to oral replacement therapy. There are only a few well-documented reports of patients falling into this category.

Increased Requirements. INFANCY AND CHILDHOOD. At birth the average, full-term infant possesses about 250 mg of iron, most of which is in hemoglobin; the storage compartment is small (approximately 35 mg). During the first year of life normal growth and an expanding red cell mass entail the accruement of at least 150 mg of iron. Erythropoiesis decreases promptly after birth, and the elevated peripheral erythroid values characterizing the fetus fall rapidly to normal postnatal levels. As a result, sufficient iron is made available to the infant to supply his needs for the first six months. After this age about 0.8 mg of iron must be assimilated from dietary sources each day to end the first year of life in positive iron balance. Several factors influence iron metabolism in infancy. Too early clamping and failure to strip the cord can deprive the infant of erythrocytes containing as much as 40 mg of iron. Infants born with peripheral erythroid values at the lower limits of normal may require exogenous iron (about 0.8 mg/day) as early as three months of age. A birth weight less than normal is another contributing factor because of the infant's smaller red cell mass. The status of the maternal iron stores may also play a limited role, but an infant ordinarily receives his complement of iron at the mother's expense. In cases of severe maternal iron deficiency infants may be born with less than an optimal amount of iron.

Prematurity is perhaps the most important factor affecting iron balance throughout the first few months of life. Since most of an infant's iron is acquired during the last few weeks of gestation, premature birth will deprive him of this much-needed iron. If iron deficiency is to be prevented, exogenous iron will be needed by the end of the second month. It is virtually impossible for premature infants to obtain enough iron (about 0.8 mg/day) from food alone, and their diet should be supplemented with inorganic iron.

All young children (even normal, full-term infants) are in jeopardy of developing iron deficiency, for the best of diets barely fills an infant's needs. It is not surprising, therefore, that iron deficiency anemia, the commonest anemia of childhood, occurs in about 30 per cent of children between the ages of six months and three years. Blood loss or gross dietary inadequacy will, of course, increase the incidence and severity of such anemias. After the age of one or two years, iron requirements are less acute. However, adult iron stores must be acquired during the ensuing 14 to 18 years (about 0.5 mg of iron is needed each day in addition to the minimal daily requirements to accomplish this task). Most children eating normal diets have little difficulty in enlarging their storage compartments.

ADOLESCENCE. Rapid growth at puberty obligates about 200 to 300 mg of iron to take care of the augmentation in red cell mass and increase in muscle tissue. In adolescents with suboptimal dietary intakes or in those with inadequate stores, there may not be sufficient iron available to meet this increased need. Clinically, few adolescent males become iron-deficient on this basis, even though their growth rate is rapid. In girls, however, the additive effect of blood loss consequent to menarche increases the likelihood that an iron deficiency anemia will develop.

PREGNANCY AND LACTATION. The iron requirements of a normal pregnancy amount to about 500 mg, with half going to the fetus, around 75 mg to the placenta and cord, and approximately 175 mg in blood lost at the time of delivery or shortly thereafter. Because of the iron conserved by amenorrhea, the actual drain amounts to about 250 to 300 mg above the daily requirements of a normal menstruating female or approximately 3 mg/day during pregnancy. This daily requirement usually exceeds that which can be obtained from normal dietary sources. Furthermore, the need for iron is not evenly distributed throughout pregnancy but is most marked during the last few weeks of gestation. Most pregnant women are in negative iron balance before delivery. As iron stores are depleted, absorption of food iron increases, but daily requirements (especially during the last trimester) generally exceed the maximal amount that can be gleaned from a normal diet even by iron-deficient persons. In addition, inadequate intake or suboptimal iron stores resulting from earlier pregnancies or excessive blood loss often contribute importantly. For these reasons iron deficiency anemia (or at least negative iron balance and contraction of the storage compartment) can be expected in virtually all pregnant women who are not given supplemental inorganic iron. Lactation requires additional iron amounting to about 1 mg/day, but amenorrhea usually counteracts this deficit and daily requirements remain essentially what they are in a normal menstruating female.

Excessive Loss. Chronic recurrent bleeding is the commonest cause of an iron deficiency anemia and the only way that the metal can be lost from the body in sufficient amounts to deplete stores. There is no normal excretory mechanism whose overactivity might be implicated in iron loss. Although certain data suggest that the ferritin content of mucosal cells shed into the lumen of the gastrointestinal tract may constitute an excretory mechanism, its capacity is quite limited (probably less than 5 mg/day); furthermore, it appears to operate only in case of iron overload. Consequently, such a process cannot be implicated in the pathogenesis of iron deficiency. The iron content of blood is high (each milliliter of whole blood contains about 0.5 mg of elemental iron). Therefore even slight bleeding constitutes a significant loss of iron. The maximal amount of food iron that can be absorbed from a normal diet by a person with depleted iron stores is only 3 to 6 mg (30 per cent of total dietary iron amounting to 10 to 20 mg). If daily blood loss exceeds 6 to 12 ml, negative iron balance occurs. If bleeding persists for a long enough time, an iron deficiency anemia is inevitable. Hence even occult bleeding can lead to profound iron deficiency, and it is *not* necessary to demonstrate massive or even overt hemorrhage in order to implicate chronic bleeding as the cause of an iron deficiency anemia (about 80 ml of blood are required to produce a black, tarry stool). It is readily apparent from these figures that an increase in menstrual bleeding so slight as to pass unnoticed by the patient is quite capable of depleting body iron stores. An iron deficiency anemia is usually a manifestation of chronic bleeding. Self-limited, acute hemorrhage in a patient with normal iron stores causes a temporary normocytic, normochromic anemia (p. 69). However, if acute bleeding recurs often enough or is sufficiently massive, iron deficiency will result.

Since any disease process associated with bleeding can cause an iron deficiency anemia, a complete listing of all such disorders is purposeless. The gastrointestinal and genitourinary tracts are the most frequent sites of blood loss. Some of the commoner causes of iron deficiency anemia are peptic ulcer, hiatus hernia, gastrointestinal carcinoma, hookworm infestation, hemorrhoids, esophageal varices, ulcerative colitis, functional menorrhagia, and uterine fibroids. Although unusual, iron deficiency caused by excessive loss need not always reflect external bleeding. Patients with a disorder such as paroxysmal nocturnal hemoglobinuria may develop iron deficiency secondary to hemoglobinuria and hemosiderinuria (p. 151). In most instances bleeding into body cavities or tissues will not produce a microcytic, hypochromic anemia, for the iron will eventually be reabsorbed. However, in idiopathic pulmonary hemosiderosis (a rare disorder characterized by bleeding into the pulmonary parenchyma) anemia may occur because iron sequestered in the lungs is not physiologically available.

CLINICAL MANIFESTATIONS

The true incidence of iron deficiency anemia is not known, but it is the commonest type of anemia in the world and one of the most frequent problems encountered in clinical medicine. *An iron deficiency anemia is never a primary diagnosis and is always evidence of some underlying disorder.* The clinical manifestations of iron deficiency are the same regardless of cause; however, the actual clinical pictures vary considerably, for they also reflect the basic disease that is responsible for the depleted iron stores. Both sexes and all ages are susceptible. Iron deficiency anemia occurs in every race and in all parts of the world, although its prevalence depends on a number of contributory factors such as diet and extent of gastrointestinal parasitic infestation.

Symptoms. An iron deficiency anemia is a chronic disorder. Its onset is insidious and symptoms develop slowly over a period of several months. For the most part, complaints are relatively nonspecific and can be attributed to anemia; that is, weakness, ease of fatigue, tachycardia, and exertional dyspnea. Severity of symptoms varies directly with the magnitude of the anemia. In view of the chronicity of an iron deficiency anemia, normal physiologic adjustments to a decrease in the oxygen-carrying capacity of the blood may obscure symptoms until the peripheral erythroid values reach quite low levels. Headache is particularly common. Some patients with marked deficiency complain of a sore tongue or mouth, and dysphagia is prominent in a few. Nail changes (brittleness, deformities) generally accompany long-standing, severe iron deficiency. Anorexia and gastrointestinal disturbances may be secondary to iron deficiency alone, but more often than not they are manifestations of the primary underlying disease (e.g., weight loss, diarrhea, and melena may reflect a carcinoma of the colon). Since chronic blood loss is the usual cause of an iron deficiency anemia, patients often complain of abnormal bleeding (e.g., black tarry stools, menorrhagia, and hematuria). It should be re-emphasized, however, that bleeding is often occult or hidden.

Physical Findings. Pallor of the skin and mucous membranes is the most consistent physical manifestation of iron deficiency. Some patients with moderate to marked anemia exhibit blotchy, irregular denudation of the tongue. Less often there is evidence of generalized glossitis, cheilosis, stomatitis, or even proctitis or vaginitis. Slight splenomegaly (2 to 4 cm below the left costal margin on deep inspiration) occurs in 10 per cent or less of the patients (splenic enlargement is most likely to accompany the more marked deficiency states). Abnormalities of the nails (koilonychia) have been stressed but are not ordinarily observed; these changes include longitudinal ridging, brittleness, and flattening or concavity. Other physical findings reflect either the long-standing anemia (e.g., tachycardia and cardiac murmurs) or the primary disorder responsible for the negative iron balance such as an abdominal tumor mass, skin or mucous membrane lesions of hereditary telangiectasia (p. 482), and so forth.

Laboratory Findings. PERIPHERAL BLOOD. Iron deficiency is characterized by a microcytic, hypochromic anemia (Fig. 5-1). Early, the peripheral erythroid values are only slightly below normal, but patients with long-standing, severe iron deficiency can be markedly ane-

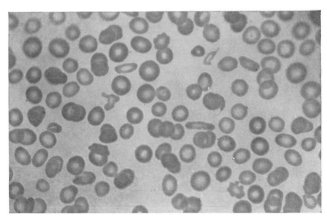

Figure 5-1. Peripheral blood film from a patient with an iron deficiency (microcytic, hypochromic) anemia (× 650).

mic with hemoglobin levels of 3 to 4 gm/100 ml of blood or even less. Morphologic abnormalities (hypochromia and microcytosis) affect most cells when the deficiency and the anemia are marked. In patients with mild iron deficiency, normal-appearing erythrocytes predominate and hypochromic microcytes may be few in number. At this stage in the development of an iron deficiency anemia, the cell indexes are usually normal and hypochromic cells may be easily overlooked. However, a trained observer has little difficulty making a correct morphologic classification on the basis of the peripheral blood film, regardless of the level of the erythroid values or the number of abnormal red cells present. Hypochromic erythrocytes are not normal constituents of the peripheral blood, and even rare cells displaying true hypochromia (an accentuation of the central area of pallor or achromia) are diagnostically significant. Microcytosis is another prominent feature (most hypochromic cells are smaller than normal). Anisocytosis varies from mild to marked, depending on the level of the erythroid values. Poikilocytosis is also common with pencil-shaped, tear-drop, and other bizarre-appearing erythrocytes. Leptocytes and target cells may be numerous. In markedly anemic patients an occasional nucleated red cell may be encountered in the peripheral blood. The reticulocyte count is most often normal or low; if increased, it usually reflects recent hemorrhage. Patients with an iron deficiency anemia are still able to respond (at least in an abortive fashion) to such stimuli as acute blood loss, for the lack is relative and never absolute. The plasma in an iron-deficient patient is unusually clear and almost colorless. The circulating leukocyte and platelet counts do not show consistent or uniform aberrations, although thrombocytosis is fairly common. In some patients with severe iron depletion, the leukocyte count may be slightly below normal.

BONE MARROW. There is a relative and absolute increase in erythropoiesis with an erythroid:granulocyte (E:G) ratio of 1:1 or higher. The degree of hypercellularity varies from slight to moderate (it is rarely marked) and is dependent on the severity of the anemia. Erythropoiesis is orderly without evidence of defective maturation; however, it is characterized by impaired hemoglobinization with late rubricytes and metarubricytes displaying scant basophilic cytoplasm and irregular cell borders (Fig. 5-2). There is a relative but no absolute decrease in

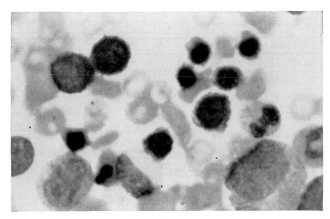

Figure 5-2. Bone marrow aspirate from a patient with an iron deficiency anemia; the nucleated red cells exhibit impaired hemoglobinization with scant basophilic cytoplasm.

granulopoiesis, which is orderly and normal. Megakaryocytes are present in normal to slightly increased numbers and are actively budding platelets. Hemosiderin granules (golden-yellow in unstained preparations, blue-black in Wright-stained films, and bright blue when stained with Prussian blue) are typically absent. The marrow sideroblast count is drastically reduced (normally, erythrocytic precursors contain one or more stainable iron granules in their cytoplasm).

OTHER LABORATORY FINDINGS. *Plasma iron* does not exceed 50 μg/100 ml and is ordinarily less than 35; values of 10 or below indicate profound deficiency. *Plasma iron-binding capacity* is elevated (generally above 450 μg/100 ml), but only 10 per cent or less is saturated with iron. *Free erythrocyte protoporphyrin* is increased. *Erythrocyte osmotic fragility* is usually decreased. *Achlorhydria* is a common finding when tested for in the usual manner, but free acid is excreted in the augmented histamine test. Biopsies of the tongue or stomach may reveal nonspecific atrophic changes. *Plasma ^{59}Fe clearance* is increased, that is, a half time of less than one hour. *Hypercupremia is usual.* Other laboratory examinations yield normal values or reflect the cause of the iron deficiency; for example, positive fecal guaiac reactions; x-ray evidence of a peptic ulcer, hiatus hernia, esophageal varices, or a gastrointestinal neoplasm; and hookworm ova in the feces. The anemia per se may be responsible for additional findings such as nonspecific electrocardiographic changes (p. 57).

DIAGNOSIS

The diagnosis of an iron deficiency anemia is predicated on depleted iron stores. With few exceptions, however, a microcytic, hypochromic anemia is the result of iron deficiency. Consequently, evaluation of the peripheral blood film is the single most valuable diagnostic procedure; the finding of small hypochromic erythrocytes is tantamount to the demonstration of inadequate iron stores. The hematologic manifestations of moderate to marked iron deficiency are readily apparent and easily recognized. The striking accentuation of the central pale area, microcytosis, and poikilocytosis are typical and hard to miss. Artifact caused by delayed drying of the blood film or Wright's stain contaminated with small amounts of water may cause confusion, but it can be distinguished from true hypochromia without much difficulty. Such artifact affects all cells (an unusual finding even in patients with severe iron deficiency anemia) and consists of a sharply demarcated, punched-out center surrounded by a well-stained peripheral rim. Artifactual "hypochromia" can be largely prevented by fixing the blood film with absolute methanol before exposing it to Wright's stain. A careful search of well-made, adequately stained blood films is required to detect characteristic red cell abnormalities in mild deficiency states, but a diligent observer rarely goes unrewarded. The presence of hypochromic microcytes is a finding of considerable diagnostic significance, even though normal-sized, well-colored erythrocytes predominate and cell indexes indicate a "normocytic, normochromic anemia."

In the face of such obvious causes for iron depletion as positive stool guaiacs, a history of excessive menstrual bleeding, or dietary inadequacy in an infant, the morphologic diagnosis of a microcytic, hypochromic anemia may be considered synonymous with the etiologic diagnosis of an iron deficiency anemia. No other hematologic studies are needed unless the patient fails to respond to adequate replacement therapy. Because of the rarity of the other causes for a microcytic, hypochromic anemia, a therapeutic trial is also justified in patients without an apparent reason for negative iron balance; however, demonstration of a depleted storage compartment places the diagnosis on a firmer footing. Iron stores can be assessed in a variety of ways. Evaluation of the hemosiderin content of the bone marrow is the simplest; a low plasma iron and an increased plasma iron-binding capacity are also pathognomonic of iron deficiency. Iron tolerance tests (changes in plasma iron after an oral loading dose) and marrow sideroblast counts provide additional evidence of iron deficiency, but these procedures are more involved and less reliable indicators. Although ferrokinetic studies with radioiron have yielded invaluable data pertaining to iron metabolism, they play no significant role in the diagnosis of iron deficiency anemia.

Diagnosis of the underlying disease may not be so easy a task as recognition of the anemia. An iron deficiency anemia is *never* a primary diagnosis and is *always* a secondary manifestation of some other disorder. Consequently, the work-up is not complete until the precise cause of the iron deficiency is found. In this regard the history often provides valuable clues (e.g., abnormal bleeding, inadequate diet, multiple pregnancies, symptoms of a peptic ulcer, or some other gastrointestinal lesion that may be responsible for chronic blood loss). Physical examination may also be informative. If the history and physical findings fail to suggest a likely cause for depleted iron stores, careful evaluation of the gastrointestinal and genitourinary tracts is indicated because of the statistical frequency with which bleeding from these sites can be implicated in the pathogenesis of an iron deficiency anemia. In fact, a microcytic, hypochromic anemia in an adult male connotes chronic gastrointestinal bleeding until proved otherwise.

The importance of establishing the etiology of an iron deficiency anemia cannot be overemphasized. Since this type of anemia will respond to iron salts regardless of cause, treatment will restore normal erythroid values and may obscure the nature of the primary disease until remedial therapy is precluded; for example, surgical removal of an early, well-localized colonic carcinoma that has been bleeding. Failure to respond to oral therapy in the face of depleted iron stores indicates impaired absorption. If the explanation for an iron deficiency anemia cannot be found, the patient should be followed closely in view of the potential seriousness of many of the diseases associated with this secondary hematologic disorder.

Because great diagnostic significance is attached to the morphology of the red cells in iron deficiency anemia, it is important to consider the other causes of a microcytic, hypochromic anemia. Because of the clearcut relationship between iron deficiency and hypochromia, it has often been assumed erroneously that this morphologic abnormality must be the result of iron lack or a block in iron incorporation. Any quantitative impairment in an erythrocytic precursor's ability to synthesize hemoglobin will cause hypochromia. Consequently, a hypochromic anemia may reflect iron deficiency (by far the most common cause), impaired synthesis of globin, limited production of protoporphyrin, or interference with the utilization of iron. A hypochromic anemia due to some cause other than iron lack is rarely encountered and can be distinguished with relative ease from a true iron deficiency anemia. *Only* an iron deficiency anemia is associated with depleted body iron stores, and *only* an iron deficiency anemia will respond to iron-replacement therapy. The demonstration of either one provides absolute proof that a microcytic, hypochromic anemia is due to iron deficiency. Therefore some other explanation for such an anemia need be sought only in the face of normal or increased iron stores or a therapeutic failure.

Thalassemia Syndromes. These disorders are the result of genetically determined, quantitative defects in the synthesis of globin; they are discussed in detail elsewhere (p. 268). Pertinent manifestations that serve to separate thalassemia from iron deficiency anemia include such obvious differences as a normal or increased plasma iron, abundant stainable iron in the bone marrow, a similar abnormality in some other member of the patient's family, moderate splenomegaly, increased levels of Hgb F or Hgb A_2, and lack of response to the administration of iron.

Anemia of Infection, Rheumatoid Arthritis, and Malignant Disease. A mild to moderate anemia is commonly associated with a variety of chronic infections. It is usually normocytic and normochromic (p. 289), but some patients exhibit slight hypochromia. Plasma iron and iron-binding capacity are both decreased (plasma iron-binding capacity is increased in iron deficiency anemia); tissue iron, for example, stainable iron in the bone marrow, is increased. Plasma radioiron clearance is shortened and plasma iron turnover is slightly increased, despite the decreased plasma iron levels. Erythrocyte uptake of radioiron is moderately decreased. Free erythrocyte protoporphyrin is increased. Current evidence favors the hypothesis that this type of anemia reflects a defect in the release of iron from reticuloendothelial cells and impaired reutilization of iron contained in senescent, nonviable red cells. Although most patients with rheumatoid arthritis or malignant disease have a normocytic, normochronic anemia, some manifest an anemia characterized morphologically by minimal microcytosis and hypochromia. Such anemias appear to belong to the same general category as the hypochromic anemia of infection. These patients do not respond to oral iron.

Pyridoxine-Responsive Anemia. Pyridoxine (vitamin B_6) plays an important role in the biosynthesis of protoporphyrin (p. 20). A microcytic, hypochromic anemia develops in pigs, dogs, cats, and certain other animals maintained on pyridoxine deficient diets; the anemia is corrected by the administration of pyridoxine. A similar type of pyridoxine-responsive anemia has been reported in about 100 human subjects, but the precise pathogenesis has not been elucidated (it is not the result of a dietary deficiency). These patients manifest a microcytic, hypochromic anemia that is often severe, a normal or increased plasma iron, a nearly saturated plasma iron-binding capacity, and tissue hemosiderosis. They respond, at least partly, to large doses of pyridoxine (100 to 200 mg/day) but not to iron; relapse occurs when the pyridoxine is stopped. Diagnosis rests on an adequate therapeutic response following the administration of pyridoxine.

Lead Poisoning. Patients with plumbism have an anemia that is often slightly hypochromic. In vitro lead blocks porphyrin production; in vivo lead affects adversely several aspects of hemoglobin formation. Its major effect is on the synthesis of porphyrin (perhaps by inactivating the sulfhydryl groups necessary for the activity of certain enzymes) and is reflected by several abnormalities, most notably increased quantities of delta-aminolevulinic acid and coproporphyrin, type III in the urine. In addition, lead apparently interferes with the combination of iron and protoporphyrin to form heme, and free erythrocyte protoporphyrin is increased. Lead also appears to retard globin synthesis in some still unexplained way. Plasma iron and tissue iron stores are normal or increased in patients with lead poisoning. Other differences serving to distinguish the hypochromic anemia of plumbism from that of iron deficiency include: (1) a history of excessive exposure to lead, (2) moderate to marked basophilic stippling of erythrocytes (probably precipitated or altered RNA), (3) slight reticulocytosis (erythrocyte life-span is decreased, p. 147), (4) abdominal pain, (5) a stippled, dark line at the gingival margin, and (6) neuromuscular abnormalities such as paresthesias or wrist or foot drop.

Sideroachrestic or Sideroblastic Anemia. These designations have been used for severe microcytic, hypochromic anemias that are refractory to iron and all other types of therapy and do not seem to be related to the thalassemia syndromes (p. 268). Tissue hemosiderosis is usually marked. Plasma iron is high, and the iron-binding protein is almost completely saturated. Nucleated erythrocytic precursors contain increased numbers of iron granules (sideroblasts), as do circulating, nonnucleated red cells (siderocytes). This category of hypochromic anemias is probably a heterogeneous one. The nature of the block in hemoglobin synthesis is not known. In a few patients, the anemia appears to be hereditary and sex-linked (transmitted by females with overt disease occurring in males); in others there is no evidence that it is genetically determined. The only treatment consists of transfusions as needed to maintain satisfactory erythroid values, a procedure that contributes to tissue hemosiderosis. In the past certain patients with pyridoxine-responsive anemia were undoubtedly classified in this category. Because there is nothing else to offer a patient with a sideroblastic anemia and because it is a diagnosis of exclusion, a therapeutic trial with pyridoxine is indicated in all persons in whom this diagnosis is being entertained.

TREATMENT AND COURSE

Treatment of iron deficiency anemia consists of supplying the missing substance, that is, iron. The response is prompt, dramatic, predictable, and completely effective. A microcytic, hypochromic anemia resulting from iron deficiency is the *only* type of anemia that will respond to iron; therefore it is the *only* type of anemia for which iron is indicated. With the possible exception of an acute hemorrhagic anemia, all other anemias are associated with normal or increased iron stores. Under these circumstances there is no rational basis for the administration of iron; in fact, it is actually contraindicated. Because an anemic subject absorbs greater quantities of iron than a nonanemic person, iron therapy in a patient with an anemia that is not due to iron deficiency (e.g., a chronic hemolytic anemia) may lead to tissue hemosiderosis and serious dysfunction of the liver, heart, and so forth. On the other hand, iron is specific in patients with depleted iron stores and evokes one of the most rewarding and gratifying responses in clinical medicine. All patients with an iron deficiency anemia, regardless of cause, will respond to adequate replacement therapy. It is not enough, however, for the physician to recognize the presence of an iron deficiency anemia and to begin appropriate therapy, even though a complete hematologic response ensues. As previously stressed, an iron deficiency anemia is always *secondary* to some primary disorder (usually one that causes chronic bleeding). Every physician who institutes iron therapy has an obligation to the patient to uncover the cause for the negative iron balance and to take steps to eliminate or correct it; *this obligation must be met.*

Oral Therapy. PREPARATION AND DOSE. An inorganic, bivalent iron salt given by mouth is the treatment of choice. Ferrous sulfate is the standard with which other iron preparations should be compared. No other form of iron has been shown to be superior to ferrous sulfate, which is readily absorbed, usually well tolerated, and completely effective. In addition, ferrous sulfate is the least expensive iron preparation available and in therapeutic amounts has one of the widest margins of safety of any potent medicinal. The hydrated salt (20 per cent elemental iron) is available in 0.3 gm tablets and the exsiccated salt (29 per cent iron) in 0.2 gm tablets. Tablets are coated to prevent oxidation and exposure to moisture; however, there is no place for the use of enteric coated tablets or "prolonged-release" preparations, for most of the iron contained therein would not be made available for absorption until it had bypassed the most efficient absorptive sites (i.e., the duodenum and proximal jejunum). Liquid preparations are made for use in children and in certain patients, such as those with gastroenterostomy, in whom tablets may not dissolve before they have gone beyond the absorptive mucosa of the upper small intestine.

A normal person will absorb about 20 per cent and an iron-deficient subject as much as 60 per cent of a physiologic dose of inorganic iron, that is, a quantity of iron equivalent to that contained in a normal diet. As the dose of iron is increased from physiologic to pharmacologic levels, there is a progressive increment in the amount retained, although the percentage absorbed falls. In adults an optimum daily dose for the treatment of iron deficiency anemia is 180 mg of elemental iron (0.9 gm of hydrated ferrous sulfate or 0.6 gm of the exsiccated salt); an iron-deficient patient treated according to this schedule will assimilate about 15 to 30 mg of iron a day. Since absorption is rendered less efficient for approximately four hours after a single large dose of iron, ferrous sulfate should be given in divided doses (one tablet three times daily). Infants and young children should be treated with 60 to 90 mg of elemental iron a day; special formulas to calculate dosage are not needed, and children over the age of two may be given adult doses.

Larger amounts of ferrous sulfate offer no advantage, for the rate of response is determined by the capacity of the marrow; the aforementioned dose provides more than enough iron to support maximal erythropoietic activity. Even though most patients will respond to smaller doses, they constitute suboptimal replacement and cannot be recommended. Although more iron is absorbed in the fasting state, ferrous sulfate should be given during or immediately after meals to minimize gastrointestinal side effects.

Despite the many evident advantages of ferrous sulfate, the physician is confronted by dozens of proprietary iron compounds, each with a dubious claim to superiority and to more effectiveness or better toleration than ferrous sulfate. Since ferrous sulfate is totally effective, it is impossible for another agent to evoke a better therapeutic response. The widely held concept that ferrous sulfate is poorly tolerated appears to be largely iatrogenic. Only 5 to 10 per cent of these patients complain of significant gastrointestinal symptoms when ferrous sulfate is given in the manner and dose prescribed here. Furthermore, those individuals who do attribute side effects (anorexia, nausea, vomiting, abdominal pain, constipation, or diarrhea) to ferrous sulfate will ordinarily have similar complaints with other iron compounds. There is no scientific basis for the continuing search for a "better iron preparation." Moreover, the increased cost to the patient cannot be justified without his gaining any advantage, therapeutic or otherwise. For those few persons who cannot (or more likely *will* not) take ferrous sulfate, there is certainly no dearth of substitutes. However, the physician should be aware that therapeutic effectiveness has, in some instances, actually been sacrificed for such tenuous advantages as improved palatability. Should another preparation be needed, the best one to select is in general a simple one (e.g., ferrous gluconate or ferrous fumarate).

RESPONSE TO THERAPY. The response to iron-replacement therapy is prompt and orderly. The patient often reports symptomatic improvement (decreased fatiguability and an increased sense of well-being) within three to five days after iron is started and well before the erythroid values start to increase. There is some experimental support for the contention that this early response is the result of repletion of certain iron-containing enzymes. The reticulocyte count begins to increase within two to four days and reaches a peak in about 10 days. The height of the reticulocyte response varies inversely with the pretreatment erythroid values and may reach levels of 20 per cent or more in severely anemic patients. As the reticulocytosis subsides, the circulating hemoglobin increases at a rate of about 0.2 gm/100 ml of blood each day. Normal erythroid values are restored within four to eight weeks, although hypochromic erythrocytes formed before treatment may be detectable in the peripheral blood for a longer period of time. If the hemoglobin deficit is at least 5 gm/100 ml of blood and the patient is not actively bleeding, the hemoglobin content of the peripheral blood should increase 2 gm/100 ml or more during the first three weeks of therapy. In patients failing to show such a response, alternative explanations include an abnormality in absorption, the presence of some other disorder limiting marrow activity, or an incorrect diagnosis.

INDICATIONS FOR ORAL IRON. The foremost indication for iron therapy is an iron deficiency anemia; *all* such patients should be treated. Iron should also be given to those individuals who have depleted iron stores consequent to hemorrhage (e.g., gastrointestinal bleeding or too frequent donation of blood) even though they still have enough iron to maintain a normal circulating hemoglobin level; these persons will have trouble repleting their storage compartments from dietary iron alone. Because of the precarious state of iron balance in pregnant women and premature infants, prophylactic iron supplementation is recommended.

Ferrous sulfate should be started as soon as an iron deficiency anemia is recognized. There is no reason to withhold treatment pending diagnosis of the primary disease responsible for the depleted iron stores. Although inorganic iron salts will turn the stools black and thereby obscure this manifestation of gastrointestinal bleeding, chemical tests (guaiac reaction) for blood are not affected. The guaiac reaction is not dependent on the presence of iron but on the peroxidaselike activity of hemoglobin. This property of hemoglobin catalyzes the oxidative action of hydrogen peroxide on guaiaretic acid to yield a blue compound of unknown composition. Therefore the administration of therapeutic doses of iron will not cause false positive reactions for occult blood in the stool.

DURATION OF TREATMENT. If the mechanism responsible for negative iron balance cannot be eliminated, inorganic iron should be continued indefinitely. Even if the cause can be corrected (e.g., a hysterectomy in a patient with bleeding uterine fibroids), treatment should be continued for 9 to 12 months. Since it is virtually impossible to replenish iron stores from dietary sources alone, therapy should extend beyond the time required to restore normal circulating hemoglobin levels. There is no accurate way to determine when the storage compartment has been repleted. Available data indicate that iron stores are rebuilt quite slowly. Although the anemic, iron-deficient subject retains 10 to 15 per cent of the iron in therapeutic doses of ferrous sulfate, the proportion absorbed declines after the anemia has disappeared. Thus prolonged administration of supplemental inorganic iron is indicated to ensure the re-establishment of normal iron stores.

Therapeutic Adjuncts. Additional therapy consists only of that needed to treat the primary disease (e.g., a bleeding peptic ulcer). Insofar as the anemia is concerned, iron and iron alone is sufficient. If dietary inadequacy is responsible for negative iron balance, the diet should obviously be improved. There is no reason, however, to advise any type of special diet in the iron-deficient patient. Increasing dietary iron does nothing to hasten recovery or replenishment of iron stores, for inorganic iron is absorbed more easily than food iron and is already being given in excess to patients receiving therapeutic doses of ferrous sulfate. Ascorbic acid will enhance the absorption of physiologic amounts of organic and inorganic iron; but the iron in ferrous sulfate is absorbed so well that any slight increase attributable to ascorbic acid is inconsequential and does not warrant the increased cost or bother of such supplementation.

From time to time other substances (e.g., copper, molybdenum, arsenic, and cobalt) have been advocated as additions to iron. *None can be recommended.* There is no established place in the physician's therapeutic armamentarium for any iron compound other than a simple, inorganic salt such as ferrous sulfate. Rare infants have been described with a syndrome characterized by hypocupremia, hypoferremia, and hypoproteinemia, but all other persons with iron deficiency anemia have increased blood copper levels. Therefore copper plays no role in the treatment of the usual patient. Although cobalt has been widely used, there is no rational basis for it. Cobalt enhances erythropoiesis in normal experimental animals, most likely by inactivating certain enzymes concerned with the transport and utilization of oxygen; histotoxic hypoxia ensues and is apparently responsible for enhanced humoral erythropoietic factor activity (p. 11). The patient who has an iron deficiency anemia already has increased humoral erythropoietic activity, and the bone marrow of an iron-deficient subject who is receiving ferrous sulfate is hyperplastic and functioning at full capacity. It would serve no useful purpose to aggravate tissue hypoxia or to augment further the already increased humoral factor activity. These facts, together with the potential dangers associated with the administration of cobalt (angina, goiter production, and skin lesions), are such that the use of iron-cobalt preparations cannot be condoned.

Blood Transfusions. There are few reasons to transfuse a patient with an iron deficiency anemia. Although each unit of whole blood contains about 250 mg of elemental iron, the risks associated with transfusions (p. 530) warrant their use only under exceptional circumstances. An iron deficiency anemia is chronic and develops slowly. Consequently, most patients adjust well, even to a very severe anemia. The administration of one or two transfusions to a well-compensated patient with an iron deficiency anemia for the sole purpose of rapid restoration of the hemoglobin or hematocrit level to one that is more acceptable to the physician is to be deplored. Unless there is a straightforward indication for a transfusion, such as active hemorrhage, the prospect of immediate surgery, circulatory instability, or air hunger (acute, severe anemic hypoxia), iron-deficient patients should not be transfused. Properly administered oral iron is harmless and the erythropoietic response is prompt.

Parenteral Iron Therapy. Most patients can and should be treated with oral iron. Because of the body's tenacious hold on iron and because excess iron is harmful to the tissues, parenteral therapy must *never* be used if there is any doubt of the status of iron stores. Parenteral iron may evoke adverse reactions, whereas oral iron in therapeutic amounts is innocuous and just as effective therapeutically. For these reasons only a few situations warrant parenteral iron, even in patients who are known to be iron deficient. Convenience is not a valid indication.

INADEQUATE ABSORPTION. If a suitable preparation is given orally in sufficient amounts, most deficient persons absorb enough iron to restore normal circulating hemoglobin levels and replete stores. The majority of patients with malabsorption syndromes also respond to pharmacologic doses given orally. On the other hand, lack of response to oral iron in the face of an unequivocal deficiency is a clear-cut indication for parenteral therapy. Exceptional patients may bleed so actively and persistently that the maximum amount of iron that can be assimilated from therapeutic doses of ferrous sulfate is less than that being lost. Under these circumstances, both oral and parenteral therapy may be needed to provide enough iron to maintain normal peripheral erythroid values.

RAPID REPLETION OF IRON STORES. Although the reticulocyte response to parenteral iron reaches a slightly higher peak a day or so before it does with oral therapy, the subsequent daily increments in the circulating hemoglobin are comparable. What little difference there may be in the time required to restore normal erythroid values is of no practical significance. However, parenteral iron does permit more rapid restoration of iron stores, a process that requires several months with oral therapy. For this reason it may be of value in the severely iron-depleted pregnant woman who is first seen during the last trimester of pregnancy. Parenteral iron has also been recommended for the iron-deficient subject who requires immediate surgery, but this type of patient will undoubtedly be transfused to near normal values. Enough iron will be gained in this fashion to tide the patient over until oral therapy can be started postoperatively.

GASTROINTESTINAL INTOLERANCE. Most patients who are "unable" to take oral iron because of gastrointestinal side effects have no organic basis for their complaints. Psychogenic intolerance to oral iron is rarely, if ever, a valid reason to give iron parenterally. For the most part, even patients with gastrointestinal disease (e.g., a bleeding peptic ulcer) tolerate oral iron well. However, a few individuals with such disorders as regional enteritis and ulcerative colitis are better treated with parenteral iron. Although the iron does not appear to irritate these disease processes directly, it is capable of altering normal gastrointestinal physiology, which may, in turn, adversely affect the primary gastrointestinal disease.

The most widely parenteral iron preparations are *saccharated iron oxide* (Proferrin) and *iron dextran* (Imferon). Both are effective in the treatment of iron deficiency anemia. Saccharated iron oxide is given intravenously and is removed from the plasma by reticuloendothelial cells within three to six hours. Iron dextran, given intramuscularly, is released slowly over a period of days to weeks into the blood, from which it is also removed by the reticuloendothelial cells. These cells split off the iron, which is then carried by transferrin to the marrow. Several formulas have been devised to determine the total amount of parenteral iron (usually between 1500 and 3000 mg), which is given in a series of divided doses. Average daily doses are 100 mg of saccharated iron oxide and 200 mg of iron dextran. The initial injections should be smaller and gradually increased as tolerated.

Parenteral iron evokes a small but significant number of adverse reactions. Even death has been attributed to such therapy in one or two instances. Saccharated oxide of iron is commonly associated with local venospasm and pain as well as with thrombophlebitis. About 10 per cent of the patients with this preparation exhibit systemic manifestations (fever, chills, nausea, vomiting, pain in the back and extremities, tachycardia, bronchospasm, urticaria, faintness, convulsions, hypotension, and even shock). Reactions may occur immediately or be delayed for several hours. Iron dextran is less likely to evoke a generalized reaction, but pain at the injection site is common, and local staining of the skin may occur unless special precautions are taken to prevent subcutaneous leakage. The indication for parenteral iron therapy must justify the added risk. Although of great value in selected cases, it should be re-emphasized that few patients require such treatment.

Iron Poisoning.   Because of the frequent occurrence of iron deficiency anemia and the widespread practice of giving iron prophylactically during pregnancy, it is an unusual household that does not possess a readily available bottle of iron tablets. Inasmuch as many iron preparations are sugar coated, they are particularly appealing to small children. Although there is a wide margin of safety between therapeutic and toxic doses, iron frequently causes death when ingested in excess. It has been estimated that the lethal dose of ferrous sulfate in man is approximately 900 mg/kg, or about sixty 0.3-gm tablets in a 20-kg child. Initially, iron poisoning is manifested by nausea and vomiting, followed by lassitude, drowsiness, metabolic acidosis, hyperventilation, and shock. If the patient survives, he may improve temporarily, only to have shock recur 12 to 24 hours later. Plasma iron levels may reach several thousand μg/100 ml. Treatment consists of gastric lavage and the prompt administration of large doses of a chelating agent such as ethylenediamine tetraacetate (edathamil; EDTA) or diethylenetriamine pentaacetate (desferrioxamine; DTPA); the latter appears to be more effective.

Vitamin B₁₂ and Folic Acid
Deficiency Anemias
(Megaloblastic Anemias)

A megaloblastic anemia is the hematologic manifestation of faulty proliferation of blood cell precursors. Fully developed cases are characterized by a normochromic anemia with oval macrocytes and irregularly shaped microcytes, leukopenia with large hypersegmented neutrophils, thrombocytopenia with giant platelets, and distinctive morphology of bone marrow cells. The abnormality in mitotic activity, which most likely reflects improper or defective nucleoprotein synthesis, also affects other proliferating cell systems such as the gastrointestinal tract. More than 95 per cent of the megaloblastic, macrocytic anemias are the result of a deficiency of vitamin B₁₂ or folic acid. Although the metabolic functions of these compounds are closely related, they do differ; for example, vitamin B₁₂ is needed to maintain the integrity of nerve tissue, a role not shared by folic acid. However, the hematologic pictures brought about by their respective deficiencies are identical. Therefore the precise etiology of a macrocytic anemia with a megaloblastic marrow cannot be determined on the basis of hematologic criteria alone.

HISTORY

In 1824 Combe of Edinburgh published the first clinical account including autopsy findings of a patient who probably died of a megaloblastic anemia. However, Thomas Addison of Guy's Hospital in London deserves the credit for establishing this type of anemia as a clinical entity ("idiopathic anemia") in his publications of 1849 and 1855. In 1872 Biermer of Zurich focused attention on this disorder by accurately describing many of the clinical manifestations under the heading of "progressive pernicious anemia." It is of interest that Biermer included patients who were pregnant or infested with *Diphyllobothrium latum* as well as those who appear to have had what would now be classified as addisonian pernicious anemia. Thus it was emphasized (but not widely appreciated) at an early date that a multiplicity of etiologic factors could produce a megaloblastic anemia. The bone marrow abnormalities were first described by Pepper (1875), Cohnheim (1876), and Ehrlich (1880). Eichhorst pointed out the presence of macrocytic and microcytic red cells in the peripheral blood in his monograph published in 1878. Fenwick demonstrated gastric atrophy in 1870, and, near the close of the nineteenth century, numerous observers called attention to achlorhydria. At about the same time the clinical and pathologic features of the neurologic component of this disorder were accurately described. The progressive nature of pernicious anemia and its fatal outcome were apparent soon after the entity was recognized.

The third decade of the twentieth century witnessed a dramatic victory in man's fight against disease. Prompted by Whipple's investigations in dogs on the role of liver and other foods in blood-loss anemia, Minot and Murphy began to treat pernicious anemia patients with a special diet that was "rich in complete proteins and iron—particularly liver." The effectiveness of this treatment and the value of the reticulocyte count as an indicator of hematologic recovery were demonstrated conclusively in their first report in 1926; a "pernicious," that is, deadly, disease had been conquered. For their epochal discovery Whipple, Minot, and Murphy were awarded the Nobel Prize in 1934. In 1928 Cohn, Minot, and their associates introduced a potent liver extract, and by 1936 relatively purified extracts of liver were available for intramuscular injection.

Although completely effective therapy was now available, important questions pertaining to etiology and pathogenesis remained unanswered and served as a stimulus to many investigators. Since his initial studies in 1929, Castle has contributed greatly to our knowledge of pernicious anemia by clarifying the nature of the gastric defect in the causation of this disease. He demonstrated that the gastric secretions of patients with pernicious anemia were deficient in a substance (intrinsic factor) that interacted with an extrinsic factor in such foods as beef muscle and liver to yield the active antipernicious anemia principle. The search for the active principle in liver and for the extrinsic factor led first to the synthesis of folic acid in 1945 and ended in 1948 with the isolation of vitamin B_{12} and the demonstration that vitamin B_{12} was both the extrinsic factor *and* the antipernicious anemia principle. The cobamide coenzymes, which are probably the naturally occurring and biologically active forms of vitamin B_{12}, were discovered by Barker and associates in 1958. The biosynthesis in 1950 of ^{60}Co-labeled vitamin B_{12} permitted the development of valuable research tools. Intense investigative activity continues, and the final chapter on this subject has yet to be written. The literature is voluminous and often confusing because of the failure, until recently, to recognize that vitamin B_{12} and folic acid deficiencies produce identical hematologic pictures and that supraphysiologic doses of folic acid evoke hematologic responses in patients with vitamin B_{12} deficiency and vice versa.

PHYSIOLOGY OF VITAMIN B_{12} AND FOLIC ACID

Vitamin B_{12}. Vitamin B_{12} (cyanocobalamin) was isolated from liver in 1948; its chemical structure ($C_{63}H_{88}O_{14}N_{14}PCo$) was revealed in 1955 by x-ray crystallographic analysis. This red crystalline substance, which is active in extremely minute amounts, contains one cobalt atom and a cyanide group. The cyanide moiety (–CN) may be replaced by other radicals, for example, –OH or –NO$_2$, to yield such compounds as hydroxycobalamin and nitrocobalamin. All these substances possess comparable biologic activity and are referred to collectively as the *cobalamins.* Naturally occurring forms differ chemically from the cobalamins. Several *cobamide coenzymes* have been identified and are most likely the only biologically active compounds. The cobamide coenzymes are unstable and easily changed into cyanocobalamin, hydroxycobalamin, and so forth. Therefore the latter compounds may be artifacts induced by extracting procedures, an important point, for present knowledge is based largely on observations on cyanocobalamin, which is chemically stable and easily obtained. There is good evidence, however, that these data are applicable to the cobamide coenzymes.

Vitamin B_{12} is synthesized solely by certain bacteria and other microorganisms; all other living things depend on these sources for their supply of this essential substance. Some microorganisms, for example,

Euglena gracilis and *Lactobacillus leichmannii*, are unable to synthesize vitamin B_{12} and can be used to quantify the amount contained in serum and other test materials. Vitamin B_{12} is obtained commercially as a byproduct in the production of certain antibiotics, most notably streptomycin. Although a significant amount of vitamin B_{12} is synthesized by bacteria in the large intestine, it cannot be absorbed in the colon and is therefore not available to the organism. Rabbits and certain other animals obtain their vitamin B_{12} by coprophagy; man depends on food-stuffs of animal origin, such as meat, fish, milk, cheese, and eggs. The average daily diet in the United States contains about 2 to 8 μg of vitamin B_{12}. Approximately 50 to 70 per cent of dietary vitamin B_{12} is absorbed; the rest is lost in the feces.

Absorption of physiologic amounts of vitamin B_{12}, that is, the content of a normal diet, is highly complex; it takes place in the distal ileum and requires the presence of intrinsic factor. The precise nature and mode of action of intrinsic factor are unknown. It appears to be a mucoprotein elaborated independently of acid or pepsin by the chief secreting cells scattered throughout the fundus and cardia of the stomach. Facilitation of vitamin B_{12} absorption by intrinsic factor is a species-specific phe-nomenon, although there is some overlap; several heterologous intrinsic factor preparations are active in man. During the first phase of absorp-tion intrinsic factor competes successfully with other vitamin B_{12}-binding substances contained in food. As a result, it preferentially removes and firmly binds dietary B_{12}. An acid medium facilitates this binding, which appears to take place in the stomach.

The second step involves the adherence of the intrinsic factor-vitamin B_{12} complex to the mucosal cells of the ileum. Calcium plays an essential but not a unique role in this process (bivalent cationic dependency is evident in the absorption of a variety of substances). The manner by which vitamin B_{12} traverses the intestinal epithelium is poorly under-stood. Membrane vesiculation (pinocytosis) is a possible but still unproved mechanism of absorption. There is some evidence that vitamin B_{12} may be released at the surface of or within the wall of the ileum consequent to enzymatic conversion of the calcium-dependent bond. However, the fate of intrinsic factor is unknown, and the possibility that the intrinsic factor-vitamin B_{12} complex may be absorbed intact cannot be entirely excluded. Transmucosal migration is slow. Vitamin B_{12} begins to appear in the plasma at about 4 hours and does not reach a peak until 8 to 10 hours after ingestion. Depending on the technique, normal serum vitamin B_{12} levels range from as low as 100 to as high as 900 μμg/ml. Approximately 80 to 85 per cent of the vitamin B_{12} in the blood is bound to plasma proteins, primarily an α_1 globulin. Re-cently absorbed vitamin B_{12} is detectable in about equal amounts in a variety of tissues, such as the spleen, kidneys, and liver. After two days almost all of a physiologic dose of vitamin B_{12} is found in the liver where it has a biologic half-life of around one year.

Massive or supraphysiologic amounts of vitamin B_{12}, that is, 0.5 to 1.0 mg, are absorbed by a different mechanism. Under these circumstances absorption apparently takes place by "mass action" and simple diffusion; the assistance of intrinsic factor is not required. Peak plasma levels are reached in four hours in contrast to the delayed appearance of physiologic quantities of vitamin B_{12}. This type of absorption is inefficient. Although a normal subject absorbs 90 per cent or more of a 0.5-µg dose, 40 per cent of 2 µg, and about 20 per cent of 5 µg, only 1.5 per cent of a 1000-µg dose is absorbed. Such an absorptive mechanism is probably not physiologically operative. However, it does possess pharmacologic significance, and large oral doses have been effectively used in the treatment of vitamin B_{12} deficiency resulting from deficient intrinsic factor elaboration.

The normal human body contains approximately 4 mg of vitamin B_{12}. Daily attrition amounts to about 0.2 per cent of body stores or around 8 µg in a normal adult. Most of the daily loss is in the feces (a very small amount is excreted in the urine). Gastric and pancreatic secretions contain a little vitamin B_{12}, and a relatively large quantity is present in the bile. Much of the vitamin B_{12} in bile is reabsorbed (the enterohepatic circulation) by way of the intrinsic factor mechanism, but a significant amount is lost. The minimal adult daily requirement is 1 µg. Manifestations of deficiency are not evident until body stores are reduced to nearly 5 per cent of normal or to about 200 µg. At this level approximately 0.4 µg is lost each day. Therefore 1 µg of vitamin B_{12} per day is adequate to prevent the development of overt clinical deficiency.

The physiologic functions of vitamin B_{12} are poorly understood. It appears to participate in a number of metabolic systems and is probably concerned with the *de novo* synthesis of one-carbon fragments. Although it has long been assumed to play an important role in the biosynthesis of DNA and RNA, there is little evidence that vitamin B_{12} significantly influences RNA production. Rather compelling support is given to the thesis that vitamin B_{12} contributes to DNA formation by affecting the synthesis of deoxyribotides. Additional functions of vitamin B_{12} include a role in the synthesis of certain proteins as well as in folic acid metabolism by promoting the conversion of folic acid to its biologically active forms. It should be emphasized, however, that the precise biochemical functions of vitamin B_{12} remain to be elucidated and most of its apparent activities have been demonstrated in bacteria only.

Folic Acid. Folic acid (pteroylglutamic acid) is a synthetic substance consisting of a pteridine grouping linked by *p*-aminobenzoic acid to a single glutamic acid residue (Fig. 8-11, p. 355); however, the term is also used to refer to a group of naturally occurring substances (conjugated polyglutamates). Some authors prefer to designate all compounds with folic acid-like activity as *folates*. A folate was first isolated from spinach leaves in 1941 and from liver in 1943; pteroylglutamic acid was synthesized in 1945. Folates are widely distributed in nature and occur most abundantly in fresh green, leafy vegetables, liver, kidney, eggs, yeast, dried beans, nuts, grains, and certain fruits. Milk is uniquely low in folate activity. Although precise data are not available, the normal dietary requirement appears to be about 50 µg/day. Normal body stores are estimated to be around 6 to 8 mg. In the United States the average diet supplies a great excess of folates; however, considerable activity (as much as 95 per cent) is lost in cooking. Folic acid is absorbed readily and passively in the "jejunum." Microbiologic assay of the folate content of such test materials as serum is possible by using one of several organisms; for example, *Lactobacillus citrovorum, Lactobacillus casei,* or *Streptococcus fecalis,* but the technique is difficult and relatively insensitive. Furthermore, some organisms respond only to monoglutamates, whereas others measure polyglutamates as well. Therefore the exact range of normal serum folate activity is not known. Relatively little information is available concerning the transport, storage, and excretion of folic acid. The recent introduction of tritium-labeled folic acid may clarify many of these points similar to the elucidation of cyanocobalamin metabolism made possible by radioactive cobalt-labeled vitamin B_{12}.

The physiologic functions of folic acid are not entirely understood. In order to become biologically active, folic acid must be reduced to such forms as N5-formyl-tetrahydrofolic acid (folinic acid, citrovorum factor) and N5-methyl-tetrahydrofolic acid, a monoglutamate, which appears to be the most important source of folate activity in human blood and tissue. The active forms of folic acid function as coenzymes in a number of metabolic systems in which they affect the donation or movement of preformed one-carbon compounds, for example, methyl [–CH_3] and formyl [–CHO] groups, from one site or acceptor to another. In this manner folic acid influences, among other things, the biosynthesis of purines and pyrimidines, most notably the anabolism of DNA. Available data indicate that the primary function of folic acid is probably in the synthesis of a DNA precursor, perhaps thymidylic acid. Although "activation" of folic acid appears to require vitamin B_{12}, there is no evidence that folic acid directly influences vitamin B_{12} metabolism; however, certain of the functions of these two substances are closely related.

PATHOPHYSIOLOGY OF VITAMIN B₁₂ AND FOLIC ACID DEFICIENCY

Vitamin B$_{12}$. The major clinical manifestations of vitamin B$_{12}$ deficiency are due to defective cell mitosis (presumably a result of impaired DNA synthesis) and to neurologic disease (presumably a result of impaired protein synthesis).

ABNORMAL CELL PROLIFERATION. Vitamin B$_{12}$ deficiency affects all dividing cells, but abnormalities are most evident in those cell systems, such as the bone marrow, that have the fastest rates of growth. Therefore the clinical picture is dominated by hematologic aberrations involving all cells derived from the myeloid reticulum. The bone marrow is hypercellular and has distinctive *megaloblastic* morphology. The primary defect appears to be decreased mitotic activity consequent to lengthening of the intermitotic interval. Although the cells contain normal or even slightly increased quantities of DNA, they are apparently unable to synthesize enough DNA to permit the replication needed for cellular division. As a result, the marrow becomes "crowded" with cells awaiting mitosis. During the prolonged resting phase the chromatin is dispersed diffusely throughout the nucleus to yield the characteristic megaloblastic pattern, which shows accentuation of parachromatin, a finely reticulated or lacework appearance of the basichromatin, and a sharp differentiation between the two.

Marrow cells contain increased quantities of RNA, probably because of their inability to convert appropriate portions of RNA to DNA (RNA is the principal source of the extra DNA needed for cell division). The RNA:DNA and uracil:thymine ratios in the marrow are increased (RNA contains uracil; DNA contains thymine). Although the proclivity of megaloblastic cells to reduplicate is impaired, they retain specialized, cytoplasmic functions such as the ability to synthesize hemoglobin. Therefore cells grow large and nuclear-cytoplasmic asynchronism becomes evident, that is, hemoglobinization in an otherwise immature erythrocytic precursor. In addition to these morphologic changes, there is evidence of defective marrow cell maturation with increased numbers of immature elements. All aspects of myelopoiesis are affected by a deficiency of vitamin B$_{12}$. Although marrow hypercellularity reflects an increase in all cell lines, erythrocytic precursors usually predominate. Morphologic abnormalities are also most evident in the erythrocytic series, but comparable changes occur in granulocytic precursors and in megakaryocytes.

Despite erythrocytic hyperplasia and a severalfold increase in heme turnover, marrow output is less than normal. Ineffective erythropoiesis prevails and "marrow hemolysis" (destruction of immature erythrocytic precursors) contributes significantly to hyperbilirubinemia and increased fecal and urine urobilinogen levels. In addition, the mature products of megaloblastic erythropoiesis have shortened survival times because of intrinsic and extrinsic defects. The nature of the extrinsic defects is not known; the intrinsic defects are most likely related to the deformed cells produced in the face of inadequate supplies of vitamin B_{12}. As a result, anemia develops and is accompanied by those symptoms and findings attributable to a reduction in red cell mass regardless of cause (e.g., weakness and dyspnea). Leukopenia and thrombocytopenia also occur but are less marked than the reduction in circulating hemoglobin.

The products of a megaloblastic marrow are qualitatively abnormal. Large oval red cells are characteristic, but microcytic poikilocytes are equally prominent. There is some support for the thesis that these small cells may result from fragmentation of the ovalocytic macrocytes. Since the synthesis of hemoglobin is not impaired, red cells are well colored and have a normal concentration of hemoglobin. The reticulocyte count is low and not a reliable index because of the asynchronism between nuclear and cytoplasmic maturation and the frequent loss of reticulum before extrusion of the nucleus and release of the cell from the bone marrow. Large hypersegmented neutrophils and atypical platelets are manifestations of the defects in granulopoiesis and thrombopoiesis. The neutrophils, which undoubtedly reflect the block in cell division, possess five or more lobes and are of considerable diagnostic significance. Morphologic abnormalities are not detectable in lymphocytes.

Bone marrow dysfunction and the subsequent changes in the peripheral blood (anemia, thrombocytopenia, and leukopenia) account for many of the symptoms and other manifestations of vitamin B_{12} deficiency. However, all proliferating cells require vitamin B_{12} and the deficiency is generalized. Therefore, changes in other cell systems contribute to the clinical picture. Morphologic abnormalities are demonstrable in epithelial cells from the mucosa of the mouth, stomach, vagina, and urinary bladder. These cytologic changes are analogous to those in the marrow, that is, giant cells with diffusely dispersed nuclear chromatin. They are responsible for such manifestations as a sore and/or smooth, uncoated tongue and gastrointestinal symptoms (anorexia, nausea, and diarrhea).

NEUROLOGIC DISEASE. Involvement of the nervous system characteristically accompanies vitamin B_{12} deficiency. Although most often termed subacute combined degeneration of the cord, *vitamin B_{12} neuropathy* is preferred, for the brain and peripheral nerves are also affected. Furthermore, the process is more likely to be chronic than subacute. The pathogenesis of these neurologic lesions is obscure. DNA turnover in nerve cells is slow; however, RNA content is high and intense protein synthesis is required to maintain the integrity of the axons. Vitamin B_{12}

neuropathy was once believed to reflect defects in RNA synthesis, but there is little experimental support for this contention. On the other hand, vitamin B_{12} does appear to play an important role in the synthesis of certain other proteins. Pending further clarification, it may be logically inferred that the protein synthesis needed to preserve the functional and histologic integrity of nerve cells cannot take place without vitamin B_{12}; the typical lesions of vitamin B_{12} neuropathy ensue.

Histologically, there are multiple, irregularly distributed foci of spongy degeneration in the white matter of the spinal cord involving both myelin sheaths and axis cylinders. There is relatively little proliferation of fibrous glia. Involvement of the posterior or dorsal columns (ascending fibers) is responsible for weakness, numbness, tingling, decreased vibratory sense, impaired position sense, ataxia, hypotonicity, hyporeflexia, and bladder disturbances. Lesions affecting the lateral columns or pyramidal tracts (descending fibers) produce hyperactive deep tendon reflexes, positive Babinski signs, and muscular spasticity. Symptoms and findings are characteristically symmetrical and affect the distal portions of the extremities first. Impaired superficial sensation and hyperesthesias may be the result of peripheral nerve abnormalities, but it should be pointed out that the evidence for a peripheral neuropathy in vitamin B_{12} deficiency is more clinical than pathologic. Because of the diverse findings produced by lesions of the cord and peripheral nerves, the final clinical picture is subject to considerable variation and depends on the location of the areas of degeneration.

Cerebral involvement is less common than that of the spinal cord and is most often associated with marked, long-standing deficiency states. Brain lesions resemble those in the spinal cord, that is, scattered foci of degeneration in white matter. Mental depression, irritability, and memory loss are the usual clinical manifestations, but delusions, hallucinations, and frank psychotic behavior have been observed as well as electroencephalographic abnormalities.

Folic Acid. The major manifestations of folic acid deficiency are attributable to altered cell proliferation consequent to impaired DNA synthesis. Although vitamin B_{12} and folic acid affect different metabolic systems in nucleoprotein synthesis, the end result is the same, that is, defective DNA production. Furthermore, vitamin B_{12} appears to play an important role in normal folate metabolism. Hence a vitamin B_{12} deficiency is physiologically tantamount to folic acid deficiency. In fact, it seems quite likely that an inadequate supply of the tetrahydrofolates is basically responsible for megaloblastic proliferation, whether because of a lack of folic acid or vitamin B_{12}. It is not surprising, therefore, that the findings in the marrow and peripheral blood in folic acid deficiency are identical with those of vitamin B_{12} deficiency. Folic acid deficiency also produces changes in other proliferating cell systems similar to those caused by vitamin B_{12} inadequacy. Thus a macrocytic, normochromic anemia with ovalocytes, leukopenia with hypersegmented neutrophils, thrombocytopenia with giant platelets, a megaloblastic marrow, and a sore and/or uncoated tongue characterize the clinical picture of both vitamin B_{12} and folic acid deficiencies.

In another respect the pathophysiologic manifestations of folic acid deficiency differ strikingly from those caused by lack of vitamin B_{12}. Vitamin B_{12} *is* required to maintain the functional integrity of nervous tissue; folic acid *is not*. Neurologic disease similar to vitamin B_{12} neuropathy has *never* been observed as a manifestation of folic acid deficiency alone. Other pertinent differences between vitamin B_{12} and folic acid deficiencies include in folic acid deficiency decreased serum folate activity, normal serum vitamin B_{12} levels, and increased excretion of formiminoglutamic acid (FIGLU) in the urine. FIGLU is a normal catabolite in the degradation of histidine to glutamic acid, a process requiring N5-formyl-tetrahydrofolic acid (the citrovorum factor). In the face of an inadequate supply of folates, FIGLU accumulates and is excreted in the urine. It should be noted, however, that a significant number of patients with addisonian pernicious anemia (vitamin B_{12} deficiency) also have increased quantities of FIGLU in their urine and that all folic acid deficient subjects do not excrete excessive amounts.

Response to Replacement Therapy. Vitamin B_{12}. The abnormalities in cellular division induced by vitamin B_{12} deficiency respond promptly and dramatically to replacement therapy. In the marrow cells DNA synthesis is increased, RNA content is decreased, and a normal RNA:DNA ratio is restored. Megaloblastic cells that have already reached a postmitotable stage continue to mature along megaloblastic lines; however, more immature, mitotable megaloblastic cells undergo mitosis and yield two normoblastic cells at a comparable stage of development. Therefore, morphologic changes are demonstrable in the bone marrow within a few hours after replacement therapy has been started, and all evidence of megaloblastic maturation usually disappears within two to four days. In the peripheral blood reticulocytosis heralds the return of normal myelopoiesis. The magnitude of the reticulocyte response varies inversely with the pretreatment erythroid values. When given parenterally, vitamin B_{12} is effective in very small doses, that is, 1 μg or less daily. It will cause reversion to normal morphology when instilled directly into the marrow cavity as well as in cultures of megaloblastic cells growing in vitro.

Certain pyrimidine precursors also evoke hematologic responses in vitamin B_{12}-deficient subjects, presumably by bypassing the block in DNA synthesis. Such substances include uracil, thymine, and a mixture of uridylic and cytidylic acids. Less predictable have been responses to orotic acid and thymidine. Of more clinical significance is the complete hematologic response induced in the vitamin B_{12}-deficient patient by pharmacologic doses of folic acid. Although physiologic amounts of folic acid (100 or 200 µg/day) are without effect, larger quantities (400 µg or more daily) will restore hematopoietic normalcy. Therapeutically, doses of 5 to 15 mg/day are commonly used. Although the metabolic functions of vitamin B_{12} and folic acid differ, their physiologic effects are closely related and in certain reactions they act jointly. Larger doses of folic acid apparently correct the block in cellular division caused by vitamin B_{12} deficiency, perhaps by diverting the limited amounts of vitamin B_{12} into metabolic activities dealing with folic acid and DNA synthesis. Since vitamin B_{12} deficiency is always relative and never absolute, normal or near normal mitotic activity is restored by pharmacologic doses of folic acid, at least temporarily. However, there are other functions of vitamin B_{12} independent of folic acid; for example, its role in maintaining the integrity of nerve tissue. Because of "shunting" of the already depleted stores of vitamin B_{12} into other metabolic systems, vitamin B_{12} neuropathy will therefore often progress despite hematologic improvement. If massive doses of folic acid are continued, hematologic relapse eventually ensues when the limited supplies of vitamin B_{12} become exhausted.

After the administration of vitamin B_{12} to deficient patients, other evidences of altered cell division also subside promptly; for example, tongue abnormalities and gastrointestinal symptoms. However, the minimal regenerative powers of nerve cells are such that complete recovery from the neurologic manifestations of vitamin B_{12} deficiency cannot always be expected.

FOLIC ACID. Very small amounts of folic acid, that is, 100 µg or less daily, evoke prompt and complete clinical recovery in folic acid-deficient patients. The hematologic response is comparable to that induced by vitamin B_{12} in vitamin B_{12}-deficient subjects. Thymine will also bring about a hematologic response, but uracil will not. These observations lend support to the thesis that folic acid plays a fundamental role in the methylation of uracil (a component of RNA) to 5-methyl uracil or thymine (a constituent of DNA). Physiologic amounts of vitamin B_{12}, that is, less than 1 µg/day, will not affect hematopoiesis in a folic acid-deficient person. However, massive doses, 500 to 1000 µg and perhaps as little as 30, will cause hematologic responses, probably consequent to increased utilization of the remaining folate stores similar to the response induced by pharmacologic doses of folic acid in patients with vitamin B_{12} deficiency.

ETIOLOGY OF THE MEGALOBLASTIC ANEMIAS

The various causes of a megaloblastic anemia are listed in Table 5-3. More than 95 per cent are due to a deficiency of vitamin B_{12} or

Table 5-3. *Causes of Megaloblastic, Macrocytic Anemias*

I. *Deficiency of Vitamin B$_{12}$ or Folic Acid*
  A. Decreased intake
    1. Nutritional deficiency   *Folic acid*
                                           Vitamin B$_{12}$
  B. Impaired absorption
    1. Pernicious anemia   *Vitamin B$_{12}$*
    2. Gastrectomy   *Vitamin B$_{12}$*
    3. Severe gastric disease   *Vitamin B$_{12}$*
    4. Small bowel resection   *Vitamin B$_{12}$*
    5. Intestinal blind loops,
        diverticulae, or strictures   *Vitamin B$_{12}$*
    6. *Diphyllobothrium latum* infestation   *Vitamin B$_{12}$*
    7. Malabsorption syndromes (sprue)   *Folic acid*
                                             Vitamin B$_{12}$
  C. Increased requirements   *Folic acid*
    1. Pregnancy
    2. Hemolytic anemias
    3. Malignant tumors *e. g. hypersplenism*
II. *Impaired Utilization*   *Folic acid*
  A. Folic acid antagonists
  B. Anticonvulsant drugs
  C. Liver disease
  D. Ascorbic acid deficiency (?)
III. *Miscellaneous Causes*
  A. Cytotoxic therapy (alkylating agents, ionizing radiation, antipurines)
  B. Congenital orotic aciduria ?
  C. Myelomonocytic leukemia ("megaloblastoid" marrow)

folic acid. Combined deficiencies exist, especially in certain of the malabsorption syndromes. In most patients, however, there is a single deficiency in which complete response follows the administration of one agent. Classification of the megaloblastic anemias has been confused because it was once thought that a hematologic response to folic acid meant folic acid deficiency and that a response to vitamin B$_{12}$ clearly implicated this substance in the pathogenesis of a megaloblastic anemia. Such an assumption is no longer tenable; in pharmacologic amounts vitamin B$_{12}$ and folic acid are each capable of evoking a hematologic response in a patient who is deficient in the other substance.

Decreased Intake of Folic Acid or Vitamin B$_{12}$. FOLATE NUTRITIONAL DEFICIENCY. Megaloblastic anemias resulting from a dietary deficiency of folates are common. The nature of the foodstuffs with high folate content (e.g., green leafy vegetables) and the loss of activity with cooking contribute to the frequency of this nutritional deficiency. Normal body stores are adequate to prevent clinical evidence of folate deficiency for only four to five months. This type of megaloblastic anemia is encountered most often in chronic alcoholics (wine contains very small amounts of folates; hard liquor has none). Megaloblastic anemia of infancy is another example of nutritional deficiency (all kinds of milk are uniquely low in folates).

Vitamin B$_{12}$ Nutritional Deficiency. Megaloblastic anemias caused by a dietary deficiency of vitamin B$_{12}$ are quite rare. Even patients with grossly inadequate diets, such as chronic alcoholics, ordinarily ingest sufficient quantities of meat or milk to forestall the development of this form of megaloblastic anemia. Furthermore, body stores of vitamin B$_{12}$ are sufficient to prevent clinical evidence of deficiency for three or more years. Therefore patients with nutritional vitamin B$_{12}$ deficiency are usually diet faddists who ingest *no* animal food (most vegetarians eat eggs, milk, and cheese and obtain enough vitamin B$_{12}$ from these sources). Because an adequate intake of folates may obscure the hematologic manifestations of vitamin B$_{12}$ deficiency as the neurologic disease is allowed to progress, neuropathy is particularly likely to dominate the clinical picture.

Impaired Absorption of Vitamin B$_{12}$ or Folic Acid. Pernicious Anemia. The basic defect in pernicious anemia (often called addisonian pernicious anemia to distinguish it with certainty from the other causes of a megaloblastic anemia) is deficient elaboration of intrinsic factor by the stomach. As a result, absorption of dietary vitamin B$_{12}$ is impaired and leads eventually to a generalized vitamin B$_{12}$ deficiency. The cause of the gastric abnormality is not known. The increased incidence of achlorhydria, impaired absorption of vitamin B$_{12}$, and even overt pernicious anemia in other members of a patient's family attest to the importance of genetic factors; however, the precise mode of inheritance has not been elucidated. Because pernicious anemia rarely has its onset before the fifth decade of life, it has been suggested that anatomic and functional degeneration subsequent to aging is necessary to potentiate a congenital defect and permit the development of clinical disease. Although most unusual, there are a few well-documented reports of addisonian pernicious anemia in children and young adults. The hypothesis has been advanced that some of these occurrences may reflect the presence of two abnormal genes, that is, one from each parent, but proof is lacking.

Numerous other pathogenic mechanisms have been advanced; none has been proved and most are no longer tenable. A recent suggestion is that pernicious anemia may be an example of an autoimmune disorder. Proponents of this thesis cite such observations as the demonstration of intrinsic factor, gastric parietal cell, and thyroid antibodies in a significant number of patients with pernicious anemia. In addition, there appears to be a relationship between pernicious anemia and thyroid disease (there is rather convincing support for the autoimmune nature of thyroiditis). It should be stressed that, although attractive, this explanation of the pathogenesis of pernicious anemia remains highly speculative.

The nature of the gastric defect is obscure. In the typical adult patient achlorhydria (in fact, achylia gastrica) and gastric atrophy invariably accompany the decreased intrinsic factor production; but neither of these findings would appear to constitute the primary defect. Progressive gastric atrophy will eventually affect intrinsic factor formation and failure to secrete free hydrochloric acid in an augmented histamine test is *prima facie* evidence of overt or latent pernicious anemia. However, gastric atrophy or decreased acid production is not always associated with inadequate intrinsic factor elaboration. Rare children and young adults with pernicious anemia have been shown to secrete acid normally and to have a histologically normal gastric mucosa. Thus intrinsic factor elaboration appears to be independent of acid production or atrophic anatomic change. Because all the manifestations of pernicious anemia except achlorhydria and gastric atrophy disappear after adequate replacement therapy, it seems unlikely that these findings could be caused by the vitamin B_{12} deficiency.

GASTRECTOMY. Intrinsic factor is secreted by the stomach and plays an essential role in the absorption of the physiologic amounts of vitamin B_{12} contained in a normal diet. Therefore total gastrectomy will always be followed by vitamin B_{12} deficiency and a megaloblastic anemia, provided sufficient time elapses. Body stores are such that they will prevent the development of overt deficiency for about three years. Because total gastrectomies are usually done for extensive malignant disease, few patients live long enough after surgery to develop a megaloblastic anemia. After partial gastrectomy megaloblastic anemia occurs in less than 1 per cent of the patients, although serum vitamin B_{12} levels are depressed following this procedure. As little as 10 per cent of the fundus of the stomach appears capable of elaborating sufficient intrinsic factor to prevent the development of clinical vitamin B_{12} deficiency. Iron deficiency anemia is much more common in gastrectomized patients (p. 168) than a megaloblastic anemia.

SEVERE GASTRIC DISEASE. Extensive involvement of the stomach by carcinoma, that is, malignant linitis plastica, is accompanied by deficient intrinsic factor production. However, body stores of vitamin B_{12} ordinarily prevent the development of a megaloblastic anemia before the patient succumbs to the neoplastic disease. Corrosive chemical gastritis or marked atrophic gastritis also interfere with the secretion of intrinsic factor and the absorption of vitamin B_{12}. Differentiation between severe atrophic gastritis and addisonian pernicious anemia appears to be largely a problem in semantics.

SMALL BOWEL RESECTION. Vitamin B_{12} is absorbed in the ileum, and extensive ileal resection eliminates the intestinal receptors for the intrinsic factor–vitamin B$_{12}$ complex. Absorption of physiologic amounts of vitamin B$_{12}$ is thereby impaired and a megaloblastic anemia develops after body stores have been depleted by normal attrition.

INTESTINAL BLIND LOOPS, DIVERTICULAE, OR STRICTURES. These abnormalities of the small intestine are rare causes of a megaloblastic anemia due to vitamin B$_{12}$ deficiency. Intrinsic factor elaboration is normal. Available data indicate that the primary defect is stasis with an ecologic change that permits alterations in the normal bacterial flora. Blind loops are usually the result of surgery involving the distal small intestine. In most of the reported cases of megaloblastic anemia associated with diverticulae, the lesions have been in the jejunum. Intestinal strictures (e.g., tuberculosis or postoperative) have ordinarily affected the lower small intestine. The "foreign" bacteria appear to compete successfully for dietary vitamin B$_{12}$. As a result, this vitamin B$_{12}$ is no longer available to the host and deficiency ensues. Considerable support for this pathogenic mechanism is derived from the hematologic responses induced in such patients by certain antibiotics.

Diphyllobothrium latum INFESTATION. In the United States the fish tapeworm is an extremely rare cause of a megaloblastic anemia; however, in other parts of the world (most notably Finland) this type of anemia is encountered more often. By using radioactive vitamin B$_{12}$ it is possible in an infected person to demonstrate preferential uptake of dietary vitamin B$_{12}$ by the worm. Although 20 to 30 per cent of the population in Finland harbor this parasite, less than 0.1 per cent of these individuals actually have a megaloblastic anemia. Because body stores can prevent the development of clinical vitamin B$_{12}$ deficiency for three years or more, the length of time that an individual has been infested is undoubtedly of paramount importance. Other contributing factors include the position of the worm in the gastrointestinal tract (anemia is more likely to occur if the worm is in the proximal small intestine) and the amount of vitamin B$_{12}$ contained in the diet.

MALABSORPTION SYNDROMES. Tropical sprue, idiopathic steatorrhea (nontropical sprue), and celiac disease are clinical syndromes characterized by impaired absorption of a variety of substances. Malabsorption also accompanies such small intestinal disorders as tuberculosis, amyloidosis, and regional enteritis. These patients frequently have defective absorption of folic acid, vitamin B$_{12}$, or both, and a significant number develop a megaloblastic anemia. Folic acid is most often at fault; however, vitamin B$_{12}$ deficiency may occur when the ileum is extensively involved. The increased excretion of fat so typical of these malabsorption syndromes brings about excessive loss of calcium in the form of insoluble soaps. Since absorption of the intrinsic factor-vitamin B$_{12}$ complex is dependent on a calcium bond, such a mechanism may contribute to impaired vitamin B$_{12}$ absorption. Iron deficiency often complicates the hematologic picture, especially in patients with celiac disease (p. 169).

Increased Requirements (Folic Acid). There is no proof that increased vitamin B_{12} requirements play a significant role in the pathogenesis of megaloblastic anemias. Body stores of folic acid are more limited, and increased need for this nutrient can lead to such an anemia, especially when coupled with decreased intake.

MEGALOBLASTIC ANEMIA OF PREGNANCY. Pregnancy causes a drain on body folate stores which may eventuate in the last trimester in a megaloblastic anemia. Complete recovery follows delivery. The incidence of megaloblastic anemia of pregnancy varies in different parts of the world, but it is not particularly common. An increase in folic acid requirements does not by itself appear to be an adequate explanation, and decreased (or at least marginal) dietary intake is probably a requisite for the development of clinical folate deficiency. Decreased absorption has also been mentioned as an additional pathogenic factor, but this mechanism is conjectural. It is unlikely that vitamin B_{12} deficiency contributes to the usual megaloblastic anemia of pregnancy. Of course, other causes of vitamin B_{12} deficiency such as pernicious anemia can exist in a pregnant woman and must be excluded.

HEMOLYTIC ANEMIAS. Rarely, a megaloblastic anemia complicates chronic hemolysis [e.g., hereditary spherocytosis (p. 111) or a hereditary hemoglobinopathy (p. 257)]. In these patients folic acid deficiency appears to be the result of increased need for nucleoprotein synthesis (occasioned by the accelerated erythropoiesis) in the face of suboptimal nutritional intake.

MALIGNANT DISEASE. Another uncommon cause of a megaloblastic anemia due to increased folate requirements is a malignant growth. The explanation is similar to that for the megaloblastic anemias accompanying chronic hemolysis, that is, increased growth requirements of the malignant cells acting jointly with inadequate, or at least borderline, dietary intake.

Impaired Utilization (Folic Acid). In rare instances a megaloblastic anemia may be caused by interference with the normal metabolic functions of folic acid; no analogous situation is known to involve vitamin B_{12}.

FOLIC ACID ANTAGONISTS. These substances (p. 354) are analogues of folic acid that compete with normal substrate for the enzymes (e.g., dihydrofolic reductase) required to reduce folic acid to its metabolically active forms. In patients treated with these agents the end result, insofar as disturbed nucleoprotein synthesis is concerned, is comparable to that of a simple deficiency of folic acid. Proliferating cell systems such as the bone marrow and gastrointestinal mucosa are affected with the generation of typical megaloblastic morphology.

ANTICONVULSANT DRUGS. A megaloblastic anemia develops infrequently in patients with convulsive disorders who are receiving phenobarbital derivatives, diphenylhydantoin sodium (Dilantin), or primidone (Mysoline). Although the precise details remain to be worked out, available data indicate that the anemia results from competitive interference with the normal metabolic activities of folic acid (there is a biochemical similarity between the pyrimidine and hydantoin rings of these anticonvulsant drugs and the pteridyl portion of folic acid). However, this mechanism fails to explain why so few patients receiving these drugs manifest a megaloblastic anemia, and additional factors must be operating. Suboptimal folate intake appears to be the most reasonable contributory factor.

LIVER DISEASE. A macrocytic anemia is commonly associated with liver disease, but it is infrequently megaloblastic. Most of these megaloblastic anemias reflect superimposed nutritional folate deficiency. Some patients with advanced liver disease lack dihydrofolic reductase (an enzyme essential for the reduction of folic acid to its various tetrahydrofolic forms). The result is a block in the metabolic activities of folic acid.

ASCORBIC ACID DEFICIENCY. Evidence exists to implicate ascorbic acid in the conversion of folic acid to its metabolically active forms. It is conceivable, therefore, that an ascorbic acid deficiency might contribute to the development of a megaloblastic anemia. However, such anemias are rarely observed in patients with scurvy and, when present, are usually associated with a superimposed dietary deficiency of folic acid. Thus the role of ascorbic acid deficiency in the production of a megaloblastic anemia is quite speculative, even though ascorbic acid may contribute to the normal reduction of folic acid.

Other Causes of Megaloblastic Hematopoiesis. Any abnormality that retards DNA synthesis or cellular division will permit greater dispersion of chromatin throughout the nucleus; megaloblastic morphology results.

CYTOTOXIC THERAPY. Even though they may not interfere with the metabolic functions of folic acid or vitamin B_{12}, any cytotoxic agent affecting cell proliferation may cause megaloblastic changes in the morphology of mitotable marrow cells. Examples include ionizing radiation (p. 399), 6-mercaptopurine (p. 356), and alkylating drugs such as nitrogen mustard (p. 402).

CONGENITAL OROTIC ACIDURIA. Two case reports have been made of children with a megaloblastic anemia due to an inborn enzymatic deficiency (probably orotidylic decarboxylase and orotidylic pyrophosphorylase) which prevented the conversion of orotic acid to later pyrimidine precursors. As a result, DNA synthesis (and cellular division) was impaired, and large quantities of orotic acid appeared in the urine. One of these patients responded partially to a mixture of uridylic and cytidylic acids; the other child responded to uridine given orally. Future studies will most likely uncover similar (but perhaps quite variable) enzymatic deficiencies or blocks in the highly complex process of nucleoprotein synthesis; such individuals should manifest a megaloblastic anemia.

MYELOMONOCYTIC LEUKEMIA. When erythrocytic precursors participate in a leukemia process, that is, myelomonocytic leukemia (p. 349), they display morphologic abnormalities that resemble megaloblastic proliferation. Often termed megaloblastoid (paramegaloblastic might be more appropriate), these changes consist of accentuation of parachromatin and greater dispersion of basichromatin. Occasionally it is quite difficult to distinguish between megaloblastic and paramegaloblastic morphology, but these cells can ordinarily be separated on the basis of coarser chromatin clumps in the paramegaloblastic and a finer, reticulated chromatin network in the megaloblastic. Paramegaloblastic morphology reflects the uncontrolled, disorderly cellular proliferation that characterizes leukemia.

CLINICAL MANIFESTATIONS

Symptoms and findings attributable to vitamin B_{12} or to folic acid inadequacy are the same, regardless of the cause of the vitamin B_{12} or folate deficiency. Thus addisonian pernicious anemia and nutritional vitamin B_{12} deficiency are clinically similar, as are all the folate deficiencies. Depending on the nature of the primary disorder, however, the clinical pictures may be colored to obscure the major manifestations of the deficiency state (e.g., a megaloblastic anemia in a patient with one of the malabsorption syndromes in whom gastrointestinal symptoms predominate). It must also be borne in mind that changes in the bone marrow and peripheral blood (evidence of altered cell proliferation) are exactly the same whether caused by the lack of vitamin B_{12}, folic acid, or both. Pernicious anemia is an example of a straightforward, uncomplicated vitamin B_{12} deficiency in which all or almost all of the clinical manifestations are the direct result of vitamin B_{12} depletion. There is no analogous situation involving folic acid; even nutritional folate deficiency is likely to be complicated by inadequate amounts of other essential nutrients, underlying chronic alcoholism, and liver disease. Although the true incidence of the megaloblastic anemias is not known, they would appear to account for about 10 per cent of all anemias. Most megaloblastic anemias are the result of pernicious anemia or a nutritional folate deficiency; in the urban areas of the temperate zones their relative frequencies are about equal.

Pernicious Anemia

Addisonian pernicious anemia generally has its clinical onset in the sixth decade of life. It is infrequent under the age of 40, quite rare under the age of 30, and extremely unusual in children or adolescents. Only a few well-documented examples of pernicious anemia in children are known. Males are affected somewhat more often than females, and there may be a history of pernicious anemia in the family. This form of megaloblastic anemia is classically described as occurring in individuals of Scandinavian descent with blue eyes, large ears, and prematurely gray hair. However, the clinical significance of these physical characteristics has been overemphasized, as have possible predilections for certain ethnic groups. The once widely held concept that pernicious anemia was rare in Negroes was the result of inadequate sampling. It is now evident that the disorder occurs in all parts of the world, although it is less common among Orientals than in other races.

Symptoms. The onset of pernicious anemia is insidious, for its clinical picture evolves slowly over a period of several months. Most of the symptoms are due to the anemia, involvement of the gastrointestinal tract, or neurologic disease. Initial complaints are most often referrable to anemia and consist of the usual manifestations of a decrease in the oxygen-carrying capacity of the blood (e.g., weakness, ease of fatigue, pallor, exertional dyspnea, and tachycardia). Gastrointestinal complaints constitute the second most commonly encountered group of symptoms and include a sore tongue, anorexia, nausea, diarrhea, vomiting, perverted sense of taste, and vague abdominal pain. Weight loss is usually slight, occasionally moderate, and only rarely marked. Neurologic abnormalities are responsible for the third group of symptoms; the nature of the complaints depends on the site or sites of involvement. Paresthesias (numbness and tingling) of the feet and hands are most common. Other neurologic complaints involving the extremities are muscular weakness or stiffness, an unsteady gait (especially in the dark), awkwardness (difficulty with fine movements such as lacing shoes or buttoning clothes), and impaired superficial sensation (hypesthesia or hyperesthesia). These symptoms characteristically begin in the most distal portions and usually affect the lower extremities to a greater degree than the upper; they are symmetrical, constant, and progressive. Additional manifestations of neurologic disease include mental depression, irritability, loss of memory, bladder disturbances, impotency, and even frank psychotic behavior ("megaloblastic madness").

The nature and severity of the symptoms in pernicious anemia vary with the magnitude of the deficiency. All gradations in clinical pictures are seen, from the patient who is virtually asymptomatic to one with all the manifestations of the disease. Consequently, it serves no useful purpose to assign relative frequencies to the occurrence of certain complaints. Essentially all patients with far-advanced disease present with the classic triad of weakness, numbness and tingling of the distal portions of the extremities, and a sore tongue; on the other hand, only a few patients with early disease complain of a sore tongue. Neurologic symptoms are prominent in 95 per cent or more of the patients with long-standing disease but may be absent (or at least quite inconspicuous) early in the course. Conversely, anemia always develops at some time during the disease but may not reach a level compatible with symptoms until after neurologic disease is clearly evident. Thus the first manifestations of pernicious anemia may consist of neurologic complaints rather than those of anemia.

Physical Findings. Pallor (often with a lemon-yellow tint), an atrophic uncoated tongue, and a variety of neurologic abnormalities constitute the commonest and most significant physical findings in pernicious anemia. The form and nature of these clinical manifestations depend on the duration of the disease and the degree of vitamin B_{12} deficiency. The patient is ordinarily well nourished and, although appearing chronically ill, is rarely in acute distress, even though the peripheral erythroid values may be extremely low. Slight fever (1 or 2 degrees) is usual in markedly anemic patients. Tachycardia and tachypnea reflect the degree of anemia. In addition to pallor, vitiligo is common. Petechiae and purpura are unusual but may accompany thrombocytopenia. Retinal hemorrhages are frequently associated with severe disease. The tongue is almost always abnormal, even in patients with early disease. Most clinical descriptions of pernicious anemia emphasize the beefy red color of the tongue; however, a pale but smooth and uncoated tongue is a much more common finding (contrary to lay opinion, an adult's tongue is normally coated and an uncoated tongue is abnormal).

Neurologic findings are determined by the relative degrees of involvement of the posterior and lateral columns of the cord as well as the peripheral nerves. As a rule, changes are more pronounced in the feet and legs than in the upper extremities and especially in the distal portions. Although most often bilateral, findings may be more marked in one extremity than in the other. Loss of vibratory sense in the feet and lower legs is the most constant abnormality; occasionally it extends up over the trunk, but vibratory sense is almost always retained in the thorax. Other manifestations of posterior column involvement include loss of position sense, ataxia with a widely based gait, a positive Romberg sign, decreased to absent deep tendon reflexes, and muscle weakness. Lesions affecting the lateral columns produce muscular spasticity, hyperreflexia, and positive Babinski signs (extensor plantar responses). Decreased superficial sensation (often in a stocking or glove pattern) reflects peripheral nerve involvement; however, these lesions rarely produce motor paralysis or muscular atrophy.

It is difficult to assess the over-all frequency of splenomegaly because of its relationship to the severity of the deficiency. Slight to moderate splenomegaly (2 to 6 cm below the left costal margin on deep inspiration) is present in most patients with severe, long-standing disease. On the other hand, a palpable spleen is unusual early in the course of pernicious anemia. Minimal enlargement of the liver is to be expected. Other physical abnormalities lack specificity and, in general, reflect some underlying complication such as congestive heart failure or another associated disease.

Laboratory Findings. PERIPHERAL BLOOD. A macrocytic, normochromic anemia occurs eventually in all patients with pernicious anemia and is almost always present at the time of diagnosis. The peripheral erythroid values vary from near normal to extremely low levels (erythrocyte counts below 1,000,000/cu mm are not unusual). The hemoglobin and hematocrit levels are not proportionately so low as the red cell count because of the presence of macrocytes. The characteristic erythrocyte is large, oval, and well colored; bizarre-shaped microcytes are also prominent (Fig. 5-3). The macrocytes may appear hyperchro-

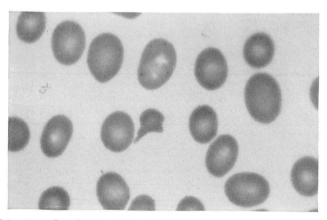

Figure 5-3. Peripheral blood film from a patient with pernicious anemia; the erythrocytes display marked anisocytosis with oval macrocytes and poikilocytic microcytes.

matic because of their increased hemoglobin content, but the concentration of hemoglobin in these cells is normal and they are not "hyperchromic." Typically, the MCV and MCH are increased, whereas the MCHC remains normal (p. 59); however, these cell indexes are particularly subject to error because of the presence of *both* macrocytes and microcytes. The reticulocyte count (both relative and absolute) is low. An occasional nucleated red cell (which usually displays megaloblastic morphology) may be found in the peripheral blood of severely anemic patients, but they are encountered with more regularity and in larger numbers shortly after the start of specific therapy. Red cells may contain a variety of inclusion bodies such as Cabot rings and Howell-Jolly bodies (p. 63). In severely anemic patients the morphologic changes in the erythrocytes are marked and pathognomonic of a vitamin B_{12} or folic acid deficiency. When the anemia is minimal, they may be slight enough to be missed by the untrained or hurried observer. However, large ovalocytes and peculiarly shaped microcytes can be found in the peripheral blood of all untreated patients and are sensitive indicators of vitamin B_{12} or folic acid deficiency.

In patients with mild disease and only slight anemia, the circulating leukocyte count is ordinarily normal. As the deficiency progresses, the leukocyte count falls. In fully developed cases leukopenia (often as low as 2000/cu mm) is as constant a finding as a macrocytic, normochromic anemia. The leukopenia reflects a relative and absolute neutropenia with a relative (but not an absolute) lymphocytosis. However, patients with pernicious anemia are capable of developing leukocytosis in response to such stimuli as acute pyogenic infections. Qualitative leukocytic abnormalities are often more obvious than quantitative changes; hypersegmented neutrophils are particularly prominent. These cells are usually large and possess five or more (sometimes as many as 10) nuclear lobes connected by filaments (Fig. 5-4). They reflect abnormal

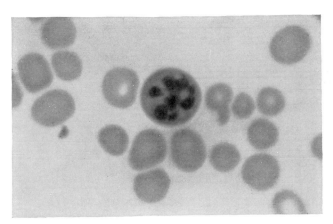

Figure 5-4. Hypersegmented neutrophil from a patient with pernicious anemia.

mitotic activity and are not, as was once thought, "hypermature" cells. The nuclear chromatin pattern is abnormal and shows accentuation of parachromatin and more finely dispersed basichromatin; cytoplasmic granules are often larger and more prominent than in normal cells. Occasional immature granulocytes (metamyelocytes, myelocytes, or, rarely, younger precursors) may be found in the peripheral blood of some patients in relapse.

The platelet count roughly parallels the erythroid values. Slight to moderate thrombocytopenia (50,000 to 150,000/cu mm) is always evident in anemic patients. In addition, the platelets are large and atypical.

Bone Marrow. The bone marrow is hyperplastic; its increased cellularity involves all myeloid elements (Fig. 5-5). However, there

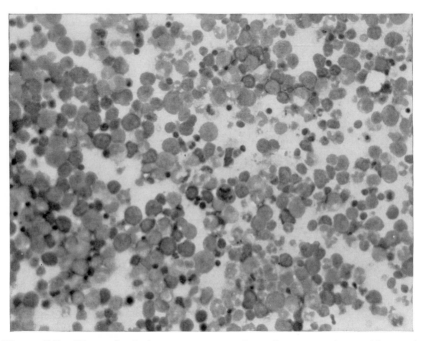

Figure 5-5. Hyperplastic bone marrow aspirate from a patient with pernicious anemia. The increased cellularity involves all marrow elements.

is a disproportionately greater increase in erythropoiesis and the E:G ratio is ordinarily around 1:1. Erythropoiesis is characterized by megaloblastic morphology; all nucleated red cells are affected (i.e., rubriblasts, prorubricytes, rubricytes, and metarubricytes), although the distinctive morphologic abnormalities are most evident in prorubricytes and rubricytes (Fig. 5-6). These cells are correctly termed megaloblastic prorubricytes, megaloblastic rubricytes, and so forth; without this qualifying adjective, names like prorubricytes and rubricytes tacitly infer normoblastic maturation. As a rule, megaloblastic red cell precursors are larger than their normoblastic counterparts (Fig. 1-4, p. 8). Nuclear chromatin is diffusely dispersed into a delicate lacework or reticulated

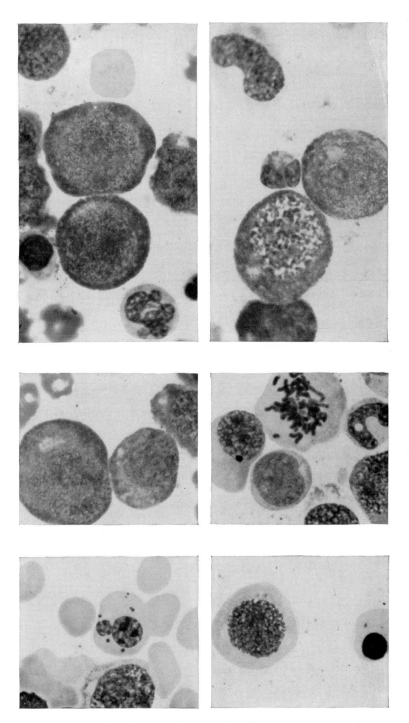

Figure 5-6. Examples of megaloblastic red cell precursors in the bone marrow of a patient with pernicious anemia.

pattern, and parachromatin is thereby accentuated. Asynchronism between nuclear and cytoplasmic maturation is evident. Although cytoplasmic maturation proceeds in an essentially normal fashion, the nuclei retain features of immature cells. Consequently, an erythrocytic precursor with the nucleus of a late prorubricyte may exhibit advanced hemoglobinization of its cytoplasm. Mitotic figures are numerous and often abnormal. In addition, there is evidence of defective maturation and a shift to the left in the ratio of immature:mature nucleated red cells; rubriblasts are especially numerous, whereas metarubricytes may be quite infrequent.

Abnormalities in granulopoiesis are sometimes overshadowed by the striking changes in erythropoiesis. However, the nuclei of developing granulocytes are also characterized by a fine network of basichromatin with accentuated parachromatin and by dissociation of nuclear and cytoplasmic maturation with the latter outdistancing the former. Immature cells are often larger than normal. Giant atypical metamyelocytes are especially prominent (Fig. 5-7), and a shift to the left in the normal ratio of immature:mature granulocytic elements occurs.

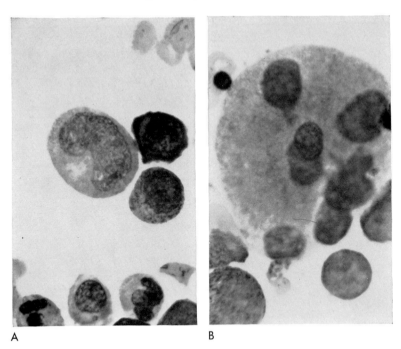

A   B

Figure 5-7. *A.* Giant metamyelocyte. *B.* Atypical megakaryocyte (marrow aspirate from a patient with pernicious anemia).

Thrombopoiesis is also abnormal. Megakaryocytes are present in normal to increased numbers but are atypical with multilobed nuclei and nuclear chromatin patterns similar to those of megaloblastic erythrocytic and granulocytic precursors (Fig. 5-7). Immature megakaryocytes are numerous, but platelet budding is decreased.

In patients with far-advanced disease the bone marrow abnormalities are striking. Under these circumstances virtually every erythrocytic precursor is megaloblastic, and it may be difficult to find a morphologically normal cell, that is, a normoblast. However, in patients with very mild deficiency, erythropoiesis is basically normoblastic with only rare megaloblastic cells. Similar gradations occur in the morphologic alterations of granulocytic elements and megakaryocytes. Thus the bone marrow may vary from one that is grossly and unequivocally abnormal to a specimen that differs only slightly from normal.

OTHER LABORATORY FINDINGS. The most consistent nonhematologic laboratory abnormalities relate to alterations in gastric secretory activity. There is a *histamine-fast achlorhydria*. In fact, the association of achlorhydria with pernicious anemia is so definite that in an adult the presence of free hydrochloric acid in the gastric secretions precludes this diagnosis. Free acid has been demonstrated in rare children or adolescents with pernicious anemia but *never* in an adult. The achlorhydria is actually a manifestation of achylia gastrica; gastric secretions are scant, and pepsin and rennin are markedly decreased to absent. Defective intrinsic factor elaboration is reflected by an abnormal *Schilling test* (p. 216). *Serum vitamin B$_{12}$* levels are decreased (less than 100 μμg/ml). *Serum folate* is normal or increased. *Plasma iron* is often elevated. *Serum bilirubin* is usually slightly increased (1.0 to 1.5 mg/100 ml, with unconjugated bilirubin predominating), as are *urine* and *fecal urobilinogen;* other liver function tests are not remarkable. *Epithelial cells* from the buccal mucosa display megaloblastic morphology, as do those from other sites such as the stomach and vagina. Gastroscopy reveals striking *atrophy of the upper two thirds of the stomach. Serum lactic dehydrogenase* and *malic dehydrogenase* levels are increased. There are no consistent x-ray abnormalities. Other laboratory findings are nonspecific (e.g., albuminuria and the electrocardiographic changes caused by anemia).

Nutritional Folic Acid Deficiency

Dietary folate deficiency occurs in all ages, affects both sexes, and is found in every race and geographic location, although it is more prevalent in certain underdeveloped areas. A careful history will reveal dietary inadequacies.

Symptoms. Symptoms are the same as those of pernicious anemia, with one notable exception; folic acid deficiency is *never* the cause of neurologic disease. Therefore complaints attributable to anemia and gastrointestinal involvement predominate (e.g., weakness, dyspnea, and a sore tongue). Inadequate intake of other essential nutrients may color the clinical picture (e.g., combined ascorbic acid and folate deficiencies). In such patients the major manifestations may be those of scurvy (e.g., abnormal bleeding and pain and tenderness in the extremities) rather than of folate deficiency.

Physical Findings.   With the exception of the neurologic abnormalities, the physical manifestations of folic acid deficiency do not differ from those of pernicious anemia. Pallor and tongue changes are the most consistent findings.

Laboratory Findings.   PERIPHERAL BLOOD AND BONE MARROW. The hematologic manifestations of nutritional folate deficiency are indistinguishable from those of pernicious anemia.

OTHER LABORATORY FINDINGS. As a rule, patients with depleted folate stores have *free acid in their gastric secretions*. Serum *folate* levels are decreased (less than 4.0 $\mu\mu g/ml$); *serum vitamin B$_{12}$* is normal. The urine contains increased amounts of *formiminoglutamic acid* (FIGLU), especially after a loading dose of histidine. Other laboratory findings are similar to those accompanying vitamin B$_{12}$ deficiency.

Other Causes of Vitamin B$_{12}$ Deficiency

The clinical manifestations of vitamin B$_{12}$ deficiency are similar, regardless of the mechanism responsible for the depleted stores. Therefore symptoms, physical abnormalities, and laboratory findings are the same in all types of vitamin B$_{12}$ deficiency and are identical with those of pernicious anemia, with the exceptions of those parameters that assess gastric secretory activity. Achlorhydria and an abnormal Schilling test are constant findings only in patients with pernicious anemia. Free acid and normal amounts of intrinsic factor in the gastric secretions are the rule in other types of vitamin B$_{12}$ deficiency. Certain other differences also serve to set pernicious anemia apart from vitamin B$_{12}$ deficiency due to other causes (Table 5-3) and include (1) the age of the patient (only pernicious anemia is "restricted" to older age groups), (2) history of dietary inadequacy, (3) past surgical procedures such as gastrectomy, resection of the small intestine, or intestinal anastomoses that might have produced blind loops, (4) x-ray evidence of a jejunal diverticulum or severe disease of the stomach, (5) *Diphyllobothrium latum* ova in the stools, and (6) manifestations of a malabsorption syndrome such as diarrhea or other absorptive defects.

Other Causes of Folic Acid Deficiency

The symptoms, physical findings, and laboratory abnormalities resulting from folic acid deficiency are the same, irrespective of its pathogenesis. Clinical manifestations differ only insofar as they are influenced by the primary disorder (Table 5-3). History is often the most important single factor serving to separate the various causes (e.g., history of taking an anticonvulsant drug or recent cytotoxic therapy).

DIAGNOSIS

Although the history and physical findings often suggest a megaloblastic anemia, a firm diagnosis is based on hematologic criteria. A macrocytic, normochromic anemia with oval macrocytes and poikilocytic microcytes, leukopenia with large hypersegmented neutrophils, and thrombocytopenia with large bizarre platelets are pathognomonic of a megaloblastic anemia. There are only a few other causes of a macrocytic, normochromic anemia (reticulocytosis and liver disease are the commonest), and they can usually be excluded by careful examination of the peripheral blood film. In each of these cases the macrocytes are round rather than oval (Fig. 5-8); furthermore, microcytes, poikilocytes,

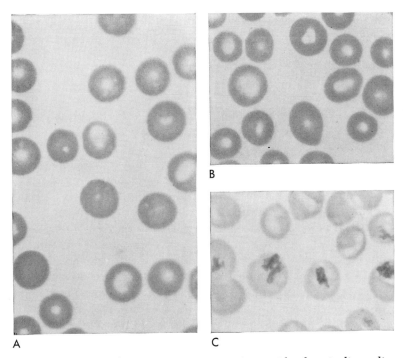

Figure 5-8. *A.* Round macrocytes in a patient with chronic liver disease. *B.* Macrocytosis due to reticulocytosis (Wright's stain). *C.* Macrocytosis due to reticulocytosis (brilliant cresyl blue film).

and hypersegmented neutrophils are not demonstrable. Other pertinent differences include increased polychromasia (and an elevated reticulocyte count), when macrocytosis is the result of reticulocytosis and the presence of target cells and hepatic dysfunction in patients with chronic liver disease. Oval macrocytes and hypersegmented neutrophils are sensitive and valid parameters of megaloblastic hematopoiesis. Large hypersegmented neutrophils are quite specific, even in small numbers; with the exception of rare patients with chronic renal disease in whom small hypersegmented neutrophils may be observed, such cells occur only in those disorders associated with a megaloblastic or megaloblastoid marrow (Table 5-3).

In the face of typical abnormalities in the peripheral blood, it can be predicted with reasonable accuracy that the marrow will exhibit megaloblastic morphology. With few exceptions, therefore, the diagnosis of a megaloblastic anemia can be established with relative ease on the basis of findings in the peripheral blood, and a marrow examination is needed only to exclude a myelomonocytic leukemia (p. 349). Problems are encountered when there is little anemia; even in these instances, however, pathognomonic cells can be found in the peripheral blood (e.g., oval macrocytes or hypersegmented neutrophils). When there are so few typical cells in the peripheral blood that they escape detection by an astute observer, a correspondingly small number of marrow cells will be megaloblastic. Consequently, it is unlikely that a bone marrow examination will supply important diagnostic information unless evidence of marrow dysfunction can be found in the peripheral blood.

Neuropathy seldom exists without the hematologic manifestations of vitamin B_{12} deficiency. Although neurologic disease may dominate the clinical picture or antedate the development of a clear-cut megaloblastic anemia, careful hematologic study will reveal at least minimal abnormalities in virtually all cases. In the untreated patient, therefore, evidence of megaloblastic hematopoiesis is the *sine qua non* of vitamin B_{12} or folic acid deficiency. It must be borne in mind, however, that patients with vitamin B_{12} deficiency respond hematologically to supraphysiologic doses of folic acid; thus hematologic normalcy may be restored in the face of persistent or even progressive neurologic involvement. Until recently most multivitamin preparations contained enough folic acid to effect a hematologic response in vitamin B_{12}-deficient patients. Because many people apparently believe that vitamin supplementation is essential, even though their diets are normal (an incorrect and unfounded assumption), numerous diagnostic pitfalls have been created.

Although the diagnosis of a megaloblastic anemia is contingent on hematologic findings, an etiologic diagnosis is based on nonhematologic data. To accomplish this task, the physician must be aware of the different causes of a megaloblastic anemia (Table 5-3) and of their varying clinical manifestations. With this information at hand, a detailed history and a careful physical examination are indispensable and may point to such obvious causes as dietary inadequacy, some underlying gastrointestinal disorder, pregnancy, a malignancy, severe liver disease, ingestion of an anticonvulsant drug, or recent cytotoxic therapy. Because an uncomplicated folate deficiency does not produce a neuropathy, symptoms or findings of neurologic disease always suggest a vitamin B_{12} deficiency and greatly narrow the list of possible etiologies.

In the absence of any other apparent cause for megaloblastic hematopoiesis, pernicious anemia becomes the most likely suspect. Gastric analysis plays an important role in the work-up of these patients. Achlorhydria is a constant finding in addisonian pernicious anemia, and free acid in the gastric secretions of an adult precludes this diagnosis. However, "histamine-fast achlorhydria," as determined by the usual technique, does not support the diagnosis of pernicious anemia as strongly as the presence of free acid militates against such a likelihood. Using a "standard" dose of histamine, about 15 per cent of otherwise normal subjects over the age of 40 and 25 per cent of those over the age of 60 fail to secrete acid. On the other hand, an augmented test appears to be quite specific for pernicious anemia. This procedure calls for a massive dose of histamine or preferably betazole hydrochloride (Histalog), which has fewer side effects. In response to such a stimulus, patients with pernicious anemia fail to secrete acid (in fact, the gastric secretions often become more alkaline); most, if not all, other individuals will secrete acid, even though the usual techniques have shown them to have "achlorhydria." Unfortunately, the augmented histamine or Histalog test is quite an ordeal for some patients and cannot be recommended as routine; it is contraindicated in the presence of asthma or other severe allergic disease or coronary insufficiency. Even a smaller dose of histamine may be hazardous in certain patients (e.g., those with coronary artery disease). In this regard a gastric analysis is not always required, and a diagnosis of pernicious anemia can generally be made on the basis of other distinctive clinical manifestations. If a problem resists solution without a gastric analysis and this procedure seems unwise because of some underlying disease, a radioactive vitamin B_{12} absorption study is the procedure of choice. A "tubeless" gastric analysis has no real place in the diagnosis of pernicious anemia.

Examples in which the diagnosis can be difficult include (1) patients with mild deficiencies and minimal hematologic findings that may be easily overlooked unless searched for by a diligent, well-trained observer, (2) patients with manifestations of vitamin B_{12} neuropathy but without clear-cut hematologic abnormalities, (3) patients who have received and responded to therapy with multiple agents (e.g., iron, vitamin B_{12}, and folic acid), in whom it is necessary to rule in or out the diagnosis of pernicious anemia and the need for lifelong maintenance therapy, (4) patients with combined deficiencies of vitamin B_{12} and folic acid or those with a megaloblastic anemia and superimposed iron deficiency, and (5) patients with myelomonocytic leukemia. It should be re-emphasized that careful study of the peripheral blood film will usually uncover typical products of a megaloblastic marrow in patients with minimal deficiency as well as in some who have been recently treated. Although their viability is impaired, abnormal red cells produced before the institution of therapy can be detected in the peripheral blood for as long as six weeks after the erythroid values have returned to normal. Hypersegmented neutrophils disappear promptly after treatment is started because of the shorter life-span of granulocytes.

Patients with combined vitamin B_{12} and folic acid deficiencies con-stitute individual problems. When there is superimposed iron deficiency, hypochromia may cause confusion by obscuring, at least partly, some of the erythrocytic changes of a megaloblastic anemia. Careful scrutiny of the peripheral blood film will usually reveal evidence of both defi-ciency states (e.g., hypochromic, oval macrocytes). Perhaps the greatest difficulty is encountered in patients with myelomonocytic leukemia (p. 344). It is commonplace for these individuals to have other manifesta-tions of a leukemic process, but in some every available means may be needed to exclude vitamin B_{12} or folic acid deficiency. Other diagnostic procedures capable of supplying relevant data are radioactive vitamin B_{12} absorption studies, microbiologic assays of blood vitamin B_{12} and folate levels, and therapeutic trials.

Radioactive Vitamin B_{12} Absorption Studies. When a small dose of radioactive cobalt-labeled vitamin B_{12} is given orally, absorption can be assessed by measuring fecal excretion, urinary excretion, uptake by the liver, and plasma levels. Although information obtained by these techniques is comparable, each method possesses certain advantages and disadvantages. The fecal excretion technique requires seven days and the likely possibility that some samples will be lost is an important disadvantage. Uptake by the liver does not depend on the collection of excreta, but it does require three to seven days and may be influenced adversely by underlying liver disease. Measurement of plasma radio-activity is quick but necessitates the use of material with high specific activity or of special counting equipment.

The urinary excretion technique (named the *Schilling test* after its originator) is most adaptable for clinical use. ^{60}Co was used initially, but ^{57}Co is now preferred; this isotope has a half-life of 270 days, as contrasted with the 5.2 year half-life of ^{60}Co. When a small amount of radioactive vitamin B_{12} is given orally and followed within one to three hours by a "flushing" dose of 1.0 mg of nonradioactive vitamin B_{12} given intramuscularly, normal subjects excrete in their urine during the following 24 hours more than 15 per cent of the ad-ministered radioactivity. Individuals with impaired absorption of vitamin B_{12} excrete less than 5 per cent (most patients with addisonian pernicious anemia excrete less than 2 per cent). If the Schilling test reveals impaired absorption, the role of intrinsic factor can be evaluated by repeating the procedure with the addition of a potent intrinsic factor preparation to the radioactive vitamin B_{12}. Persons with abnormal absorption due to inadequate intrinsic factor production should exhibit at least a fivefold increase in urinary radioactivity; excretion will not be affected significantly by the addition of intrinsic factor in patients with impaired vitamin B_{12} absorption consequent to intestinal blind loops, strictures, diverticulae, ileal resections, or one of the spruelike syndromes.

The urinary excretion technique is fast (the test can be completed in 24 hours), and a large amount of the radioactivity is "flushed" out of the body. Falsely low values may reflect incomplete collections of urine, vomiting, diarrhea, or impaired excretion caused by underlying renal disease. Although speculative and without proof, the possibility of deleterious effects on the patient or his progeny by even small amounts of radioactive materials must be reckoned with in the decision to employ clinically a diagnostic test using radioisotopes. In addition, it should be emphasized that 1.0 mg of vitamin B_{12} given parenterally will alter the clinical pictures of *both* vitamin B_{12} and folate deficiency.

Techniques such as the Schilling test have proved to be invaluable investigative tools. Most of our knowledge of the absorption, transport, storage, and excretion of vitamin B_{12} has been obtained in this manner. However, *these procedures are not essential in the work-up of all patients with a megaloblastic anemia, and their routine use cannot be condoned.* The correct diagnosis can generally be reached by using simple clinical parameters, a fortunate fact because radioisotopic tests are not universally available. Furthermore, these absorption tests are not infallible, as some authors tend to infer. In addition to laboratory error, results in some patients are quite difficult to interpret. The difference between 1 and 25 per cent excretion in the Schilling test is clear-cut; the 1 per cent value indicates greatly impaired absorption of vitamin B_{12}, whereas the 25 per cent value is obviously normal. On the other hand, excretion of 5 to 10 per cent of the administered radioactivity (a not infrequent observation) can cause confusion and equivocation.

In most patients an accurate diagnosis can (and should) be made without the use of radioisotopic techniques; however, there are certain straightforward indications for their use. Because these testing procedures do not depend on the level of the peripheral erythroid values, they are of great value in the work-up of the patient who, without benefit of a definite diagnosis, was treated with multiple agents and no longer exhibits any hematologic abnormalities. If the correct diagnosis was pernicious anemia, it is mandatory that lifelong maintenance therapy be recommended. Before the advent of radioisotopic absorption tests, the physician had to choose between continuing therapy or stopping treatment and observing the patient, thus running the risk of incurring neurologic damage from which the patient might not recover. This problem can now be solved readily with a Schilling test. Another absolute indication for such a diagnostic procedure is a person with evidence of vitamin B_{12} neuropathy but without a megaloblastic anemia (e.g., a patient with pernicious anemia who has been treated with folic acid). A Schilling test is also helpful in differentiating between impaired vitamin B_{12} absorption secondary to an intestinal disorder and that caused by deficient production of intrinsic factor, as well as in excluding with reasonable certainty vitamin B_{12} deficiency in patients with myelomonocytic leukemia. Clinically, the best rule to follow is to employ a radioisotopic technique *only* when the diagnosis cannot otherwise be made. Recent experimental observations with tritiated folic acid hold promise of providing a similar means to assess folic acid metabolism, but these procedures are not yet available for clinical use.

Blood Vitamin B_{12} and Folate Levels. It is possible to measure the vitamin B_{12} content of such test materials as serum with bioassay techniques that use microorganisms dependent on exogenous vitamin B_{12} to sustain their growth. Clinical evidence of vitamin B_{12} deficiency is accompanied by serum vitamin B_{12} levels that are less than 100 $\mu\mu g/ml$. Although the technique is accurate and of considerable diagnostic importance, such measurements are not yet generally available and can, for the most part, be obtained only in large medical centers.

Microbiologic assay of serum folate activity presents many technical problems. It is possible to distinguish between normal and low levels, but this procedure is still basically limited to a research laboratory. Formiminoglutamic acid (FIGLU) can be quantified in the urine by using microbiologic, spectrophotometric, or enzymatic techniques. Because the normal catabolism of FIGLU to glutamic acid requires tetrahydrofolic acid, patients with folic acid deficiency excrete increased amounts of FIGLU in their urine, especially after a loading dose of histidine. This technique has been used successfully as a diagnostic tool in the recognition of folic acid deficiency. However, the results must be interpreted with caution because a significant number of patients with vitamin B_{12} deficiency also excrete increased amounts of FIGLU in their urine.

Therapeutic Trials. When all other attempts at diagnosis have failed or if certain procedures such as a Schilling test are not available, a therapeutic trial will yield clear-cut data. The accuracy and diagnostic value of this time-honored technique are incontrovertible. It is essential that the patient be maintained on a diet low in folates and vitamin B_{12} for a period of seven to ten days before a therapeutic trial; daily reticulocyte counts should be obtained during this time. Treatment is then started with daily physiologic doses, administered parenterally, of the most likely suspect (i.e., 1 µg of vitamin B_{12} or 100 µg of folic acid). A positive reticulocyte response implicates the agent being given as the deficient substance.

TREATMENT AND COURSE

Treatment of a megaloblastic anemia due to vitamin B_{12} or folic acid deficiency consists of the administration of the deficient substance; the response is immediate, dramatic, and complete. Within a few hours after appropriate treatment is started, the serum vitamin B_{12} level (or folate) rises, serum iron falls, and reversion to normoblastic morphology begins in the marrow. Mitotable megaloblastic precursors undergo division, yielding two normoblastic cells of comparable maturity. Cells that have already matured to a postmitotable stage remain megaloblastic. Within two to five days all megaloblastic precursors are replaced by normal cells. During the first 48 to 72 hours the patient often reports subjective improvement in the form of an increased appetite and sense of well being. Reticulocytes begin to appear in the peripheral blood within 48 hours. The maximum reticulocyte response is reached within five to nine days with parenteral therapy and within 8 to 12 days with oral treatment. The reticulocyte response begins earlier and reaches its peak sooner in patients who are markedly anemic. The height of the reticulocytosis varies inversely with the pretreatment erythroid values. When the initial erythrocyte count is less than 1,000,000/cu mm, the maximal reticulocyte response is about 40 per cent; it is about 20 per cent with a pretreatment red count around 2,000,000 and less than 10 per cent if the count is more than 3,000,000. During the second to third week of treatment, the reticulocyte response subsides, and the erythroid values begin to increase rapidly because of the production of increased numbers of normal cells. Barring some other hematologic abnormality, normal peripheral erythroid values are restored within five to eight weeks. A few oval macrocytes may persist even after the circulating hemoglobin has returned to normal. These cells were formed before or shortly after the start of therapy and do not reflect continued megaloblastic erythropoiesis.

Concomitant with the hematologic response, the patient undergoes rapid and gratifying clinical improvement. All symptoms subside, and all physical and laboratory abnormalities disappear with the singular exception in patients with pernicious anemia of the achlorhydria and gastric atrophy, which are permanent. Patients responding in some other fashion need further study that will reveal a misdiagnosis or some additional abnormality which has prevented a full response (e.g., superimposed iron deficiency or underlying liver disease).

Insofar as possible, treatment should be deferred until an etiologic diagnosis has been made; a single agent (i.e., vitamin B_{12} or folic acid) should then be started. If the anemia is so severe that immediate therapy is deemed necessary, both vitamin B_{12} and folic acid should be given parenterally. After the patient's clinical status improves, appropriate studies can be undertaken to clarify the cause. Because adequate treatment is available, transfusions are needed only when the erythroid values are so low that life is immediately threatened. In these situations small quantities of packed red cells should be used to avoid circulatory overload, and the patient should be given *only* enough blood to tide him over. Under *no* circumstances should this patient be transfused to normal or near normal levels. If a single transfusion eliminates acute tissue hypoxia or brings about significant improvement in a patient with cardiac failure, there is no need for additional blood. Normal erythroid values can be safely and rapidly restored by replacement therapy. Because therapeutic regimens differ somewhat for the various causes of a megaloblastic anemia (Table 5-3), it is expedient to consider their treatment and courses separately.

Pernicious Anemia. Parenteral (intramuscular) vitamin B_{12} therapy is the treatment of choice and is completely effective. Patients will respond to 1 μg a day or less; however, vitamin B_{12} is nontoxic, and it is better to "overtreat" than to run the risk of progressive neurologic damage. An appropriate program consists of 100 μg of vitamin B_{12} (cyanocobalamin) intramuscularly each day for the first week, three times weekly until the erythroid values return to normal, and every two weeks for six months. The patient without significant neurologic involvement can then be placed on maintenance therapy (100 μg per month), which *must* be continued for the rest of his life. Patients with vitamin B_{12} neuropathy require more intensive therapy for longer periods of time (i.e., 100 μg twice weekly) until maximal neurologic improvement has been achieved. It is seldom worthwhile to continue this dose beyond one year, after which 100 μg every two weeks should suffice. When pharmacologic doses of vitamin B_{12} are given parenterally, a much larger proportion (as much as 70 per cent or more) is excreted in the urine than is the case with physiologic doses. Despite this loss, supraphysiologic doses are justified because actual body gain is significantly greater. Equivalent amounts of other cobalamins such as hydroxycobalamin are also effective.

Response to treatment is most gratifying. All hematologic abnormalities disappear, as do most of the other manifestations of vitamin B_{12} deficiency (e.g., tongue involvement). Achlorhydria persists and, because of the poor regenerative capacity of nerve tissue, neurologic recovery may not be complete. Neurologic improvement is most marked during the first six months of treatment, and evidence of vitamin B_{12} neuropathy persisting after a year of therapy can be considered permanent. Although all neurologic abnormalities may not disappear, neuropathy *never* progresses in the face of adequate replacement therapy.

No other therapeutic measures are indicated unless some complication is present. Iron is needed only when there is superimposed iron deficiency; folic acid is required only when there is a combined deficiency of both vitamin B_{12} and folic acid. Patients with pernicious anemia should never be given folic acid by oral or parenteral routes unless vitamin B_{12} is given simultaneously. Pharmacologic doses of folic acid (5 to 10 mg and perhaps as little as 0.5 mg/day) will temporarily restore hematologic normalcy in a patient with pernicious anemia. However, folic acid will not affect vitamin B_{12} neuropathy beneficially. In fact, neurologic involvement may actually be worsened. Folic acid is innocuous when administered with vitamin B_{12}, but combined therapy offers no advantage over vitamin B_{12} alone.

In markedly anemic patients all unnecessary manipulations should be postponed until replacement therapy has been started. These individuals are in a precarious state, and even minimal stress (e.g., gastrointestinal x-rays) may have disastrous results. The diagnosis of far-advanced disease can be made on the basis of a history, physical examination, and hematologic evaluation. All other diagnostic procedures should be deferred, pending therapeutic response. If additional studies are essential for a correct diagnosis, it is preferable to treat such patients initially with both vitamin B_{12} and folic acid.

An intensive effort has been made to find a form of oral treatment that is dependable and safe. Massive doses of vitamin B_{12} (500 µg or more daily) are effective by mouth; however, the amount that is actually absorbed is unpredictable. Physiologic amounts of vitamin B_{12} are also effective orally when given together with heterologous (e.g., porcine) intrinsic factor. Unfortunately, certain patients treated in this manner relapse in the face of continued therapy; many of these individuals have demonstrable antibodies against exogenous intrinsic factor which may play an important role in the development of therapeutic refractoriness. Furthermore, there is always the very real likelihood that asymptomatic patients may neglect to take daily oral medications. In view of these criticisms, there is little justification for the substitution of a wholly reliable form of therapy (i.e., intramuscular vitamin B_{12}) for another that is at best unpredictable.

Without treatment pernicious anemia is uniformly fatal in one to three years. In the optimally treated patient survival is comparable to that of otherwise normal persons of similar age. There is an increased incidence of gastric neoplasms (carcinoma and polyps). Data differ, but such lesions appear to occur about five times more often in patients with pernicious anemia than in others. Consequently, appropriate x-ray examinations should be repeated promptly in the event of unexplained gastrointestinal symptoms.

Other Types of Vitamin B_{12} Deficiency. The treatment of a megaloblastic anemia due to a nutritional deficiency of vitamin B_{12} consists of 5 μg of vitamin B_{12}/day orally in addition to the correction of dietary inadequacies. The vitamin B_{12} can be discontinued after normal erythroid values have been achieved, provided assurances exist of an adequate diet in the future. Patients with vitamin B_{12} deficiency consequent to gastrectomy or extensive gastric disease should be managed in the same way as those with pernicious anemia. All persons who are subjected to a complete gastrectomy should be placed on parenteral maintenance therapy prophylactically. Patients with sprue and vitamin B_{12} deficiency should be treated in a similar fashion. Megaloblastic anemias accompanying intestinal blind loops, strictures, or diverticulae also respond to parenteral therapy, as do those caused by *Diphyllobothrium latum.* Some patients in the first categories will exhibit temporary responses to antibiotics, but such an approach cannot be recommended as the sole form of treatment. If a small intestinal lesion such as a blind loop can be surgically eradicated, a permanent cure will ensue. Elimination of the fish tapeworm in patients so infested will also preclude the need for permanent maintenance therapy.

Folic Acid Deficiency.   There are few indications for parenteral folic acid. Small doses (i.e., 100 to 200 μg/day) are effective in folate-deficient patients; 1 to 5 mg/day (the amount contained in most available preparations) are more than ample even in individuals with defective absorption. All clinical manifestations caused by folate deficiency disappear promptly after replacement therapy is begun; the subsequent course and outcome depend on the nature of the underlying disease. Folic acid-deficient patients will display suboptimal and temporary hematologic responses when given supraphysiologic doses of vitamin B_{12} (i.e., 30 μg or more daily). A megaloblastic anemia will not be affected by the administration of folic or folinic acid if it is caused by congenital orotic aciduria, cytotoxic therapy, or a myelomonocytic leukemia. Persons with liver disease and a deficiency of dihydrofolic reductase will respond to folinic acid, as will recipients of folic acid antagonists (p. 355). The megaloblastic anemia associated with anticonvulsant drugs can be effectively treated with the oral administration of folic acid, and it is not necessary to discontinue the anticonvulsant.

Hypoplastic Anemias

A hypoplastic anemia is the clinical syndrome resulting from bone marrow failure; it may be idiopathic, congenital, or the result of any of a variety of marrow toxins (drugs, chemicals, or ionizing radiation). Functionally, a hypoplastic anemia is distinguished by qualitatively normal but quantitatively inadequate marrow activity. Morphologically, it is characterized by peripheral blood pancytopenia and by marrow hypocellularity without atypical precursor cells or evidence of space-occupying infiltrations. All bone marrow elements are generally affected; however, erythrocytic hypoplasia occurs singly, and instances of isolated granulocytic or megakaryocytic hypoplasia have been observed. Among the many names that have been used, *aplastic or hypoplastic anemia* and *refractory anemia* have gained widest acceptance. The latter is vague and should be discarded, for it permits inclusion of all anemias that are unresponsive to therapy, regardless of cause. Because complete marrow aplasia probably never occurs, hypoplastic anemia is the most appropriate designation. The clinically distinct syndromes caused by marrow hypoplasia are listed in Table 5-4.

Table 5-4. Classification of the Clinical Syndromes Caused by Marrow Hypoplasia

I. *Hypoplastic Anemia (Pancytopenia)*
  A. Acquired
    1. Primary (idiopathic)
    2. Secondary (due to a chemical or physical agent)
  B. Congenital (Fanconi's syndrome)

II. *Erythrocytic Hypoplasia (Anemia)*
  A. Acquired
  B. Congenital

III. *Granulocytic Hypoplasia (Neutropenia)*

IV. *Megakaryocytic Hypoplasia (Thrombocytopenia)*

In recent years there has been a growing tendency to classify, under the heading of hypoplastic (or aplastic) anemia, patients with relative bone marrow failure, that is, inadequate functional reserve to augment marrow output maximally in response to increased need, as well as those with defects in maturation and/or delivery of cells to the peripheral blood (ineffective myelopoiesis). Although these patients have peripheral blood cytopenias, their bone marrows are normocellular or hypercellular. Because of the inclusion of such disorders in the category of hypoplastic (or aplastic) anemia, the hypoplastic anemias have gradually acquired the connotation of functional marrow incompetency. This concept of physiologic rather than anatomic inadequacy has been responsible for much confusion, for it encompasses a heterogeneous group of diseases differing importantly in cause, management, and course. Discussion of the clinical manifestations of this group as a whole is meaningless. Although it is highly desirable and often essential to envisage myelopoiesis in functional rather than in purely morphologic terms, it is clinically advantageous to restrict the diagnosis of "hypoplastic anemia" to those patients whose primary abnormality is decreased blood cell production consequent to a physical lack of precursors in the bone marrow. Peripheral pancytopenia due to "functional" rather than "anatomic" hypoplasia should be classified under other headings. On careful study most cytopenic patients with normo- or hypercellular marrows will be found to be examples of hypersplenism (p. 448), subleukemic leukemia (p. 344), agnogenic myeloid metaplasia (p. 433), an atypical myeloproliferative disorder such as a "preleukemic state" (p. 353), a myelophthisic anemia (p. 240), or some systemic infection such as miliary tuberculosis or disseminated histoplasmosis. These patients should not be diagnosed as having hypoplastic anemia simply because production fails to keep pace with peripheral need.

HISTORY

Ehrlich is credited with the initial clinical description of hypoplastic anemia in 1888 and with the recognition that it was due to marrow hypocellularity. Chauffard introduced the term aplastic anemia in 1904. Although a variety of agents, such as benzene and arsenic, were soon implicated in the causation of marrow hypoplasia, it became apparent early that in many patients the precise cause could not be ascertained. In 1927 Fanconi described three siblings with congenital hypoplastic anemia and a variety of other inborn abnormalities and defects. Josephs (1936) and Diamond and Blackfan (1938) first called attention to another type of congenital hypoplastic anemia involving only red cell precursors. Subsequently acquired forms of erythrocytic hypoplasia, as well as rare patients with isolated granulocytic or megakaryocytic hypoplasia, were observed.

Acquired Hypoplastic Anemia

ETIOLOGY

Studies on the etiology of the hypoplastic anemias have been seriously limited by the inability to produce bone marrow failure in experimental animals with many chemical substances known to cause marrow hypoplasia in man and by the absence of naturally occurring animal counterparts of idiopathic acquired and congenital forms of hypoplastic anemia. Theoretically, a hypoplastic anemia could result from an inadequate stimulus to blood cell production. Such a pathogenic mechanism cannot be excluded with absolute certainty; however, the presence of increased plasma erythropoietic factor activity in patients with acquired and congenital hypoplastic anemias detracts greatly from the tenability of this hypothesis. Pending further study, it is more logical to assume that marrow hypoplasia reflects a primary cellular defect (or defects).

About 50 per cent of the patients with acquired hypoplastic anemia deny contact with any potentially injurious substance, and no reason for marrow failure can be found; they must be classified as primary or idiopathic. In the other half it is possible to implicate some chemical or physical agent. These marrow toxins can be divided into two groups (Table 5-5). The first includes those that consistently produce hypo-

Table 5-5. *Causes of Acquired Hypoplastic Anemia*

   I. *Mitotic Poisons (consistently produce marrow hypoplasia; dose-dependent)*
      A. Ionizing radiation (x-ray, ^{32}P)
      B. Radiomimetic drugs (e.g., nitrogen mustard, cyclophosphamide, busulfan, chlorambucil)
      C. Antimetabolites (methotrexate, 6MP)
      D. Mitotic inhibitors (urethane, colchicine derivatives)
      E. Miscellaneous (e.g., benzene)

   II. *Miscellaneous Drugs and Chemicals (rarely produce marrow hypoplasia)*
      A. Antimicrobials [e.g., chloramphenicol, organic arsenicals, streptomycin, sulfonamides, quinacrine (Atabrine)]
      B. Antihistaminics
      C. Antithyroid drugs
      D. Anticonvulsants (hydantoins)
      E. Tranquilizers (e.g., chlorpromazine and meprobamate)
      F. Insecticides
      G. Heavy metals (e.g., gold, bismuth, mercury, and silver)
      H. Industrial solvents

plastic anemia in man and laboratory animals, provided they have been adequately exposed. Although the modes of action of these noxious substances differ, each interferes with the proclivity of marrow precursors to undergo homeoplastic mitosis. The end result is anatomic hypoplasia, decreased marrow output, and peripheral blood pancytopenia. All dividing cells are affected by these mitotic poisons, but marrow failure dominates the clinical picture because of the greater proliferative activity of blood cell precursors. In general, the degree of marrow hypoplasia varies directly with the dose. Recovery usually follows minimal marrow injury; the severer the hypoplasia, the greater are the chances that the marrow failure will be permanent and irreversible.

The second group of etiologic agents is large and heterogeneous (Table 5-5). This list, which is growing rapidly, includes drugs (few medicinal agents have not been implicated in the pathogenesis of acquired hypoplastic anemia) as well as a variety of commonly encountered chemical substances such as insecticides, hair dyes, and cosmetics. The evidence incriminating this group of agents in the causation of hypoplastic anemia is largely circumstantial. They do not produce marrow hypoplasia in laboratory animals, and human experimentation is both infeasible and dangerous. Only rare individuals develop marrow failure on exposure, and the high mortality rate militates against rechallenging a patient who has recovered from a hypoplastic anemia. For these reasons it is virtually impossible to obtain absolute proof that a drug or chemical has caused marrow hypoplasia.

The manner by which these drugs and chemicals produce marrow hypoplasia is unknown. Since so few exposed persons develop marrow failure, it must reflect individual sensitivity. Such an idiosyncrasy, which could be acquired or genetically determined, may involve mechanisms concerned with the metabolic degradation and/or excretion of certain drugs and chemicals. There is no consistent relationship between dose or length of exposure and the development of a hypoplastic anemia. Whereas some persons manifest marrow failure after long and continued exposure, others develop fulminant and almost complete marrow aplasia after minimal contact. Occasionally, repeated exposure appears to play a role. In certain patients several weeks may elapse between contact with the offending agent and the clinical onset of a hypoplastic anemia. Possible pathogenic mechanisms include (1) a direct toxic effect on some essential enzyme system or basic cellular constituent such as DNA and (2) an immunologic reaction consequent to the elaboration of antibodies triggered by a drug, chemical, or one of their metabolites acting as a hapten. These factors could operate singly, together, or conjointly with other mechanisms (e.g., an induced deficiency of some still unknown factor necessary for normal myelopoiesis). It also seems likely that different agents may affect the marrow differently, even though the end result is the same, that is, peripheral blood pancytopenia.

Chloramphenicol deserves special mention because of the frequency with which it is associated with a hypoplastic anemia. In most parts of the world, this antibiotic appears to be responsible for more cases of hypoplastic anemia than any other single agent, and there is convincing evidence that it is a bone marrow toxin. A frank hypoplastic anemia is a rare aftermath of chloramphenicol therapy. However, erythropoietic depression is common and is dependent on the blood chloramphenicol level which reflects dose, duration of treatment, and liver or renal disease (the latter interfere, respectively, with inactivation by glucuronide conjugation and excretion of chloramphenicol and its metabolities). Functional erythropoietic suppression precedes other abnormalities and is manifested by an elevated plasma iron, increased saturation of the iron-binding protein, and decreased ^{59}Fe incorporation in hemoglobin. Continued administration of the drug evokes reticulocytopenia and morphologic abnormalities in the marrow, which include clear, round vacuoles in the cytoplasm (they often form a collar around the periphery of the cell) and nuclei of red cell precursors (Fig. 5-9).

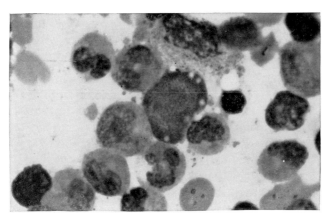

Figure 5-9. Vacuoles in the cytoplasm of an erythrocytic precursor in the bone marrow of a patient with erythropoietic suppression caused by chloramphenicol.

In addition, immature nucleated red cells increase in number. If the drug is continued after the onset of these ferrokinetic and morphologic aberrations, the peripheral erythroid values begin to fall in 10 to 14 days. Further evidence of the suppressive effect of chloramphenicol on erythropoiesis has been obtained in patients with pernicious anemia or iron deficiency anemia, in whom it prevents the typical reticulocyte response to replacement therapy with vitamin B_{12} or iron.

Chloramphenicol appears to act by interfering with the attachment of messenger or template RNA to ribosomes, thereby impairing protein synthesis. The erythropoietic manifestations of chloramphenicol therapy are usually reversible when the drug is stopped. Still unanswered is the question pertaining to the relationship between the frequently encountered erythropoietic toxicity and the infrequent development of a hypoplastic anemia with peripheral blood pancytopenia. There are two schools of thought. One maintains that erythropoietic suppression presages generalized marrow toxicity. The opposing view contends that a chloramphenicol-induced hypoplastic anemia is the result of an idiosyncratic reaction and reflects a different pathogenic mechanism than that responsible for such abnormalities as hyperferremia and vacuolated erythrocytic precursors. The striking disparity between the frequency of erythropoietic suppression and the incidence of hypoplastic anemia, as well as the occasional patients who manifest marrow hypoplasia after a short course of therapy, favors an idiosyncratic reaction. However, most patients who develop a hypo-plastic anemia do so only after prolonged administration of large doses, and some patients with erythropoietic suppression exhibit vacuoles in marrow granulocytic elements, even though their leukocyte counts are normal. It is obvious that further study is needed before this problem can be resolved.

PATHOPHYSIOLOGY

The fundamental abnormality in the acquired hypoplastic anemias is reduced myelopoiesis consequent to anatomic hypoplasia. The bone marrow is characterized by increased amounts of fat with a variable number of hematopoietic foci. Marrow aspirates or open biopsies are typically hypocellular; however, a fortuitous aspiration from an island of active blood cell formation may yield a normocellular or even a hypercellular specimen. Although quantitatively decreased, marrow func-tion is qualitatively normal and the marrow cells do not exhibit specific morphologic aberrations. Maturation proceeds in an orderly manner. Since there are comparable decreases in erythropoiesis and granulo-poiesis, the E:G ratio remains normal. There is generally a relative (but not an absolute) increase in marrow lymphocytes and plasmacytes.

The quantitative curtailment in marrow output is reflected in the peripheral blood by a pancytopenia, that is, anemia, leukopenia, and thrombocytopenia. The cells formed are morphologically normal and physiologically competent. Therefore, the anemia is normocytic, normo-chromic, without significant alterations in erythrocyte morphology. The reticulocyte count is decreased, and red cell survival times are normal. Slightly increased amounts of an alkali-resistant hemoglobin (presum-ably Hgb F) have been found in a few patients (both acquired and congenital forms of the disease), but the precise significance of these observations is not known. The leukopenia reflects a relative and ab-solute neutropenia with a relative (but not an absolute) lymphocytosis. Typically, the leukocytes in the peripheral blood are mature and mor-phologically normal, although BGN is often increased. The thrombo-cytopenia is not associated with other platelet abnormalities; it is responsible for a prolonged bleeding time, impaired clot retraction, and a positive capillary resistance test.

The manifestations of an acquired hypoplastic anemia are directly attributable to bone marrow failure; dysfunction of other organs is not apparent. Thus the clinical picture is a composite of or is dominated by the symptoms and physical findings of anemia, a hemorrhagic dia-thesis (thrombocytopenia), and frequent infections (neutropenia). The pathogenic mechanism(s) responsible for the marrow hypoplasia also appears to affect the pluripotential reticulum cells in other tissues, and extramedullary hemopoiesis is notably absent. Consequently, splenomegaly, hepatomegaly, and adenopathy are not characteristic of hypoplastic anemia and, when present, point to another diagnosis or to some superimposed disorder such as transfusion hemosiderosis, serum hepatitis or its aftermath postnecrotic cirrhosis), or an acute bacterial infection with secondary lymphadenitis.

CLINICAL MANIFESTATIONS

About half of the patients with acquired hypoplastic anemia have secondary disease; that is, they give a history of recent exposure to some toxic agent; the remainder have no discernible cause and must be classified as primary or idiopathic. The clinical manifestations are the same in both groups. Acquired hypoplastic anemia is a rare cause of anemia. Although its exact frequency is unknown, these patients are scarce even in institutions with active clinical hematology services. Few reported series include more than 50 cases; however, it is entirely reasonable to anticipate a rising incidence. During the last two decades an impressive array of potentially toxic drugs has been introduced into clinical medicine. In addition, man's chemical environment has become exceedingly complex because of the widespread use of insecticides, food preservatives and additives, and so forth. As a result, the entire population is now more or less constantly exposed to a variety of substances capable of inflicting severe marrow damage in susceptible persons. Acquired hypoplastic anemia affects all ages from the very young to the elderly. It occurs in all parts of the world but is slightly more common in males than in females and is somewhat less common in Negroes than in other races.

Symptoms. As a rule, the onset of an acquired hypoplastic anemia is insidious, but it may be acute and fulminant. The presenting complaints are contingent on the degree of marrow hypoplasia and the speed with which it develops. Symptoms of anemia (e.g., weakness, ease of fatigue, and exertional tachycardia and dyspnea) may predominate in patients with chronic, slowly progressive disease, but when severe marrow hypoplasia develops suddenly, the first manifestations are more likely to be abnormal bleeding or an enhanced susceptibility to infections. Initially, the symptoms always reflect one or more aspects of bone marrow failure and other systemic complaints are unusual. As the disease progresses, additional symptoms may have their onset consequent to the development of transfusion hemosiderosis or serum hepatitis. Because the manifestations attributable to hemorrhage and infection depend on the location of the bleeding and the site and nature of the infectious process, the clinical picture is far from stereotyped.

Physical Findings. Physical findings are nonspecific and protean, for they reflect bleeding or intercurrent infections. Pallor and hemorrhagic phenomena (e.g., petechiae, purpura, epistaxis, gingival bleeding, and retinal hemorrhages) are the most consistently encountered physical abnormalities. Patients with acquired hypoplastic anemia are well nourished and fail to exhibit evidence of other organ dysfunction. Splenomegaly, hepatomegaly, and adenopathy are not characteristic. Early in the course of the disease an enlarged spleen or liver suggests some other diagnosis; however, splenomegaly and/or hepatomegaly secondary to hemosiderosis are fairly common in patients with longstanding hypoplastic anemia who have received multiple transfusions.

Laboratory Findings. PERIPHERAL BLOOD. Patients with acquired hypoplastic anemia invariably have a moderate to marked normocytic, normochromic anemia. It is not uncommon for the peripheral erythroid values to reach extremely low levels. When the erythrocytes are evaluated before transfusions, their morphology is essentially normal (red cells formed by the patient do not manifest significant anisocytosis or poikilocytosis). However, most patients depend on transfusions for the maintenance of a satisfactory red cell mass. Therefore transfused cells comprise the bulk of the circulating erythrocytes and greatly influence the over-all picture in regard to red cell morphology. Indeed, the spheroidal configuration of many transfused cells contrasted with normal-sized cells probably accounts for the once widely held view that most or at least many hypoplastic anemias were "macrocytic." There is little evidence of active blood cell regeneration, and both relative and absolute reticulocyte counts are decreased. Nucleated red cells in the peripheral blood occur so rarely, if ever, that their presence casts grave doubt on the validity of the diagnosis. Red cell life-span is normal in patients with early disease, as are osmotic and mechanical fragilities. Decreased erythrocyte viability caused by extrinsic factors is demonstrable in some patients who have received numerous transfusions, but an overt hemolytic anemia is unusual, even in these situations. Increased quantities (5 to 10 per cent) of an alkali-resistant hemoglobin (presumably Hgb F) may be found.

Leukopenia and thrombocytopenia accompany the anemia. The severity of these cytopenias parallels the degree of anemia. The leukopenia reflects a relative and absolute neutropenia with a relative (but not an absolute) lymphocytosis. Some patients also manifest a lymphopenia. Immature leukocytes are not present in the peripheral blood. BGN (p. 309) is often moderately to strikingly increased. In patients with severe hypoplasia, the leukocyte count may be less than 1000/cu mm and the neutropenia, literally absolute. Platelet morphology is normal but thrombocytopenia is ordinarily marked.

BONE MARROW. Typically, the marrow is diffusely hypocellular with increased amounts of fat (Fig. 5-10). Because this quantitative abnormality chiefly affects erythrocytic precursors, granulocytic elements,

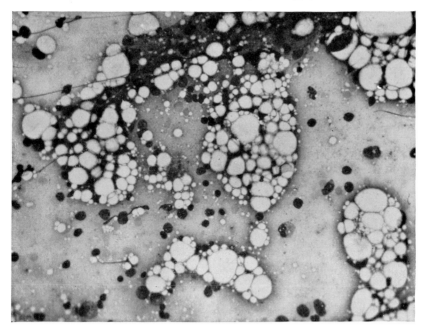

Figure 5-10. Bone marrow aspirate from a patient with an acquired hypoplastic anemia, showing decreased cellularity and increased fat.

and megakaryocytes, there is a relative (but not an absolute) lymphocytosis. There is a relative and occasionally a slight absolute increase in plasmacytes, and mast cells are often increased in number. Bone marrow cells display normal morphology, but BGN is generally quite evident. Stainable marrow iron is often increased, especially in patients with long-standing disease or in those who have received multiple transfusions. Because the residual myelopoietic activity is usually present in small islands of active blood cell formation, a fortuitous aspiration or open biopsy (this technique is often needed in order to procure an adequate specimen) may yield cellular clumps which exhibit normal maturation, morphology, and differential counts. Thus a cellular marrow is not necessarily incompatible with the diagnosis of a hypoplastic anemia; however, it would be distinctly unusual for repeated sampling to reveal similar findings

OTHER LABORATORY FINDINGS. *Plasma iron* is increased, whereas the *plasma iron-binding capacity* is normal or decreased (saturation is therefore increased). *Plasma ^{59}Fe clearance and ^{59}Fe incorporation into circulating hemoglobin* are both decreased. Other laboratory findings are nonspecific and include diverse abnormalities attributable to anemia, hemorrhage, intercurrent infection, transfusion hemosiderosis, and serum hepatitis. A complete listing serves no useful purpose.

DIAGNOSIS

The diagnosis of acquired hypoplastic anemia is based on the findings of peripheral blood pancytopenia and myeloid hypoplasia in the absence of any other disorder affecting the marrow. A history of recent exposure to some drug, chemical, or physical agent known to be capable of causing hypoplastic anemia is often helpful. However, it is impossible to elicit a history of significant contact with a bone marrow toxin in about half the patients. Absolute proof of the diagnosis of an acquired hypoplastic anemia demands the demonstration of recurrent marrow hypoplasia following rechallenge with the suspected causative agent in a patient who has recovered fully. Such an approach is obviously impractical. Even in those individuals who recover and in whom there is good reason to suspect a single agent as being pathogenically important, deliberate re-exposure can rarely be justified because of the real danger of inducing irreversible and fatal marrow hypoplasia.

Adherence to the foregoing diagnostic criteria (pancytopenia and anatomic marrow hypoplasia) greatly simplifies this category of disease by eliminating a pathogenically heterogeneous group of disorders characterized by functional "hypoplasia." Inclusion of such entities as hypersplenism and the preleukemic state under the general heading of "hypoplastic anemia" serves only to confuse the clinical picture of hypoplastic anemia and to retard the elucidation of its cause. In general, the demonstration of one or more of the following in a patient suspected of having hypoplastic anemia points to some other diagnosis: (1) abnormal erythrocyte morphology, (2) an absolute reticulocytosis, (3) nucleated red cells or immature granulocytes in the peripheral blood, (4) a normocellular or hypercellular marrow, (5) evidence of qualitative marrow dysfunction (morphologic abnormalities and altered maturation), and (6) splenomegaly, especially if present early in the course of the disease. The manifestations of those disorders characterized by pancytopenia and most likely to simulate (at least superficially) a hypoplastic anemia (p. 224) are sufficiently distinct that they can be separated with relative ease on the basis of simple clinical parameters, that is, a history, physical examination, and careful study of the peripheral blood and bone marrow.

TREATMENT AND COURSE

No form of therapy will reverse marrow hypoplasia or impart a primary stimulus to hematopoiesis. However, acquired hypoplastic anemia is characterized by a variable tendency to undergo spontaneously partial and complete remissions. Consequently, the primary goal of treatment is to support the patient pending such a development. When first diagnosed, there is no accurate way to predict which patient will improve. About 30 per cent of adults manifest a complete remission or recover sufficiently so that medical care is no longer needed and they can lead an essentially normal life. Improvement may occur within a short time or may not be evident for months or even years. Therefore the therapeutic maxim, "never give up," is particularly appropriate for this disorder, even though the over-all mortality rate of 70 per cent remains distressingly high. Approximately 40 per cent of adult patients exhibit a fulminant and rapidly progressive course, terminating in death within six months. About 30 per cent succumb to hemorrhage or intercurrent infection (these complications are the major causes of death) after periods of time varying from a few months to as long as four to five years. Although accurate survival data must await observations in larger numbers of patients, the prognosis of acquired hypoplastic anemia is considerably better in children than in adults, primarily because of the benefit ascribable to corticosteroids and androgens (see later).

If a drug, chemical, or physical agent can be implicated in the pathogenesis of a hypoplastic anemia, it must be stopped at once. If the responsible agent falls into the group (Table 5-5) that appears to involve an idiosyncratic reaction, immediate steps should be taken to prevent re-exposure. Because contact with potential marrow toxins is becoming so widespread and because few patients are treated with a single medicinal agent, it is becoming more and more difficult to implicate one substance in the pathogenesis of a hypoplastic anemia. If any doubt exists and a person is receiving more than one drug, all medications should be stopped. A limited number of patients will improve rapidly after contact with the offending agent ceases; others will not. In the latter group, as well as in those patients in whom the cause is not apparent, intensive support is indicated. Several types of supportive therapy are available.

Transfusions. Blood transfusions constitute the cornerstone in the treatment of acquired hypoplastic anemia and should be used as needed to maintain satisfactory peripheral erythroid values. Packed red cells are preferred, for they are less likely to produce circulatory overload than are whole blood transfusions. The patient should be transfused only to the level that provides adequate tissue oxygenation commensurate with his activity and metabolic requirements (usually a hemoglobin of 9 to 10 gm/100 ml of blood). It is foolhardy to transfuse beyond this level, for it will not improve physiologic function or ameliorate symptoms. Furthermore, unnecessary transfusions will hasten the development of transfusion hemosiderosis. Since many patients depend on transfusions for the rest of their lives (or at least for many years), the complications of repeated transfusions figure importantly in the management of acquired hypoplastic anemia.

Transfusion hemosiderosis (p. 537) is to be expected after 100 or more transfusions and contributes directly to death in a significant number of patients. Chelating agents such as desferrioxamine B (p. 186) offer a promising but still inadequately evaluated means of ridding the body of excess iron, and forestallment of the development of serious tissue hemosiderosis by the judicious use of transfusions remains the best positive approach to this problem. Multiple transfusions also increase the risk of such undesirable side effects as serum hepatitis (p. 535) and sensitization to minor blood group factors with resultant hemolytic transfusion reactions (p. 532). In large part, however, these adverse effects are unavoidable and the risks are clearly justified, for transfusions are essential to sustain the patient's life.

Because their red cell mass can be augmented with relative ease by transfusions, patients do not succumb to anemia. Neutropenia and thrombocytopenia are the commonest causes of death, for they are not benefited by blood that has been collected and administered in accordance with standard blood bank and transfusion protocol. Techniques are now available in most large medical centers for the procurement and administration of platelets, but to date many important problems have resisted solution. Although the initial effect is usually dramatic (the circulating platelet count increases and bleeding often ceases), survival of donor platelets in the recipient leaves much to be desired. Viability decreases rapidly with subsequent platelet transfusions, presumably a reflection of the elaboration of antiplatelet immunoglobulins in response to the stimulus provided by platelets possessing different antigenic factors from those of the recipient. Consequently, the indications for platelet transfusions are more clear-cut in certain acute, self-limited thrombocytopenias than in chronic hypoplastic anemia, although they are rapidly assuming an indispensable role in tiding over the chronic patients during severe hemorrhagic episodes. It is reasonable to predict that basic knowledge to be derived from current and future experimental studies will greatly improve the effectiveness of platelet transfusions. Such developments will permit much more optimism insofar as the ultimate prognosis of hypoplastic anemia is concerned. Preliminary observations on the feasibility of leukocyte transfusions are now underway in several laboratories. Granulocytes from patients with chronic granulocytic leukemia and from normal subjects have been shown to survive in neutropenic recipients and appear to lessen their susceptibility to infection; however, much work remains to be done before the therapeutic potentiality and practicality of leukocyte transfusions can be ascertained. At the moment these studies constitute the most promising approach to lengthening survival and decreasing mortality in patients with acquired hypoplastic anemia.

Antibiotics. Infections are an ever-present threat to neutropenic patients. Modern antimicrobials have done much to lessen morbidity and mortality. Emergence of resistant organisms and superinfection with fungi militate against the use of antibiotics prophylactically. However, immediate antibiotic coverage (including a bactericidal agent) in greater than usual doses is indicated at the first sign of an infectious process. After appropriate cultures and when in vitro sensitivity studies are available, empirically chosen drugs can be changed, but delay in instituting antibiotics must be avoided.

Corticosteroids. Corticosteroids have little to offer the adult with primary (idiopathic) or secondary acquired hypoplastic anemia. Thus the undesirable side effects of prolonged corticosteroid therapy (especially an increased susceptibility to infection in a person who is already prone to develop serious infectious complications) must figure importantly in the decision to use these compounds. Most of the favorable reports that attribute improvement to corticosteroids appear to involve patients falling into the heterogeneous group of disorders characterized by functional hypoplasia. It is logical to assume that a certain number of these patients would respond [e.g., those with pancytopenia due to hypersplenism (p. 462)]. Unfortunately, inclusion of these patients under the heading of acquired hypoplastic anemia has been responsible for the erroneous inference that all individuals so diagnosed have a reasonably good chance of responding to corticosteroids. If one adheres to the diagnostic criteria already outlined and excludes all patients except those with bone marrow failure caused by anatomic hypoplasia, the ineffectiveness of this therapy becomes quite apparent. Therefore the diagnosis of acquired hypoplastic anemia in an adult is not in itself an indication for corticosteroids; the potential disadvantages outweigh what little, if any, benefit might accrue. However, the high mortality rate justifies a trial of corticosteroids in certain selected patients, especially those with marked thrombocytopenia and a severe hemorrhagic diathesis. If improvement is not evident after four to six weeks, there is virtually no hope that continued therapy will accomplish anything other than to increase the likelihood that the patient will develop one or more of the adverse effects of corticosteroids. In contrast to the poor results attributable to corticosteroids in adults, a significant number of children with acquired hypoplastic anemia respond slowly (but often dramatically) to long-term therapy with androgens and corticosteroids.

Androgens. During the last few years much interest has developed in the erythropoietic effects of testosterone (p. 16), especially in patients with hypoplastic anemia. Scanty observations in adults are not encouraging, and controlled studies in a large group of patients are needed before androgens can be assigned a precise role in the therapy of acquired hypoplastic anemia. In children, however, rather striking improvement has been attributed to a combination of androgens and corticosteroids. Various forms of testosterone have been used. Parenteral testosterone enanthate (weekly injections of 300 to 600 mg) has several potential advantages, including sustained action and a relative lack of serious complications (e.g., cholangiolitic jaundice). Although few series are large, a significant number of children treated in this manner have manifested a delayed and sustained reticulocytosis after several weeks to months of therapy, followed by an increase in the peripheral erythroid values. Less often, the leukocyte and platelet counts have also increased. Responses have varied from none to slight to complete remissions that tend to persist even after the testosterone and corticosteroids are discontinued. Certain data are quite persuasive, but it must be borne in mind that acquired hypoplastic anemias (both primary and secondary) are characterized by a tendency to undergo partial or complete remissions spontaneously. Occasionally, complete remissions occur after hypoplasia has persisted for several years. Consequently, the results of specific therapy must be interpreted with caution. Although the final answer is not known, guarded optimism is justified. Pending the introduction of some other agent of undoubted therapeutic superiority, most children with acquired hypoplastic anemia deserve a trial of testosterone and corticosteroids. Certain unwanted effects are to be expected with massive doses of testosterone (e.g., masculinization in females, virilization in males, and fluid retention); however, the lack of alternative therapeutic agents and the generally poor prognosis detract considerably from their importance.

Splenectomy. The role of splenectomy in the treatment of hypoplastic anemia is a controversial subject about which much has been written. There is little doubt that certain patients have improved following removal of the spleen. On close scrutiny, however, few of these patients have had true marrow hypoplasia. Instead, they appear to have had some disease associated with functional hypoplasia [e.g., hypersplenism (p. 462)] or some complication such as transfusion hemosiderosis with splenomegaly and decreased red cell survival. Since patients with hypoplastic anemia are poor surgical risks, splenectomy is indicated only in the presence of overt hypersplenism. With a normal blood volume of about 5000 ml, the red cells contained in approximately 500 ml of blood would be destroyed by natural destructive processes every 12 days. Therefore failure of one unit of blood to maintain the level of the circulating hemoglobin for this period of time points to decreased viability of erythrocytes (autologous and homologous). Such a patient is a potential candidate for splenectomy, but the decision to operate can be made only after careful consideration of each individual case. In most patients with hypoplastic anemia, splenectomy is hazardous and without benefit.

Other Therapeutic Measures. Numerous agents have been recommended from time to time; none has been consistently effective and scattered reports of therapeutic successes have not been confirmed. In this regard, it should be re-emphasized that acquired hypoplastic anemia is a capricious disease that displays a tendency to undergo spontaneous remissions after variable periods of time. Cobaltous chloride deserves special mention because it has been widely used. However, there is no proof that cobalt stimulates blood cell production in this disorder and it cannot be recommended (the potential toxicity of cobalt far outweighs any hope for benefit). To date, the results of bone marrow transplantation have been quite disappointing. For the most part, graft failure is probably similar to rejection of homologous transplants in other situations, but persistence of the pathogenic mechanism responsible for the marrow hypoplasia may also play a role and might preclude success even with an isologous or autologous graft.

Congenital Hypoplastic Anemia

This syndrome (approximately 75 patients have been reported) is characterized by multiple congenital anomalies, including marrow hypoplasia and peripheral blood pancytopenia. It is often termed Fanconi's syndrome. Sporadic cases have been observed; however, the hereditary nature appears to be clear-cut, and the majority of the patients give a history of hypoplastic anemia or some congenital anomaly in other members of their families. There is also an increased incidence of leukemia in the families of children with congenital hypoplastic anemia, but the significance of this observation is not apparent. The syndrome appears to reflect multiple defects of closely linked, autosomal recessive genes; the precise abnormality (or abnormalities) is not known. Bone marrow failure usually does not manifest itself until the child is several years old. Occasionally, the hematologic aspects of this congenital disorder are not evident until adolescence.

The clinical manifestations are similar to the acquired hypoplastic anemias plus those attributable to one or more congenital defects. Some of the more commonly observed anomalies are skin pigmentation, small stature, a variety of skeletal abnormalities, hypogenitalism, strabismus, renal defects, mental retardation, and deafness. Diagnosis is based on the demonstration of peripheral blood pancytopenia and marrow hypoplasia plus one or more congenital anomalies. A positive family history provides additional helpful information. Some observers have classified separately a second type of congenital hypoplastic anemia without other associated anomalies; however, such an entity is difficult to delineate from idiopathic acquired hypoplastic anemia. Even in the presence of a positive family history, the possibility of similar environmental exposure cannot be excluded.

In general, the prognosis of congenital hypoplastic anemia is poor. The course is generally progressive, and death in childhood is due to bleeding, infection, or transfusion hemosiderosis. Rare patients have survived to adulthood and spontaneous remissions and relapses have been observed. Improvement has been attributed recently to the simultaneous, long-term administration of corticosteroids and androgens. In the relatively few patients who have been treated in this manner relapse has followed discontinuation of these agents. Although the exact role of this therapeutic regimen must await evaluation in more patients, the rareness and severity of congenital hypoplastic anemia are such that a trial is indicated. Transfusions and antibiotics play the same important roles in the management of these patients as they do in those with acquired hypoplastic anemia.

Congenital Erythrocytic Hypoplasia

Pure red cell anemia, aregenerative anemia, erythrogenesis imperfecta, and the Diamond-Blackfan syndrome are other names that have been applied to this rare disorder, characterized by anemia and marrow erythrocytic hypoplasia. Circulating platelet and leukocyte counts are normal, and granulopoiesis and thrombopoiesis remain active. Anemia usually appears around the age of four months, but it has been observed at birth and has not had its onset until several years of age in a few patients. The cause is unknown. Although its appearance in infancy suggests strongly that this syndrome is congenital, there is little support for the concept that it is hereditary or genetically transmitted. Limited observations point to a defect in tryptophan metabolism (increased amounts of anthranilic acid, a metabolite of tryptophan, have been found in the urine of some but not all children with this anemia). The pathogenic importance of this biochemical abnormality is quite speculative, but it represents a promising lead and should be subjected to further study.

Initially, the clinical manifestations are those of anemia. The peripheral blood reveals a normocytic, normochromic anemia and reticulocytopenia without other abnormalities. There is a striking paucity of nucleated red cells in the bone marrow, whereas other myeloid elements are present in essentially normal numbers. The course is variable with spontaneous remissions occurring in as many as 30 per cent of the patients, even after several years have elapsed. Transfusions as needed to maintain satisfactory erythroid values constitute the most important therapeutic measure; however, a significant number of patients will respond to corticosteroids (beginning response is usually evident within two weeks), and every patient deserves such a therapeutic trial. The development of transfusion hemosiderosis is often a serious problem. Reports of splenomegaly and a hemolytic component in patients with congenital erythrocytic hypoplasia most likely reflect hemosiderosis rather than the basic disease. If superimposed hemolysis becomes an important contributing factor, splenectomy may be worthwhile.

Acquired Erythrocytic Hypoplasia

In adults the clinical manifestations of erythrocytic hypoplasia are similar to those in children with congenital erythrocytic hypoplasia, although the etiologic factors appear to be much more variable. About 50 such patients have been reported. Approximately half of the adult patients with erythrocytic hypoplasia have had associated thymic tumors; this relationship cannot be ascribed to chance and must be of pathogenic importance. The histologic appearances of the thymomas have been varied and inconstant. Because of the basic role of the thymus in the body's immunologic milieu, that is, a source of immunologically competent cells, it has been suggested (but not yet proved) that the thymic tumor may be responsible for the elaboration of antibodies directed against marrow erythrocytic precursors. In those patients in whom a thymoma cannot be found the etiology has rarely been detected. In a few cases a drug or some other bone marrow toxin has been implicated in the causation of acquired erythrocytic hypoplasia, but most of these patients have to be classified as idiopathic.

The clinical manifestations are predominately those of anemia. Splenomegaly has been observed in some patients, but it most likely reflects transfusion hemosiderosis or perhaps some unrecognized myeloproliferative disorder such as a preleukemic state (p. 353). Most patients have a normocytic, normochromic anemia with a cellular marrow characterized by the presence of few (if any) nucleated red cells. Occasional patients have been reported to have neutropenia and/or thrombocytopenia, but these hematologic abnormalities may be secondary to some complication such as a transfusion hemosiderosis.

Diagnosis is based on the demonstration of selective erythrocytic hypoplasia in the bone marrow. The course is variable and typically chronic. Transfusion hemosiderosis is a common terminal event. If a thymoma can be demonstrated, thymectomy is indicated and may be curative. If erythrocytic hypoplasia is caused by a drug, the medicinal agent must, of course, be stopped. Corticosteroids are generally without effect, but a therapeutic trial may be in order; the same applies to treatment with androgens. Splenectomy is indicated only in those patients who have definite evidence of superimposed hypersplenism. A few patients have been observed to develop acute leukemia as a terminal event. Rather than reflecting the natural course of acquired erythrocytic hypoplasia, it seems more likely that the initial diagnosis was probably in error and that the erythrocytic hypoplasia was an early manifestation of an atypical myeloproliferative disorder.

Granulocytic Hypoplasia

Isolated granulocytic hypoplasia is usually due to some drug with a predilection for granulocytic precursors [e.g., phenothiazines (especially chlorpromazine), certain antithyroid drugs, and phenylbutazone]. A few patients have been described with idiopathic acquired granulocytic hypoplasia (analogous to acquired erythrocytic hypoplasia), but insufficient data preclude etiologic speculations. Neutropenia and an increased susceptibility to infection characterize the clinical picture. If caused by some drug or chemical, contact with the offending agent must be eliminated at once. Treatment consists of those measures designed to combat the neutropenia in acquired hypoplastic anemia and is purely supportive.

Megakaryocytic Hypoplasia

Megakaryocytic hypoplasia rarely occurs as an isolated finding. Although megakaryocytes are especially sensitive to certain medicinal agents, such as gold salts, erythrocytic and/or granulocytic hypoplasia usually accompanies megakaryocytic hypoplasia. A few patients have been described with idiopathic megakaryocytic hypoplasia analogous to congenital or acquired erythrocytic or granulocytic hypoplasia. These patients exhibit thrombocytopenia and a hemorrhagic diathesis. Therapy is supportive and consists of platelet transfusions and corticosteroids.

Myelophthisic Anemias

The abnormalities in the peripheral blood associated with space-occupying lesions of the marrow are referred to collectively as a *myelophthisic or leukoerythroblastic anemia*. The causes are multiple and the manifestations are variable. Nonetheless, the hematologic picture is sufficiently well defined to warrant its consideration as a separable syndrome. Metastatic tumor is the usual cause. Lung, breast, prostate, thyroid, and stomach carcinomas, melanocarcinoma, and neuroblastoma are the most common offenders because of their tendency to metastasize early via vascular channels to bone. Marrow involvement is typically focal but may be diffuse. Red marrow-containing bones are affected most often without predilection for a particular site (the sternum and iliac crests are involved with about

equal frequency). Some hematologic neoplasms also produce myelophthisic anemias, especially plasmacytic myeloma (p. 418). Less often,
lymphomatous involvement of the marrow evokes similar findings. Certain
of the manifestations of leukemia, such as a slight reticulocytosis and a
few nucleated red cells in the peripheral blood, may also be explicable on
a myelophthisic basis, but they are ordinarily obscured by the more
striking leukocyte abnormalities ascribable directly to the leukemic process. The peripheral blood picture of agnogenic myeloid metaplasia is
characteristically that of a myelophthisic anemia (p. 433). Less prevalent
causes include Gaucher's disease, Niemann-Pick disease, and granulomatous infections of the marrow (e.g., tuberculosis or histoplasmosis).

The pathogenesis of the myelophthisic anemias is not clear. Although
customarily attributed to "crowding out" of normal marrow elements by
abnormal cells, this explanation is rarely tenable. Correlation between the
degree of marrow involvement and the magnitude of the hematologic
findings is poor, and striking changes in the peripheral blood may be associated with minimal marrow metastases. In occasional patients with
widely disseminated malignant disease, extensive marrow replacement by
tumor cells is reflected in the peripheral blood by a moderate to marked
pancytopenia. More often, however, the anemia is slight and the leukocyte
and platelet counts are normal or increased. In most patients with malignant space-occupying lesions of the marrow, the anemia appears to reflect the pathogenic mechanisms responsible for the anemia of malignant
disease without marrow metastases (p. 290). The other hematologic
manifestations of a myelophthisic anemia might best be described as
"irritative phenomena" consequent to some poorly defined disturbance in
the normal homeostatic milieu of the bone marrow.

CLINICAL MANIFESTATIONS

Because of its diverse etiologies, myelophthisic anemias affect both
sexes and occur in all ages and races. The symptoms and physical findings
lack specificity and are determined by the nature of the underlying primary disease. The rarity of splenomegaly in patients with nonhematologic
neoplasms deserves emphasis. Although microscopic metastases can be
found in a significant number of persons dying of metastatic carcinoma, a
palpably enlarged spleen consequent to splenic metastases is distinctly
unusual.

Laboratory Findings. PERIPHERAL BLOOD. The hematologic manifestations of space-occupying lesions of the marrow are the same, regardless of their cause. Typically these patients have a mild to moderate
normocytic, normochromic anemia. Not uncommonly, however, the peripheral erythroid values are at the lower limits of normal or only slightly
decreased. Increased polychromasia, a reticulocyte count of 3 to 6 per
cent, and 1 to 5 nucleated red cells/100 leukocytes are characteristic

findings; very rare patients exhibit a large number of circulating nucleated red cells (10 to 50 or more/100 leukocytes). Increased rouleau formation and elevated erythrocyte sedimentation rates are common (a reflection of the marrow plasmacytosis and hyperglobulinemia that accompany many types of malignancies).

The leukocyte count is normal, slightly decreased, or more often slightly increased (10,000 to 20,000/cu mm); marked leukocytosis is unusual but has been observed. Of greater diagnostic significance than these variable quantitative changes is the rather consistent finding in the peripheral blood of small numbers of immature granulocytes. All stages of immaturity may be represented, including myeloblasts. Other peripheral leukocyte abnormalities include basophilic granulation of the neutrophils (BGN), occasional irritation lymphocytes (p. 312), and even rare plasmacytes. As a rule, the platelet count is normal or increased (sometimes quite strikingly so); thrombocytopenia occurs in a few patients but is a much less common finding. In general, the platelets are morphologically normal, although large, bizarre forms may be noted as well as an occasional circulating, atypical megakaryocyte.

Bone Marrow. The bone marrow may be normal or may contain diagnostically specific cells or exhibit nonspecific changes such as increased number of mature plasmacytes. Because most space-occupying lesions are focal rather than diffuse, routine marrow aspirates are often negative even in patients with proved marrow involvement. "Aimed punctures" (aspirations at sites of pain, tenderness, or bony deformity) are most likely to produce specific cells. Introduction of the needle into a relatively large tumor nodule may yield a uniform population of abnormal cells. More often, however, tumor cells are scattered among normal marrow elements, either singly or in small clumps or syncytia. A trained observer has little difficulty recognizing malignant cells that have originated from an extramedullary site, but with few exceptions it is impossible to ascertain the location of the primary tumor on the basis of individual cell morphology. The widely differing appearances of malignant cells are contingent on the nature of the primary lesion, although they possess several common morphologic attributes, including hyperchromicity and prominent nucleoli. The presence of small clumps or syncytia of abnormal cells is a particularly helpful finding. Since a marrow specimen may contain only a rare clump of malignant cells, it is necessary to examine with care many preparations before concluding that an aspirate is negative. Examples of several types of malignant cells in Wright-stained marrow aspirates are shown in Figure 5-11. Although this technique permits retention of detailed cell morphology and greatly facilitates the recognition of malignant cells, examination of serial fixed tissue sections is generally more productive because of the greater amount of material available for study. Patients with myelophthisic anemias secondary to hematologic ma-

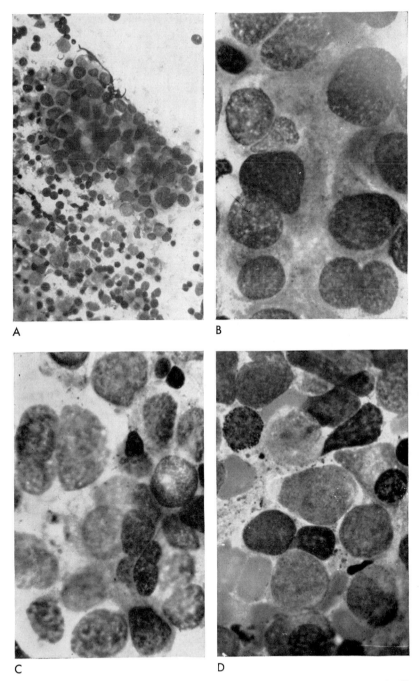

Figure 5-11. Examples of carcinoma cells in bone marrow aspirates. *A.* Carcinoma of the stomach. *B.* High-power view of tumor cells shown in *A.* *C.* Bronchogenic carcinoma. *D.* Carcinoma of the prostate.

lignancies display marrow abnormalities unique to the type of neoplastic disease (e.g., myeloma cells in plasmacytic meloma, Reed-Sternberg cells in Hodgkin's disease, and lymphosarcoma cells in lymphosarcoma). Gaucher (Fig. 12-1, p. 459) and Niemann-Pick cells are fairly distinctive and not easily confused with normal marrow elements or with metastatic carcinoma cells. As a rule, granulomatous infections cannot be recognized in marrow aspirates, and their diagnosis ordinarily requires marrow biopsy and/or cultures. However, exceptions occur, and such organisms as *Histoplasma capsulatum, Leishmania donovani,* and *Myobacterium tuberculosis* have been observed in routine marrow aspirates.

OTHER LABORATORY FINDINGS. Other laboratory findings are quite variable and depend on the primary disease. Bone x-rays are of particular interest; however, it must be borne in mind that about one third of patients with known bone marrow metastases have negative bone x-rays. In contrast to the lesions of plasmacytic myeloma, which are purely lytic, most bone metastases are mixed (osteolytic and osteoblastic) or predominately osteoblastic (e.g., carcinoma of the prostate).

DIAGNOSIS

The diagnosis of a myelophthisic anemia is suggested by a combination of hematologic abnormalities that is not characteristic of any other better-defined disorder (e.g., nucleated red cells and immature granulocytes in the peripheral blood, slight reticulocytosis, and very little if any anemia). The presence of some disease such as carcinoma, which is known to be associated with space-occupying marrow lesions, is, of course, helpful information. A positive diagnosis is based on the actual histologic demonstration of the marrow lesions (e.g., carcinoma cells). However, a significant number of patients with a myelophthisic anemia will have negative marrow aspirates or biopsies, even on repeated examinations. It seems likely that all patients with peripheral blood manifestations of a myelophthisic anemia have marrow involvement, even though it may resist demonstration. There are insufficient data to determine whether bone marrow metastases or proliferation in the marrow cavity of other "foreign cells," such as Gaucher cells, can be associated with an entirely normal peripheral blood. Such an occurrence would appear to be unlikely but cannot be excluded with certainty.

In general, a myelophthisic anemia can be diagnosed (or at least strongly suspected) with relative ease. Elucidation of the nature (and site) of the basic disease is often much more difficult; for example, where is the primary tumor? Hematologic abnormalities, that is, a myelophthisic anemia, may first call attention to the presence of disseminated malignancy. Of even greater pertinence, however, is the demonstration of a myelophthisic anemia in a patient with a known malignancy, because it negates the possibility of a localized tumor and confirms the presence of metastatic disease. Such an observation contraindictates "curative" or radical surgery. All patients with a malignant process and hematologic findings suggesting a myelophthisic anemia deserve one or more marrow examinations before definitive surgery. On the other hand, the chances of obtaining a diagnostic specimen in a patient with an entirely normal peripheral blood are so slight that routine preoperative marrow examination cannot be justified in all patients with malignant disease.

Although the peripheral blood manifestations of a myelophthisic anemia may resemble superficially a number of primary hematologic disorders (e.g., agnogenic myeloid metaplasia, leukemia, and hemolytic anemia), other clinical findings (especially the marrow examination) readily point to the correct diagnosis and eliminate confusion. In this regard it should be emphasized that any discussion of the differential diagnosis of myelophthisic anemia is largely a problem in semantics. A myelophthisic anemia is defined as the peripheral hematologic manifestations of the proliferation of abnormal cells (hematologic and nonhematologic) in the marrow or, in the case of agnogenic myeloid metaplasia, in the deposition of excess fibrous tissue. It is not a well-defined or sharply delineated entity. Thus it should be viewed as a reflection of some other disorder and not as a disease *sui generis*. Whether the space-occupying lesion consists of carcinoma cells, fibrous or bony tissue (agnogenic myeloid metaplasia or marble bone disease), or Gaucher cells, the end result is the same—a leukoerythroblastic blood picture. Consequently, diagnosis of the primary disease must rest on criteria other than changes in the peripheral blood.

TREATMENT AND COURSE

The course and prognosis of a myelophthisic anemia are those of the underlying disease. Since the primary disorder is most often disseminated malignancy, the outlook is grave. There is no treatment other than that indicated for the basic disease (e.g., cytotoxic therapy). Transfusions are rarely needed, for the anemia is usually not severe. There are no indications for any type of antianemic therapy unless the patient manifests an additional superimposed defect such as iron deficiency, folic acid deficiency, or hypersplenism. Because many types of neoplasm are associated with blood loss, iron deficiency often accompanies a myelophthisic anemia. The clinical manifestations are then colored by those of iron deficiency (p. 172), and treatment with iron is indicated. A few patients with malignant disease develop folic acid deficiency consequent to increased requirements coupled with inadequate intake; a megaloblastic, macrocytic anemia (p. 201) then contributes to the clinical abnormalities caused by bone marrow metastases, and these patients should be treated with folic acid. Less often patients with certain malignant disorders develop hypersplenism; the manifestations and treatment are then those of hypersplenism, regardless of cause (p. 461). In the absence of any of these treatable complications, most patients with a myelophthisic anemia show progressive worsening of their hematologic abnormalities. However, improvement does accompany control of the underlying disease (e.g., treatment of metastatic breast carcinoma with androgens or prostatic carcinoma with estrogens). In these patients serial hematologic evaluations may provide relevant information regarding the efficacy of the oncolytic therapy.

Hereditary Hemoglobinopathies

The *hemoglobinopathies* are clinical syndromes caused by defective hemogloblin synthesis consequent to genetically determined abnormalities in the formation of the globin moiety of the molecule. These disorders can be divided into *qualitative* and *quantitative hemoglobinopathies*. The qualitative are characterized by the production of structurally abnormal hemoglobin molecules. The quantitative reflect deficient production of normal hemoglobin and are usually referred to as the *thalassemia syndromes*. Occasionally qualitative and quantitative hemoglobinopathies coexist. The heterozygous state (a single abnormal gene) is associated with few, if any, clinical abnormalities; however, homozygosity or double heterozygosity (an abnormal gene inherited from each parent) causes serious and often fatal disease.

NORMAL GLOBIN SYNTHESIS

Knowledge of the structure of the hemoglobin molecule and of the genetic factors controlling globin synthesis are requisite for a discussion of the etiology and pathophysiology of the hereditary hemoglobinopathies. The composition of hemoglobin is described elsewhere (Fig. 1-7, p. 18); the following points deserve re-emphasis. The hemoglobin molecule is made up of heme (iron protoporphyrin 9, type III) and globin. The globin moiety consists of four polypeptide chains composed of amino acids arranged in a definite sequential and spatial pattern. The predominant normal human hemoglobin (Hgb A) contains two types of globin chains. The α chains constitute 141 amino acids and have a molecular weight of 15,126; β chains contain 146 amino acids and have a molecular weight of 15,866. Each molecule of Hgb A has two α chains and two β chains. Two other hemoglobins, Hgb F (fetal hemoglobin) and Hgb A₂, are present in small amounts in the normal adult. Each contains two α chains that are identical with those in Hgb A. Replacing the β chains of Hgb A are γ chains (Hgb F) and δ chains (Hgb A₂). Although γ- and δ-peptide chains contain the same number of amino acids as β chains, their amino acid composition differs. β and δ chains bear the closest resemblance and differ by fewer than 10 amino acids; β and γ chains differ by more than 30 amino acids. β, γ, and δ chains are more closely related in structure to one another than to α chains, which differ from normal β chains by more than 70 amino acids.

Since the heme moieties of the normal hemoglobins are identical, it is appropriate to designate them according to the structural formulas of their globin moieties. Thus Hgb A is written as $\alpha_2\beta_2$, Hgb F as $\alpha_2\gamma_2$, and Hgb A_2 as $\alpha_2\delta_2$. The absence of a superscript denotes a structurally normal globin chain; the addition of a superscript indicates a qualitatively abnormal chain (e.g., $\alpha_2\beta_2^S$ is the formula for Hgb S or sickle cell hemoglobin).

During the first few months of gestation, only α- and γ-peptide chains are synthesized. Therefore the normal fetal hemoglobin is Hgb F ($\alpha_2\gamma_2$). At about the fifth month β-chain synthesis begins, and Hgb A ($\alpha_2\beta_2$) appears. At birth Hgb F normally makes up 60 to 80 per cent of the hemoglobin. By the age 12 to 18 months, Hgb F has decreased to less than 5 per cent; by the age of four years, normal adult levels (less than 2 per cent) are reached. δ-chain production begins at about the same time β chains make their appearance; however, Hgb A_2 normally does not exceed trace amounts (less than 2.5 per cent), even in adult life. The precise physiologic significance of Hgb F is not known. In vivo it appears to have a greater affinity for oxygen than Hgb A; however, this difference is not demonstrable in vitro. The γ chains of Hgb F are the only human globin chains that contain isoleucine; Hgb F can be identified and readily separated from other hemoglobins on the basis of its resistance to alkali and acid denaturation. Some evidence suggests that δ chains may represent a fairly recent evolutionary development from β-peptide chains and that Hgb A_2 ($\alpha_2\delta_2$) may be destined to replace Hgb A ($\alpha_2\beta_2$).

Synthesis of each of the normal globin chains (α, β, γ, and δ) is controlled by two structural genes (allelomorphic cistrons on a pair of autosomal chromosomes). The β and δ loci are closely linked and are near the gene controlling γ-chain production; however, the locus for α-chain formation appears to be on a different chromosome. The genetic control of normal hemoglobin synthesis is depicted schematically in Figure 5-12. Each structural gene makes messenger RNA, which transmits the basic genetic code from the nucleus to the cytoplasm. Molecules of messenger RNA attach in template fashion to ribosomes and direct peptide bond formation. Amino acids are added in the precise order determined by the messenger RNA, and a complete globin chain is produced in about 90 seconds. Although every red cell precursor is able to synthesize α, β, γ, and δ chains, there appears to be room for only one template on each polyribosome unit, with the resultant synthesis of a single kind of peptide. The hemoglobin molecule consists of two subunits made up of a pair of identical polypeptide chains (e.g., $\alpha_2\beta_2$); hybrid molecules (e.g., $\alpha_2\beta\gamma$) have not been demonstrated as occurring normally or in any of the hemoglobinopathies. Thus globin chains are apparently dimerized before they are liberated into the solution of the cell. Therefore it is permissible to consider one gene responsible for the synthesis of one subunit composed of two similar globin chains. The mere presence of two like polypeptide

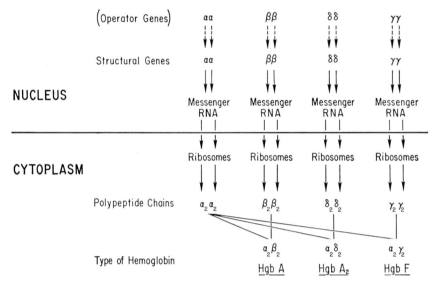

Figure 5-12.   Genetic control of hemoglobin synthesis.

chains is apparently sufficient for their combination, which appears to take place without any known energy, enzymatic, or genetic requirements.

Many facets of the control of hemoglobin synthesis remain to be clarified, including the mechanisms that are responsible for "turning off" γ-chain production and for "turning on" β- and δ-chain synthesis as well as those that determine the quantitative relationship between the normal hemoglobins; for example, why is there more than 40 times as much Hgb A formed as Hgb A$_2$? A popular, but unproved, thesis concerns the possible role of regulatory or operator genes (Fig. 5-12). Although there is no genetic proof of such genes in mammalian cells, it seems likely that the activity of many structural genes may be controlled in this manner. Operator or regulatory genes could be responsible for "turning on" β-chain production shortly before birth. It is also possible that such a δ-chain regulator might be set at a much lower level than the hypothetical β-regulator gene, thus explaining the discrepancy between β- and δ-chain synthesis. Some sort of feedback mechanism affecting a γ regulator could be responsible for the reciprocal relationship between γ- and β-chain production.

Qualitative Hemoglobinopathies

The clinical syndromes caused by structural changes in the peptide chains that make up the globin moiety of the hemoglobin molecule are termed, collectively, the *qualitative hemoglobinopathies*. Abnormal hemoglobins, such as Hgb Bart's and Hgb H, are composed of four γ and four β

chains and do not fall into this category, for the individual polypeptide chains are structurally normal. These tetramers reflect suppression of
α-chain synthesis and are therefore associated with the quantitative hemoglobinopathies (p. 273). A single change in the amino acid sequence of a
globin chain can cause marked alterations in the chemical and physical
properties of the hemoglobin molecule; a variety of clinical manifestations
ensues. Most of the clinically significant qualitative hemoglobinopathies
are the result of mutations of the structural genes controlling β-peptide-
chain synthesis. Although the heterozygous state is associated with the
presence of an abnormal hemoglobin, it rarely causes significant alterations in bodily function. On the other hand, homozygosity is reflected by
serious disease, characterized in most instances by a chronic, progressive
hemolytic anemia. In general, a double heterozygote, that is, a person
with two different abnormal genes, displays clinical manifestations midway between those of the heterozygote and homozygote.

H I S T O R Y

The first qualitative hemoglobinopathy to be recognized clinically was
sickle cell anemia. The initial description of this disorder was made in
Chicago by Herrick in 1910; his patient, a 20-year-old Negro male, pre-
sented with marked anemia and peculiar crescent-shaped erythrocytes in
his peripheral blood. Emmel described the development of sickling
in vitro five years later. Mason suggested the name sickle cell anemia in
1922. In 1923 Talifero and Huck pointed out the hereditary nature of
this disease. It soon became evident that there were two kinds of sickle
cell disease of varying severity (one was distinguished by the presence
of sickle cells in vivo, severe anemia, and early death; the other was associated with the development of sickle cells in vitro, normal peripheral
erythroid values, and normal longevity). The first evidence that the hemoglobin molecule in sickle cell anemia was structurally altered consisted
of the demonstration of its abnormal electrophoretic behavior by Pauling
and his associates in 1949. This structurally different hemoglobin was designated Hgb S. Credit for the initial description of a globin abnormality
belongs to Hörlein and Weber, who made such an observation in 1948
in a patient with congenital methemoglobinemia (seven years later this
abnormal hemoglobin was named Hgb M). However, it was the report of
Pauling and his group that generated a great burst of enthusiasm. The
tempo of investigative activity increased strikingly with the finding in
rapid succession of Hgb C (Itano and Wells, 1950), Hgb D (Itano, 1951),
and Hgb E (Itano and associates, Chernoff and associates, 1954). In 1956
Ingram discovered that the abnormality in Hgb S lay in the β-peptide
chain and that it consisted of a single amino acid substitution (valine for
a glutamic acid). Despite this slight difference, the amino acid substitution appears to be responsible for all the manifestations of sickle cell

anemia. For the first time in the history of medicine, a disease complex had been explained on the basis of a single genetically determined molecular abnormality. Activities in this field continue to be brisk, and many more structurally abnormal hemoglobins have now been discovered. In addition to uncovering new diseases and clarifying the pathogenesis of previously recognized clinical syndromes, observations on the quantitative hemoglobinopathies have provided invaluable opportunities to extend our basic knowledge of genetics and of protein chemistry and synthesis.

ETIOLOGY

The qualitative hemoglobinopathies are due to point mutations on one or more of the four structural genes that control the synthesis of α and β chains. The mutant gene behaves as a nonsex-linked incomplete dominant. An individual who is heterozygous (one defective gene) produces an abnormal hemoglobin but can also synthesize Hgb A (Fig. 5-13). In fact,

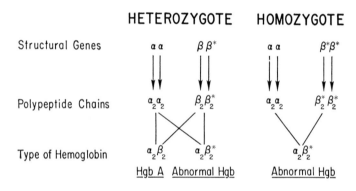

* Indicates mutant genes and structurally abnormal globin chains

Figure 5-13. Genetic abnormalities underlying the qualitative hemoglobinopathies.

Hgb A predominates under these circumstances, and the abnormal hemoglobin always makes up less than 50 per cent of the hemoglobin. These heterozygotes are often classified as having the trait of a qualitative hemoglobinopathy. Homozygotes possess a pair of mutant genes; they cannot synthesize Hgb A and essentially all of their hemoglobin is abnormal (Fig. 5-13). A double heterozygote with two different defective genes is unable to synthesize Hgb A when both members of a pair of structural genes are affected and produces equal amounts of two abnormal hemoglobins (Fig. 5-14). In the presence of a mutant α and a mutant β gene, about one fourth of the hemoglobin is Hgb A; such a person has comparable amounts of three abnormal hemoglobins (Fig. 5-14).

DOUBLE HETEROZYGOTES

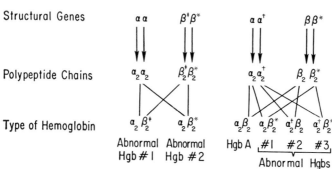

$\overset{*}{\underset{+}{^{+}}}$ Indicate mutant genes and structurally abnormal globin chains

Figure 5-14. Hemoglobin synthesis in double heterozygotes with two different mutant structural genes.

Because the hemoglobin molecule always contains pairs of like polypeptide chains, it is theoretically possible for four major abnormal hemoglobins to coexist in a single individual. In addition, one would expect trace amounts of other abnormal hemoglobins in those cases in which one or both of the α-structural genes are defective [the α chains of Hgb F $(\alpha_2\gamma_2)$ and A_2 $(\alpha_2\delta_2)$ are the same as those of Hgb A $(\alpha_2\beta_2)$]. Actually, complete proof of this genetic pattern is not yet available because of the rarity of most of these abnormal genes. Statistically, the chances of more than two mutant genes operating in a single person are almost nonexistent. There are scattered reports of individuals with three abnormal hemoglobins plus Hgb A, but it is distinctly unusual to find more than two major hemoglobins, that is, Hgb A and one abnormal hemoglobin or two abnormal hemoglobins.

The defective structural gene is responsible for the formation of abnormal messenger RNA which directs the polyribosome units to fabricate polypeptide chains that are different from normal α or β chains (Figs. 5-13 and 5-14). An amino acid substitution or change in the normal amino acid sequence is reflected by abnormalities in the chemical and physical attributes of the hemoglobin molecule containing the altered globin chains. These properties, in turn, determine the clinical manifestations characterizing the qualitative hemoglobinopathies. In Hgb S the formation of sickle-shaped erythrocytes with thromboses and infarcts reflects the tendency of reduced Hgb S to form tactoids or paracrystalline aggregates. On the other hand, methemoglobinemia distinguishes the presence of Hgb M α Boston. Tyrosine replaces histidine at such a spot in the Hgb M α Boston molecule that the sixth coordination valence of the iron atom in heme binds firmly to the neighboring phenol side chain of tyrosine. As a result, a stable phenolate complex, which cannot be reduced by the erythrocyte's normal complement of enzymes, is formed. Thus the α chains of Hgb M α Boston remain in the methemoglobin form and cannot carry oxygen. It is readily apparent, from these two examples, why the clinical syndromes associated with the different qualitative hemoglobinopathies are so variable.

CLASSIFICATION

Nomenclature has proved to be a problem in this rapidly expanding field. Most of the abnormal hemoglobins have been assigned a letter (e.g., Hgb S or Hgb C). Although more cumbersome, the designation of hemoglobin type by its globin structure is more informative, for such formulas indicate which globin chain is defective (e.g., $\alpha_2\beta_2^S = $ Hgb S; $\alpha_2^I\beta_2 = $ Hgb I). Recognition of numerous hemoglobins in rapid succession resulted in different hemoglobins being assigned the same letter by different investigators. Therefore it has been necessary to qualify further the designation of certain abnormal hemoglobins by indicating the globin chain involved and the geographic location in which they were described (e.g., Hgb M α Boston, Hgb M β Milwaukee, and Hgb M β Saskatoon). To date some 50 to 60 qualitatively abnormal hemoglobins have been described, in about two thirds of which the involved globin chain has been identified. In at least 22 the precise structural defect is known. It seems quite likely that many more abnormal hemoglobins will be found. Recognition of some may be difficult if the structural change is in the interior of the molecule, for it would not be reflected by electrophoretic abnormalities. Mutations affecting the gene locus that governs β-peptide chain synthesis are responsible for most of the clinically significant qualitative hemoglobinopathies. Discussions of the pathophysiology and clinical manifestations of all the qualitative hemoglobinopathies are beyond the scope of this book. Hgbs S, C, E, and D cause almost all of the problems encountered clinically, and consequently these hemoglobinopathies are considered in detail. The incidence of the other abnormal hemoglobins is extremely low; furthermore, they occur chiefly in heterozygotes without clinically apparent disease.

Hemoglobin S Disease

Hgb S ($\alpha_2\beta_2^S$) is synthesized consequent to a defect in one or both of the structural genes that control the formation of β-peptide chains. β^S chains differ from normal β chains by only one amino acid (the glutamic acid in the sixth position from the end of the normal β chain is replaced by valine in the β^S peptide). The heme moieties and α chains of Hgb S are normal. Thus a molecule of Hgb S, which contains two β^S chains, differs from one of Hgb A by only two amino acids out of a total of 574.

The genetic determinant of hemoglobin S disease behaves as a nonsex-linked, incomplete dominant. The heterozygous state (only one abnormal β gene) is characterized by erythrocytes that contain 20 to 40 per cent Hgb S and 60 to 80 per cent Hgb A. Individuals who are homozygous for the $β^S$ or sickle cell gene synthesize no Hgb A (Fig. 5-13) and their red cells contain 90 to 100 per cent Hgb S (the remainder is Hgb F).

The incidence of the $β^S$ gene varies greatly in different parts of the world. It is largely restricted to the Negro race, but it has been observed in other peoples, most notably natives of Greece, India, and Turkey. In the United States about 8 to 10 per cent of the Negro population are heterozygous for the $β^S$ gene; about 0.3 per cent are homozygotes; a smaller number are double heterozygotes and possess the $β^S$ gene plus a gene for some other hemoglobinopathy. In certain parts of Africa, the incidence of the sickle cell trait is as high as 40 per cent. Genetic mutations are much more likely to be harmful than useful and because homozygosity for the $β^S$ gene is usually lethal before the individual reaches the reproductive age, the gene would be expected to decrease in frequency and eventually disappear. Therefore a persistently high incidence of heterozygosity must indicate some potential advantage. Although still the subject of dispute, there are cogent reasons to believe that it may reflect interaction between the $β^S$ gene and malaria (*Plasmodium falciparum* infection). Hgb S appears to confer a certain degree of protection from malaria, especially in children, and areas with the highest incidence of the $β^S$ gene are also areas in which malaria is endemic. Explanations for a decrease in the morbidity and mortality from malaria remain conjectural. However, such protection could impart an advantage to the person who is heterozygous for the $β^S$ gene not held by a normal person, thereby serving to maintain a high incidence of sickle cell trait. It is worthy of note that any gain to be derived from such balanced polymorphism would be offset by loss brought about by homozygosity when the incidence of the trait exceeds 40 per cent of the population.

PATHOPHYSIOLOGY

Hemoglobin S disease is a striking example of a complex disorder, the diverse manifestations of which can be explained on a simple molecular basis. The single amino acid substitution in the $β^S$-peptide chain is responsible for marked alterations in the physicochemical properties of the Hgb S ($α_2β_2^S$) molecule. Because Hgb S possesses a higher net electrical charge (an excess of two positive charges—one for each abnormal β chain), its electrophoretic mobility differs clearly from that of Hgb A (Fig. 5-17, p. 267). More important are the changes induced by deoxygenation. In the reduced form Hgb S is much less soluble than deoxygenated Hgb A and forms birefringent tactoids or paracrystalline aggregates consequent to the attraction and resultant parallel orientation of the long chains of the hemoglobin polymers (true three-dimensional crystals are not formed). These changes, which are demonstrable in stromal free solutions of Hgb S and reversible on reoxygenation, are the architectural basis for the formation of sickle cells, the hallmark of Hgb S disease. With few, if any, exceptions, all the manifestations of hemoglobin S or sickle cell disease can be explained by this unique property of Hgb S to be transformed into a viscous, semisolid gel on deoxygenation.

In vivo the following sequence of events make up the pathophysiology of sickle cell disease. Reduced Hgb S undergoes tactoid formation which distorts the red cells and causes them to assume sickle, oat-shaped, filamentous, and other bizarre forms (Fig. 5-15). These deformed erythro-

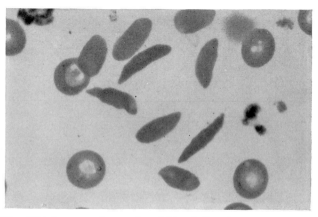

Figure 5-15.   Wright-stained peripheral blood film from a patient with homozygous hemoglobin S disease (sickle cell anemia).

cytes have increased mechanical fragility and impaired viability. Because there is no quantitative marrow defect (only a qualitative abnormality in globin chain synthesis), decreased red cell survival is followed by a reduction in circulating hemoglobin, marrow stimulation via the humoral erythropoietic regulatory mechanism, erythrocytic hyperplasia, and increased marrow output (polychromasia, reticulocytosis, and nucleated red cells in the peripheral blood). When increased production fails to keep pace with peripheral destruction, an overt hemolytic anemia develops. Because the concentration of hemoglobin in the erythrocytes is normal (the defect is qualitative *not* quantitative), the cells are normochromic. Other morphologic abnormalities of the red cells (target cells and Howell-Jolly bodies) most likely reflect hyposplenism and are probably secondary to the tendency of patients with sickle cell anemia to undergo an autosplenectomy as the result of repeated splenic infarcts.

Because sickle cells cannot readily form the small aggregates needed for erythrocytes to settle, the sedimentation rate is falsely low.

The presence of sickle cells greatly increases blood viscosity. As a result, a vicious circle is initiated, and decreased blood flow causes increased deoxygenation of Hgb S, which in turn increases sickle cell formation and viscosity (stasis also brings about a decrease in pH of blood and tissues which further facilitates the sickling process). The aftermath of these events is vascular occlusion and infarction. However, vascular occlusion cannot be attributed solely to increased blood viscosity. The lower the hematocrit, the less marked is the increase in viscosity brought about by sickle cells. Because patients with homozygous hemogloblin S disease are anemic (most severely so) and are still prone to frequent infarcts, mechanisms other than increased blood viscosity must participate. In this regard it should be noted that the peculiar rigid shape of the sickle cell can in itself initiate occlusion of small vessels because of the cell's inability to adjust its shape and successfully navigate the smaller capillaries (pliability is an important attribute of the normal red cell).

The clinical manifestations of sickle cell disease are divisible into two major categories. The *hematologic manifestations* are characterized by the singular morphology of the red cells and by a hemolytic anemia. The anemia causes such additional findings as cardiac hypertrophy, dilatation, and eventual failure; the frequent occurrence of cholelithiasis (pigment stones); osteoporosis of marrow-containing bones; and tissue hemosiderosis (the chronic anemia is responsible for increased assimilation of dietary iron as well as the need for frequent transfusions). The second group of manifestations is caused by *vascular occlusions.* Because any organ may be affected, the symptoms and findings attributable to infarctions are multiple and diverse. Abdominal pain (mesenteric, intestinal, and splenic infarcts) is quite common, as are repeated pulmonary infarcts. In fact, splenic infarcts occur with such frequency that patients with homozygous hemoglobin S disease who survive to adulthood possess only small nubbins of scar tissue to mark the sites of their spleens. Bone infarcts cause pain and may be demonstrable roentgenographically as areas of localized osteoporosis. Bone infarcts also appear to contribute to an increased incidence of osteomyelitis. (*Salmonella* organisms are most often the cause of such infections and probably reflect capillary thromboses in the gastrointestinal tract that permit bacteria to enter the blood and localize in ischemic and necrotic bone.) Neurologic abnormalities are prominent in patients with sickle cell anemia and, for the most part, are the result of thrombotic complications.

The pathogenesis of the renal abnormalities attributable to Hgb S deserve separate consideration. Hyposthenuria and hematuria are common findings in patients with sickle cell disease and appear to be explicable on the basis of the hyperosmolality of the renal medulla (about four times that of plasma). The countercurrent mechanism creates a graded osmolality from the base of the medulla to the tip of the papillae where the most marked hypertonicity occurs. Although the oxygen tension of maximally concentrated urine is slightly above the level at which sickle cell formation begins, exposure to a hypertonic medium will cause cells containing Hgb S to sickle even in the presence of high oxygen tensions (this effect is probably a reflection of cellular dehydration). Thus the hypertonic milieu of the renal medulla provides an ideal environment for sickle cell formation, which is then responsible for increased blood viscosity, circulatory stasis, hypoxia, and tissue injury. The end result is dysfunction of tubular cells and decreased tonicity of the urine. The latter serves to decrease the tendency for sickle cell formation in the kidneys. In heterozygotes the lesion does not progress beyond hyposthenuria, for the lack of hypertonicity precludes further sickling. In patients with homozygous hemoglobin S disease, sickling occurs at physiologic oxygen tensions; therefore renal ischemia persists despite the loss of the kidneys' concentrating ability and eventually leads to fibrosis and obliteration of glomeruli and tubular elements.

Sickle cell formation is primarily dependent on the amount of Hgb S in the erythrocyte. The concentration of Hgb S in the red cells of homozygotes is such that sickling occurs at physiologic oxygen tensions. Consequently, these persons manifest a progressive, ultimately fatal course characterized by a severe chronic hemolytic anemia and recurrent infarctions; the majority succumb to their disease before they reach the third decade of life. On the other hand, the heterozygote, that is, the individual with sickle cell trait or one β^S gene, has such a low concentration of Hgb S in his erythrocytes that sickle cell formation occurs only at unphysiologic oxygen tensions. Therefore he exhibits virtually no evidence of his hemoglobinopathy under normal conditions. Red cell morphology is normal, and these individuals have normal peripheral erythroid values with no evidence of a hemolytic component. However, red cells from individuals with the sickle cell trait can be made to sickle (extreme deoxygenation will cause sickling of 100 per cent of these cells), and this tendency is responsible for occasional vascular occlusions (e.g., splenic infarcts brought about by flying in unpressurized aircraft). The occurrence of sickling under certain unphysiologic conditions plus the genetic implications of the heterozygous state contribute to the significance of what is otherwise a benign, asymptomatic abnormality compatible with normal longevity.

Hgb F will not enter into molecular aggregates or polymer formation with Hgb S as will Hgb A and Hgb C. Therefore Hgb F protects an erythrocyte against the sickling phenomenon (30 per cent Hgb F will prevent sickle cell formation). For this reason homozygous hemoglobin S disease (sickle cell anemia) is not evident at birth (60 to 80 per cent of a newborn infant's hemoglobin is Hgb F) and rarely manifests itself before the age of three months. Methemoglobin will also prevent sickle cell formation in a cellular concentration of about 20 per cent.

The sickling phenomenon may be accentuated in persons who are heterozygous for the β^S gene and also possess some other mutant gene that affects globin chain synthesis. For example, patients with one β^S and one β^C gene have about equal amounts of Hgb S and Hgb C and will exhibit sickling in vivo. Individuals with one β^S gene and the trait of β thalassemia also display sickling in vivo because of the quantitative decrease in Hgb A synthesis and the consequent increase in cellular concentration of Hgb S (p. 281).

Although the course of homozygous hemoglobin S disease is unremitting and progressive, it is characterized by episodes of increased activity, or "sickle cell crises." These crises have been classified in the past as hemolytic, aplastic, and painful or thrombotic. There is no convincing evidence that the first occurs. Aplastic crises are most unusual; their pathogenesis is obscure but some may be the result of superimposed folic acid deficiency which has progressed to a stage of marrow hypoplasia (increased folic acid need in the face of inadequate intake, p. 201). Almost all crises are associated with episodes of pain (often quite severe) and appear to reflect vascular occlusive complications. Such episodes may occur without apparent cause, but most often they are triggered by fever, an infection, or exposure to cold. Each of these factors contributes to the formation of reduced Hgb S (e.g., fever increases tissue oxygen requirements and cold leads to vasoconstriction and circulatory stasis). Thus a sickle cell crisis may result from any set of conditions that enhances or aggravates tactoid formation.

CLINICAL MANIFESTATIONS

Homozygous Hemoglobin S Disease (Sickle Cell Anemia). SYMPTOMS. Sickle cell anemia rarely has its onset before the age of three months; however, it usually becomes evident some time during the first two years of life and appears before the age of one in about 50 per cent of the patients. Almost all individuals with this hemoglobinopathy are Negroes. The predominant symptoms at the onset and throughout the course of the disease reflect either hemolytic anemia (weakness, tachycardia, dyspnea, pallor, jaundice, and dark urine) or thrombotic episodes. Since vascular occlusions can affect any organ, symptomatology attributable to this manifestation of the sickling phenomenon is too diverse and lengthy to warrant listing. Abdominal pain is particularly common, as is pain in the chest (pulmonary infarction) and bones. Hematuria is another frequent complaint. Although some patients adjust fairly well to low peripheral erythroid values, the activity of most is definitely curtailed by the limitations imposed by the persistent anemia. Variable neurologic symptoms (e.g., manifestations of a cerebrovascular accident, convulsions, or meningeal signs) occur in about 30 per cent.

PHYSICAL FINDINGS.   Conjunctival icterus and pallor are the most consistent physical abnormalities. These patients are often physically underdeveloped, and individuals who survive until puberty usually manifest a shortened trunk with disproportionately long extremities and evidence of hypogenitalism. During crises or episodes of more active disease, patients are febrile and appear quite toxic and acutely ill. Tachycardia, cardiomegaly, and a variety of murmurs (usually systolic) are common findings. Although the spleen may be enlarged in young children, it is rarely, if ever, palpable in adolescents or adults. In fact, patients with sickle cell anemia are prone to undergo autosplenectomy as the result of repeated splenic infarcts, and a palpable spleen in a patient over the age of 10 virtually excludes the diagnosis of homozygous hemoglobin S disease. Minimal to moderate hepatomegaly is usual. Vascular abnormalities (increased tortuosity, venous saccular dilatations, and capillary microaneurysms) are often demonstrable, especially in the conjunctivae or retinae. Bone deformities may follow bone infarcts; aseptic or avascular necrosis of the femoral head is fairly common, but pathologic fractures are quite rare. Bony swelling and tenderness generally reflect osteomyelitis, the incidence of which is increased. Many patients have indolent ulcers over their lower legs or scars of previous ulcerations. Other physical abnormalities lack specificity and include such findings as friction rubs over the chest (pulmonary infarction) or left upper abdomen (splenic infarction). Abdominal tenderness and muscle spasm are frequent findings; however, bowel sounds are usually normal, even though other evidence may suggest an acute surgical abdomen. Priapism occurs in a small number of patients. Neurologic abnormalities are diverse, for they reflect varied thrombotic episodes.

LABORATORY FINDINGS.   A normocytic, normochromic anemia is characteristic of homozygous hemoglobin S disease; the hematocrit is typically between 20 and 30 per cent. Sickle cells are evident in routine peripheral blood films (Fig. 5-15), and sickle cell preparations are markedly positive (p. 266). Manifestations of hemolysis include reticulocytosis (up to 20 per cent or higher), increased polychromasia, and nucleated red cells in the peripheral blood. Target cells are often present but rarely exceed 30 per cent; they are most likely to be prominent in older individuals in association with Howell-Jolly bodies (a probable reflection of hyposplenism more than the hemoglobinopathy per se). Hemoglobin electrophoresis reveals a single component (Hgb S) migrating more slowly than Hgb A (Fig. 5-17, p. 267). Erythrocyte osmotic fragility may be normal or even decreased, but mechanical fragility is increased. The erythrocyte sedimentation rate is less than normal. Slight to moderate leukocytosis and thrombocytosis are additional manifestations of the hemolytic process (p. 89). Bone marrow morphology is normal. Although cellularity is increased largely because of erythrocytic hyperplasia, maturation is orderly. In older children and adults marrow iron is increased.

Nonhematologic laboratory abnormalities include hyposthenuria (urine specific gravity fixed at about 1.010) as a rather consistent finding. Hematuria occurs in many patients. Serum bilirubin is usually increased (the unconjugated fraction predominates), as are fecal and urinary urobilinogen; plasma haptoglobin is markedly decreased (all of these findings are manifestations of hemolysis, p. 85). In patients with long-standing disease, hepatocellular dysfunction is characteristic. Most of the x-ray findings are nonspecific and include manifestations of marrow hyperplasia or bone infarcts (osteoporosis or aseptic necrosis) as well as the effects of chronic anemia (cardiomegaly or cholelithiasis) or vascular occlusions (pulmonary infarction). Electrocardiographic abnormalities occur in most patients but for the most part are vague and attributable to the anemia (p. 57).

TREATMENT AND COURSE.   There is no treatment for homozygous hemoglobin S disease other than transfusions. Since the anemia is ordinarily tolerated fairly well, there is little need for frequent transfusions. A hemoglobin of 8 to 9 gm/100 ml of blood is quite adequate. These patients should never be transfused to normal or even to near normal levels because of the very real dangers of serum hepatitis (most patients already have significant liver damage consequent to hepatic infarcts or cholelithiasis with obstruction), transfusion hemosiderosis, and the development of minor blood group incompatibilities (patients with sickle cell anemia will be dependent on transfusions to prevent acute anemic hypoxia throughout the rest of their lives). Because vascular occlusions are unusual when the number of sickle cells falls to about 60 per cent or less, regularly scheduled, periodic transfusions have been advised to dilute the patient's cells with normal cells. Although this approach will decrease thrombotic episodes and hemolytic activity, the possible hazards associated with this regimen militate against its routine use. In general, transfusions should be reserved for markedly anemic patients, for those rare individuals who develop an aplastic crisis, and for those with severe, persistent thrombotic (or painful) crises.

No other form of treatment is effective. Attempts to prevent sickling by the formation of methemoglobin with such agents as sodium nitrite or para-amino-propriophenone have not proved to be clinically useful. Oxygen therapy and endeavors at alkalinization have also failed. Splenectomy is worthwhile only if the patient develops clear-cut, superimposed hypersplenism (a most unusual complication). Evidence of folic acid deficiency is, of course, an indication for the administration of folic acid. Otherwise, treatment is purely symptomatic.

Sickle cell anemia runs a progressive course characterized by a chronic, unremitting hemolytic anemia, episodes of severe pain (crises), and a fatal outcome. Many individuals die in infancy or early childhood, a few survive until adolescence, and occasional persons reach the third decade. Although exceptions occur, survival until middle age (into or beyond the fourth decade of life) is most unusual. It seems likely that most of the long-term survivals reported were double heterozygotes for Hgb S and Hgb D. Those persons who reach the reproductive age constitute a special problem. All of their offspring will receive β^S genes. In addition, pregnancy poses a threat, for both fetal and maternal morbidity and mortality are increased. Cholelithiasis, renal insufficiency, and hepatic dysfunction are common. Infections are frequent and contribute importantly as a cause of death. Differentiation between an acute surgical abdomen and an intra-abdominal vascular occlusion is difficult at best and often taxes the ingenuity of the most experienced clinician. Since fever and leukocytosis are common to both, these parameters are of little use.

Heterozygous Hemoglobin S Disease (Sickle Cell Trait). The concentration of Hgb S in the erythrocytes of a person with a single β^S gene is so low (20 to 40 per cent) that sickling does not occur at physiologic oxygen tensions. Since the clinical manifestations of hemoglobin S disease are contingent on the sickling phenomenon, the sickle cell trait is not associated with symptoms or physical abnormalities. These persons are not anemic, their erythrocyte morphology is normal (sickle cells are not demonstrable in routine blood films), and they have no reticulocytosis, increased polychromasia, or nucleated red cells in their peripheral blood. The laboratory manifestations of heterozygous hemoglobin S disease are (1) the presence of both Hgb S (less than 50 per cent) and Hgb A (more than 50 per cent), (2) a positive sickle cell preparation (extreme deoxygenation will evoke sickling in all red cells containing Hgb S), and (3) hyposthenuria (inability to concentrate urine occurs in about 70 per cent of persons with sickle cell trait).

With few exceptions, sickle cell trait is a benign disorder compatible with a normal life-span. Its chief clinical importance concerns its genetic implications. Fifty per cent of the offspring of a Hgb S heterozygote will have a β^S gene; the union of two such persons will produce heterozygotes (50 per cent) and homozygotes (25 per cent). Unless detected as part of a routine survey or a genetic work-up of a patient with hemoglobin S disease, the sickle cell trait may go unrecognized. However, rare persons will exhibit clinical manifestations. Hematuria occurs in some and may be quite severe. Vascular occlusions have also been observed. In most cases thrombosis follows exposure to unphysiologic conditions (e.g., a splenic infarct induced by flying in an unpressurized aircraft), but some reports indicate that as many as 10 to 15 per cent of individuals with sickle cell trait can expect to have one or more infarcts at some time during their lives. Even aseptic necrosis of the femoral head has been attributed to heterozygous hemoglobin S disease. Other deleterious effects of heterozygosity for the β^S gene include an increased likelihood of a urinary tract infection as a complication of pregnancy. Thus the designation heterozygous hemoglobin S *disease* would appear to be appropriate.

Hemoglobin SC Disease. In this qualitative hemoglobinopathy the erythrocytes contain about 50 per cent Hgb S and 50 per cent Hgb C. Sickling occurs at physiologic oxygen tensions and the abnormalities attributable to it characterize this disorder. Consequently, the clinical manifestations of hemoglobin SC disease are similar to but less severe than those of homozygous hemoglobin S disease. This qualitative hemoglobinopathy occurs almost exclusively in Negroes.

SYMPTOMS. About half of the persons with hemoglobin SC disease are well until the second decade of life or later. Weakness, ease of fatigue, tachycardia, and exertional dyspnea (symptoms of a reduction in the oxygen-carrying capacity of the blood) occur in most, but are rarely marked, for the anemia is usually minimal. The majority are aware of conjunctival icterus and dark urine. Episodic abdominal pain is typical and pain in the chest and bones is common. Neurologic complaints are prominent in about one fourth of the patients. Other symptoms include hematuria, priapism, and bony deformities (e.g., aseptic necrosis of the femoral head).

PHYSICAL FINDINGS. The physical manifestations of hemoglobin SC disease differ from those of homozygous hemoglobin S disease in two respects: physical habitus is normal and most patients have splenomegaly. Otherwise it is not possible to distinguish between these hemoglobinopathies on the basis of physical abnormalities, although quantitative differences are apparent; for example, cardiac murmurs are uncommon in patients with hemoglobin SC disease because the anemia is less severe.

LABORATORY FINDINGS. Persons with hemoglobin SC disease have a slight to moderate normocytic, normochromic anemia (the hematocrit is usually above 30 per cent). Target cells are always present in large numbers (30 to 80 per cent or more of the erythrocytes), and there are a few sickle cells in the routine peripheral blood films of most patients. Sickle cell preparations are positive. The reticulocyte count is slightly elevated but rarely exceeds 8 to 10 per cent. Increased polychromasia and occasional nucleated red cells in the peripheral blood are frequent findings, but Howell-Jolly bodies are not demonstrable. Hemoglobin electrophoresis reveals about equal amounts of Hgb S and Hgb C (Fig. 5-17, p. 267). Hgb F is not increased. The leukocyte and platelet counts are normal, and erythrocytic hyperplasia in the bone marrow is slight to moderate. Hyposthenuria is present in most patients. Hyperbilirubinemia (unconjugated fraction) and increased fecal and urinary urobilinogen reflect the hemolytic process. Other laboratory findings lack specificity and include such abnormalities as x-ray evidence of aseptic necrosis of the femoral head.

Treatment and Course. With few exceptions hemoglogin SC disease does not impair longevity. There is no specific treatment, and blood transfusions are rarely indicated. In most cases symptomatic therapy will suffice (e.g., analgesics during episodes of pain). Persons with hemoglobin SC disease have a higher incidence of complications during pregnancy and in the puerperium. Genetic counseling is always indicated for half the offspring of an individual with hemoglobin SC disease will inherit β^S genes and the other half will receive β^C genes.

Hemoglobin S—High Hemoglobin F Syndrome. Although it appears to be an uncommon occurrence, hereditary persistence of high fetal hemoglobin deserves comment. The genetic mechanism underlying this hemoglobinopathy is obscure. It has been suggested (but not yet proved) that the "high F" syndrome may reflect failure of an operator gene to "turn on" β-chain production (Fig. 5-12); as a result, γ-chain synthesis continues, and fetal levels of Hgb F persist into adult life. Homozygosity for this abnormality has been observed in at least one patient whose red cells contained just Hgb F. Double heterozygosity (Hgb S and hereditary persistence of high Hgb F) is characterized by the presence of Hgb S and Hgb F. Phenotypically, these findings are indistinguishable from those of homozygous hemoglobin S disease; however, there are clear-cut quantitative and clinical differences. In the double heterozygotes about 70 per cent of the hemoglobin is Hgb S and the rest is Hgb F. Since Hgb F will not enter into molecular aggregates with Hgb S (a cellular concentration of Hgb F of approximately 30 per cent or more will prevent sickling), these individuals have few, if any, clinical manifestations despite the fact that Hgb S is the predominant hemoglobin. It seems likely that some patients who have been classified in the past as mild or atypical forms of sickle cell anemia may actually be examples of double heterozygosity for the β^S gene and hereditary persistence of high fetal hemoglobin.

Hemoglobin S—Thalassemia. This hemoglobinopathy reflects both qualitative and quantitative defects in globin synthesis and is discussed separately (p. 281).

Hemoglobin C Disease

Hgb C ($\alpha_2\beta_2^C$) is the qualitatively abnormal hemoglobin produced as the result of a mutant gene that is allelomorphic to the normal β and β^S genes. The structural defect consists of lysine in the sixth position rather than glutamic acid. Thus the amino acid substitution in Hgb C and Hgb S involves the same locus in the normal β-chain peptide sequence. The β^C

gene occurs almost exclusively in the Negro race. About 2.5 per cent of American Negroes are heterozygotes; that is, they possess one normal β gene and one β^C gene. In certain areas of west Africa, however, heterozygosity for the β^C gene reaches an incidence as high as 20 per cent. In the United States homozygous hemoglobin C disease is quite rare (about 0.01 per cent of the Negro population). There is no evidence that the Hgb C imparts any selective advantage insofar as resistance to malaria is concerned. On paper electrophoresis, at pH 8.6, Hgb C migrates more slowly than Hgb S (Fig. 5-17, p. 267). Reduced Hgb C is more soluble than Hgb A, but Hgb C has a tendency to undergo crystallization in vitro subsequent to dehydration. As a result, erythrocytes containing Hgb C may become distorted by rod-shaped crystals. Target cells are the *sine qua non* for the presence of Hgb C (Fig. 5-16).

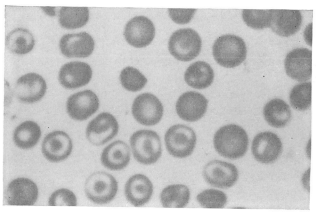

Figure 5-16. Target cells in the peripheral blood of a patient with heterozygous hemoglobin C disease.

Heterozygous Hemoglobin C Disease (Hemoglobin C Trait). Heterozygosity for the β^C gene is a benign disorder without symptoms or physical abnormalities. It is not associated with significant morbidity or decreased longevity. Laboratory findings are normal, with the exception of a variable number of target cells (usually less than 40 per cent) and an abnormal hemoglobin electrophoretic pattern (20 to 40 per cent Hgb C, 60 to 80 per cent Hgb A). Hgb F is not increased. The erythroid values are normal, and there is no evidence of a hemolytic component. With the exception of its genetic implications, heterozygosity for the β^C gene is clinically significant only when the abnormal gene coexists with another gene that affects globin synthesis (e.g., hemoglobin SC disease).

Homozygous Hemoglobin C Disease. This qualitative hemoglobinopathy is characterized by splenomegaly, the presence of numerous target cells (40 to 100 per cent of the erythrocytes), and a mild to moderate hemolytic anemia. The anemia is reflected by slight reticulocytosis, increased polychromasia, and appropriate pigment changes. Occasionally, the hemolytic process may be compensated with normal peripheral erythroid values. The red cells contain almost 100 per cent Hgb C; some patients have been reported to have a slight increase in Hgb F. Most patients with homozygous hemoglobin C disease have few complaints and live out a normal life-span.

Hemoglobin C—Thalassemia. This rare hemoglobinopathy is discussed in another section (p. 282).

Hemoglobin E Disease

Hgb E ($\alpha_2\beta_2^E$) is another β-chain defect. The abnormality involves the twenty-sixth amino acid from the end of the β-peptide chain and consists of the substitution of lysine for the glutamic acid that normally occupies this locus. The β^E gene is most common in southeast Asia, where heterozygosity occurs in as many as 15 per cent of certain ethnic groups (e.g., the Thai). The electrophoretic mobility of Hgb E on paper at pH 8.6 is between that of Hgb C and Hgb S (Fig. 5-17, p. 267).

Heterozygous Hemoglobin E Disease (Hemoglobin E Trait). Heterozygosity for Hgb E is manifested clinically by a few target cells in the peripheral blood and an abnormal hemoglobin electrophoretic pattern (20 to 40 per cent Hgb E; 60 to 80 per cent Hgb A). Hgb F is not increased. The trait of Hgb E is not associated with symptoms, physical abnormalities, or other laboratory findings; it does not affect longevity.

Homozygous Hemoglobin E Disease. Homozygosity for the β^E gene is reflected by a mild hemolytic anemia. Target cells are prominent, but splenomegaly is unusual. The erythrocytes contain almost 100 per cent Hgb E; Hgb F is present in normal to slightly increased amounts (up to 6 per cent). Patients with homozygous hemoglobin E disease have few complaints and usually live out a normal life-span.

Hemoglobin E—Thalassemia. This double heterozygous state is discussed elsewhere (p. 282).

Hemoglobin D Disease

Three varieties of Hgb D have been observed: Hgb Dα, Dβ, and Dβ Punjab. The first is an α-chain defect; the other two involve β chains. All these hemoglobins have an electrophoretic mobility indistinguishable on paper at pH 8.6 from that of Hgb S. Therefore Hgb D assumes clinical importance because of the confusion it may cause in the diagnosis of the various types of hemoglobin S disease. Because reduced Hgb D is soluble, Hgb S can be distinguished from Hgb D on the basis of solubility determinations. Hgb D does not cause sickling. Heterozygosity for Hgb D occurs in about 0.5 per cent of American Negroes and in as many as 2 per cent of the populations in certain other areas, most notably Algeria and north central India.

Heterozygous Hemoglobin D Disease (Hemoglobin D Trait). Hemoglobin D trait is a benign asymptomatic condition. Its clinical importance lies in the electrophoretic pattern, which is identical to heterozygous hemoglobin S disease or sickle cell trait. Unless correlated with a negative sickle cell preparation or appropriate solubility determinations, heterozygosity for Hgb D may be incorrectly diagnosed as sickle cell trait.

Hemoglobin SD Disease. Persons who are doubly heterozygous for Hgb S and Hgb D exhibit sickling and all the manifestations of homozygous hemoglobin S disease, although their clinical course is much more benign. Since hemoglobin electrophoresis reveals a single component migrating as Hgb S, these patients may be incorrectly classified as sickle cell anemia. It seems likely that most of the published reports of long-term survival in patients with sickle cell anemia represent individuals with hemoglobin SD disease.

Homozygous Hemoglobin D Disease. This hemoglobinopathy is extremely rare and can be distinguished readily from sickle cell anemia by the absence of sickling and the minimal clinical manifestations. However, routine hemoglobin electrophoresis will not permit this distinction.

Other Qualitative Hemoglobinopathies

Although the incidence of *hemoglobin Lepore* is quite low, this abnormal hemoglobin is of special interest. The globin moiety of Hgb Lepore consists of two normal α chains and a pair of abnormal polypeptide chains. The first third of the latter appears to be identical with the first third of a normal δ chain; the amino acid sequence of the last two thirds is similar to the comparable portion of a normal β chain. In addition to the presence of a structurally abnormal hemoglobin with an abnormal electrophoretic pattern (Fig. 5-17, p. 267), heterozygosity for Hgb Lepore is characterized by deficient hemoglobin synthesis and a microcytic, hypochromic anemia. This finding is in distinct contrast to the heterozygous forms of the other qualitative hemoglobinopathies, which are not accompanied by anemia. Although it lacks proof, an attractive hypothesis contends that the abnormal structural gene controlling the synthesis of Lepore polypeptide chains may be subject to δ-regulator genes which appear to be set at much lower levels than β-regulator genes (p. 248).

More than 50 other abnormal hemoglobins have been discovered; however, the genes responsible for these defects in globin chain structure occur with such low frequency that inadequate observations preclude formulation of well-defined clinical pictures. Available data neither permit nor do they warrant detailed clinical discussion of these rarely encountered qualitative hemoglobinopathies. Furthermore, most abnormal hemoglobins exist in the asymptomatic heterozygous state and lack clinical significance.

DIAGNOSIS OF THE QUALITATIVE HEMOGLOBINOPATHIES

A qualitative hemoglobinopathy is often suggested by the history (chronic anemia, recurrent or persistent jaundice, anemia in other members of the family, and/or cholelithiasis at an early age), physical findings (habitus, leg ulcers, and splenomegaly), and routine laboratory determinations (e.g., anemia, reticulocyosis, poikilocytosis, and target cells). Such a diagnosis must be excluded in any patient with an unexplained chronic hemolytic anemia, especially in a Negro. Although these clinical parameters may point to a qualitative hemoglobinopathy, the diagnosis is contingent on the demonstration of the abnormal hemoglobin molecule and, insofar as possible, should have appropriate genetic confirmation. A variety of techniques is available for the recognition and quantification of normal and abnormal hemoglobins. Attempts to demonstrate the sickling phenomenon, hemoglobin electrophoresis, and alkali denaturation are essential in the work-up of every patient suspected of having a qualitative hemoglobinopathy. Solubility determinations, amino acid analysis of peptide fragments by a combination of electrophoresis and chromatography ("fingerprint patterns"), and immunologic studies are some of the other techniques that can provide important information; however, these procedures, which are complex, technically difficult, and not universally available, are basically research tools and are not needed to solve most clinical problems.

Sickle Cell Phenomenon. The demonstration of sickle cells is virtual proof that the erythrocytes in question contain Hgb S. Sickle cells are usually evident in routine peripheral blood films of patients with homozygous hemoglobin S disease, hemoglobin SC disease, hemoglobin SD disease, and hemoglobin S-thalassemia. Under these circumstances further tests along these lines are superfluous. However, if sickle cells are not found in the routine peripheral blood film, special techniques are required to enhance deoxygenation and promote sickling. This procedure is designated a "sickle cell preparation." A simple test consists of placing a drop of blood on a slide, covering it with a coverslip, and sealing it with petroleum jelly. The preparation is then examined periodically for the presence of sickle cells; if no sickle cells are seen at the end of 24 hours, the test is negative. In order to hasten the formation of sickle cells, a rubber band may be placed around the finger for three to four minutes before the blood is obtained. An alternative technique is to add a reducing agent such as sodium metabisulfite or sodium bisulfite to the blood. These variations permit completion of the test within 15 to 20 minutes. The speed with which sickling occurs may be some indication of the concentration of Hgb S in the cells, but the number of sickle cells is irrelevant, for each erythrocyte contains Hgb S, even in a heterozygote, and can be made to sickle in vitro.

There are few exceptions to the rule that sickle cells denote the presence of Hgb S. Sickle cells have been described in individuals with Hgb I and Hgb C Georgetown. Otherwise, sickling has been observed only in human beings who synthesize the abnormal β-globin chains that characterize Hgb S. Sickling of cells containing Hgb I occurs only in the presence of a high concentration of sodium metabisulfite and appears to reflect a specific interaction between Hgb I and sodium metabisulfite. Thus the pathogenesis of this type of sickling differs significantly from that of Hgb S. It is of interest along these lines that certain species of deer exhibit sickling but none of the pathophysiologic manifestations attributable to this phenomenon in man.

Hemoglobin Electrophoresis. Because of alterations in electrical charge consequent to amino acid substitutions, most abnormal hemoglobins display a characteristic electrophoretic pattern that differs clearly from Hgb A and from most other structurally abnormal hemoglobins. Hemoglobin electrophoresis is indispensable in the work-up of all patients suspected of having a qualitative hemoglobinopathy. Paper electrophoresis at pH 8.6 is a simple procedure that permits positive identification of most of the clinically important abnormal hemoglobins (Fig. 5-17). A few hemo-

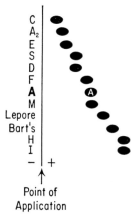

Figure 5-17. Schematic representation of the electrophoretic behavior of a variety of hemoglobins on paper at a pH of 8.6.

globins (e.g., S and D) exhibit similar electrophoretic behavior and must be differentiated by other means such as solubility determinations (reduced Hgb S is insoluble, whereas reduced Hgb D is soluble). Separation of Hgb A and Hgb F by paper electrophoresis is also difficult;

however, Hgb F resists alkali denaturation, whereas Hgb A does not. It is essential that the electrophoretic mobility of each unknown hemoglobin be compared with those of Hgb A and the abnormal hemoglobin(s) in question. Therefore, a variety of abnormal hemoglobins must be available. In this regard it should be noted that most hemoglobins show blurring on electrophoresis after storage for a few weeks, even at temperatures of minus 20°C. Paper electrophoresis is not a reliable technique for the detection of a hemoglobin present in a concentration of less than 10 per cent. Numerous modifications have been devised to sharpen the electrophoretic definition of the different hemoglobins, such as varying the pH of the buffer and the use of media other than paper (e.g., starch block and agar gel). In general, these technical variations have proved to be of greatest value in the research laboratory.

Alkali Denaturation. Hgb F resists denaturation by alkali and can, because of this property, be separated from other hemoglobins and quantified. Although variations in the concentration of Hgb F are of greater diagnostic significance in the quantitative hemoglobinopathies (p. 276), this hemoglobin is often slightly increased in certain qualitative hemoglobinopathies.

By utilizing the foregoing laboratory procedures in conjunction with the other pertinent clinical manifestations, we can easily recognize and accurately categorize most qualitative hemoglobinopathies. Family studies provide additional relevant data and should be obtained if possible. On occasion, it may be necessary to use other techniques (e.g., Hgb S and Hgb D exhibit identical electrophoretic mobilities but different solubilities). The type of abnormal hemoglobin can generally be predicted with reasonable certainty on the basis of routine preliminary observations; for example, numerous target cells and splenomegaly suggest hemoglobin C disease; a few target cells, Howell-Jolly bodies, sickle cells, and the absence of a palpable spleen point to hemoglobin S disease; sickle cells, target cells, no Howell-Jolly bodies, and splenomegaly indicate hemoglobin SC disease; and so on. It should be re-emphasized, however, that a positive diagnosis rests on the precise identification in the laboratory of a structurally abnormal hemoglobin.

Quantitative Hemoglobinopathies
(Thalassemia Syndromes)

The *quantitative hemoglobinopathies* are genetically determined disorders characterized by deficient hemoglobin synthesis and impaired red cell viability. They are manifested clinically by a chronic microcytic, hypochromic anemia, overt hemolysis, numerous leptocytes and target cells, and splenomegaly. Despite the hypochromia, body iron stores are normal or increased. As far as can be ascertained, all moieties of the hemo-globin molecules are structurally normal. Heterozygosity for the mutant gene responsible for this type of hemoglobinopathy is reflected by mild disease and normal longevity, whereas homozygosity causes severe anemia and early death. This disease category includes several closely related abnormalities that may affect either α or β globin chain production. Be-cause of the high incidence of such hemoglobinopathies in the area surrounding the Mediterranean Sea, these disorders have been named "thalassemia" from the Greek word meaning the sea. Hereditary leptocy-tosis, target cell anemia, Cooley's anemia, and Mediterranean anemia are among the other names that have been suggested or used. Because of its general acceptance and pertinence, *thalassemia syndromes* appears to be a particularly appropriate designation and is used in a generic sense throughout the rest of this discussion to refer to all the quantitative hemo-globinopathies.

HISTORY

In 1889 and 1890 von Jaksch described three patients with severe anemia and proposed the name "anaemia infantum pseudoleucaemica." Although it seems unlikely that these patients had thalassemia as we know it today, the terms "von Jaksch's anemia" and "pseudoleukemic anemia" quickly gained wide usage. For the next 50 years many patients who un-doubtedly had thalassemia were classified under these headings. In the early part of the twentieth century, numerous references appeared in the Italian literature to hereditary anemias which probably were quantitative hemoglobinopathies. However, it was not until the clinical descriptions by Cooley and Lee (U.S.) in 1925 that the existence of thalassemia as a specific entity (or entities) became evident. In this same year Rietti pub-lished in Italy reports of three patients with a similar but much less severe disease. This form of thalassemia was first recognized in the United States by Wintrobe and by Dameshek in 1940. Significant developments in the last two decades include clarification of the pattern of inheritance of the thalassemia syndromes and cognizance of the fact that the quantita-tive hemoglobinopathies are not restricted to the Mediterranean basin but occur in many other geographic locations and ethnic groups. More re-cently the interaction (or coexistence) of qualitative and quantitative hemoglobinopathies has been recognized. Silvestroni and Bianco first described sickle cell thalassemia or microdepranocytic disease. Numerous other abnormal hemoglobins have since been shown to exist in a double heterozygous state with the gene causing thalassemia.

ETIOLOGY

The thalassemia syndromes reflect the inability of an erythrocytic pre-cursor to synthesize its full complement of hemoglobin. Current data indicate that these disorders are caused by an abnormality (or abnormalities) in the gene (or genes) which exerts regulatory control over the formation of normal adult hemoglobin (Hgb A). Theories of pathogenesis include (1) mutations in the structural genes controlling globin synthesis that lead to the formation of a qualitatively abnormal polypeptide chain, (2) defects in heme synthesis, and (3) deficient hemoglobin synthesis consequent to curtailed production of normal globin chains.

To date, all attempts have failed to reveal a structurally abnormal hemoglobin in patients with this form of hereditary hemoglobinopathy. The possibility of changes in the interior of the molecule which might not be detectable by the usual parameters (e.g., electrophoretic behavior) cannot be excluded with absolute certainty. However, the existence of such structural defects appears quite unlikely and, in any event, could not explain all the manifestations of thalassemia. There is no quantitative impairment in hemoglobin synthesis in the qualitative hemoglobinopathies with unequivocal defects in globin structure. Erythrocytes containing an abnormal hemoglobin such as Hgb S have a normal concentration of hemoglobin, and these red cells *do not* appear hypochromic. On the other hand, hypochromia (and microcytosis) is a consistent feature of the thalassemia syndromes. Normochromic erythrocytes are maximally saturated with hemoglobin, and hypochromia always reflects a decreased cellular concentration of hemoglobin (p. 60). Conversely, a less than normal hemoglobin concentration is always manifested by hypochromia. Therefore it is impossible to explain the presence of hypochromia solely on the basis of a qualitative abnormality in the hemoglobin molecule. Even if a structurally abnormal hemoglobin could be demonstrated in the thalassemia syndromes, it would still be necessary to postulate an additional quantitative defect.

Because of the prominence of hypochromia and the recognition that this finding usually indicates an abnormality in iron metabolism (most hypochromic anemias are the result of iron deficiency), a popular theory has been that of impaired heme synthesis (either decreased porphyrin production, a defect in iron utilization, or the formation of a structurally abnormal porphyrin). There is little experimental support for this hypothesis, and those changes that have been described probably reflect secondary phenomena. Available evidence indicates that heme is structurally normal and, since the nucleated red cells in the thalassemia syndromes contain increased amounts of both iron and free protoporphyrin, there is obviously no inadequacy of these two components of heme. The possibility of some block in the insertion of iron into the porphyrin nucleus or in the combination of heme and globin cannot be excluded with certainty, but several observations militate against the likelihood. The heme moieties of Hgb A, Hgb F, and Hgb A_2 are identical. Patients with thalassemia are unable to synthesize normal amounts of Hgb A but are able to produce normal to increased quantities of Hgb F and/or Hgb A_2. It is hard to envisage a defect in heme synthesis as playing a significant role in the causation of a cellular deficiency of Hgb A without affecting the production of these other hemoglobins.

Existent observations are in accord with the theory that the thalassemia syndromes are caused by a defect in one or more of the genes (either operator or structural) that normally control the synthesis of α or β peptide chains. Every molecule of hemoglobin contains four atoms of iron, four protoporphyrin structures, and four polypeptide chains. If there is a deficiency of any component (globin chains, iron, or porphyrin), *no* hemoglobin is formed (an "incomplete" molecule of hemoglobin cannot be synthesized). Globin inadequacy could reflect a ribosomal abnormality, defective messenger RNA, or a deficiency of messenger RNA. There is no evidence that the polyribosomes in the erythrocytic precursors of patients with thalassemia are in short supply or that their function is impaired. The possibility of an abnormal messenger RNA which fails to bring about polypeptide chain formation even though it attaches in template fashion to a polyribosome unit cannot be discarded; however, deficient messenger RNA production seems somewhat more likely. Inadequate amounts of messenger RNA could be the result of the deletion of one or both of the structural genes that control α or β globin chain synthesis, or it could be a manifestation of a mutant operator or regulator gene. The majority of workers in this field favor the latter possibility. Regardless of the nature of the genetic abnormality, the end result would be the same, that is, the synthesis of Hgb A would be curtailed.

Although the complex genetic mechanisms underlying the thalassemia syndromes continue to defy precise definition, the pattern of inheritance is fairly clear. The abnormal genes appear to be allelomorphic to the genetic loci that normally control the formation of α or β polypeptide chains. Therefore it is permissible for the purposes of discussion to refer to the genes that cause the thalassemia syndromes as $α^{Thal}$ or $β^{Thal}$, even though it is not known whether the affected gene is an operator or a structural gene. The quantitative hemoglobinopathies can then be subdivided into α *thalassemia* or β *thalassemia*, depending on the globin chain affected. The thalassemia genes behave as nonsex-linked mendelian dominants. Heterozygotes with one thalassemia gene exhibit mild disease (thalassemia minor or thalassemia trait); half their offspring will acquire the abnormal gene and will exhibit a similar hemoglobinopathy. Homozygosity is manifested by severe disease and early death (thalassemia major); all their offspring should be heterozygotes, but death before the reproductive age prevents proof of this genetic pattern. One fourth of the children born to a couple who are heterozygous for the same type of thalassemia will have thalassemia major; 50 per cent will be heterozygous, and the rest will be normal. Although theoretically feasible, double heterozygosity (one α^{Thal} and one β^{Thal} gene) has not been recognized.

Among the questions still to be answered is that of varying severity of the disease. Some heterozygotes have virtually no evidence of their hemoglobinopathy, whereas others have relatively severe disease. It has been suggested that thalassemia minor consists of two categories of disease, thalassemia intermedia and thalassemia minima. However, it is difficult to reconcile such a classification with the known genetic behavior of the thalassemia syndromes. Variations in gene expressivity or the existence of several different thalassemia genes are more logical explanations for the dissimilitude of the clinical manifestations in heterozygotes.

It must be emphasized that the foregoing pathogenic mechanisms are in large part conjectural. Furthermore, they do not take into consideration the decrease in red cell survival time. Despite a great deal of investigative effort, the hemolytic component, which contributes so importantly to the clinical manifestations of the thalassemia syndromes, remains enigmatic. Impaired hemoglobin synthesis and a decreased cellular concentration of hemoglobin (i.e., hypochromia) should not affect erythrocyte viability (patients with marked hypochromia secondary to iron deficiency do not manifest significant abnormalities in red cell life-span). For this reason the quantitative hemoglobinopathies are not explicable on the basis of a single genetic defect as are the qualitative hemoglobinopathies. Other defects, most notably coarseness of the erythrocyte surface structure when viewed by electron microscopy, indicate that additional genetic abnormalities may play important roles in the pathogenesis of this group of hereditary hematologic disorders.

PATHOPHYSIOLOGY

The thalassemia syndromes reflect the combined effects of the erythrocytic precursors' inability to synthesize a normal complement of hemoglobin and of impaired red cell viability. The "block" in globin synthesis curtails marrow output and contributes to an anemia distinguished by hypochromia, microcytes, target cells, and leptocytes. The hemolytic component, which plays the major role in the causation of the anemia of thalassemia, consists of intramedullary hemolysis (ineffective erythropoiesis) and shortened survival of circulating erythrocytes. It is responsible for increased polychromasia, reticulocytosis, and nucleated red cells in the peripheral blood as well as for erythrocytic hyperplasia in the marrow. Together these two mechanisms result in a chronic hypochromic, hemolytic anemia, the hallmark of the thalassemia syndromes. Symptoms, physical findings, and other laboratory abnormalities are directly attributable to the anemia, which is likely to be particularly severe, for it reflects both increased blood loss and impaired production. Plasma erythropoietic factor (erythropoietin) activity is increased. Because the proliferation of marrow cells, synthesis of porphyrin, and absorption and utilization of iron appear to be essentially normal, the thalassemia syndromes are associated with myeloid erythrocytic hyperplasia, increased free erythrocyte protoporphyrin, and augmented iron stores (the chronic anemia and hyperactive marrow serve to enhance the assimilation of dietary iron; transfusions also contribute to tissue hemosiderosis).

The clinical picture of the thalassemia syndromes is dominated by the nonspecific symptoms and findings of anemia (e.g., weakness, cardio-respiratory manifestations, and pallor), together with evidence of hemolysis (e.g., acholuric jaundice and cholelithiasis). Splenomegaly reflects the chronic hemolysis, that is, work hypertrophy (p. 88), as well as extramedullary myeloid metaplasia. The erythrocytic hyperplasia in the marrow is responsible for skeletal x-ray abnormalities (widening of medullary cavities and cortical atrophy). Erythrocyte survival time is decreased. Ineffective erythropoiesis (intramedullary hemolysis) is manifested by accelerated plasma iron turnover and decreased red cell ^{59}Fe uptake. The severity of the process depends on whether the patient is a homozygote or heterozygote, and certain other abnormalities are contingent on the globin chain affected.

Thalassemia Minor (Heterozygous Disease). ALPHA THALASSEMIA. All the normal hemoglobins contain α polypeptide chains. Therefore heterozygosity for α thalassemia affects the synthesis of each in a like manner and the normal ratio between Hgb A, Hgb F, and Hgb A_2 is maintained; that is, Hgb A predominates without increases in either Hgb A_2 or Hgb F. Because α chains are in short supply, a relative over-abundance of β (or γ) chains permits four similar polypeptides to form the globin moiety of the hemoglobin molecule. In the child with α thalassemia, Hgb Bart's (γ_4) has been found. This hemoglobin, which has an affinity for oxygen 8 to 10 times that of Hgb A, is much less resistant to alkali denaturation than is Hgb F (the combination of α and γ chains evidently presents a less accessible target for denaturation). The adult counterpart of Hgb Bart's has a globin structure consisting of four β chains and has been designated Hgb H. This fast-moving hemoglobin (Fig. 5-17) readily undergoes irreversible denaturation and is precipitated in the form of intraerythrocytic inclusion bodies. A number of patients have been observed with 5 to 40 per cent Hgb H and the manifestations of thalassemia minor. It has been suggested that these persons might be double heterozygotes with a thalassemia gene and one which brings about the formation of Hgb H. However, Hgb H does not possess structurally abnormal globin chains, and, furthermore, this hemoglobin has never been found in the absence of thalassemia. It seems most likely, therefore, that individuals with Hgb H reflect heterozygosity for an α^{Thal} gene that causes a more marked shortage of α chains than is usually observed. Recently, a third hemoglobin made up of four δ chains has been described. Because persons who are heterozygous for α thalassemia can synthesize a significant amount of Hgb A, the clinical manifestations of this quantitative hemoglobinopathy vary from mild to moderate but are never severe.

Beta Thalassemia. A single β^{Thal} gene causes a deficiency of β chains and curtails Hgb A ($\alpha_2\beta_2$) production. Under these circumstances there should be a relative overabundance of α chains and a hemoglobin molecule made up of four α chains might be anticipated. Although recent observations suggest that such a tetramer may exist, it has not been identified with certainty. It is possible that the release of α_2 subunits from the polyribosomes may be contingent on the presence of β_2, γ_2, or δ_2 dimers. Because the β^{Thal} gene does not affect the synthesis of γ or δ chains, increased cellular concentrations of Hgb A_2 and Hgb F might be expected. Most β thalassemia heterozygotes have elevated levels of Hgb A_2 (about 5 to 7 per cent); however, these persons usually have normal amounts of Hgb F. A smaller number of heterozygotes have slight increases in Hgb F with normal Hgb A_2 levels. The explanation for this reciprocal relationship between Hgb A_2 and Hgb F is not known. These findings probably reflect different genetic mutations and point again to the heterogeneity of this category of thalassemia syndromes. The other clinical manifestations of heterozygous β thalassemia do not differ significantly from those caused by a single α^{Thal} gene.

Thalassemia Major (Homozygous Disease). Alpha Thalassemia. Homozygosity for the α^{Thal} gene affects the formation of all normal hemoglobins (Hgb A, Hgb F, and Hgb A_2) and is apparently incompatible with life. Several cases of hydrops fetalis have been attributed to homozygous α thalassemia; available data indicate that these infants possessed only Hgb Bart's (γ_4).

Beta Thalassemia. Homozygosity for the β^{Thal} gene drastically curtails synthesis of Hgb A and causes a severe, progressive, hemolytic anemia with death in the first or second decade of life. In contrast to the rather consistent elevation of Hgb A_2 in heterozygous β thalassemia, the concentration of Hgb A_2 in homozygotes is quite variable and ranges from normal to slightly increased (up to about 10 per cent). On the other hand, Hgb F is typically increased and usually accounts for 50 to 90 per cent of the hemoglobin. However, Hgb F is not increased in every patient with the major form of β thalassemia, and the precise significance of these variable findings remains to be clarified. In general, it is not possible to correlate clinical severity with either Hgb F or Hgb A_2 levels.

CLINICAL MANIFESTATIONS

The thalassemia syndromes constitute a problem of considerable magnitude (millions of individuals throughout the world possess these abnormal genes). Although particularly common in the inhabitants of the countries surrounding the Mediterranean Sea or in their descendants, thalassemia has been observed in essentially all races, ethnic groups, and geographic locations. In certain areas (e.g., portions of Italy, Sardinia, and Sicily) there is a 10 to 20 per cent incidence of heterozygosity, and approximately 0.2 per cent of these populations have thalassemia major. In some isolated regions the mutant gene is even more common. Since homozygosity is ordinarily lethal before the individual reaches the reproductive age, an explanation must be sought for the persistence of this high incidence of heterozygosity. Increased fertility of thalassemia heterozygotes has been suggested, but this hypothesis lacks proof. Balanced polymorphism with increased resistance to malaria is a more popular view and does possess significant support, although it remains unproved. The quantitative hemoglobinopathies affect both sexes equally and are usually apparent at birth or shortly thereafter. With few exceptions, thalassemia major produces severe disease during the first year of life; however, the diagnosis of thalassemia minor may not be made until the patient reaches adulthood or even old age. Since homozygosity for the α^{Thal} gene appears to cause death *in utero* or at birth, the following discussion of thalassemia major pertains only to β thalassemia.

Thalassemia Major (Homozygous Disease). SYMPTOMS. Pallor, listlessness, retarded growth, and jaundice generally have their onset during the first few weeks of life. In an older child the predominant complaints are attributable to anemia (dyspnea, tachycardia, and markedly reduced tolerance to physical activity). Some patients have pressure symptoms secondary to greatly enlarged spleens.

PHYSICAL FINDINGS. Marked pallor and moderate to massive splenomegaly are the most consistent physical abnormalities. Hepatomegaly is usual, but lymphadenopathy is not characteristic. Although conjunctival icterus is common, marked jaundice is unusual. Most patients manifest retarded growth and enlargement of the skull with mongoloid facies; those few individuals who survive until puberty exhibit hypogenitalism. Chronic leg ulcers occur but are quite rare in contrast to the frequency with which they are associated with certain other chronic hemolytic anemias.

LABORATORY FINDINGS. A severe microcytic, hypochromic anemia is characteristic of thalassemia major (Fig. 5-18). Anisocytosis and poikilocytosis are marked, and leptocytes and target cells are numerous. Increased polychromasia, basophilic stippling of the erythrocytes, and reticulocytosis (5 to 15 per cent) are conspicuous findings. There are usually 10 to 20 nucleated red cells per 100 leukocytes in the peripheral blood. Erythrocyte osmotic fragility is decreased; that is, resistance to lysis in hypotonic media is increased. Slight leukocytosis is the rule (10,000 to 20,000/cu mm), and there may be occasional immature

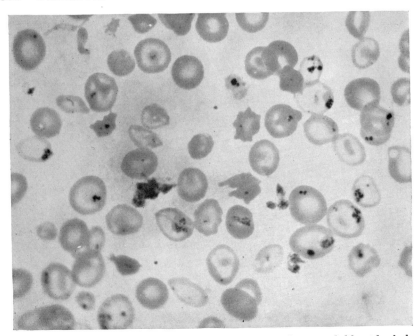

Figure 5-18. Wright-stained peripheral blood film from a child with thalassemia major who had been splenectomized; note the marked anisocytosis, poikilocytosis, and hypochromia with target cells, leptocytes, Pappenheimer bodies, and Howell-Jolly bodies. (Courtesy of Dr. Muriel C. Meyers.)

granulocytes in the peripheral blood. Most patients exhibit slight thrombocytosis. Bone marrow is hypercellular. Although all marrow elements are increased, there is a disproportionately greater increase in erythropoiesis, which is orderly and characterized by impaired hemoglobinization of the late rubricytes and metarubricytes. Stainable marrow iron is increased. Plasma iron is normal to increased, and most of the iron-binding protein is saturated. Plasma iron turnover is increased, but ^{59}Fe incorporation in circulating hemoglobin is decreased. Serum bilirubin (unconjugated fraction) is slightly to moderately increased, as are fecal and urinary urobilinogen levels. ^{51}Cr-tagged survival studies reveal impaired viability of circulating erythrocytes. Plasma haptoglobin is markedly decreased to absent. Hgb F is usually (but not always) increased and may be as high as 50 to 90 per cent. Hgb A$_2$ varies from normal to slightly increased amounts. Hemoglobin electrophoresis is most often interpreted as normal (Hgb A and Hgb F have very similar mobilities when electrophoresed on paper at pH 8.6; see Fig. 5-17). Free erythrocyte protoporphyrin is increased. Bone x-rays reveal generalized demineralization and cortical atrophy; these changes are particularly prominent in the skull, in which the diploic space may be greatly widened. Spontaneous fractures are quite rare. Other laboratory findings are nonspecific (e.g., the electrocardiographic changes attributable to anemia).

Thalassemia Minor (Heterozygous Disease). SYMPTOMS. Some patients are asymptomatic, but most complain of slight weakness, ease of fatigue, tachycardia, and exertional dyspnea. A few individuals are aware of pallor and slight jaundice, but in general thalassemia minor is tolerated well and interferes little, if at all, with the patients' activities or daily routines. Episodes of abdominal pain reflect an increased incidence of cholelithiasis.

PHYSICAL FINDINGS. Slight to moderate splenomegaly is the most consistent physical abnormality. Other frequent findings include minimal pallor and icterus. Habitus is usually normal, although some skull enlargement may occur. Leg ulcers are most unusual.

LABORATORY FINDINGS. The hematologic manifestations of thalassemia minor are similar to those of thalassemia major, although they are much less marked. The hemoglobin and hematocrit typically range from about 10 gm/100 ml of blood and 30 per cent, respectively, to almost normal levels. Because of microcytosis, the erythrocyte count is disproportionately higher than the other erythroid measurements and may actually be slightly increased or at the upper limits of normal, even though the circulating hemoglobin is decreased. The erythrocytes always display morphologic abnormalities, although the changes may be quite slight in patients with little anemia. Hypochromia, microcytes, target cells, leptocytes, increased polychromasia, basophilic stippling, slight reticulocytosis (3 to 5 per cent), and occasional nucleated red cells characterize the peripheral blood (Fig. 5-19). Erythrocyte osmotic fragility is decreased; leukocyte and platelet counts are normal. There is slight to moderate erythrocytic hyperplasia in the bone marrow and impaired

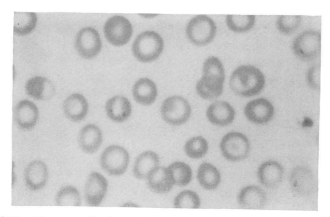

Figure 5-19. Target cells, hypochromia, and microcytes in the peripheral blood of a patient with thalassemia minor.

hemoglobinization of the more mature erythrocytic precursors. Stainable marrow iron is present in normal to increased amounts, and plasma iron is normal or slightly increased. Serum bilirubin is usually normal, but the unconjugated fraction may be slightly increased. Plasma haptoglobin reflects the magnitude of the hemolytic process and varies from near normal to markedly subnormal levels. In some patients bone x-rays reveal minimal osteoporosis. In α thalassemia heterozygotes Hgb F and Hgb A_2 are not increased, and hemoglobin electrophoresis is normal. In most patients with the trait of β thalassemia, Hgb A_2 comprises 5 to 7 per cent of the hemoglobin; a smaller number of these patients exhibit slightly increased concentrations of Hgb F (2 to 5 per cent), but, as a rule, do not show increased concentrations of Hgb A_2. Other laboratory findings lack specificity.

DIAGNOSIS OF THE QUANTITATIVE HEMOGLOBINOPATHIES

Thalassemia Major (Homozygous Disease). The diagnosis of thalassemia major rarely presents a problem. Severe anemia with its onset in infancy, jaundice, splenomegaly, marked hypochromia without iron deficiency, numerous leptocytes and target cells, and evidence of hemolysis (nucleated red cells in the peripheral blood, increased polychromasia, and reticulocytosis) are so characteristic that there is little chance for confusion. The following laboratory procedures provide additional relevant data: (1) measurement of alkali-resistant hemoglobin (Hgb F is usually increased), (2) hemoglobin electrophoresis (this technique is needed to exclude a mixed quantitative-qualitative hemoglobinopathy), and (3) determination of plasma iron or marrow iron content (iron stores are increased). Superficially, thalassemia major may resemble a number of other hematologic disorders, such as acute leukemia, severe iron deficiency anemia, or other forms of hemolytic anemias. However, these possibilities can be eliminated with relative ease; for example, acute leukemia has typical marrow findings, body iron stores are decreased in iron deficiency, and other hemolytic anemias are not associated with hypochromia. Hematologic evaluation of other members of the patient's family affords a means to confirm the diagnosis with certainty. Each of the parents of a patient with thalassemia major should have thalassemia minor, and three out of four siblings should also be affected (one with homozygous and two with heterozygous disease). Thus genetic studies contribute significantly to this diagnosis.

Thalassemia Minor (Heterozygous Disease). Recognition of thalassemia minor is often a difficult job and the diagnosis is frequently not made until middle or even old age. Thalassemia minor is most likely to be confused with iron deficiency anemia or some other form of hemolytic anemia. The demonstration of a normal or increased plasma iron and/or adequate amounts of stainable iron in the marrow of a patient with a microcytic, hypochromic anemia should immediately point to the possibility of thalassemia minor. Insofar as other hemolytic anemias are concerned, a patient with thalassemia minor who has a hemolytic component severe enough to be recognized as such will also exhibit hypochromia without evidence of iron deficiency. Thus the history, physical findings, and study of the peripheral blood provide the first clues to the diagnosis. Some measure of iron stores (plasma iron or evaluation of stainable iron in the marrow) and hemoglobin electrophoresis are mandatory in the work-up of all patients suspected of having thalassemia minor in order to exclude iron deficiency and a qualitative hemoglobinopathy. Determination of Hgb F and Hgb A_2 levels contributes additional important information. Because a slight increase in Hgb A_2 cannot be quantified with simple paper electrophoresis, other techniques (e.g., starch block electrophoresis) are needed to assess accurately the levels of Hgb A_2. Increased amounts of Hgb A_2 provide strong presumptive evidence of the diagnosis of thalassemia minor. With the exception of occasional patients with thalassemia major, elevated Hgb A_2 levels have been observed only in patients with heterozygous β thalassemia. Although the majority of the latter (perhaps as many as 85 to 90 per cent) have Hgb A_2 concentrations of 5 to 7 per cent, a few do not fall into this category and instead have slight increases in Hgb F. In addition, Hgb A_2 is not increased in patients with heterozygous α thalassemia. Therefore failure to demonstrate an increase in Hgb A_2 does not preclude the diagnosis of thalassemia minor. Last, but by no means least, are genetic studies. As is true for all hereditary disorders, absolute confirmation of the diagnosis of thalassemia minor and exclusion of such remote possibilities as pyridoxine-responsive or sideroachrestic anemias (p. 178) are contingent on the demonstration of a similar disorder in another member of the patient's family.

TREATMENT AND COURSE

Thalassemia Major (Homozygous Disease). Thalassemia major runs a progressive unremitting course; few patients live beyond childhood or early adolescence and many die in infancy. Survival beyond adolescence is such a rare occurrence that it suggests another diagnosis. There is no effective therapy. Blood transfusions constitute the only treatment. Since these patients ordinarily adapt well to the chronic anemia, there is no need to transfuse them to normal or even to near normal values. A hemoglobin after transfusion of 8 to 9 gm/100 ml of blood is quite satisfactory and will prevent significant symptoms or physiologic disadvantage consequent to the reduced oxygen-carrying capacity of the blood. In fact, attempts to maintain higher values by transfusions are contraindicated. Tissue hemosiderosis is an important feature of untreated thalassemia major, and transfusions add greatly to the already overabundant iron stores. Hemosiderosis always develops if the patient lives long enough and often contributes to or causes the patient's death. Newer chelating agents such as desferrioxamine B (p. 186) may afford a means of hindering (but probably not of preventing) the development of serious hemosiderosis; however, further evaluation is needed before the exact role of this agent in the over-all management of the patient with thalassemia major can be ascertained.

There is rarely any need or indication for other treatment. Occasionally, a patient with thalassemia major will develop a superimposed megaloblastic, macrocytic anemia secondary to folic acid deficiency brought about by increased requirements in the face of suboptimal intake (p. 201). These persons should receive folic acid supplementation. Otherwise, there is no reason to administer any other "antianemic" agent. In a few cases rapidly increasing anemia has been associated with marrow hypoplasia. The explanation for this unusual occurrence is not known, but the possibility of profound folic acid deficiency cannot be excluded.

Much has been written about the role of splenectomy in thalassemia major. A few patients develop overt hypersplenism (thrombocytopenia, neutropenia, and/or aggravation of anemia) consequent to hemosiderosis or the "big spleen" syndrome; under these conditions improvement may follow removal of the spleen. In most instances, however, splenectomy offers nothing and should be reserved for those patients in whom clear-cut evidence of superimposed hypersplenism can be obtained. Cholelithiasis is to be expected in the older patient. Intercurrent infection, the complications of excess body iron, and the effects of severe anemia are the usual causes of death.

Thalassemia Minor (Heterozygous Disease). In general, thalassemia minor is tolerated well and is compatible with a normal life-span. Therapy (i.e., blood transfusions) is rarely needed, for these patients adjust well to their chronic anemia. Under no circumstances should an asymptomatic (or nearly asymptomatic) patient be transfused just to allay the physician's (or the patient's) concern over the decreased peripheral erythroid values. The incidence of cholelithiasis is increased in patients with thalassemia minor and may necessitate cholecystectomy. The physician's primary responsibility in the management of the patient with thalassemia minor is to reassure the patient, to explain the nature of his disease, and to offer appropriate genetic counseling (one fourth of the offspring of two persons with thalassemia minor can be expected to have a lethal disease, i.e., thalassemia major).

Mixed Hemoglobinopathies

Geographically, those areas in which the qualitative hemoglobinopathies are most frequent overlap significantly with those in which the incidence of the thalassemia genes is high. Therefore it is not surprising that these mutant genes should coexist in a doubly heterozygous state. Hemoglobin S-thalassemia was the first mixed hemoglobinopathy to be described. Examples of many other structurally abnormal hemoglobins have been observed. However, the rarity of most of these hemoglobinopathies precludes the formulation of precise clinical pictures. It is now evident that most (if not all) of the patients with suspected thalassemia intermedia actually had a mixed hemoglobinopathy. Combinations of thalassemia with Hgb S, Hgb C, Hgb E, and Hgb Lepore warrant consideration.

The mixed hereditary hemoglobinopathies can be subdivided into two groups. *Interacting hemoglobinopathies* involve the same globin chain and produce clinical manifestations midway in severity between those characterizing the heterozygous and homozygous states. For example, a person possessing one β^S and one β^{Thal} gene is at a distinct physiologic disadvantage. Because of the β^{Thal} gene, production of β^S peptide chains exceeds that of normal β chains. Therefore the red cells contain a greater concentration (more than 50 per cent) of Hgb S than Hgb A. As a result, sickling and all the pathophysiologic manifestations attendant thereto occur at physiologic oxygen tensions. Since Hgb C, Hgb E, and Hgb Lepore are also β chain defects, the genes controlling the synthesis of these qualitatively abnormal hemoglobins can also interact with the β^{Thal} gene. The second category of mixed hemoglobinopathies involves different globin chains; these disorders are designated as *noninteracting*. In an individual with one β^S and one α^{Thal} gene, α globin chains are in short supply, but β-chain production is quantitatively normal. Under these circumstances there is comparable curtailment of Hgb A and Hgb S synthesis, and the cellular ratio of Hgb A:Hgb S will be the same as in persons with heterozygous hemoglobin S disease or the sickle cell trait. Because the concentration of Hgb S is too low for sickling to occur at physiologic oxygen tensions, the clinical manifestations are similar to but no worse than those of thalassemia minor and sickle cell trait existing alone. For similar reasons a hemoglobin with a structurally abnormal α polypeptide chain (e.g., Hgb I) will not interact with a β^{Thal} gene.

HEMOGLOBIN S-THALASSEMIA (MICRODEPRANOCYTIC DISEASE)

Double heterozygosity for β^S and β^{Thal} genes produces a clinical picture identical with although less severe than that of homozygous hemoglobin S disease (p. 257). These individuals manifest sickling and all the hematologic and vascular occlusive phenomena that it causes. In most patients the clinical manifestations are more suggestive of sickle cell anemia than of thalassemia major. Important differences serving to separate hemoglobin S-thalassemia from sickle cell anemia include both hypochromia and splenomegaly. Hemoglobin electrophoresis reveals 50 to 80 per cent Hgb S; the rest is chiefly Hgb A (Hgb A_2 or Hgb F may be slightly increased). Genetic studies are especially helpful because one parent will have hemoglobin S disease and the other will have thalassemia. Although many patients reach adult life, morbidity is marked; few patients have a normal life-span and most succumb to their hemoglobinopathy. Noninteracting hemoglobin S-thalassemia, that is, α^{Thal} and β^S, is characterized by the combined clinical manifestations of thalassemia minor and heterozygous hemoglobin S disease. The physiologic disadvantages of this doubly heterozygous state are no greater than those of single heterozygosity. It is of interest that most of the American Negroes with hemoglobin S-thalassemia have this noninteracting form.

HEMOGLOBIN E-THALASSEMIA

This mixed hemoglobinopathy was first described in Thailand. It is associated with clinical manifestations similar to but less severe than those of thalassemia major. These double heterozygotes possess Hgb E, Hgb A, and Hgb F. Theoretically, Hgb E would be expected to predominate, a situation analogous to the relationship between Hgb S and Hgb A in hemoglobin S-thalassemia. However, most reports indicate that Hgb F makes up more than 50 per cent of the hemoglobin. Observations on more patients, including genetic data, are needed to clarify this point. With the exception of the demonstration of small amounts of Hgb E on electrophoresis, the clinical manifestations of Hgb E-α thalassemia do not differ from those of thalassemia minor.

HEMOGLOBIN C-THALASSEMIA

Only a few of these double heterozygotes have been described. Most have had a concentration of Hgb C greater than 50 per cent. The clinical manifestations are basically those of thalassemia and are severer than thalassemia minor but less severe than thalassemia major. Some observers have stressed the presence of microspherocytes, although their pathogenesis and pathophysiologic significance are conjectural.

HEMOGLOBIN LEPORE-THALASSEMIA

A person who is heterozygous for Hgb Lepore synthesizes decreased numbers of abnormal globin chains in contrast to individuals with the other qualitative hemoglobinopathies in whom normal numbers of abnormal chains are formed. Clinically, heterozygosity for Hgb Lepore resembles thalassemia minor (p. 265). It is not surprising, therefore, that the few double heterozygotes (Hgb Lepore and β thalassemia) who have been reported have had disease similar in severity to thalassemia major.

Secondary Anemias of Unknown Cause

The causes of the anemias discussed in Chapter 4 and in the preceding sections of Chapter 5, as well as those caused by leukemia (Chap. 8), plasmacytic myeloma (Chap. 10), and the other myeloproliferative and lymphoproliferative disorders (Chap. 11), are clear-cut. Several forms of anemia remain, the pathogeneses of which are obscure. Although "secondary" to a variety of primary diseases, these anemias generally exhibit similar hematologic manifestations. Consequently, they often present a problem in differential diagnosis, and it is appropriate to consider them as a unit. With few exceptions these anemias are chronic, slight to moderate, and normocytic, normochromic. As a rule they are not associated with any other abnormalities in the peripheral blood. The bone marrow is either normal or reveals changes lacking diagnostic specificity (e.g., erythrocytic hyperplasia). These anemias presumably reflect depressed or inadequate erythropoiesis, and in most cases a hemolytic component also contributes.

Although the precise incidence of these secondary anemias is not ascertainable, they constitute a clinical problem of considerable magnitude. In the presence of a normocytic, normochromic anemia, without other associated hematologic abnormalities, renal insufficiency, liver disease, chronic infection, and malignancy, as well as the "anemias" of certain endocrinopathies [e.g., hypothyroidism (p. 154)], must be considered and excluded. There may be occasional hematologic clues such as thin macrocytes and/or target cells in patients with chronic liver disease, but the diagnosis is primarily dependent on nonhematologic data (e.g., abnormal liver function tests, an elevated blood urea nitrogen, pyuria, or evidence of thyroid dysfunction). The normocytic, normochromic anemia commonly dominates the clinical picture and may effectively hide the underlying basic disease. If careful study of the peripheral blood fails to uncover any hematologic abnormalities other than a normocytic, normochromic anemia, there is no reason to obtain a marrow specimen. Under these circumstances it can be predicted with virtual certainty that the marrow will be normal or display nonspecific changes. Neither can the performance at random of specialized laboratory procedures be condoned (e.g., hemoglobin electrophoresis, Schilling test, or red cell survival studies). The proper approach to this clinical problem is based on knowledge of the causes of the anemia and their elimination by appropriate studies; for example, a careful urinalysis, evaluation of renal and hepatic function, attempts to uncover a chronic infection or occult neoplasm, and assessment of thyroid function.

ANEMIA OF RENAL INSUFFICIENCY

Regardless of cause, chronic renal insufficiency is consistently accompanied by an anemia the severity of which correlates well with the degree of azotemia. In general, anemia does not appear until the blood urea nitrogen (BUN) reaches concentrations of about 50 mg/100 ml. The peripheral erythroid values exhibit a progressive decline as the BUN increases from 50 to around 250 mg/100 ml; however, more marked azotemia is not accompanied by severer anemia, and, in the absence of some complicating factor(s), the hemoglobin rarely drops below 6 gm/100 ml of blood. The anemia is typically normocytic, normochromic.

The pathogenesis of the anemia of chronic azotemia remains obscure, despite recent observations that implicate the kidneys as a major site of elaboration (or activation) of erythropoietin (p. 11). There is compelling support for the thesis that the anemia of renal insufficiency is basically the result of decreased erythropoiesis, and it is entirely logical to assume that erythropoietic suppression reflects, at least in part, decreased erythropoietin production. However, the relative insensitivity of existent assay techniques precludes accurate quantification of less than normal levels of plasma erythropoietic factor (erythropoietin) activity. Available data indicate that uremic, anemic patients do not show increased levels of plasma erythropoietic activity as do most other anemic patients. Instead, their plasma erythropoietic activity is similar to (or less than) that present normally. These findings are in accord with the suggestion that decreased erythropoietin production is the major cause of the anemia of chronic renal insufficiency. Further studies are required to clarify the precise role of erythropoietin in the pathogenesis of this type of anemia, most notably the therapeutic response to the administration of erythropoietin if and when it becomes available for human use.

Even though decreased erythropoietin production can be proved to exist, other etiologic mechanisms also appear to contribute. For example, there is some evidence favoring the existence of an erythropoietic inhibitory factor (or factors) in the plasma of anemic uremic subjects. Furthermore, marrow erythrocytic hypoplasia is not a consistent finding, as would be expected if the anemia were solely the result of depressed erythropoiesis. In addition, many patients manifest slight impairment in red cell viability because of a poorly defined extracorpuscular factor. Thus the anemia of azotemia appears to reflect both decreased production and increased peripheral destruction. In most cases decreased production predominates, but in a few patients overt hemolytic activity is demonstrable. Therefore, pending further elucidation, it can be concluded that the pathogenesis of the anemia of chronic renal insufficiency is complex and involves the interaction of several factors affecting cell production and survival.

Anemia often dominates the clinical picture, and it is not uncommon for the nonspecific manifestations attributable to a reduction in the oxygen-carrying capacity of the blood (weakness, exertional dyspnea and tachycardia, and pallor) to call attention to the presence of renal disease, the primary abnormality. There are few hematologic findings other than a normocytic, normochromic anemia. The erythrocytes frequently show little variation in size and shape, although some patients with moderate to marked azotemia will exhibit "burr cells" (Fig. 3-2, p. 63). The exact significance of these poikilocytes, which are characterized by several blunt, spinelike projections, is not known. Since their marrow precursors display the same morphologic abnormality, it must reflect a formative defect rather than an injury following release into the circulation. Although most commonly observed in uremic patients, burr cells lack specificity and have also been associated with gastrointestinal bleeding and gastric neoplasms. The reticulocyte count is typically less than normal, but rare patients manifest overt hemolytic activity with slight polychromasia and reticulocytosis. A nucleated red cell in the peripheral blood is a most unusual finding.

The leukocyte and thrombocyte counts are characteristically normal. Small hypersegmented neutrophils are demonstrable in a few patients; their pathogenesis and significance are not apparent. There are no other qualitative abnormalities in the peripheral blood. The bone marrow varies from patient to patient; deviations from normal are never specific and involve only quantitative differences. In some patients the marrow appears to be essentially normal; in others slight to moderate erythrocytic hypoplasia is evident (marked erythrocytic hypoplasia is seldom encountered); a few individuals display erythrocytic hyperplasia. Quantitative changes in other myeloid elements are, for the most part, relative rather than absolute. Marrow stainable iron is often increased.

With the exception of the manifestations of renal insufficiency (e.g., an elevated blood urea nitrogen), other laboratory findings are nonspecific. Plasma iron is somewhat variable, though generally normal with a slightly decreased iron-binding capacity. ^{59}Fe uptake is decreased; ^{51}Cr red cell survival studies commonly reveal a slight to moderate reduction in erythrocyte life-span.

The diagnosis of the anemia of renal insufficiency is based on nonhematologic data and is largely one of exclusion and association, that is, a normocytic, normochromic anemia without other important hematologic abnormalities and without evident cause in a patient with proved azotemia. Renal failure must be excluded in all patients with an unexplained anemia. Treatment is basically that of the primary disease; improved renal function and a fall in the blood urea nitrogen level are followed by increased erythropoiesis and augmentation in the peripheral erythroid values. Transfusions are rarely needed, for most of these patients adapt well to their chronic anemia. Furthermore, it is unusual for chronic renal insufficiency to cause marked or progressive anemia (the hemoglobin is most often between 8 to 10 and rarely falls below 6 gm/100 ml of blood). Unless the decreased oxygen-carrying capacity of the blood causes significant symptoms or interferes with the patient's activity, transfusions should be avoided. Because many uremic patients are in borderline or frank congestive heart failure, circulatory overload is a common aftermath of transfusions.

In a few patients improvement in the anemia has been attributed to the administration of cobalt. In normal recipients the cobaltous ion does stimulate erythropoiesis, apparently by interfering with cellular oxygen utilization, producing histotoxic hypoxia, and thereby augmenting plasma erythropoietic factor activity (p. 11). However, anemic, uremic patients already have anemic hypoxia, and the erythropoietic effect of an additional tissue oxygen deficit would appear to be nugatory. Because the response to cobalt is inconstant, infrequent, and, at best, inconsequential, the potential toxicity of this metal precludes its routine use. Furthermore, the clinical manifestations attributable to anemia are rarely limiting factors in the return of a patient with chronic renal insufficiency to a normal mode of living.

Acute renal insufficiency is also associated with anemia and profound alterations in erythropoiesis. Following acute renal shutdown, the peripheral erythroid values ordinarily drop precipitously as the result of acute hemolysis consequent to an ill-defined extracorpuscular defect. Suppressed marrow activity often contributes to the severity of the anemia, and acute erythroblastopenia or virtual aplasia of erythrocytic precursors has been observed. Other patients exhibit a typical response to increased blood loss with reticulocytosis and nucleated red cells in the peripheral blood and erythrocytic hyperplasia in the bone marrow. The other pathophysiologic manifestations of acute renal failure generally take precedence over the anemic component, which rarely requires any form of specific therapy, that is, transfusions. If acute renal shutdown is followed by prolonged renal insufficiency and persistent azotemia, the anemia of chronic uremia will ensue.

ANEMIA OF CHRONIC LIVER DISEASE

Few persons with chronic liver disease have normal peripheral erythroid values. In many patients the major cause of the anemia is well defined and includes (1) iron deficiency (patients with chronic liver disease are prone to bleed from such lesions as esophageal varices, peptic ulcerations, and hemorrhoids), (2) folic acid deficiency (dietary inadequacies are common in alcoholics with cirrhosis), and (3) hypersplenism (chronic congestive splenomegaly and Banti's syndrome occur frequently in patients with portal hypertension secondary to intrahepatic obstruction, and hyperlipemic hemolysis is frequently associated with early cirrhosis and fatty infiltration of the liver). In these cases the predominant hematologic manifestations are those of iron deficiency (p. 174), folic acid deficiency (p. 212), Banti's syndrome (p. 457), or hemolysis (p. 85). Certain of these anemias will respond to specific therapy (e.g., ferrous sulfate or folic acid). However, few patients will have normal erythroid values after these other causes of anemia have been corrected. Furthermore, most individuals with chronic hepatic disease are anemic in the absence of any of the complications cited. Thus it is evident that chronic liver disease per se is a cause of anemia.

The pathogenesis of the anemia of chronic liver disease is speculative and obscure. Available data indicate that it is the result of both impaired red cell viability and decreased marrow activity. The hemolytic component reflects a poorly defined extracorpuscular defect. Even though there may be myeloid erythrocytic hyperplasia, relative marrow failure is a major cause of the decrease in circulating red cell mass; that is, the response is inadequate to compensate for the increased peripheral loss. In a few patients (especially those with esophageal varices) hypervolemia with resultant hemodilution accentuates the reduction in the venous hematocrit. Because the anemia of chronic liver disease bears no relationship to the type of hepatic disease, it would appear to be a relatively specific response to varied and nonspecific hepatic abnormalities. Cirrhosis (alcoholic or postnecrotic) is the commonest cause.

In the absence of some complication such as iron or folic acid deficiency, the anemia of chronic liver disease is slight to moderate, with a circulating hemoglobin most often between 9 and 12 and seldom below 8 gm/100 ml of blood. There is rather poor correlation between the severity of the hepatic dysfunction and the degree of anemia. Although patients with the most advanced hepatic disease tend to have the lowest erythroid values, a clear-cut anemia is frequently attributable to liver disease, even in the face of minimal disturbance of hepatic function. In this regard it should be noted that a significant number of patients with histologically proved cirrhosis (perhaps as many as 10 to 15 per cent) have normal to only slightly increased bromsulphalein (BSP) retention. Thus careful evaluation of several parameters of liver function is required before it can be concluded with any certainty that an unexplained anemia is not the result of chronic liver disease.

As a rule, the anemia of chronic liver disease is not severe enough to produce significant complaints or physical findings. Other than minimal pallor, the clinical picture is ordinarily dominated by the manifestations of liver disease (e.g., hepatomegaly, splenomegaly, spider angiomata, and jaundice). In about 60 per cent of patients with uncomplicated anemia secondary to chronic liver disease, the anemia is macrocytic and normochromic; in the rest it is normocytic, normochromic. The macrocytes are characteristically round and thin (i.e., leptocytes) and appear to be the result of abnormal formation, for their marrow precursors are also large; however, the precise explanation for the production of these macrocytes is conjectural. Target cells are evident in a smaller number of patients. Thick macrocytes have also been described in patients with chronic liver disease, but these cells probably reflect superimposed folic acid deficiency rather than the liver disorder per se. The erythrocytes show little variation in shape. In the absence of significant hypersplenism, the reticulocyte count is usually normal and there are no nucleated red cells or increased polychromasia in the peripheral blood. The leukocyte count is typically low normal or below; the platelet count is most often normal. A slight relative and absolute monocytosis is characteristic of chronic liver disease. The bone marrow reveals variable quantitative changes; minimal erythrocytic hyperplasia with large precursors (macronormoblasts) and increased numbers of mature plasmacytes are frequent findings. Thus, with the exception of thin macrocytes, the hematologic manifestations of chronic liver disease are nonspecific. It must be reemphasized, however, that superimposed complications (iron lack, folic acid deficiency, hypersplenism, and acute hemorrhage) contribute to the peripheral blood and marrow abnormalities in many of these patients and greatly influence the clinical picture. Other laboratory findings reflect the underlying liver disease and lack hematologic specificity.

The diagnosis of the anemia of chronic liver disease is mainly one of association (the presence of a normocytic or macrocytic anemia in a patient with some type of liver disease). Round macrocytes with or without target cells and monocytosis are quite suggestive of liver disease, but they are by no means specific findings. Because of the frequency with which these patients develop other forms of anemia (folic acid deficiency, iron deficiency, or hypersplenism), the physician must be prepared to recognize these abnormalities superimposed on the underlying anemia of chronic liver disease. Some assessment of hepatic function is indicated in all patients with an unexplained anemia.

There is no treatment for the "uncomplicated" anemia of chronic liver disease other than therapy directed at improving hepatic function. Because the anemia is chronic and rarely severe (barring hemorrhage or the development of some other complication), transfusions are seldom indicated. The erythroid values will increase if and when liver function improves. Iron and folic acid are of value only in the presence of deficiencies. Other antianemic agents have no place in the management of these patients. In particular, the administration of vitamin B_{12} or liver extract is valueless because chronic liver disease is not in itself associated with a deficiency of vitamin B_{12}.

ANEMIA OF CHRONIC INFECTION

Chronic infections are commonly associated with anemia, the severity of which varies with the nature of the infection and type of organism. Empyema, lung abscess, subacute bacterial endocarditis, bronchiectasis, osteomyelitis, chronic urinary tract infections, pelvic inflammatory disease, brucellosis, and fungal infections are the commonest offenders. Localized tuberculosis is an exception and is at best associated with a minimal anemia. The anemia of chronic infection is typically modest (9 to 12 gm/100 ml of blood), and unless there is some superimposed complication, the peripheral erythroid values are not markedly depressed. The pathogenesis of this form of anemia is obscure. Plasma iron is decreased, as is the plasma iron-binding capacity. Plasma iron turnover is normal or slightly increased, and radioiron incorporation in new erythrocytes is consistently decreased. Current data favor the hypothesis that these ferrokinetic abnormalities reflect impaired release by reticuloendothelial cells of iron derived from senescent erythrocytes, thus interfering with the availability of this iron to be transported by transferrin to the marrow for the synthesis of new hemoglobin. Iron stores are normal to increased (there are abundant amounts of stainable iron in the bone marrow). Free erythrocyte protoporphyrin is increased.

These alterations in iron metabolism probably explain those cases in which the anemia of chronic infection is microcytic and hypochromic (p. 178). In most patients, however, the anemia is normocytic and normochromic, and it becomes necessary to postulate some impairment in cell production and/or viability in addition to defective hemoglobin synthesis. Although red cell survival is slightly decreased in patients with the anemia of chronic infection, a normal marrow would be able to compensate without difficulty for such a slight decrease in erythrocyte lifespan. Therefore impaired cell production of unknown cause appears to play a major role in the pathogenesis of the anemia of chronic infection. Overt hemolysis accompanies certain types of acute infection (p. 149).

The clinical manifestations in patients with the anemia of chronic infection are primarily those of the infection; however, the anemia dominates the clinical picture in some patients and may first call attention to the underlying infection. The anemia is usually normocytic and normochromic without significant anisocytosis or poikilocytosis. The reticulocyte count is normal to low. In a few patients hypochromia and microcytes are evident. These individuals have hypoferremia, but, in contrast to persons who are iron deficient, their iron-binding protein is also decreased and iron stores are normal to increased. The leukocyte and platelet counts are most often normal (leukocytosis is not a characteristic manifestation of chronic infections). BGN (basophilic granulation of the neutrophils) may be increased. The bone marrow is normal or reveals nonspecific changes; for example, erythrocytic precursors may be present in normal, decreased, or increased numbers. Other laboratory findings reflect the basic disease (i.e., the infection).

The diagnosis of the anemia of chronic infection is based on association (an unexplained normocytic, normochromic anemia in a patient with a chronic infection, especially of the forms described). This particular anemia is refractory to all known antianemic agents and improves only when the chronic infection is eradicated. Even those patients who manifest hypochromia fail to respond to iron therapy, for they are not really iron deficient. When facilities for ferrokinetic measurements are available, the abnormalities that distinguish an inflammatory process may provide a clue to the correct diagnosis, but these findings are not specific and accompany other anemias such as the anemia of malignancy.

ANEMIA OF MALIGNANCY

Most malignant neoplasms are associated with an anemia. Because of the propensity of malignant disorders to cause abnormal bleeding, the anemia is often microcytic and hypochromic as a consequence of iron deficiency (p. 174). Certain malignancies are accompanied by a megaloblastic macrocytic anemia secondary to folic acid deficiency (increased requirements in the face of dietary inadequacy, p. 201). Other complications of malignancy that may eventuate in anemia include superimposed hypersplenism with overt hemolysis (p. 460), and, of course, bone marrow metastases with a myelophthisic anemia (p. 240). However, even in the absence of these causes for anemia, the majority of patients with malignant neoplasms of one kind or another exhibit a slight to moderate anemia (the hemoglobin seldom falls below 9 gm/100 ml of blood in these patients). This form of anemia is generally normocytic, normochromic without other significant hematologic abnormalities; bone marrow is normal or reveals nonspecific changes. Occasionally the anemia is slightly hypochromic and microcytic, with ferrokinetic abnormalities similar to those that characterize the anemia of chronic infection (decreased plasma iron and iron-binding capacity with normal or increased body iron stores).

The pathogenesis of the anemia of malignancy is also obscure. It resembles in many respects the anemia of chronic infection. A modest decrease in erythrocyte survival time is present, but a normal marrow would be able to compensate for such a minor degree of hemolysis without detectable change in the peripheral erythroid values. Therefore depressed erythropoiesis appears to be of paramount importance in the production of the anemia. In the absence of treatable complications, such as superimposed iron or folic acid deficiency, the anemia of malignancy is refractory to all forms of therapy except those directed at the neoplasm. Control (or eradication) of the malignant growth is followed by an increase in the circulating hemoglobin. Transfusions are seldom needed, unless complicating factors such as extensive marrow metastases or massive hemorrhage are present.

ANEMIA OF RHEUMATOID ARTHRITIS

Rheumatoid arthritis is rather consistently associated with a mild to moderate anemia that varies in severity with the extent and activity of the arthritic process. The anemia is most often normocytic, normochromic and is unaccompanied by other significant hematologic abnormalities. Rarely, the anemia may be slightly hypochromic. This form of anemia resembles that of chronic infection and appears, predominantly, to reflect marrow failure. Although a slight decrease in red cell survival times is often demonstrable, overt hemolysis is unusual, and so minimal a hemolytic component is an inadequate explanation for the anemia. The anemia of rheumatoid arthritis is refractory to the usual antianemic agents. Some severely anemic patients have been reported to respond to iron (especially parenteral iron); however, it seems likely that most of these patients were actually iron deficient. Transfusions are seldom indicated, for the anemia as a rule is not severe enough to interfere significantly with the patient's activity or normal physiologic functions.

The diagnosis of the anemia of rheumatoid arthritis is basically one of association and exclusion (an unexplained normocytic, normochromic anemia without other pertinent hematologic abnormalities in a patient with rheumatoid arthritis). Those patients who exhibit slight hypochromia have normal to increased iron stores and can be distinguished from persons who are iron deficient by such readily accessible parameters as marrow iron content.

Polycythemia
(*Erythrocytosis*)

An increase above normal with respect to age and sex in the peripheral erythroid values (erythrocyte count, hemoglobin level, and hematocrit) is commonly designated *polycythemia* but might more appropriately be termed *erythrocytosis.* It may be relative or absolute (Fig. 6-1). When relative, it is the result of a decrease in the fluid portion of the blood and is usually transient; when absolute, it reflects an actual increase in red cell mass and may be primary or secondary (Table 6-1).

Relative Erythrocytosis

DEHYDRATION

Because the blood cells are suspended in a liquid medium, their concentration in an aliquot of blood will vary inversely with the quantity of plasma present. Thus a decrease in plasma volume subsequent to dehydration (e.g., decreased fluid intake, persistent vomiting, severe diarrhea, and diabetic acidosis) will be manifested by increases in the red cell count, circulating hemoglobin level, and venous hematocrit. Total red cell mass is not increased. Differentiation from an absolute polycythemia is most often clear-cut, with obvious dehydration or symptoms of the primary disease pointing to the correct diagnosis. Even though some confusion may exist initially, the rapid restoration of plasma volume following hydration quickly establishes the nature of the polycythemia.

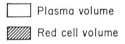

Plasma volume
Red cell volume

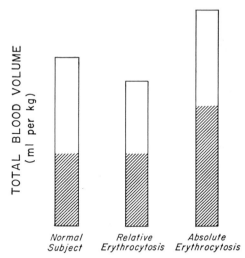

| Normal Subject | Relative Erythrocytosis | Absolute Erythrocytosis |

Figure 6-1. Schematic representation of changes in plasma volume and red cell mass in relative and absolute erythrocytosis.

Table 6-1. *Types and Causes of Polycythemia (Erythrocytosis)*

I. *Relative*
   Dehydration
   "Stress" erythrocytosis

II. *Absolute*
   Secondary
      A. Due to hypoxemia
         1. Residence at high altitude
         2. Chronic pulmonary disease
         3. Obesity
         4. Acquired cardiac disease
         5. Venoarterial shunts
         6. Decreased oxygen-carrying capacity (abnormal hemoglobins)
      B. Without hypoxemia
         1. Renal disease
         2. CNS disease
         3. Miscellaneous tumors
         4. Cushing's syndrome
   Primary (polycythemia vera)

STRESS ERYTHROCYTOSIS

Although less common, this form of relative erythrocytosis is more important because of its chronicity and the increased likelihood that it may be mistaken for polycythemia vera. This entity appears to reflect a decrease in plasma volume; however, a shift in the vascular distribution of red cells may also play a role. Total red cell volume is normal, as are all parameters that assess rates of erythropoiesis. The etiology is obscure; it has been attributed to "nervous stress" analogous to the temporary fall in plasma volume and resultant hemoconcentration induced by acute "hypoxic stress."

Stress erythrocytosis is encountered most often in hyperactive, hard-driving, middle-aged males. Symptoms are vague and suggest a psychoneurotic origin and underlying anxiety. The patients are ruddy, usually obese, and frequently hypertensive. There is no evidence of cardiac or pulmonary disease, and the arterial oxygen saturation is normal. The spleen and liver are not enlarged. The peripheral erythroid values are slightly to moderately increased (the hematocrit is rarely above 60 per cent). In contrast to the findings in polycythemia vera, the leukocyte and thrombocyte counts are not elevated, and granulocyte alkaline phosphatase activity is not increased. There are no immature leukocytes or nucleated red cells in the peripheral blood. Bone marrow is normal.

Diagnosis is dependent on these clinical findings in the presence of a normal total red cell mass. Phlebotomies and myelosuppressive therapy are not indicated. The course is benign and consists of reassurance and periodic re-evaluation. Although the venous hematocrit may remain elevated for long periods, rapid fluctuations are observed occasionally. Certain patients with stress erythrocytosis formerly were classified as Gaisböck's syndrome (erythrocytosis and hypertension without splenomegaly).

Secondary Polycythemia

ERYTHROCYTOSIS DUE TO HYPOXEMIA

The erythropoietic response to hypoxic hypoxia, initially described by Bert in 1878, has been studied extensively and today is indisputable. Hypoxia is now generally accepted as the fundamental stimulus for erythropoiesis which is mediated by the humoral erythropoietic regulatory mechanism (p. 13). Oxygen content of the blood (volumes per cent) is the product of the oxygen capacity and the oxygen saturation. Oxygen capacity (volumes per cent) is determined by multiplying the hemoglobin (grams/100 ml) by 1.34 (each gram of hemoglobin can carry 1.34 ml of oxygen); oxygen saturation (per cent of hemoglobin present as oxyhemoglobin) is primarily dependent on oxygen tension (Fig. 1-9, p. 21). In arterial blood the pO_2 is normally about 90 mm of mercury; at this tension approximately 96 per cent of the hemoglobin is saturated with oxygen. Therefore the oxygen content of normal arterial blood with 15 gm of hemoglobin/100 ml is 19.3 volumes per cent ($15 \times 1.34 \times 0.96 = 19.3$). Any disorder that affects arterial oxygen saturation or the capacity of hemoglobin to carry oxygen will sequentially reduce oxygen content of the blood, produce tissue hypoxia, enhance humoral factor activity, stimulate erythrocyte production, and augment red cell mass.

Decreased Arterial Oxygen Saturation. The sigmoidal oxyhemoglobin dissociation curve (Fig. 1-9, p. 21) affords a distinct physiologic advantage, and minor changes in oxygen tension do not significantly affect oxygen saturation. Reduction in oxygen tension sufficient to yield an oxyhemoglobin of less than 85 to 90 per cent constitutes a potent erythropoietic stimulus, regardless of the cause of hypoxemia. In general, the degree of erythrocytosis varies inversely with the oxygen saturation, although it is not possible to relate precisely the level of the erythroid values with oxygen saturation. A decrease in arterial oxygen tension may be the result of decreased oxygen tension in the inspired air, hypoventilation, an alveolar-capillary block, or an admixture of venous and arterial blood. Specific causes are listed in Table 6-1.

RESIDENCE AT HIGH ALTITUDE. Because atmospheric pressure decreases with altitude, oxygen tension of inspired air falls and arterial hypoxemia ensues. For this reason residence at high altitude is invariably associated with erythrocytosis. Shortly after arrival at high altitudes, plasma volume falls and a relative erythrocytosis is demonstrable. The explanation for this finding is not apparent, but it probably represents a physiologic compensatory mechanism that temporarily increases the oxygen content per unit volume of blood. This relative erythrocytosis is soon replaced by an absolute increase in red cell mass which persists as long as residence at high altitude is maintained. The level of the erythroid values usually varies directly with the altitude; that is, the higher the altitude, the greater the erythrocytosis. There is a limit, however, and above 20,000 feet red cell production is impaired. Following descent the erythroid values return to normal. After residence at high altitude for many years, certain patients develop chronic mountain sickness or Monge's disease with marked erythrocytosis, dyspnea, and cyanosis. This disorder is probably the result of superimposed pulmonary disease.

CHRONIC PULMONARY DISEASE. Pulmonary disease of varied etiology may produce arterial hypoxemia as a result of alveolar hypoventilation or an alveolar-capillary block. Emphysema is an example of the former and interstitial fibrosis, the latter. Although emphysema is a common form of chronic pulmonary disease and a frequent cause of arterial hypoxemia, few of these patients exhibit erythrocytosis. The reason these individuals do not develop an increased venous hematocrit needs further study. It may reflect the depressive effect of chronic pulmonary infection.

Obesity. Extreme obesity may cause hypoventilation and arterial hypoxemia, thus leading to erythrocytosis. Hypoventilation is secondary to mechanical factors and periodic respirations brought about by somnolence and decreased sensitivity of the respiratory center. Because these patients resemble the fat boy described by Dickens, this entity has been termed the "Pickwickian syndrome." The erythroid values decrease with weight reduction.

Acquired Cardiac Disease. Chronic congestive heart failure may be associated with erythrocytosis regardless of the nature of the cardiac lesion. The increase in peripheral erythroid values is modest.

Venoarterial Shunts. Disorders that permit venous blood with an oxygen tension of about 35 mm of mercury to bypass the lungs and mix directly with arterial blood produce marked hypoxemia and may be associated with profound erythrocytosis. Examples include pulmonary arteriovenous aneurysms and certain types of congenital heart disease, such as the tetralogy of Fallot, Eisenmenger's complex, transposition of the great vessels, or a patent ductus arteriosus with reversed flow.

Patients with erythrocytosis secondary to decreased arterial oxygen saturation ordinarily present with symptoms and findings of their primary disease. Other points that aid in distinguishing these patients from those with polycythemia vera include cyanosis and the absence of splenomegaly. The erythrocytosis more often than not is mild. In general, a hematocrit above 60 per cent indicates a venoarterial shunt, a severe pulmonary abnormality such as Ayerza's disease, or polycythemia vera. Total blood volume is increased consequent to an expanded red cell mass, and plasma volume is normal or slightly decreased. Leukocytosis and thrombocytosis are not seen. Arterial oxygen saturation is low. Bone marrow shows only erythrocytic hyperplasia.

Treatment is correction of the environment or of the underlying cardiovascular disorder. Since hypoxic polycythemia reflects a physiologic corrective mechanism, myelosuppressive therapy is contraindicated. The role of phlebotomies is more disputable. Even though arterial oxygen saturation remains low, a normal oxygen content may be maintained by an increased oxygen capacity. With a hemoglobin of 18 gm/100 ml and an arterial oxygen saturation of 80 per cent, the oxygen content of the blood is normal ($18 \times 1.34 \times 0.80 = 19.3$ volumes per cent). In such a patient phlebotomy would produce the same effect as in a normal subject and arterial oxygen content would fall. When arterial hypoxemia is severe, an increase in the oxygen-carrying capacity of the blood fails to correct the oxygen deficit. Under these circumstances the stimulus to erythropoiesis persists, and a physiologic response becomes an unphysiologic secondary polycythemia. The viscosity of the blood varies directly with the magnitude of the erythrocytosis and may further impair oxygenation of blood in the lungs or delivery of oxygen to the tissues. In certain patients the deleterious effect of the increased viscosity outweighs the beneficial effect of the increased oxygen-carrying capacity. There is no exact level above which this situation can be anticipated; many individual factors, such as the nature of the underlying disease, are involved. Therefore the decision to employ phlebotomies may require a trial-and-error approach. Patients with moderate to marked erythrocytosis who fail to respond to treatment of their primary disease or those for whom no treatment is available should be observed closely following the cautious removal of 300 to 500 ml of blood. If improvement occurs, phlebotomies may be repeated daily until the optimal level of the erythroid values is established. One should never try to restore "normal" peripheral erythroid values because they would in effect be "abnormal" for the hypoxemic patient.

Decreased Oxygen-Carrying Capacity (Abnormal Pigments). The presence of methemoglobin or sulfhemoglobin is frequently listed as a cause of secondary polycythemia. Because these pigments are incapable of carrying oxygen, the oxygen capacity and content of the blood are reduced in their presence. In addition, the oxyhemoglobin dissociation curve is shifted to the left in the presence of methemoglobinemia. Tissue hypoxia results and accelerated erythropoiesis would be expected. In susceptible individuals these pigments may be produced by such drugs as nitrites, sulfonamides, and analine derivatives. However, it is doubtful that significant erythrocytosis ever occurs in patients with acquired methemoglobinemia or sulfhemoglobinemia. Approximately 100 cases of hereditary methemoglobinemia have been reported. Some have been caused by a deficiency of an erythrocyte enzyme that catalyzes the reduction of methemoglobin by DPNH (p. 78); other patients have had an abnormal hemoglobin, Hgb M (p. 251). An occasional patient with congenital methemoglobinemia has been reported to have increased erythroid values, although measurements of red cell mass are not available. Spectroscopic examination will confirm the presence of abnormal pigments but their importance as causes of secondary polycythemia has been overrated.

ERYTHROCYTOSIS WITHOUT ASSOCIATED HYPOXEMIA

Renal Disease. Recent studies implicating the kidneys in erythropoietic factor elaboration (p. 11) have served to emphasize the relationship between erythrocytosis and renal disease. Increasing numbers of these patients are being observed; the majority have renal carcinoma, but some have relatively benign disorders, including hydronephrosis, renal cysts, and nephrosis. Splenomegaly, leukocytosis, and thrombocytosis do not accompany the increased red cell mass; arterial oxygen saturation is normal. Few patients with elevated erythroid values exhibit renal lesions; however, the possibility of a renal etiology must always be considered in patients with erythrocytosis because nephrectomy might be curative. Enhanced erythropoietic stimulatory activity has been demonstrated in the plasma and tumor extracts or cyst fluid of some, but not all, patients studied to date. It is reasonable to conclude that the erythrocytosis is the result of enhanced humoral factor activity most likely originating in the diseased kidney.

Central Nervous System Disease. Polycythemia also accompanies certain brain diseases, most notably cerebellar hemangioblastoma. Although rare (fewer than 40 patients have been reported), such lesions should be considered in the presence of erythrocytosis and a normal arterial oxygen saturation. Papilledema is often an important clue. The leukocyte and platelet counts are not elevated and the spleen is not enlarged. The erythroid values have fallen to normal in a significant number of these patients after surgical removal of the tumor. Although sketchy, available data indicate that the erythrocytosis is due to an erythropoietic substance produced by the tumor. Polycythemia has also been attributed to encephalitis, Parkinson's disease, and other brain disorders, but so few patients have been observed that the relationship is not clear-cut. Occasionally, abnormalities of the respiratory center may produce hypoventilation, arterial hypoxemia, and erythrocytosis.

Other Tumors. In a few patients erythrocytosis without leukocytosis, thrombocytosis, or splenomegaly has accompanied such tumors as uterine fibroids, hepatic carcinoma, pheochromocytoma, and bronchogenic carcinoma. The pathogenesis of the erythrocytosis in these cases has not been elucidated.

Cushing's Syndrome. Slight erythrocytosis occurs in some patients with Cushing's syndrome and probably reflects the increased oxygen consumption brought about by increased corticosteroid secretion.

Polycythemia Vera

Polycythemia vera is a chronic disease of unknown cause characterized by an absolute erythrocytosis, leukocytosis, thrombocytosis, and splenomegaly.

HISTORY

Polycythemia vera was described initially by Vasquez in 1892 and established as a specific disease entity in case reports by Saundby and Russell in 1902 and by Osler in 1903. In 1904 Türk pointed out the presence of leukocytosis and of immature granulocytes and nucleated red cells in the peripheral blood. Hutchinson and Miller described marrow megakaryocytic hyperplasia in 1906. By 1908 more than 70 case reports had appeared. The clinical picture was completed in 1910 with the recognition of thrombocytosis by Lesourd and Pagniez.

ETIOLOGY

The pathogenesis of polycythemia vera is unknown. Theories of causation include hypoxia, an abnormality of the midbrain, a neoplastic process, and a derangement in normal physiologic regulatory mechanisms. In view of the potent erythropoietic stimulus imparted by hypoxia, its possible role in the pathogenesis of polycythemia vera has been stressed. Despite many attempts to confirm this hypothesis, there is no evidence of an oxygen deficit. Arterial and marrow blood oxygen saturations are normal, and pulmonary hyperoxia fails to reduce the rate of erythropoiesis. The possibility that vascular lesions of the bone marrow may produce localized hypoxia has not been entirely excluded; however, the leukocytosis, thrombocytosis, and splenomegaly suggest a pathogenic mechanism other than simple hypoxia.

Attempts to assign the central nervous system a primary role in the etiology of polycythemia vera have also failed. Although the hypophyseal-hypothalamic system most likely exerts a modifying effect on erythropoiesis, abnormalities in this area are not demonstrable in patients with the characteristic findings of polycythemia vera. The widely held concept that polycythemia vera is a neoplastic disease is supported by the increased incidence of leukemia and other myeloproliferative disorders developing in these patients. However, polycythemia vera does not fulfill the criteria of a malignant process. It is not uniformly fatal unless some complication intervenes, and the histologic picture is not one of uncontrolled growth with tissue infiltration.

The theory that polycythemia vera may be the result of some derangement in basic regulatory mechanisms is no longer without experimental support. Enhanced erythropoietic, thrombopoietic, and leukopoietic activities have been demonstrated in plasmas from some patients with polycythemia vera. Although available data do not constitute proof, they support the thesis that polycythemia vera may be caused by a metabolic imbalance that results in an overproduction of humoral factors or, conversely, in the failure to inactivate such materials at rates sufficient to maintain hemopoietic equilibrium. Future studies along these lines should provide relevant information in regard to the causation and pathogenesis of polycythemia vera.

PATHOPHYSIOLOGY

The basic abnormality in polycythemia vera is the overproduction of all bone marrow elements with increased numbers of erythrocytes, platelets, and granulocytes in peripheral blood. Extramedullary hemopoiesis may be present, but there is no evidence of disorderly cell proliferation or tissue invasion. *Blood volume is increased because of an absolute increase in red cell mass; plasma volume is little changed.* Capillary dilatation and vascular engorgement are responsible for most of the clinical manifestations. Since all tissues are plethoric, the symptoms are many and varied. The elevated hematocrit serves to increase blood viscosity and decrease blood flow, thereby contributing, together with the thrombocytosis, to a high incidence of thromboses. Overdistention of the vascular bed plays an important role in the causation of hemorrhage as do other factors such as thrombocytosis (p. 503) and defective clot retraction with erythrocyte "fall out." Peptic ulcer is increased, apparently as the direct result of the erythrocytosis and vascular engorgement. Increased nucleic acid catabolism consequent to hyperactive hemopoiesis is responsible for hyperuricemia and occasional instances of overt gout.

Plasma iron turnover is about two to three times greater than that brought about by arterial hypoxemia. This increased rate of erythrocytic iron renewal is out of proportion to the red cell mass. Certain data indicate that it may be a manifestation of a double cell population comprised of normal cells and of short-lived cells. The short-lived cells, which are microcytic and display decreased resistance to lysis in hypotonic media, appear to reflect the excessive effect of the thermostable plasma erythropoietic factor that probably affects erythroblastic cellular division (p. 12). In polycythemia vera plasma a disproportionately greater effect is attributable to this humoral erythropoietic agent than to erythropoietin, the glycoprotein factor that enhances hemoglobin synthesis (p. 11). The thermostable fraction of plasmas from patients with polycythemia vera quite consistently induces in normal rats erythrocytosis due to the production of microcytes with abnormal osmotic behavior; remarkably similar cells are found in the blood of patients with polycythemia vera. On the other hand, increased erythropoietin activity (an enhancing effect on hemoglobin synthesis) has not been demonstrable in recipients of most polycythemia vera plasmas.

There is no hypoxemia in patients with polycythemia vera, and arterial oxygen saturation is normal. The oxygen content of the blood is increased, even though clinical cyanosis may be evident because of the presence of 5 gm or more of reduced hemoglobin/100 ml of blood. Consequently, oxygen supply exceeds tissue requirements. A possible defect in pulmonary gas transfer secondary to increased blood viscosity has been proposed to explain the occasional patient with a slight decrease in arterial oxygen saturation. There is no proof, however, that polycythemia per se impairs pulmonary function. Therefore any decrease in arterial oxygen saturation may be assumed to indicate another diagnosis, that is, secondary polycythemia or an additional disease.

CLINICAL MANIFESTATIONS

Polycythemia vera is a relatively rare disorder; accurate data concerning its true incidence are not available. The disease generally has its onset in the sixth decade of life. It is uncommon below the age of 40 and virtually unheard of in children. The incidence is slightly higher in males and possibly in Jews, although preponderance in this ethnic group has been challenged. Negroes are rarely affected. Scattered instances of familial polycythemia have been described but do not permit etiologic speculations.

Symptoms. The onset is usually gradual, although an acute thrombotic episode (e.g., a myocardial infarction) or abnormal bleeding (especially postoperatively) may first call attention to the disease. Occasionally, elevated erythroid values or redness of the skin may suggest the diagnosis in an otherwise asymptomatic person. Most often the initial complaints are vague and include weakness, ease of fatigue, headache, dizziness, visual difficulties, and syncope. Sometimes nondescript symptoms suggest a functional disorder and lead to an erroneous psychiatric diagnosis. Vascular engorgement, thromboembolic phenomena, or a hemorrhagic diathesis may affect any organ or tissue. Consequently a listing of the multiple symptoms is without value; however, certain complaints deserve emphasis. Generalized pruritus, which is aggravated by heat and is most noticeable after a hot bath, occurs in about 25 per cent of patients with polycythemia vera and is perhaps the most singular complaint attributable to this disorder. Abdominal pain is another common symptom (peptic ulceration is four to five times more common in patients with polycythemia vera than in the general population). Joint symptoms may be a manifestation of secondary gout. Although weight loss is rarely stressed, it is a prominent manifestation in about 20 per cent of the patients.

Physical Findings. The most characteristic physical findings are directly attributable to the enhanced red cell mass. Increased coloration of the skin and mucous membranes is evident in 90 per cent or more of the patients. It is a distinctive "ruddy cyanosis" caused by the admixture of increased amounts of oxyhemoglobin (red) and reduced hemoglobin (blue). The predominant color is dependent on the rate of peripheral blood flow, but the reddish hue is always evident and serves to differentiate this finding from the cyanosis of arterial hypoxemia. Because peripheral blood flow is affected by external temperature, Osler's description of these patients as being "red as a rose" in summer and "blue as indigo" in winter is especially appropriate. Exposed skin surfaces (face, ears, and fingertips) are involved most often. Engorgement of retinal veins is another common manifestation of the increased blood volume and generalized vascular distention.

The spleen is enlarged in three fourths or more of the cases and the liver in about one third. The spleen usually descends less than 5 cm below the costal margin on deep inspiration; however, massive enlargement (below the level of the umbilicus) is encountered occasionally. Most of the patients with massive splenomegaly have long-standing disease which may actually be evolving into myeloid metaplasia (p. 430). There is no reason to classify separately patients with cirrhosis and polycythemia (the so-called Mosse's syndrome).

Blood pressure is elevated in approximately 50 per cent of the patients. Sternal tenderness has been described, but it is not particularly common. Clubbing of the fingers and toes does not occur in uncomplicated polycythemia vera. Other physical abnormalities lack diagnostic specificity and are dependent on the presence of hemorrhage or thromboses (e.g., evidence of thrombophlebitis, residual of a cerebral vascular accident, or congestive heart failure consequent to a myocardial infarction).

Laboratory Findings. PERIPHERAL BLOOD. The erythroid values are invariably greater than normal. The red count ordinarily does not exceed 9 million/cu mm, the hemoglobin 25 gm/100 ml, or the hematocrit 80 per cent; however, higher values have been recorded. Total blood volume is increased because of a two- to threefold increase in red cell mass; as a rule plasma volume is normal but may be slightly increased or slightly decreased. The erythrocytes exhibit moderate anisocytosis but little poikilocytosis. The anisocytosis reflects the presence of a bimodal cell population consisting of normocytic and microcytic erythrocytes. The small cells are discernible on stained films and demonstrable graphically by Price-Jones measurements. The red cells are normochromic, unless repeated phlebotomies have produced iron deficiency and hypochromia. Minimal polychromasia and a slight reticulocytosis (up to 4 per cent) are common, as is an occasional nucleated red cell in the peripheral blood. The erythrocyte sedimentation rate is decreased because of the elevated hematocrit and shorter distance for the red cells to fall. When measured with quantitative photocolorimetric techniques, osmotic fragility patterns do not deviate significantly from normal; when determined with a direct cell enumeration technique employing red cell pipettes and hypotonic salt solutions as diluents, decreased osmotic resistance of the microcytes can be demonstrated.

Leukocytosis is present in approximately 70 per cent of the patients. Counts usually range between 10,000 and 20,000/cu mm; however, values of 50,000 or more do occur. The leukocytosis is largely the result of a relative and absolute neutrophilia, but eosinophils, basophils, and monocytes are also increased. Occasional immature granulocytes in the peripheral blood are not uncommon. Morphologically, the leukocytes appear normal; the alkaline phosphatase content of the mature granulocytes is increased in many patients but may be normal or even decreased.

Thrombocytosis occurs in 60 per cent or more of the patients, and platelet counts may reach levels of several million per cubic millimeter. The platelets are most often morphologically normal. On rare occasions atypical megakaryocytes or fragments are found in the peripheral blood. Bleeding and coagulation times are generally normal, but clots may be fragile and retraction impaired. Several other abnormalities in the coagulation mechanism have been described, but none is consistent.

Bone Marrow. The bone marrow is hyperplastic with increased numbers of all normal myeloid elements, that is, nucleated red cells, granulocytes and their precursors, and megakaryocytes. Proliferation is orderly, and normal ratios of immature to mature cells are maintained. Therefore the only deviation from normal is quantitative.

Other Laboratory Findings. Slight to moderate hyperuricemia is found in about 30 per cent of the patients. Most patients have mild to moderate elevations in their basal metabolism rates. Arterial oxygen saturation and pulmonary function tests are normal. Plasma ^{59}iron turnover is about five times the normal. Other laboratory findings are nonspecific and reflect complications of the disease (e.g., the electrocardiographic abnormalities of a myocardial infarction).

DIAGNOSIS

The demonstration of an absolute erythrocytosis is requisite for the diagnosis of polycythemia vera. Measurement of the peripheral erythroid values will suffice if they are clearly elevated and if there are other findings such as splenomegaly, leukocytosis, and thrombocytosis. Otherwise, it is mandatory to determine total red cell and plasma volumes. Following the establishment of an absolute erythrocytosis, secondary polycythemia must be excluded. In most cases the symptoms, physical findings (splenomegaly, ruddy cyanosis, and absence of cardiac or pulmonary disease), and routine examination of the peripheral blood (leukocytosis and thrombocytosis) will confirm the diagnosis of polycythemia vera. However, some patients do not exhibit leukocytosis, thrombocytosis, or splenic enlargement. Differentiation then requires knowledge of the arterial oxygen saturation which is normal in polycythemia vera and reduced in most types of secondary polycythemia. Patients with erythrocytosis secondary to certain renal lesions, cerebellar hemangioblastomas, and so forth, also have normal arterial oxygen saturations but do not manifest leukocytosis, thrombocytosis, or splenomegaly. In these rare cases other findings such as hematuria or papilledema will ordinarily suggest the need for pyelography or other diagnostic procedures. The absence of a leukemic marrow and the increased alkaline phosphatase content of the mature granulocytes help to differentiate polycythemia vera with minimal erythrocytosis from early chronic granulocytic leukemia.

TREATMENT AND COURSE

If the patient does not succumb to a thrombotic episode or hemorrhage, polycythemia vera is characterized by a relatively benign course lasting 10 to 20 years. However, these complications occur with such frequency that few untreated patients survive longer than three to five years. Properly treated, the median survival time is almost normal for the age of the patients involved, that is, 12 to 13 years, and compares favorably with the life expectancy of the treated patient with pernicious anemia. The treatment of choice is *radioactive phosphorus* (^{32}P), supplemented as needed by *phlebotomies*. Since first used by Lawrence in 1939, substantial clinical experience involving thousands of patients has clearly established the efficacy of radioactive phosphorus. This radioisotope with a half-life of 14.3 days participates extensively in a number of biochemical processes. It is widely distributed in bone and nucleoproteins of rapidly growing hemic precursors in which its beta emissions interfere with mitotic proliferation of all marrow cells.

The initial diagnosis of polycythemia vera is an indication for treatment. All patients should be considered for myelosuppressive therapy, unless the diagnosis is in doubt or the hematocrit is less than 60 per cent and thrombocytosis and leukocytosis are not present. Under these circumstances it is best to remove 300 to 500 ml of blood daily until the venous hematocrit is below 55 per cent in males and less than 50 per cent in females. If satisfactory control can be maintained by infrequent phlebotomies (i.e., every two to three months), additional treatment may be deferred. The development of thrombocytosis or leukocytosis or the need for more frequent phlebotomies are indications for myelosuppressive therapy. Most patients require radioactive phosphorus at the time of or shortly after diagnosis. Depending on the height of the erythroid values, the imminence of a thrombotic episode, or the need for surgery, phlebotomies are usually needed for rapid control. Radioactive phosphorus is then given orally in a dose of 4 to 6 mc or intravenously in a dose of 3 to 4.5 mc. Patients should be rechecked at six-week intervals and additional radioactive phosphorus given as needed. Retreatment should never be given unless six weeks or more have elapsed. Because of the life-span of an erythrocyte, maximal reduction in red cell mass may not occur for several weeks; leukocyte and platelet counts usually begin to fall within three weeks. Many patients respond satisfactorily after a single dose of radioactive phosphorus; some require two, but few need more. Remissions lasting months to years may be expected in 85 to 90 per cent of the patients treated in this way. During therapeutic remissions patients should be checked at two- to three-month intervals; recurrent activity of the disease is an indication for retreatment.

This therapeutic regimen has been criticized because (1) the erythrocytic response is slow, (2) excessive bone marrow depression may occur, (3) all patients do not respond, and (4) radioactive phosphorus may increase the incidence of leukemic transformation. None of these potential disadvantages outweighs the beneficial effects of such treatment. An equally slow erythrocytic effect would be expected with any other myelosuppressive agent. Furthermore, the red cell mass can be rapidly and simply reduced by phlebotomies. In the past it was assumed that phlebotomies would act as an additional stimulus to an already hyperactive marrow, but current data indicate that this is not the case. Acute hemorrhage enhances red cell production in a normal subject because of the resultant tissue hypoxia and its effect on humoral erythropoietic factor activity (p. 13). Patients with polycythemia vera have increased oxygen-carrying capacities and are still capable of maintaining normal tissue oxygenation, even though the circulating hemoglobin is reduced. Acute blood loss also evokes thrombocytosis, presumably through a humoral mechanism (p. 70). In view of the role of thrombocytosis in the pathogenesis of thrombosis and hemorrhage, such a stimulus would not be desirable in a patient with polycythemia vera. However, these patients already have increased thrombocytosis-promoting activity in their plasma and urine, and it would seem quite unlikely that phlebotomies would further increase the activity. Therefore there is no valid reason to avoid phlebotomies.

The degree of marrow suppression is directly related to the dose of radioactive phosphorus. Excessive radiation will produce thrombocytopenia, leukopenia, and anemia; however, irreversible marrow hypoplasia is virtually unheard of, unless the patient is overtreated or treated too often. In fact, the toxic manifestations of radioactive phosphorus are unequivocally less than those associated with any of the other myelosuppressive drugs that have been used to treat polycythemia vera. Radioactive phorphorus is not 100 per cent effective, but the number of patients failing to respond is small. In most instances these patients will also fail to respond to other forms of therapy. Therefore occasional therapeutic failures do not constitute a valid reason to discard a method that is effective in most.

Despite numerous attempts, the question of the leukemogenic effect of radioactive phosphorus has not been answered. It is first necessary to define clearly the natural course of the disease; unfortunately, this information is not available. The relationship among polycythemia vera, granulocytic leukemia, primary thrombocythemia, and agnogenic myeloid metaplasia (the myeloproliferative disorders) is well known. It is not unusual for one disorder to follow or to blend subtly with another, thus suggesting a common or similar pathogenic mechanism. Granulocytic leukemia, agnogenic myeloid metaplasia, or, less often, myelomonocytic leukemia may be the terminal event in a patient with polycythemia vera. Rarely, a leukemic picture may evolve into polycythemia. Although known to occur prior to the introduction of radioactive phosphorus, there is little doubt that leukemia (usually acute granulocytic) is seen more often in patients treated with this radioisotope. The precise incidence is difficult to ascertain, but leukemia can be expected to develop in 10 per cent and myeloid metaplasia in another 10 per cent of patients treated with radioactive phosphorus. However, this fact does not necessarily militate against such treatment. Polycythemia vera appears to progress slowly, but its course is characterized by frequent serious and often fatal thromboembolic or hemorrhagic complications. In the untreated patient the incidence of these complications is high and survival is short, that is, five years or less. If the development of leukemia or myeloid metaplasia represents part of the natural course of polycythemia vera, premature death from bleeding or a thrombotic episode would prevent their occurrence. Therefore prolongation of life with appropriate therapy may permit survival of the patient long enough for transformation to a disorder such as leukemia to be manifested. Thus the incidence of leukemia in radioactive phosphorus-treated patients may be "increased" only as it relates to that previously observed and not to the true incidence, had the patients been spared death from thromboembolic or hemorrhagic complications.

Debate continues but there is increasing support for the foregoing thesis. Despite the possibility that radioactive phosphorus may exert a leukemogenic effect (a logical speculation in view of the malignancies induced experimentally by this type of radiation), the striking benefit following its use warrants the risk of enhancing the likelihood that a given patient may develop leukemia or some other myeloproliferative disorder. This form of treatment is effective, simple, and hematologically sound. It presents less risk to the patient than any other type of therapy and remains, together with phlebotomies as needed, clearly the treatment of choice.

Failure to respond to radioactive phosphorus or unavailability of this radioisotope constitutes an indication for other types of therapy. There are three basic approaches to such a patient: (1) production of iron deficiency by serial phlebotomies with or without an iron-deficient diet, (2) destruction of red cells by phenylhydrazine, and (3) use of some other myelosuppressive agent. Although once popular, deliberate attempts to produce iron deficiency cannot be condoned. Iron deficiency may lower the erythroid values, but it introduces symptoms of its own and fails to affect the leukocytosis and thrombocytosis. Phenylhydrazine is an effective form of treatment that is capable of lowering the red cell mass. However, its over-all toxicity and failure to depress granulopoiesis and thrombopoiesis are such that phenylhydrazine can no longer be recommended.

Of the other myelosuppressive agents that have been employed, total body x-radiation is perhaps the safest and most dependable. Treatment with 10 to 12 r daily to a total of 100 to 120 r anteriorly and posteriorly exerts a therapeutic effect comparable to that of radioactive phosphorus. The duration of therapy constitutes an important disadvantage. Several chemotherapeutic agents have been applied successfully, and among them *busulfan* (Myleran) has been most widely used (p. 367). This drug is given orally in initial doses of 6 to 9 mg per day until the desired effect is achieved or undesirable toxicity is produced. The toxicity, chiefly bone marrow depression, has been observed more often with busulfan than with radioactive phosphorus; however, further experience may eliminate such occurrences. Because of the minimal depressant effect on erythropoiesis, phlebotomies are usually needed to maintain satisfactory erythroid values. If radioactive phosphorus is unavailable or if the patient does not respond to ionizing radiation, treatment with busulfan is justified and is effective in most. A commonly mentioned reason for its use, that is, fear of leukemia induction with radioactive phosphorus, does not justify the added risk (patients have developed irreversible marrow aplasia) and added trouble (close followup is mandatory); furthermore, busulfan has also been shown to be leukemogenic in experimental animals.

Leukocyte Responses

Relatively little is known about the fundamental mechanisms that control the production, delivery to and removal from the peripheral blood, and destruction of leukocytes. Furthermore, only a small fraction of the total body leukocytes is present in the peripheral blood at one given time. Even so, quantitative and/or qualitative alterations in the circulating leukocytes characterize many diverse diseases and are often diagnostically significant. Since the first white blood cell count was performed by Welcker in 1853, this procedure has become a routine part of all clinical evaluations. Consequently, every physician must be familiar with normal findings and with the type, magnitude, and significance of leukocyte responses to both physiologic and pathologic stimuli.

In the adult the normal circulating leukocyte count is 4000 to 10,000/cu mm. At birth the white count ranges between 15,000 to 25,000 and falls, by the fourth day, to about 12,000. By the fourth year the average count decreases to around 8000, with the upper limit of normal at 12,000. Normal adult values are ordinarily reached by the age of 12. At birth there is a preponderance of neutrophils, but by the end of the second week lymphocytes make up 60 per cent or more of the circulating leukocytes and predominate throughout infancy and early childhood. By the age of 4 the circulating lymphocyte and granulocyte counts are about equal; granulocytes then become more numerous, and the normal adult distribution (Table 7-1) is reached by the age of 14 or 15. Although clinical discussions often refer to the relative numbers of circulating leukocytes (i.e., the differential count), the absolute numbers are more important. Thus a total count of 300,-000 with 1 per cent neutrophils constitutes a relative but not an absolute neutropenia; under these circumstances the absolute neutrophil

Table 7-1. *Normal Adult Circulating Leukocyte Counts*

CELL TYPE	RANGE OF NORMAL VALUES	
	PER CENT	PER CU MM
Neutrophils	38–70	1520–7000
(band)	(3–5)	(120–500)
(segmented)	(35–65)	(1400–6500)
Lymphocytes	15–45	600–4500
Monocytes	1–8	40–800
Eosinophils	1–5	40–500
Basophils	0–2	0–200

count is within normal limits (3000/cu mm). It should also be borne in mind that a circulating "leukocyte" count is actually a "nucleated" cell count. If there are 10 or more nucleated red cells per 100 leukocytes, the count should be corrected accordingly.

QUALITATIVE RESPONSES

Immature Leukocytes. In a normal peripheral blood film the youngest cells are band neutrophils, although occasional metamyelocytes and even myelocytes can be found in concentrated preparations of leukocytes from normal subjects. The presence of immature cells in the peripheral blood is in itself a rather nonspecific finding. They are most characteristic of leukemia but are also associated with other myeloproliferative disorders such as polycythemia vera and agnogenic myeloid metaplasia. Immaturity commonly accompanies neutrophilic leukocytosis, irrespective of cause or the height of the white count. In general, however, the stage of maturity varies inversely with the severity of the stimulus. A mild infection is reflected by increased numbers of band neutrophils and occasional metamyelocytes, whereas a fulminant septicemia often calls forth progranulocytes or even myeloblasts. Tuberculosis of the bone marrow may evoke a striking monocytic reaction with immature monocytes in the peripheral blood. Immature cells (usually granulocytic) also characterize a myelophthisic process (e.g., metastatic carcinoma) as well as the abnormal cell proliferation brought about by deficiencies of folic acid or vitamin B_{12}. During recovery from drug-induced marrow depression, a few immature granulocytes are common in the peripheral blood.

Basophilic Granulation of the Neutrophils (BGN). Blue-black cytoplasmic granules of variable size are found in the neutrophils of patients with a variety of "toxic" states, such as acute infections, poisoning with drugs or heavy metals, and severe burns (Fig. 7-1). Toxic granules are most evident in segmented and band neutrophils but may be observed in younger cells. They are often associated with increased cytoplasmic vacuolation and probably reflect cellular damage. BGN is rated from +

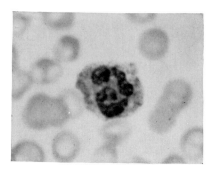

Figure 7-1. Segmented neutrophil showing toxic or basophilic granulation (BGN).

to + + + +, depending on the extent of the granulation and the number of cells involved. Although it is not a specific finding, BGN varies directly with the severity of the basic disease and provides valuable information in regard to the intensity of the underlying process and to the body's reaction to it.

Hypersegmented Neutrophils. Neutrophilic nuclei with five or more lobes are indicative of abnormal mitotic activity. Such cells are most characteristic of vitamin B_{12} or folic acid deficiency (Fig. 5-4, p. 207) but can also reflect treatment with a myelosuppressive drug like an alkylating agent or an antimetabolite. Similar cells may be observed in some patients with granulocytic leukemia or renal failure. The explanation for the occasional finding of hypersegmented neutrophils in uremic patients is not apparent.

Asynchronous Maturation. In response to a gross abnormality in granulopoiesis, cytoplasmic and nuclear maturation may be dissociated (e.g., cytoplasmic maturity of a segmented neutrophil with the nuclear structure of a myelocyte). This finding is generally a manifestation of leukemia or a reflection of impaired proliferation caused by a deficiency of vitamin B_{12} or folic acid.

Degranulation. The granules of all types of granulocytes contain a variety of enzymes and other substances that are vital to the cells' normal physiologic functions. Granules rupture and disappear on release of their contents. Therefore degranulated cells reflect normal cell function. For example, degranulation of basophils in allergic disorders and after alimentary lipemia probably reflects, respectively, the release of histamine and heparin.

Giant Neutrophils. An inherited anomaly characterized by neutrophils that are about twice normal size, with nuclei possessing six to ten lobes, has been observed in a few patients. These cells have not been associated with other clinical manifestations.

Döhle Bodies. Round or oval cytoplasmic inclusion bodies that stain blue-green with a Romanowsky stain were first described in granulocytes of patients with scarlet fever, but they also occur in a variety of other disorders, including leukemia, lymphoma, polycythemia vera, severe burns, tuberculosis, measles, and diphtheria. They appear to be identical with *Amato bodies.* Döhle bodies probably represent RNA and most likely reflect an abnormality in cytoplasmic maturation.

Pelger-Huet Anomaly. The Pelger-Huet anomaly is a benign abnormality which consists of a defect in nuclear segmentation of granulocytes. It is most noticeable in neutrophils, the majority of which have band, rodlike, or, less often, bilobed nuclei. The nuclear chromatin is coarsely clumped. This anomaly may be inherited as a simple dominant or associated with such disorders as myxedema or leukemia. These cells function normally.

Alder's Anomaly. Numerous large, azurophilic granules in all types of leukocytes characterize this rare, hereditary condition.

Chediak-Higashi Anomaly. The Chediak-Higashi anomaly is a rare, fatal disorder which occurs in children and is characterized by atypical cytoplasmic inclusion bodies in all types of leukocytes. With a Romanowsky stain the neutrophils typically contain three to six large, irregular, blue-green masses; the inclusion bodies in the mononuclear cells stain blue-purple and appear to be made up of nuclear chromatin. The few patients who have been studied have had numerous other defects, including albinism, photophobia, and enlargement of the spleen, liver, and lymph nodes.

Hybrid Granulocytes. Cells containing both eosinophilic and basophilic granules are indicative of a marked disturbance in granulopoiesis. They are most often observed in patients with chronic granulocytic leukemia but also occur in other myeloproliferative disorders such as agnogenic myeloid metaplasia.

Phagocytic Monocytes. Atypical, ameboid-appearing monocytes or histiocytes that have phagocytized erythrocytes (Fig. 7-2) are highly

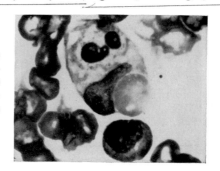

Figure 7-2. A phagocytic monocyte containing an erythrocyte and a neutrophil from a patient with subacute bacterial endocarditis (film was prepared from the first drop of ear-lobe blood).

suggestive of subacute bacterial endocarditis and are often designated SBE cells. Although similar cells are occasionally observed in patients with other infectious diseases, hemolysis, or leukemia, they are sufficiently characteristic to demand the exclusion of bacterial endocarditis. Because of the greater selective filtering effect of the capillary vasculature of the ear lobes, these cells, which do not circulate freely, may be found only in films prepared from the first drop of ear lobe blood.

Virocytes. Atypical lymphocytes are characteristic of infectious mononucleosis (Fig. 7-5, p. 318). Smaller numbers of identical cells can be found in the peripheral blood of patients with a variety of infectious diseases, including virus pneumonia, infectious hepatitis, herpes zoster, rubeola, rubella, roseola infantum, influenza, and the common cold. These cells most likely reflect the lymphocytic response to a virus infection; hence the term virocyte.

Irritation Lymphocytes (Türk cells). Türk cells are hyperchromatic lymphocytes with plasmacytoid features (Fig. 7-3). They lack specificity

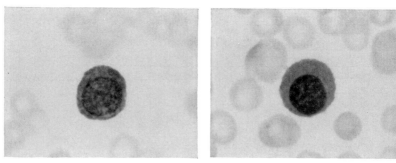

Figure 7-3. Irritation lymphocytes (Türk cells) showing plasmacytoid features.

and may be observed in the peripheral blood of patients with a variety of acute and chronic infections.

Auer Bodies. Rodlike cytoplasmic inclusion bodies in myeloblasts or monoblasts (but not in lymphoblasts) are virtually pathognomonic of acute granulocytic or monocytic leukemia (Fig. 8-7, p. 347).

Abnormal Cells. On occasion, a variety of abnormal cellular elements can be found in the peripheral blood, including carcinoma cells, Reed-Sternberg cells, hemohistiocytes, and megakaryocytes. They are more readily detectable in leukocyte concentrates but have been observed in routine blood films. Fragments of megakaryocyte nuclei are often discernible in buffy coat preparations of normal blood.

L.E. Cells. These cells are not found in the circulating blood and are dependent on (1) an antinuclear antibody (the L.E. factor—a gamma globulin), (2) naked nuclei (DNA is necessary for the reaction to occur), and (3) viable, phagocytic cells. A minimum of 30 minutes incubation in vitro is needed for the formation of the L.E. cell (Fig. 7-4), which is typically a neutrophil (less often an eosinophil) that

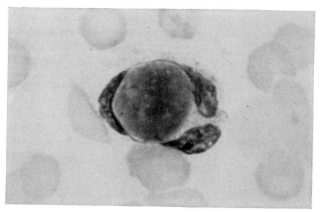

Figure 7-4. L.E. cell (× 1700). (Courtesy of Dr. Gertrude L. Pease.)

contains a homogeneous, structureless inclusion body consisting of nucleoprotein (usually derived from lymphocyte nuclei) altered by the L.E. factor. The L.E. factor probably depolymerizes DNA or combines directly with it, causing the nucleoprotein to become chemotactic; it is then engulfed by a neutrophil or evokes the formation of a "rosette" (an extracellular mass of altered nuclear material surrounded by a group of neutrophils). Only the serum factor is unique to the patient with systemic lupus erythematosus; the phagocytic cells and nuclear material can be derived from other sources (i.e., a normal donor). The L.E. cell must be distinguished from monocytes that have phagocytized nuclear material. Such nucleophagocytosis is a common finding without pathologic significance. In contrast to the L.E. cell, this nuclear material always retains a structural pattern with a condensed peripheral chromatin ring. The L.E. phenomenon is highly specific for systemic lupus erythematosus but not absolutely diagnostic. Similar cells have been observed in other disorders, especially rheumatoid arthritis and hypersensitivity reactions.

QUANTITATIVE CHANGES

A circulating leukocyte count of more than 10,000/cu mm is termed *leukocytosis;* a count below 4000 is designated *leukopenia.* Although an occasional normal subject will have counts outside the normal range, these findings should be considered abnormal until proved otherwise.

Leukocytosis

There are no clinical manifestations attributable solely to leukocytosis. An increase in the number of circulating leukocytes is tolerated without untoward effects and is significant only insofar as it may provide a clue to the nature of some underlying disorder and of the body's response to it. The pathogenesis of most types of leukocytosis is obscure and poorly understood. They probably reflect increased production and/or release of cells from the marrow or sites of capillary sequestration; the latter mechanism is undoubtedly responsible for prompt (and usually short-lived) leukocytosis. Although there is no compelling support for the thesis, prolonged cell survival is another possible explanation. With the exception of leukemia, the leukocyte count seldom exceeds 30,000; however, exceptions have been observed in every category. In most cases the height of the leukocyte count varies directly with the severity of the basic disease.

Neutrophilia. Leukocytosis is most often the result of a relative and absolute increase in circulating neutrophils. The causes of neutrophilia may be divided into the following broad categories.

Hormonal. The secretions of the adrenal gland exert profound effects on the circulating leukocyte count. Epinephrine induces a prompt leukocytosis, and prolonged administration of the corticosteroids evokes a neutrophilia. Enhanced elaboration of these substances as a physiologic response to stress is most likely the explanation for the neutrophilic leukocytosis that occurs normally in pregnant women and the newborn and that which follows strenuous exercise, emotional upsets, parturition, surgical procedures, fractures and other trauma, burns, anesthesia, protracted vomiting, convulsions, and paroxysmal tachycardia. It should be recognized that these hormones may also contribute, at least in part, to neutrophilia classified as due to other causes. The leukocytosis accompanying Cushing's syndrome is undoubtedly a manifestation of hypercorticosteroidism.

Acute Infections. Acute bacterial infection (especially with pyogenic cocci such as staphylococci, streptococci, pneumococci, and meningococci) is the commonest cause of neutrophilia. Infections with other bacteria, certain protozoa, fungi, and even some viruses (e.g., poliomyelitis and rabies) also evoke a neutrophilia. Neutrophilia accompanies both localized and generalized acute infections but not long-standing processes such as chronic bronchitis or chronic urinary tract infections. Slight leukocytosis, minimal neutrophilic immaturity, and little basophilic granulation of the neutrophils (BGN) point to a mild infection and a good host response; a higher leukocyte count with many immature cells suggests a severer process; little or no increase in the leukocyte count, many immature cells, and marked BGN indicate an overwhelming infection and/or impaired host response.

NEOPLASTIC DISEASE. All types of rapidly growing malignancies with or without marrow metastases may be associated with a neutrophilia.

NONINFLAMMATORY CONDITIONS. A myocardial infarction is regularly followed in two to three days by a neutrophilic leukocytosis. Poisoning with certain drugs, chemicals, heavy metals, carbon monoxide, and so forth, also evokes a neutrophilia, as do hypersensitivity reactions (serum sickness) and metabolic intoxications (diabetic acidosis, uremia, hepatic failure, eclampsia, and gout).

ACUTE BLOOD LOSS. A neutrophilic leukocytosis follows acute hemorrhage and some types of acute hemolysis. Although sudden hemolysis is most likely to be associated with a leukocytosis, a persistent neutrophilia may accompany certain types of chronic hemolytic activity (e.g., hereditary spherocytosis or sickle cell anemia).

MYELOPROLIFERATIVE DISORDERS. Chronic granulocytic leukemia, polycythemia vera, and agnogenic myeloid metaplasia are examples of neutrophilia due to enhanced granulopoiesis. The nature of the stimuli to such increased cell proliferation is unknown.

Eosinophilia. An absolute eosinophilia is seldom sufficient to elevate the total leukocyte count. It is a relatively nonspecific finding and occurs in a number of seemingly unrelated disorders, including (1) *parasitic infections* (e.g., certain types of gastrointestinal infestation, trichinosis, and echinococcus disease), (2) *skin disorders* of varied cause, (3) *allergic phenomena* (bronchial asthma, allergic rhinitis, urticaria, angioneurotic edema, and drug reactions), (4) *primary hematologic disorders* (polycythemia vera, chronic granulocytic leukemia, Hodgkin's disease, and, rarely, eosinophilic leukemia), (5) *malignant disease* (especially involving bone, liver, or serosal surfaces), (6) *hypopituitarism* or *Addison's disease* (due to decreased adrenal corticosteroid production), (7) *tropical eosinophilia* and *Loeffler's syndrome*, and (8) *polyarteritis nodosa. Familial eosinophilia* has been observed in a few families.

Basophilia. Increased numbers of circulating basophils are seldom encountered except in chronic granulocytic leukemia, polycythemia vera, and basophilic leukemia.

Monocytosis. A monocytosis does not, as a rule, cause leukocytosis. Increased numbers of these cells accompany (1) *chronic bacterial infections* (e.g., subacute bacterial endocarditis, tuberculosis, and brucellosis), (2) *protozoal and rickettsial infections* (e.g., malaria, kala-azar, and Rocky Mountain spotted fever), (3) *liver disease* (e.g., cirrhosis), (4) *monocytic leukemia,* and (5) *Hodgkin's disease.*

Plasmacytosis. Plasmacytes are not normal constituents of the peripheral blood, but an occasional cell may be found in some patients with liver disease, chronic infections, malignancies, rubella, rubeola, or varicella. In plasmacytic myeloma circulating atypical plasmacytes are common, but they are rarely present in sufficient number to cause leukocytosis.

Lymphocytosis. Because of the relatively small numbers of lymphocytes present normally, an absolute lymphocytosis is not always associated with leukocytosis. Lymphocytosis is normal in infants and young children and is characteristic of certain lymphoproliferative disorders such as chronic lymphocytic leukemia and primary macroglobulinemia. Although rarely marked, a slight increase in circulating lymphocytes is a common finding in patients with hyperthyroidism and myasthenia gravis and during convalescence from an acute infection. Lymphocytosis typically accompanies a variety of infections, including, among others, pertussis, mumps, rubeola, varicella, influenza, brucellosis, infectious hepatitis, infectious mononucleosis, and infectious lymphocytosis. Lymphocytosis is ordinarily the major manifestation of infectious mononucleosis and infectious lymphocytosis, which are, for this reason, generally classified as hematologic disorders. Consequently, it is pertinent and appropriate to consider them in detail.

Infectious Mononucleosis

Infectious mononucleosis is an acute, self-limited illness characterized by fever, lymphadenopathy, atypical lymphocytes, and heterophil antibodies.

HISTORY

Credit for recognizing this entity is customarily given to Pfeiffer, who described Drüsenfieber or glandular fever in 1889; however, Filatoff referred to such a disorder in 1885 in a Russian textbook of pediatrics. Ozawa described the same disease in 1891 and called it Tokushima fever. West published the first article in the United States in 1896. Confusion regarding the nature of this disorder persisted for the next two decades; several reports of "cured leukemia" were undoubtedly examples of what we now call infectious mononucleosis. This term was introduced in 1920 by Sprunt and Evans, who also emphasized the presence of atypical lymphocytes in the peripheral blood. Shortly thereafter Longcope (1922) and Downey and McKinley (1923) published detailed and accurate descriptions of these cells. The demonstration of heterophil antibodies by Paul and Bunnell in 1932 and the introduction of the differential absorption technique by Davidsohn and Walker in 1935 constituted major advances.

ETIOLOGY

Infectious mononucleosis is presumably a viral infection, although the responsible agent has eluded detection. There is no convincing evi-

dence for the contention that epidemic and sporadic infectious mononucleosis differ etiologically or that these disorders are different from
glandular fever. The clinical manifestations and natural course suggest
an infectious etiology; however, epidemiologic studies indicate a very
low grade of contagiousness. Sporadic cases predominate. Under natural
circumstances direct transmission is infrequent; intimate oral contact is
a common but not an exclusive feature. It has not been possible to
transmit the disease to experimental animals or human subjects, and
numerous attempts to culture a virus in vitro have been unsuccessful.
Possible explanations for the failure to isolate the responsible agent
or to infect others include (1) an organism that is easily destroyed, (2)
widely distributed immunity due to subclinical or unrecognized disease,
and (3) the use of unnatural modes of transmission (e.g., blood transfusions). The type of lymphocytic reaction provides indirect support
for a viral etiology. Lymphocytosis is a typical manifestation of virus
infections, and atypical lymphocytes identical to those in infectious
mononucleosis are found in a number of other diseases known to be
caused by viruses. "Viruslike" inclusion bodies in the lymphocytes of
patients with infectious mononucleosis have been observed by electron
microscopy. There is no convincing support for the hypothesis that
infectious mononucleosis may reflect an autoimmune or hypersensitivity
phenomenon.

PATHOPHYSIOLOGY

The hallmark of infectious mononucleosis is widespread lymphoid
hyperplasia characterized by the presence of morphologically distinctive
mononuclear cells. There is general agreement that these cells are
atypical, mature lymphocytes. They exhibit rather marked polymorphism
(Fig. 7-5). Although these cells vary in size, most are equal to or larger
than a normal large lymphocyte; they are often irregularly shaped, and
cell margins are frequently indented by adjacent erythrocytes. The
nuclei are usually oval or kidney-shaped but may be round or lobulated;
they are frequently eccentric, and a perinuclear clear zone is often
evident, especially in the hof of the nucleus. The nuclear chromatin
pattern is typically lymphocytic with scattered dense clumps superimposed on a rather homogeneous background. Occasionally, the nuclear
chromatin is more finely dispersed (suggesting a more immature cell),
and a nucleolus may be present. The abundant, basophilic cytoplasm
is characteristically (but not always) vacuolated or "foamy," and a
few reddish granules are commonly encountered. Some authors recognize three types of cell in accordance with the suggestion of Downey
and McKinley that there are three varieties of disease. However, such
an arbitrary classification is always difficult and often impossible because
of the cells' variable morphology and subtle differences. Clinically, there
is no need for more detailed separation than between normal and atypical

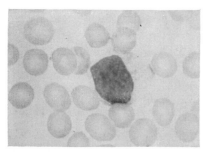
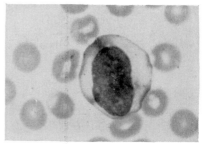

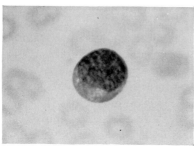

Figure 7-5. Examples of atypical lymphocytes from patients with infectious mononucleosis.

large lymphocytes, and it should be re-emphasized that these abnormal lymphocytes are not unique to infectious mononucleosis.

Because few patients die, opportunities to observe the pathologic features of infectious mononucleosis have been limited. However, study of excised nodes and spleens and of percutaneous liver and bone marrow biopsies has supplemented available necropsy data and a fairly characteristic picture has evolved. Although differing in degree, the distribution of the lymphocytic infiltrates is fairly constant. Lymph nodes, spleen, and liver reveal the most marked abnormalities. Atypical lymphocytes similar to those in the peripheral blood are always evident. *Lymph nodes* manifest follicular hyperplasia, and, although the pattern is often blurred and may simulate lymphoma superficially, normal architecture is not obliterated. The *spleen* typically reveals moderate to marked lymphocytic hyperplasia, with infiltration of the capsule and trabeculae; as a result, normal architectural features are obscured but not eradicated. The *liver* shows lymphocytic infiltrates in the periportal areas and sinusoids; foci of necrotic liver cells are unusual in contrast to the frequency with which they occur in infectious hepatitis. The *bone marrow* is less abnormal. Atypical lymphocytes are evident in aspirated specimens, but they probably reflect dilution with peripheral blood. Focal granulomatous lesions have been observed in serial marrow sections. Other tissues are involved to a lesser degree, but perivascular aggregates of atypical mononuclear cells are demonstrable in the gastrointestinal tract, central nervous system, kidneys, myocardium, and so forth.

The pathophysiologic manifestations of infectious mononucleosis are divisible into the following categories.

Systemic Symptoms. These nonspecific manifestations are characteristic of all types of acute infections and include fever, malaise, and anorexia.

Lymphocytic Hyperplasia. Proliferation of atypical lymphocytes is reflected by lymphocytosis in the peripheral blood, adenopathy, splenomegaly, and hepatomegaly. Infiltration of the capsule appears to be responsible for the increased incidence of splenic rupture. Liver involvement is manifested by evidence of hepatic dysfunction and, occasionally, by clinical jaundice. Acute pharyngitis may reflect a "portal of entry"; however, a local lymphocytic reaction cannot be excluded (atypical lymphocytes are readily identified in pharyngeal exudates). Lymphocytic proliferation in other tissues causes symptoms and findings unique to that organ; for example, neurologic manifestations, hematuria (secondary to lymphocytic infiltrates in the kidneys), gastrointestinal bleeding (ulcerations of mucosal lymphocytic infiltrates), and electrocardiographic abnormalities. In view of the widespread distribution of lymphoid tissue, the effects of lymphocytic hyperplasia are many and varied. Bone marrow dysfunction (anemia, neutropenia, and/or thrombocytopenia) is noticeably absent.

Cellular Dysfunction. Infectious mononucleosis is associated with serologic abnormalities—most notably the presence of heterophil antibodies. Because of the role of lymphocytes in protein synthesis and immunoglobulin elaboration, it is reasonable to attribute the production of heterophil antibodies to the "infectious mononucleosis cell." Heterophil antibodies were first described by Forssman in 1911. These substances react with antigens that are different from and phylogenetically unrelated to those that evoked the antibody response; for example, the blood from a patient with infectious mononucleosis contains sheep erythrocyte agglutinins which are the basis for the agglutination test used in the diagnosis of this disease. The heterophil antibodies in infectious mononucleosis differ from those that occur in some normal subjects and in certain patients with serum sickness and a variety of other disorders, including leukemia, lymphoma, and other malignancies. Infectious mononucleosis heterophil antibodies are completely removed by beef red cells but not by guinea pig kidney antigen. Other antisheep agglutinins are removed by guinea pig kidney; serum sickness antibodies are also completely absorbed by beef cells. These differences permit the differential absorption test described later. Aberrant protein synthesis is also reflected by hyperglobulinemia, abnormal electrophoretic patterns (usually an increase in γ or α_2 globulins), and false positive serologic tests for syphilis. Although it is not a common complication, hypersplenism (hemolysis, neutropenia, and/or thrombocytopenia) occurs in some patients. It seems likely that these occurrences are examples of "autoimmune" hypersplenism (p. 453) brought about by abnormal globulins synthesized by the atypical lymphocytes. Positive Coombs' and bromelin tests and the demonstration of platelet and leukocyte agglutinins in some but not all patients with these hematologic complications attest to the validity of this explanation.

CLINICAL MANIFESTATIONS

Infectious mononucleosis is predominantly a disease of children and young adults. The peak incidence is in the second and third decades of life, and more than three fourths of the patients are between the ages of 15 and 25. It is rare above the age of 35, and only five or so reports of unequivocal infectious mononucleosis occurring in patients over the age of 60 have been published. Because of widely differing diagnostic criteria, the precise incidence is unknown. The high frequency with which it occurs in hospital personnel and on college campuses (about 5 per cent of all admissions to college infirmaries are attributable to infectious mononucleosis) probably reflects, for the most part, more readily available diagnostic facilities. Subclinical and undiagnosed cases may be numerous. Infectious mononucleosis occurs in all races and all parts of the world. The once widely held view that it rarely affected Negroes has been disproved. Although the manifestations of infectious mononucleosis are often described as protean, most patients present a rather characteristic and uniform picture.

Symptoms. As a rule, malaise, headache, generalized muscle aches, anorexia, and fever develop gradually over a period of several days, and few patients can accurately delineate the day of onset. Chilliness is common, but frank chills are unusual. Fever is invariably present at some time during the course of the disease. About 75 per cent of the patients complain of a sore throat, but nasal symptoms and cough are infrequent. Most patients are aware of enlarged and tender lymph nodes. Rarely, the predominant symptoms are those of some complication such as a ruptured spleen (acute abdominal pain), neurologic involvement (evidence of meningeal irritation or ascending paralysis), severe hepatitis (jaundice), or hypersplenic thrombocytopenia (a hemorrhagic diathesis).

Physical Findings. Fever and peripheral lymph node enlargement are found in virtually all patients. The temperature elevation is generally moderate (101 to 102°F). Cervical nodes are most commonly enlarged, especially the posterior chain. The nodes vary considerably in size, but most are 1 to 3 cm in diameter; they are discrete, movable, firm but not hard, and often tender. Overlying skin is not involved, and the nodes do not suppurate. The spleen is palpable 2 to 4 cm below the costal margin in approximately 60 per cent of the patients; occasionally, it is tender. Minimal to moderate hepatomegaly occurs in about one third of the patients. Pharyngeal inflammation is present in approximately 85 per cent. A palatal exanthem occurs in about one fourth and is a finding of some diagnostic value. Typically, 10 or more 0.5- to 1.0-mm petechial lesions appear at the junction of the hard and soft palate about three to ten days after onset of the disease and gradually disappear over the ensuing few days. Edema of the eyelids is rather common. Nondescript skin lesions are present in less than 5 per cent. About one out of 20 patients is clinically icteric. Physical findings attributable to the "complications" of infectious mononucleosis are considered later.

Laboratory Findings. PERIPHERAL BLOOD. The erythroid values and platelet count are almost always normal. The leukocyte count is variable, but normal levels or slight leukocytosis predominate. At the onset about 10 per cent of the patients are leukopenic; these individuals rarely develop leukocytosis. The leukocyte count is between 4000 and 10,000/cu mm in approximately 40 per cent, 10,000 and 15,000 in a similar number, and more than 15,000 in 10 per cent or less. It is quite unusual for the leukocyte count to exceed 40,000/cu mm. In general, the leukocyte count is lowest at the onset and increases slowly during the first two to five days. A relative and absolute lymphocytosis resulting from the presence of atypical cells (Fig. 7-5) characterizes the peripheral blood. There is a relative but not an absolute neutropenia; slight eosinophilia (4 to 8 per cent) is common, especially during convalescence. Atypical lymphocytes make up 20 to 90 per cent of the circulating leukocytes. These cells are always present, and, if serial observations are made, they will at some time during the disease exceed 1500/cu mm. In most patients more than half of the leukocytes in the peripheral blood are atypical lymphocytes. Their number increases slowly for several days; maximum levels, which are reached by the fifth to tenth day, are maintained for several days. Atypical cells ordinarily persist for only two to three weeks, but, in some patients they are still discernible three months or more after the acute illness has subsided.

SEROLOGY. Heterophil antibodies are demonstrable in significant titers in 90 per cent or more of patients with infectious mononucleosis. These antibodies are completely absorbed by beef erythrocytes but not by guinea pig antigen. The titer reaches a peak in the second or third week of illness. Infectious mononucleosis heterophil antibodies usually persist for two to eight weeks, or about twice as long as the atypical lymphocytes; however, they are still detectable in occasional persons several months after the acute illness. About 5 per cent of the patients will exhibit a transiently positive serologic test for syphilis.

BONE MARROW. In the average case myelopoiesis is qualitatively and quantitatively normal. Marrow aspirates often contain increased numbers of atypical lymphocytes as a result of dilution with peripheral blood.

OTHER LABORATORY FINDINGS. An abnormality in one or more liver function tests is a consistent finding. *Alkaline phosphatase* is increased in more than 80 per cent of the patients; in most, *cephalin flocculation, thymol turbidity,* and *bromsulphalein (BSP) excretion* are abnormal and *serum lactic dehydrogenase* and *glutamic oxalic transaminase* are increased. *Serum bilirubin,* however, is usually normal. Other laboratory findings reflect certain complications (e.g., electrocardiographic abnormalities) and are discussed separately.

DIAGNOSIS

The diagnosis of infectious mononucleosis is based on the clinical picture, peripheral blood findings, and heterophil agglutination test. Bone marrow examination is rarely needed and serves only to exclude such disorders as acute leukemia. The symptoms and physical findings often suggest the diagnosis, but they lack specificity. Atypical lymphocytes are present in all patients and heterophil antibodies occur in most. However, small numbers of similar cells can be found in other viral infections, and heterophil antibodies are often demonstrable in normal subjects in titers of 1:56 and reach levels of 1:224 or higher in a variety of diseases, including serum sickness, leukemia, lymphoma, and other malignancies. Therefore neither atypical lymphocytes nor heterophil antibodies are pathognomonic. If the atypical lymphocyte count exceeds 3000/cu mm, or if lymphocytes account for 50 per cent or more of a circulating leukocyte count of more than 8000 and most are atypical, a diagnosis of infectious mononucleosis is justified in the presence of compatible symptoms and physical findings. If there are fewer atypical lymphocytes, a heterophil agglutination test is needed. In the presence of a typical clinical picture, a titer of 1:224 is diagnostic. If the titer is less than 1:224, or if other manifestations are absent or not convincing even though the heterophil titer is more than 1:224, a differential absorption test is indicated (Table 7-2). Persistence of antibodies in a titer of at least 1:56 after absorption with guinea pig kidney and complete removal by beef erythrocytes constitutes a positive test. It should be noted that a dynamic response (a changing titer) during the course of an illness may be highly significant even if the titers just given are never reached.

Table 7-2. Properties of Heterophil Antibodies
(Basis for Differential Absorption Test)

	ANTIGENS	
TYPE OF ANTIBODIES	GUINEA PIG KIDNEY	BEEF ERYTHROCYTES
Normal	Absorbed	Not absorbed
Serum sickness	Absorbed	Absorbed
Miscellaneous diseases	Absorbed	Not absorbed
Infectious mononucleosis	Not absorbed	Absorbed

Controversy has revolved around the significance of a positive or negative heterophil agglutination test. A positive test is not unequivocal proof that an acute illness is due to infectious mononucleosis. Other explanations include antibodies persisting after a remote episode of infectious mononucleosis or an anamnestic reaction brought about by some other infection. Technical factors must also be considered; for example, cold agglutinins may be responsible for a false positive test unless the specimens are warmed before they are read. Conversely, a negative test does not exclude the diagnosis, for maximum titers are reached at different times and persist for variable periods. It seems likely that heterophil antibodies may escape detection in some patients even if serial tests are obtained. Furthermore, a few individuals appear to be truly seronegative, perhaps as a manifestation of varying responses with seropositivity reflecting a severer process. Other vagaries of this serologic test, such as the loss of agglutinability of sheep red cells with storage and differing reactions of cells from different sheep, weaken its reliability as the sole diagnostic parameter. Thus a diagnosis of infectious mononucleosis is justified in the presence of typical symptoms and physical findings, together with a significant number of atypical lymphocytes even if the heterophil agglutination test is negative. On the other hand, a positive agglutination test (as already defined) confirms the diagnosis, even in the presence of small numbers of atypical lymphocytes. However, the failure of a trained observer to detect any atypical lymphocytes excludes, for practical purposes, the diagnosis of infectious mononucleosis, even though the heterophil test is positive.

Strict adherence to these diagnostic criteria will eliminate most sources of confusion. The importance of serial studies deserves emphasis because diagnostically significant hematologic and serologic abnormalities may occur at different times during the illness. Because these findings persist for relatively long periods of time, it is unlikely that they will be missed if repeated observations are made.

Infectious mononucleosis is most likely to mimic the following disorders:

Acute Lymphocytic Leukemia. The age of the patient, mode of onset, symptoms, and physical findings (enlargement of spleen, liver, and nodes) all suggest acute leukemia. Leukocytosis and/or atypical mononuclear cells in the peripheral blood are other common findings. Heterophil antibodies also occur in a number of patients with acute leukemia. At this point, however, the similarity ends. The heterophil antibodies in patients with acute leukemia are removed by guinea pig kidney, and the atypical lymphocytes in infectious mononucleosis differ clearly from the lymphoblasts in acute lymphocytic leukemia. In addition, anemia and thrombocytopenia are most unusual manifestations of infectious mononucleosis, whereas they are invariably present in acute leukemia. Should doubt exist, a marrow examination is mandatory. In infectious mononucleosis the marrow *never* displays the abnormalities in proliferation and maturation that are the *sine qua non* of leukemia (p. 337).

Infectious Hepatitis. Liver involvement is characteristic of infectious mononucleosis, and atypical lymphocytes are usually evident in patients with infectious hepatitis. Therefore differentiation between these two disorders is often difficult. However, large numbers of atypical lymphocytes are restricted to infectious mononucleosis; the heterophil agglutination test is negative in infectious hepatitis, and hepatic dysfunction is less marked in infectious mononucleosis. Other findings such as adenopathy and pharyngitis also serve to distinguish infectious mononucleosis from infectious hepatitis.

Acute Infectious Lymphocytosis. This disorder is manifested by lymphocytosis due to small mature lymphocytes. Heterophil agglutination tests are negative and the spleen, liver, and lymph nodes are not enlarged (p. 327).

Postoperative Lymphocytic Splenomegaly. A syndrome characterized by fever, splenomegaly, and lymphocytosis with atypical cells similar to those in infectious mononucleosis has been observed in a number of patients who have had pulmonary, cardiac, or vascular surgery. Heterophil agglutination tests have been negative. This acute, self-limited illness appears to be some type of infectious process, probably viral. The history of a surgical procedure 15 to 40 days before onset serves to differentiate this syndrome from infectious mononucleosis.

Miscellaneous Disorders. Viral upper respiratory infections, viral pneumonitis, lymphoma, rubella, rubeola, roseola infantum, and aseptic meningitis are some of the other disorders that may be associated with one or more of the clinical manifestations of infectious mononucleosis. A detailed history, careful physical examination, serial evaluation of the peripheral blood, and two or more heterophil agglutination tests should clarify the diagnosis.

UNUSUAL MANIFESTATIONS

Certain rare manifestations of infectious mononucleosis deserve emphasis because of their potential seriousness and the problems they present in diagnosis and management.

Neurologic. The neurologic manifestations of infectious mononucleosis include meningitis, encephalitis, myelitis, peripheral neuropathies, and acute polyradiculoneuritis (the Guillain-Barré syndrome). Nervous involvement occurs in less than 1 per cent of the patients but has been responsible for some deaths. Infectious mononucleosis should be considered as a possible cause of acute neurologic syndromes in children and young adults. Atypical lymphocytes and heterophil antibodies have been found in the cerebrospinal fluid of some but not all patients so afflicted.

Hematologic. Anemia and/or thrombocytopenia are not typical of infectious mononucleosis; in fact, their presence detracts from the likelihood of this diagnosis. However, these hematologic abnormalities are rare manifestations of infectious mononucleosis and presumably reflect an "autoimmune" type of hypersplenism. About 30 patients with hemolysis and fewer than 40 with thrombocytopenia have been reported. In most of these patients, the hemolytic anemia is spherocytic and is associated with polychromasia, reticulocytosis, nucleated red cells in the peripheral blood, and myeloid erythrocytic hyperplasia. Thrombocytopenia is accompanied by normal or increased numbers of marrow megakaryocytes, many of which show no evidence of active platelet budding. It seems likely that certain instances of neutropenia may be similarly explained. These unusual hematologic manifestations enhance the similarity between infectious mononucleosis and acute leukemia.

Hepatic. Hepatitis is characteristic of infectious mononucleosis. It is generally mild, and only about 5 per cent of the patients are jaundiced. Severe involvement with intense icterus is very uncommon but has been observed. The hepatitis of infectious mononucleosis usually subsides in two to four weeks without residual hepatic dysfunction, but it has been known to progress into cirrhosis.

Cardiac. Transient electrocardiographic abnormalities (typically minor T-wave changes) occur in about 25 per cent of patients with infectious mononucleosis, although other evidence of cardiac dysfunction is quite unusual. Rare patients exhibit findings of pericarditis, and one or two deaths have been attributed to the cardiac manifestations of infectious mononucleosis. However, there appears to be no danger of chronic heart disease developing as an aftermath of cardiac involvement.

Respiratory System. Uncommon manifestations involving the upper respiratory tract include nasopharyngeal hemorrhage and laryngeal edema. Hilar lymph node enlargement has occurred but is most unusual. Pneumonitis is demonstrable in 2 to 3 per cent of the patients with an x-ray picture similar to that of primary atypical or viral pneumonia.

Ruptured Spleen. About 50 patients have been reported with this dramatic and serious complication of infectious mononucleosis. Splenic rupture may occur spontaneously or follow straining (defecation, coughing, or vomiting) or minimal trauma (abdominal palpation or an accidental left upper quadrant blow). It is manifested by sudden abdominal pain followed by shock and other findings of acute hemorrhage and is an indication for immediate splenectomy.

Genitourinary. On the basis of limited necropsy data, kidney involvement is common. However, renal dysfunction is not seen, and chronic renal disease does not follow infectious mononucleosis. Fewer than 5 per cent of the patients have gross hematuria.

T R E A T M E N T   A N D   C O U R S E

With rare exceptions, infectious mononucleosis runs a benign, self-limited course. Symptoms characteristically subside within one to three weeks, and abnormal findings disappear within two to four weeks. Shorter courses are not uncommon. Atypical lymphocytes and heterophil antibodies have been known to persist for two to three months after the acute episode has subsided. Although splenomegaly and/or adenopathy are often attributed to infectious mononucleosis that occurred several months or even years before, such an explanation seems untenable, for splenic and node enlargement disappear promptly. Another cause must be sought for the finding of atypical lymphocytes, splenomegaly, or peripheral node enlargement if three months or more have elapsed since an episode of infectious mononucleosis.

Therapy. *Bed rest* and *salicylates,* as needed for relief of fever and pain, usually suffice. Activity should be restricted until fever and symptoms resolve. In the jaundiced patient ambulation should be deferred pending subsidence of the acute hepatitis. Although hepatic involvement is less severe in infectious mononucleosis than in infectious hepatitis, cirrhosis has followed infectious mononucleosis. Therefore the patient with severe "infectious mononucleosis" hepatitis should be treated with bed rest and a high-protein, high-caloric intake until liver function tests improve. The unusual patient with clear-cut myocarditis (not just minor, transient T-wave changes) should remain inactive until evidence of cardiac involvement disappears.

Evaluation of the effectiveness of specific treatment is almost impossible because most patients get better whether they are treated or not. Many agents have been tried without apparent success. *Antibiotics* should be used only for secondary bacterial infections. *Corticosteroids* are indicated in patients with superimposed hypersplenism (hemolysis or thrombocytopenia) and should be tried in acutely ill patients such as those with the Guillain-Barré syndrome or laryngeal edema. Splenic rupture is an indication for emergency splenectomy.

Prognosis. With few exceptions, patients recover promptly and completely. Chronic or relapsing infectious mononucleosis appears to be a myth. Although recurrent episodes have been described, well-documented second attacks are extremely uncommon. Chronic hepatitis appears to be the only long-term aftereffect, and it is very unusual. Infectious mononucleosis has caused a few deaths (about 40 have been reported). Most of the recorded deaths have been the result of ruptured spleens; neurologic involvement (especially the Guillain-Barré syndrome) is the next most frequently encountered fatal manifestation. Other causes of death have included hemorrhage and secondary infection.

Infectious Lymphocytosis

Acute infectious lymphocytosis was first described by Smith in 1941. It is presumably a viral infection, but the responsible agent has not been isolated. Although basically a childhood disease, rare cases have been observed in young adults. There is no apparent racial predilection or seasonal variation. Some patients are essentially asymptomatic, whereas others complain of low-grade fever, persistent rhinitis, or abdominal discomfort. Occasionally central nervous system complaints are prominent. Physical examination is generally noncontributory; nodes, spleen, and liver are characteristically *not* enlarged. The most striking manifestation is leukocytosis caused by a relative and absolute lymphocytosis. Counts may reach 50,000 to 100,000/cu mm, with 90 per cent or more of the cells being small mature lymphocytes. Immature lymphocytes or atypical forms similar to those in infectious mononucleosis are not seen. There is no anemia or thrombocytopenia. Bone marrow aspirates contain increased numbers of small mature lymphocytes, most probably secondary to dilution with peripheral blood. The heterophil agglutination test is negative, and hepatic dysfunction does not occur.

Treatment is purely symptomatic; the prognosis is uniformly favorable. The lymphocytosis subsides over a period of three to five weeks. The absence of atypical lymphocytes, adenopathy, splenomegaly, and heterophil antibodies readily separates infectious lymphocytosis from infectious mononucleosis. Lymphocytosis due to normal-appearing mature cells might suggest chronic lymphocytic leukemia, but the age of the patient and the lack of other clinical manifestations preclude confusion. Other infections associated with lymphocytosis (e.g., pertussis) are easily recognized by their own unique clinical manifestations.

Leukopenia

Lymphopenia, eosinopenia, and a decreased basophil count accompany hyperadrenocorticosteroidism (exogenous or endogenous). A decrease in the circulating small lymphocyte count is characteristic of Hodgkin's disease and is the first reflection of hemopoietic depression after treatment with ionizing radiation or an alkylating agent. However, a decrease in these cells rarely causes a circulating leukocyte count less than 4000/cu mm. Because of the numerical predominance of neutrophils, a leukopenia is almost always due to a neutropenia.

Neutropenia. In contrast to neutrophilia, which does not in itself produce symptoms or altered function, neutropenia is accompanied by evidence of impaired neutrophilic activity (i.e., enhanced susceptibility to infections).

ETIOLOGY

All neutropenias are basically the result of decreased production and/ or increased destruction or removal of cells from the circulation. With certain exceptions and additions, they can be classified etiologically (Table 7-3) in a manner analogous to the anemias (Table 3-2, p. 56).

Table 7-3. Etiologic Classification of Neutropenia

I. *Increased Cell Destruction or Removal from the Circulation*
   A. Hypersplenism
      1. Immunoneutropenias
         a. drug-induced
         b. secondary—lymphoma, SLE, etc.
         c. neonatal
         d. transfusion-induced
         e. idiopathic (primary splenic neutropenia)
      2. Banti's syndrome
      3. Felty's syndrome
   B. Capillary sequestration—anaphylactoid shock

II. *Impaired Granulopoiesis*
   A. Deficiencies—vitamin B_{12}, folic acid, etc.
   B. Diversion of normal growth potential—acute granulocytic leukemia
   C. Destruction or depression—marrow granulocytic hypoplasia
   D. Displacement—lymphocytic leukemia, metastatic carcinoma, etc.

III. *Unknown Cause*
   A. Neutropenia of infection
   B. Cyclic neutropenia
   C. Myelokathexis

Increased Removal of Circulating Neutrophils. HYPERSPLENISM. It has become increasingly apparent that hypersplenism, as broadly defined (p. 448), plays an important role in the production of neutropenia. Hypersplenic neutropenia is usually associated with other hematologic abnormalities (i.e., a hemolytic anemia and/or thrombocytopenia). Most hypersplenic neutropenias appear to be *immunoneutropenias* and reflect the presence of an abnormal globulin which enhances cell destruction. They are divisible into the following categories:

1. *Drug-Induced.* Certain drugs (e.g., aminopyrine and sulfapyridine) appear to act as haptenes. These drugs, together with a plasma factor, stimulate the production of an incomplete leukocyte antibody which attaches to the surface of the cell. When the drug is readministered, cell destruction and neutropenia ensue.

2. *Secondary.* A variety of disorders associated with abnormal globu-

lins may be accompanied by neutropenia; for example, lymphoma, chronic lymphocytic leukemia, systemic lupus erythematosus, and Felty's syndrome (rheumatoid arthritis, splenomegaly, and neutropenia).

3. *Neonatal.* Although seldom encountered, neonatal neutropenia can be likened to erythroblastosis fetalis (p. 123). Because of leukocyte incompatibility, the mother elaborates leukocyte antibodies that are responsible for neutropenia in the newborn.

4. *Transfusion-Induced.* Leukocyte antibodies, formed as the result of earlier transfusions or pregnancies, are responsible for febrile transfusion reactions and, on occasion, for neutropenia.

5. *Idiopathic.* Leukocyte antibodies due to unknown cause appear to be responsible for this "autoimmune" disorder, which has also been termed primary splenic neutropenia.

In some cases neutropenia appears to be caused primarily (if not entirely) by splenomegaly. Banti's syndrome or chronic congestive splenomegaly resulting from portal hypertension of varied cause is an example (p. 457). In support of this pathogenic mechanism are the observations in patients with Banti's syndrome that all cells are equally affected (the differential pattern remains unchanged) and that the leukopenia fails to respond to corticosteroids. The pathogenesis of the profound neutropenia which characterizes Felty's syndrome is obscure (p. 459).

CAPILLARY SEQUESTRATION. Because of the removal from the circulation of large numbers of leukocytes and their sequestration in the capillaries of such tissues as the lungs, liver, spleen, and striated muscle, neutropenia occurs promptly in foreign protein reactions or anaphylactoid shock.

Impaired Granulopoiesis. DEFICIENCIES. Inadequate supplies of vitamin B_{12} or folic acid impair granulopoiesis by interfering with mitotic proliferation; neutropenia ensues. The neutropenia of hypopituitarism and Addison's disease is apparently the result of hypoadrenocorticosteroidism. Although poorly understood, nutritional deficiencies may play a role in the neutropenia associated with inanition (decreased protein intake will evoke a leukopenia in experimental animals). The slight neutropenia that accompanies iron deficiency may reflect a similar mechanism or conceivably be due to a deficiency of an iron-containing enzyme.

DIVERSION OF NORMAL GROWTH POTENTIAL. Impaired maturation and abnormal cell proliferation, characteristics of acute leukemia (granulocytic, myelomonocytic, and monocytic), will produce a deficiency of mature neutrophils and a circulating neutropenia.

DESTRUCTION. Decreased numbers of granulocytic precursors may be secondary to physical agents (ionizing radiation), chemicals (benzol), or a variety of drugs. Certain drugs regularly produce neutropenia in every patient if given in sufficient amounts (e.g., nitrogen mustard or an antimetabolite such as 6-mercaptopurine); other drugs appear to involve individual sensitivity or idiosyncrasies. Examples are many and include the phenothiazines, antithyroid agents, and chloramphenicol. It is indeed a rare drug that has never been implicated in the production of neutropenia. In most cases anemia and thrombocytopenia accompany neutropenia due to marrow hypoplasia, that is, a hypoplastic anemia (p. 222). However, certain drugs affect only granulocytic precursors (e.g., chlorpromazine which has been shown to interfere with mitotic division). A few patients have been described with decreased numbers of marrow granulocytic elements and normal erythropoiesis and thrombopoiesis (p. 240). This type of chronic idiopathic hypoplastic neutropenia is analogous to acquired erythrocytic hypoplasia (p. 239).

DISPLACEMENT. Granulocytic precursors may be displaced by lymphocytes (acute or chronic lymphocytic leukemia), carcinoma cells, Gaucher's cells, and so forth. If the marrow involvement is sufficiently marked, a circulating neutropenia will ensue.

Unknown Cause. INFECTIONS. Certain types of infection, especially viral but also bacterial (typhoid, paratyphoid, and brucellosis), protozoal (malaria and kala-azar), and rickettsial (scrub typhus and Colorado tick fever), are characterized by leukopenia rather than leukocytosis. In some cases the low count reflects primarily a decrease in lymphocytes with a normal or only slightly reduced absolute neutrophil count. In others, most notably typhoid fever, a profound neutropenia occurs. The pathogenesis of the neutropenia of infection is not known. In an overwhelming septicemia a neutropenia is a poor prognostic sign.

CYCLIC NEUTROPENIA. Cyclic neutropenia is an unusual entity of unknown cause and without evident sex or age predilections. It is characterized by recurrent or cyclic episodes of neutropenia occurring at intervals of 10 to 30 days. The neutropenia lasts for several days and is often accompanied by infection, especially oropharyngeal. Patients are asymptomatic in between the neutropenic episodes.

MYELOKATHEXIS. Myelokathexis is a term that has been used to describe a peripheral neutropenia in the face of increased numbers of mature cells in the bone marrow. A defect in the release of cells from the marrow has been postulated as a possible cause of this very rare disorder.

Agranulocytosis

The failure to include agranulocytosis as a cause of neutropenia deserves comment because of the widespread use of this term and the space devoted in most texts to this entity. The term, agranulocytosis, refers to a group of neutropenias of different causes and is a misnomer that literally means either increased numbers of cells without granules or the absence of increased numbers of granulocytes. Agranulocytosis was first described by Schultz in 1922; it increased dramatically in incidence until the mid-1930's, when it became evident that certain drugs (especially aminopyrine) were at fault. In retrospect, it is apparent that patients with all types of neutropenia were classified together under the heading of agranulocytosis. Because the clinical manifestations of neutropenia (i.e., increased susceptibility to infection) are similar regardless of basic cause, it is evident why all neutropenias were thought to be identical or closely related illnesses. Their widely differing causes, however, were responsible for marked confusion; for example, the bone marrow in agranulocytosis was variously described as hypocellular or hyperplastic with or without abnormalities in granulocytic maturation. There is no good reason to retain this category of disease or to perpetuate the confusion the use of this term has caused. Agranulocytosis should be discarded and replaced by a descriptive diagnosis such as drug-induced immunoneutropenia due to aminopyrine, neutropenia secondary to marrow hypoplasia due to chlorpromazine, and so forth.

PATHOPHYSIOLOGY

Neutrophils are the body's first line of defense against infection, for they are capable of ingesting and destroying bacteria, yeast, and fungi. When the absolute neutrophil count falls below 200/cu mm, mucous membranes are regularly invaded by microorganisms. Therefore infections of all kinds are the predominant pathophysiologic manifestations of neutropenia. Because neutrophils are needed to form pus and to wall off an infection (i.e., to form an abscess), the normal inflammatory response is altered in a neutropenic patient, and the infection progresses and spreads with remarkable speed.

CLINICAL MANIFESTATIONS

The clinical pictures associated with the neutropenias consequent to impaired granulopoiesis (Table 7-3) are dependent on or greatly affected by the nature of the basic disease and are discussed in detail elsewhere. In the hypersplenic neutropenias (also cyclic neutropenia) an acute onset with fever, chills, and prostration heralds an infectious process. Stomatitis and pharyngitis are commonest infections. Necrotic ulcerations of the oropharyngeal mucosa are characteristic, and similar lesions typically involve the rectal and vaginal mucosa as well. Physical examination is otherwise noncontributory; the spleen may or may not be slightly enlarged in the immunoneutropenias. Leukopenia due to a relative and absolute neutropenia and with a relative lymphocytosis characterizes the peripheral blood; an exception is found among patients with Banti's syndrome in whom the differential count is usually normal. The erythroid values and platelet count are normal, unless they participate in the hypersplenic process or reflect the underlying disease (e.g., the anemia of lymphoma). In patients with hypersplenic neutropenia, the bone marrow reveals normal or increased numbers of granulocytic precursors; a "maturation arrest" is often evident but does not necessarily imply a defect in cell maturation (p. 456). Leukocyte agglutinins are demonstrable in some patients with hypersplenic neutropenia, although the precise significance of this finding is not yet known. The mere presence of leukocyte antibodies does not indicate disease because such persons need not be neutropenic (leukocyte antibodies are often found in otherwise normal persons who have received multiple transfusions). Furthermore, technical factors detract from the diagnostic reliability of this procedure. Nonetheless, it may provide information of great diagnostic import in certain patients. In patients with neutropenia caused by impaired production (e.g., drug-induced marrow hypoplasia) the bone marrow will reveal decreased numbers of granulocytic precursors.

TREATMENT AND PROGNOSIS

Therapy of the neutropenic patient consists of treatment directed against the infection as well as the basic disease. Regardless of the cause of the neutropenia, infection should be treated promptly with greater than normal amounts of antibiotics and with preference given to a bactericidal agent. As soon as specimens are obtained for culture, antibiotics should be instituted; delay of even a few hours may mean the difference between death and recovery. Drugs can be changed if necessary after cultures and sensitivities are known. Before the availability of effective antibiotics, few patients survived an episode of profound neutropenia. Although it is still a dangerous situation, antibiotics have greatly improved the chances of survival. Treatment otherwise depends on the etiology (Table 7-3). If caused by a drug, the drug should, of course, be stopped at once. Corticosteroids are indicated, especially in patients with clear-cut immunoneutropenias, in doses equivalent to 60 mg of prednisone a day (15 mg every six hours). Depending on the response (and on the cause of the neutropenia), splenectomy may be indicated in selected patients with secondary or idiopathic hypersplenic immunoneutropenia (Table 7-3). Although the results are unpredictable and variable, there is generally little else to offer such patients. The leukopenia of Banti's syndrome will usually respond favorably to splenectomy (p. 458), as will the neutropenia in some patients with Felty's syndrome (p. 459).

Leukemoid Reactions

In 1926 Krumbhaar introduced the term *leukemoid reaction* to describe bizarre leukocyte responses that suggested leukemia but were actually due to other causes. Several definitions have been proposed (e.g., a circulating leukocyte count over 50,000/cu mm). It would seem more appropriate to consider any deviation in total count, that is, leukopenia or leukocytosis, or the presence of immature cells in the peripheral blood as a "leukemoid reaction," for any of these findings simulate leukemia. Leukemoid reactions are most often granulocytic and may be due to any of the causes of neutrophilia or eosinophilia already discussed. Lymphocytic leukemoid reactions characterize such infections as pertussis, acute infectious lymphocytosis, and infectious mononucleosis. Tuberculosis of the marrow evokes a monocytic reaction. In most cases other clinical manifestations indicate the correct diagnosis; for example, no splenic enlargement and increased granulocyte alkaline phosphatase activity serve to distinguish a neutrophilic leukemoid reaction from chronic granulocytic leukemia. However, the final answer lies in the marrow. The pathognomonic findings of leukemia are not present in leukemoid reactions, and, even though the marrow may be hyperplastic, maturation abnormalities characteristic of leukemia (p. 337) are not found. Miliary tuberculosis with involvement of the marrow is an exception and often can be separated from acute monocytic leukemia only with great difficulty. Such an acid-fast infection can induce a striking reticuloendothelial response; even Auer bodies have been described in a few of these patients, although it is possible that they may have had both acute monocytic leukemia and miliary tuberculosis. The concept of a leukemoid reaction warrants discussion only because it emphasizes the many causes other than leukemia of atypical leukocyte responses in the peripheral blood. It is a descriptive term only and is not a diagnosis or disease entity.

Leukemia

Leukemia is a malignant neoplasm characterized by disorderly, purposeless proliferation of hemic cells and by the overabundance of one type, usually an immature leukocyte. It is a disease of blood-forming tissue, and the bone marrow is *always* involved. Abnormalities in the peripheral blood reflect marrow dysfunction, but the circulating leukocyte count is not always elevated. Based on distinctive histologic and clinical pictures, several types of leukemia can be recognized; each runs a progressive course and is invariably fatal.

HISTORY

In 1839 Donné, a pioneer French microscopist, first observed at necropsy increased numbers of "mucous globules" in the blood of a 44-year-old woman (a patient of Barth), who apparently died from chronic granulocytic leukemia. In 1845 Bennett and Craigie in Scotland and Virchow in Germany established leukemia as a clinical entity. The case reports of Bennett, who had studied under Donné, and of Craigie were published as companion articles and antedated Virchow's by a month. However, it was Virchow who first appreciated the true nature of the disease (i.e., a primary overproduction of white blood cells). Virchow also coined the term *leukemia* and recognized the existence of two types of disease, "splenic" and "lymphatic." In 1870 Neumann pointed out the role of the marrow; "myelogenous" leukemia was subsequently shown to be the same as Virchow's "splenic" leukemia. Friedrick described the pathologic findings in a patient with acute leukemia in 1857, but this form attracted little attention before Ebstein's description of the clinical manifestations in 1889. Childhood leukemia was recognized by Biemer in 1861. Following Ehrlich's introduction of staining techniques, more precise morphologic classification was possible. Naegeli identified the myeloblast in 1900. Türk (1903) and Sternberg (1904 and 1905) were the first to call attention to lymphosarcoma cell leukemia. In 1913 Reschad and Schilling-Torgau described monocytic leukemia, and malignant proliferation of erythrocytic precursors was emphasized by Di Guglielmo in a series of articles beginning in 1923.

ETIOLOGY

Despite intensive study, the etiology of leukemia remains obscure. Numerous theories have been advanced, but none has been proved. Most promising is the thesis that leukemia is of *viral* etiology. This concept derives considerable support from animal experimentation. Spontaneous leukemia occurs in many species, with lymphocytic leukemia predominating. It has been shown conclusively that certain types of avian leukemia are caused by viruses, and there is abundant evidence implicating a similar agent in the causation of leukemia in rodents, especially mice. Viruslike particles obtained from leukemic mice will cause leukemia in strains of mice not ordinarily susceptible to the disease. These leukemogenic agents also evoke antibody production. Animal leukemia may not be strictly analogous to human leukemia, but viruslike particles have been observed by electron microscopy in patients with leukemia. In addition, cell-free extracts of human leukemic brains have been shown to enhance the development of leukemia in mice and to induce antibody formation in experimental animals and human volunteers. The increased incidence of leukemia and lymphoma in patients with agammaglobulinemia also lends some support to this theory (these patients may be less able to resist such an infection). However, numerous attempts, including cross-circulation experiments, have failed to transmit leukemia from one human to another.

Genetic factors have also been implicated in the pathogenesis of leukemia. By careful inbreeding strains of mice have been developed in which the majority manifest spontaneous leukemia; other strains are remarkably resistant to the disease. Mice with spontaneous or induced leukemia transmit the disease vertically, that is, to their offspring, rather than to their littermates (horizontal transmission). On the basis of published reports, the probability of more than one case of human leukemia occurring in the same family appears to be very small. The occurrence of leukemia in monozygotic twins greatly exceeds pure chance. On the other hand, the incidence is far less than that which would be expected if concordancy were complete. In addition, none of the mothers of the reported cases of congenital leukemia (about 50) had leukemia, and, with the exception of a single report of leukemia developing at the age of nine months, there is no published record of the disease having occurred in the offspring of leukemic mothers. Thus heredity would appear to play a relatively minor role in human leukemia, perhaps as a result of man's genetic heterogeneity. Even so, genetic factors cannot be excluded. Chromosome abnormalities have been demonstrated recently in leukemic leukocytes. Most consistent has been the presence in chronic granulocytic leukemia of the Philadelphia or Ph^1 chromosome (a small structure due to deletion or translocation of part of an arm of one of the acrocentric autosomes, probably belonging to chromosome pair No. 21 of the Denver classification). It is of considerable interest that trisomy of this chromosome is found in mongolism and that the incidence of leukemia in mongols is many times that which would be expected if there were no relationship between these disorders. A variety of abnormalities has been observed in patients with other kinds of leukemia (most notably aneuploidy); however, consistent patterns have not been evident, and their significance is not apparent. Still unanswered are such basic questions as (1) are chromosome abnormalities congenital or acquired; (2) are they prerequisites, the cause, or the result of leukemic proliferation?

Other etiologic factors include *ionizing radiation,* which is clearly leukemogenic in experimental animals and appears to play a role in the pathogenesis of some cases of human leukemia. Strongest support for such a causal relationship is the unequivocal increase in the incidence of leukemia in survivors of the atomic bomb explosions in Nagasaki and Hiroshima, Japan. There is also a definite but less marked increase in the frequency of leukemia in patients with rheumatoid spondylitis treated with x-radiation and in recipients of therapeutic doses of radioactive iodine. In addition, the incidence of leukemia in physicians (especially roentgenologists) is greater than in the general population. Less well established is the suggestion that thymic irradiation in infants and x-radiation received *in utero* may be leukemogenic. Even diagnostic roentgenography has been mentioned as contributing to the steeply rising incidence of leukemia over the last few decades. Whereas the leukemogenic effect of a single large dose of radiation has been proved in humans and experimental animals, the cumulative effect of repeated small doses and the question of a threshold dose remain to be elucidated. Since few cases of human leukemia can be causally related to ionizing radiation, its role in the pathogenesis of leukemia remains indeterminate. Even so, there is sufficient reason to implicate ionizing radiation in the induction of leukemia to warrant restriction of indiscriminate exposure.

Numerous *chemical agents* (both industrial and medicinal) have been suspected of being leukemogenic. Proof of such relationships is lacking, but, in view of the profound effect of many chemicals on the blood-forming organs, this possibility certainly cannot be excluded. Another unproved but attractive thesis is that leukemia may be the result of some *abnormality in the homeostatic controlling mechanisms* that govern cell proliferation and maturation. *Hormonal factors* also appear to exert modifying influences, especially in animal leukemia; for example, thymectomy prevents the induction of leukemia in mice as does the administration of corticosteroids or androgens.

It is apparent that the pathogenesis of leukemia must involve a complex interaction of multiple factors. Host response and resistance (perhaps conditioned by genetic endowment and hormonal environment), somatic mutations (perhaps secondary to some agent such as ionizing radiation), and a virus may all be requisites for the induction of leukemia. Future studies along these lines should be most informative. At this time, however, leukemia must be viewed as a malignant neoplasm of unknown cause. It should be noted that this conclusion is compatible with the theory that leukemia is of viral etiology; indeed, it seems quite probable that many types of neoplastic disease may reflect cellular responses to such infectious agents.

PATHOPHYSIOLOGY

The clinical manifestations of leukemia are directly attributable to uncontrolled cellular proliferation. Although the presence of increased numbers of leukemic cells was once assumed to reflect accelerated rates of growth, recent studies indicate that the time required for replication of leukemic blast cells is actually longer than normal. The major defect appears to be impaired maturation. Leukemic cells literally "live to divide," whereas normal leukocytes are expendable. Immature hemic precursors proliferate by homeoplastic mitosis; however, this attribute is eventually lost as the cell matures, and the end product is a cell with a finite life-span. Since leukemic blast cells fail to mature normally, they retain the capacity to divide for longer periods of time than normal blast cells. The result is an overabundance of leukemic cells in the marrow and other tissues; organ dysfunction ensues. Once started, the process is autonomous. The relentless progression suggests either the continued presence of the stimulus to leukemic proliferation or, alternatively, a mutant clone of abnormal cells that retain their proclivity to divide but fail to undergo normal maturation and differentiation. Numerous attempts to detect qualitative differences between leukemic cells and their normal counterparts have been inconsistent. There is good reason to believe that leukemic leukocytes are functionally abnormal; they also display certain morphologic abnormalities and quantitative differences such as the reduced alkaline phosphatase content of mature granulocytes in chronic granulocytic leukemia. However, leukemic cells have not yet been shown to possess a single constituent (e.g., an enzyme) that is not present normally and that would serve to distinguish them from normal leukocytes.

Leukemia is a generalized disease. Because of the widespread distribution throughout the body of reticuloendothelial and lymphoid tissue, no organ is immune. Although foci of leukemic cells are frequently referred to as leukemic infiltrates, proliferation might be a more accurate descriptive term. Cells that are capable of undergoing hemic differentiation are widely distributed throughout the body. Therefore the presence of immature leukocytes does not require their "infiltration" from other sites. Histology varies among the different types of leukemia, but all forms exhibit the characteristic findings of a malignant neoplasm which are uncontrolled overgrowth with predominance of a single immature cell and with obliteration and destruction of normal tissue architecture. Clinical manifestations fall into three groups.

Altered Organ Function. Anemia, neutropenia, and thrombocytopenia are the major manifestations of leukemia and reflect bone marrow dysfunction. Neutropenia contributes importantly to the increased incidence of infections; thrombocytopenia causes hemorrhage. An infection and/or abnormal bleeding, the usual presenting complaints, are also the principal causes of disability and of death in all patients with leukemia, regardless of type. Normal marrow output can be curtailed in two ways: (1) growth potential of the primitive pluripotential marrow cells may be diverted into one cell lineage at the expense of others (e.g., granulocytic leukemia) or (2) normal marrow elements may be displaced as in lymphocytic leukemia. In addition, failure of leukemic cells to undergo normal maturation brings about a deficiency of mature cells, even though their precursors are plentiful. Leukocytosis and immature cells in the peripheral blood ordinarily reflect intramedullary leukemic proliferation, but these findings are of less pathophysiologic importance than are decreased numbers of normal mature cells. Furthermore, leukocytosis is not always a true indicator of the status of the disease. The mechanisms that control the number of circulating leukemic cells are poorly understood. The leukocyte count is generally increased in the chronic leukemias, but it may be normal or decreased in the acute leukemias, even though the bone marrow is packed with blast cells. The spleen, liver, and lymph nodes are the commonest sites of extramedullary involvement, but leukemic proliferation can occur in any organ or tissue. As a result, diverse symptoms and physical findings are encountered.

Systemic Symptoms. Weight loss, fever, increased sweating, and heat intolerance predominate. Most of these complaints are common to all types of malignant diseases. However, the manifestations of hypermetabolism probably reflect the increased metabolic requirements of the excessive numbers of immature blood cells. The basal metabolic rate is often elevated and the serum cholesterol decreased, but other measures of thyroid function are normal.

Cellular Dysfunction. There are quantitative differences between normal and leukemic cells, and it is reasonable to suspect that defective leukocytic functions are responsible for certain clinical manifestations. Specific examples include delayed neutrophilic responses to infection (defective phagocytic activity has been proposed but not clearly proved) and abnormalities in immunoglobulin production. These abnormalities are encountered most often in patients with chronic lymphocytic leukemia; deficiencies of immunoglobulins contribute to frequent infections and abnormal globulins to the development of overt hypersplenism. When erythrocytic precursors participate in the leukemic proliferation, decreased survival of the abnormal erythrocytes contributes to the pathogenesis of anemia. In certain types of leukemia, functional abnormalities of platelets appear to play important roles in the causation of a hemorrhagic diathesis. Because of large numbers of immature cells, enhanced nucleic acid catabolism is responsible for hyperuricemia and hyperuricosuria. As a result, renal lithiasis is common; overt secondary gout has been observed but is rare.

CLASSIFICATION

Several types of leukemia share a common name and all involve blood-forming tissue; however, they bear about the same relationship to one another as carcinoma of the stomach does to carcinoma of the colon. The leukemias are classified on the basis of their clinical course and type of cell involved. The following definitions are pertinent to this discussion:

Acute leukemia—a rapidly progressive disease involving primitive cells or blasts with a natural course of six months or less. *Subacute leukemia* runs a somewhat longer course (up to 12 months) and exhibits more cellular differentiation. Clinically, the subacute leukemias are managed as acute forms, and there is little reason to separate the two.

Chronic leukemia—mature cells predominate in a proliferative process that runs a natural course of one to several years.

Leukemic leukemia—leukemia with a circulating leukocyte count greater than 15,000/cu mm.

Subleukemic leukemia—a leukemic process with a circulating leukocyte count less than 15,000/cu mm but with abnormal or immature cells in the peripheral blood.

Aleukemic leukemia—leukemia with a circulating leukocyte count less than 15,000/cu mm without abnormal or immature cells in a 1000-cell differential count. Strict adherence to these criteria would appear to eliminate this category of disease.

Granulocytic leukemia—uncontrolled proliferation of granulocytes and their precursors. This term includes leukemia involving neutrophils with or without participation by the other granulocytic elements. In those rare situations in which eosinophils or basophils predominate, designations of *eosinophilic* or *basophilic leukemia* are appropriate. The terms myelocytic and myelogenous, often used interchangeably with granulocytic, should be discarded. "Myeloid" refers to all phases of bone marrow activity and is not restricted to granulopoiesis.

Lymphocytic leukemia—leukemic proliferation of lymphocytes or their precursors.

Monocytic leukemia—leukemic proliferation of monocytes and their precursors. True monocytic leukemia is often referred to as the *Schilling or histiomonocytic type*. Some recognize another form, the *Naegeli or myelomonocytic type*, which involves both monocytes and granulocytes; others have considered it to be a variant of granulocytic rather than monocytic leukemia. It would seem preferable to limit the use of the term monocytic leukemia to the Schilling type and to classify the myelomonocytic type separately.

Myelomonocytic leukemia—leukemic proliferation involving two or more types of marrow cells. In the past this designation has been largely restricted to leukemia involving both monocytic and granulocytic cells; it has been classified by some as granulocytic and by others as monocytic (Naegeli type). This form of leukemia occurs mainly in adults and runs an acute or more often a subacute course. It is a specific entity and is separable from other kinds of leukemia. Inasmuch as megakaryocytes and erythrocytic precursors usually participate in the leukemic process, the term myelomonocytic ("myelo-" to indicate that all marrow elements are involved and "mono-" to emphasize the monocytoid morphology) seems to be particularly fitting.

Erythroleukemia or Di Guglielmo's syndrome—leukemic proliferation involving both erythrocytic and granulocytic precursors. This term should be discarded; myelomonocytic leukemia as already defined is more appropriate.

Erythremic myelosis or Di Guglielmo's disease—uncontrolled proliferation of nucleated red cells without participation by other marrow elements. This entity is extremely rare; most patients so classified more properly fall into the category of myelomonocytic leukemia.

Lymphosarcoma cell leukemia—leukemic proliferation involving the lymphosarcoma cell; it differs clinically and morphologically from lymphocytic leukemia.

Stem cell or hemocytoblastic leukemia—acute leukemia involving primitive, undifferentiated blast cells.

CLINICAL MANIFESTATIONS

On the basis of differences in clinical manifestations and histology, it is possible to recognize several forms of leukemia. In descending

order the most commonly encountered leukemias are chronic granulocytic, acute lymphocytic, chronic lymphocytic, acute myelomonocytic,
acute granulocytic, chronic lymphosarcoma cell, acute lymphosarcoma
cell, and acute monocytic. The chronic leukemias are almost always
leukemic, whereas the acute leukemias are often subleukemic. Because
of variability in prognosis and response to treatment, a precise diagnosis
is needed; each type of leukemia should be viewed as a separate and
distinct clinical entity.

Leukemia is no longer a rare disease. During the past few decades,
the incidence has risen sharply. Only myocardial infarction and carcinoma of the lung have shown a more rapid increase. In the United
States there were 13,507 deaths, or 7.2/100,000 population, attributed
to all types of leukemia in 1963, approximately a twofold increase over
the last 25 years. The reason(s) for the more frequent occurrence of
leukemia is not apparent; it cannot be explained solely on the basis of
improved diagnostic techniques. The greatest increase has been in those
countries that have the highest standards of living and has been especially evident in the United States and Scandinavia. The frequency of
acute leukemia in the adult has shown the sharpest rise. Many theories
have been proposed in an attempt to explain the progressive advance
in the incidence of this lethal disease. None has been proved, but the
possible role of exposure to increasing amounts of ionizing radiation
deserves careful consideration.

Information regarding the frequency of the different types of leukemia
is difficult to obtain. Variable nomenclature, failure to make morphologic classifications, and the age of the patient population act to distort
data. Although leukemia respects no age, there are certain age predilections (e.g., chronic lymphocytic leukemia is a disease of old age); acute
lymphocytic leukemia is almost limited to infants and children. About
50 per cent of the cases of leukemia are acute; the rest are chronic.
Although some data tend to indicate a somewhat greater frequency of
leukemia in certain races, the rarity of chronic lymphocytic leukemia in
Japan and other parts of Asia is the only relationship that seems definite.
Leukemia occurs in males more often than females in a ratio of about
1.5:1. The clinical manifestations and management of the acute leukemias bear sufficient similarity to justify their consideration collectively.
However, the differences between the chronic leukemias warrant separate discussions.

Acute Leukemia

Acute leukemia affects all ages. About half the cases are in children
under the age of 14; most of these are lymphocytic, and the majority
occur before the age of six. Acute granulocytic and myelomonocytic

forms predominate in adults. Acute lymphocytic leukemia is quite unusual over the age of 20; acute lymphosarcoma cell leukemia occurs, but it is not common. Accurate figures are not available for the relative frequencies in the adult of acute granulocytic, myelomonocytic, and monocytic leukemia (some have classified myelomonocytic as granulocytic disease, whereas others have considered it a monocytic variant). The incidence of acute leukemia rises toward the latter half of the second decade of life and then remains fairly constant until the sixth decade, when it again increases. As already defined, acute myelomonocytic leukemia is probably the commonest type of acute leukemia in the adult, especially in the patient over the age of 50. Acute monocytic leukemia of the Schilling type is quite rare.

Symptoms. The onset of acute leukemia is generally abrupt and is heralded in most patients by an infection or a hemorrhagic diathesis. The infection is most often a severe, atypical upper respiratory infection that fails to respond in the usual manner; the hemorrhagic diathesis is usually manifested by purpura, epistaxis, gingival bleeding, or hemorrhage following trauma or minor surgery (e.g., a tooth extraction). Less often massive gastrointestinal or genitourinary bleeding is the presenting complaint. Symptoms of anemia (e.g., weakness, ease of fatigue, exertional dyspnea, and tachycardia) are ordinarily not prominent early in the disease because of the acuteness of the onset and the relatively long life-span of erythrocytes. However, anemia develops soon thereafter. In some adults with more slowly progressing disease, these symptoms are added to other systemic manifestations of a malignant process such as loss of weight. Fever is common in acute leukemia. In many cases temperature elevations reflect underlying infections, but in some patients no suitable explanation can be found other than the leukemia itself. Increased sweating and heat intolerance are also frequent complaints.

Because hemorrhage, infection, and leukemic cell proliferation can involve all tissues, the symptomatology of acute leukemia is varied and complex. Bone pain deserves emphasis because of its diagnostic significance; it may be generalized, but it is usually more marked in flat bones such as the sternum and ribs. In children pain in the extremities and joints may be particularly troublesome. Neurologic complaints are prominent. Meningeal involvement with symptoms of increased intracranial pressure is especially common in children and young adults, and a variety of central and peripheral nerve lesions may be encountered. Visual, pulmonary, gastrointestinal, and genitourinary disturbances are but a few of the other protean manifestations of acute leukemia. The pathogenesis of these complaints is diverse. For example, dyspnea may reflect pneumonitis, laryngeal obstruction, or an alveolar-capillary block consequent to diffuse pulmonary parenchymal involvement; hematuria may be the result of leukemic proliferation in the bladder or kidneys or of renal stones. It serves no useful purpose to list all possible symptoms or to assign relative frequencies to their occurrence. It is more important to be aware of the multiplicity of complaints that may reflect the presence of acute leukemia and of the contributions to the clinical picture of hemorrhage and infection. Bizarre manifestations are to be expected.

Physical Findings. Abnormalities of the skin and mucous membranes (e.g., petechiae, purpura, ecchymoses, pallor) and fever constitute the most frequent physical manifestations of acute leukemia; they occur in virtually all patients. Bone tenderness, especially of the sternum, can be elicited in about 60 per cent. Splenomegaly occurs in the majority of cases at some time during the course of the disease, but splenic enlargement is not detectable at the time of diagnosis in 40 per cent or more of the patients who have acute granulocytic or myelomonocytic leukemia. In about 10 to 20 per cent (usually patients with rapidly progressive, fulminant disease), the spleen never becomes palpably enlarged. Splenomegaly is found most consistently in patients with acute lymphocytic or lymphosarcoma cell leukemia; enlargement is typically slight in contrast to the massive splenomegaly that characterizes the chronic leukemias. Minimal to moderate hepatomegaly occurs in most patients. Significant lymphadenopathy is rare in acute granulocytic, myelomonocytic, and monocytic leukemias. Lymph nodes are slightly enlarged in many patients with acute lymphocytic or lymphosarcoma cell leukemia. The nodes are firm, discrete, and nontender, unless involved in an acute infectious process.

Other physical manifestations are diverse and reflect varied involvement of multiple organs and tissues. Skin abnormalities include papular, nodular, and bullous lesions. In contrast to its increased incidence in persons with chronic leukemia and lymphoma, herpes zoster is unusual in acute leukemia. Gingival hypertrophy is rather common in patients with acute monocytic and myelomonocytic leukemias and may literally "bury" the teeth; the gums often take on a purplish hue and are quite friable. Bone tumors are rare, but they do occur, especially in the skull and most often in patients with granulocytic disease. Some of these tumors are green (probably because of their myeloperoxidase content) and have been termed chloromas. Involvement of other tissues is reflected by findings that are unique to the particular site and contingent on the type of lesion (i.e., hemorrhage, infection, or leukemic cell proliferation). Hemorrhage can occur anywhere; in addition to the skin and mucous membranes, the retinas and central nervous system are frequent sites of bleeding. It should be noted that patients with acute leukemia often fail to exhibit the usual physical manifestations of infections. Without normally functioning neutrophils, the body is unable to form pus or to wall off an infection. The findings produced by leukemic cell prolifera-tion are those of tumefaction and/or dysfunction of the involved organ; they lack diagnostic specificity.

Laboratory Findings. Peripheral Blood. A normocytic, normo-chromic anemia occurs in all patients with acute leukemia. Early in the disease anemia is slight, but it inevitably becomes marked as the disease progresses. Overt hemolysis is quite rare, although some shorten-ing of red cell life-span is often demonstrable, especially in patients with myelomonocytic disease in whom erythrocytic precursors partici-pate in the leukemic process. In this type of leukemia, marked anisocytosis and poikilocytosis are common (Fig. 8-1). Erythrocyte

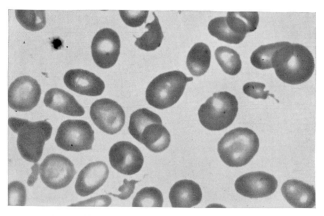

Figure 8-1. Peripheral blood film from a patient with an acute myelomono-cytic leukemia showing marked variation in the size and shape of the eryth-rocytes.

morphology is not remarkable in the other acute leukemias. Reticulo-cytopenia generally reflects a marked reduction in erythropoiesis, but there may be a slight reticulocytosis and polychromasia. It is usual to find occasional nucleated red cells in the peripheral blood in all acute leukemias; in some patients with involvement of erythropoietic tissue, nucleated red cells are numerous and display abnormal morphol-ogy similar to that in the bone marrow.

The leukocyte count is variable. About 25 per cent of the patients are leukopenic, with counts below 4000/cu mm; approximately 15 per cent have normal counts. The leukocyte count is between 10,000 and 50,000/cu mm in 25 per cent, 50,000 and 100,000 in 20 per cent, and more than 100,000 in the remaining 15 per cent. Blasts usually predomi-nate, but the number of immature cells in the peripheral blood varies. It is doubtful that immature or abnormal cells are ever totally absent from the peripheral blood. In acute lymphocytic leukemia the character-istic cell is a lymphoblast (Fig. 8-2). In granulocytic disease it is a

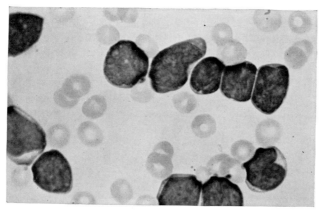

Figure 8-2. Lymphoblasts in the peripheral blood of a child with acute lymphocytic leukemia (see Table 8-1).

myeloblast (Fig. 8-3). In acute myelomonocytic leukemia the immature cells are generally quite primitive and undifferentiated (Fig. 8-4); atypical progranulocytes and promonocytes are also common in this form of acute leukemia. The presence of immature lymphosarcoma cells

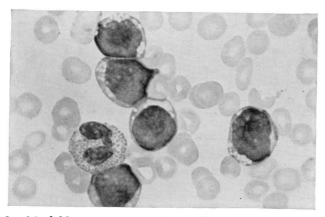

Figure 8-3. Myeloblasts in the peripheral blood of a patient with acute granulocytic leukemia (see Table 8-1).

(Fig. 8-5) distinguishes acute lymphosarcoma cell leukemia. In acute monocytic leukemia monoblasts dominate the picture (Fig. 8-6). Auer bodies (rodlike, cytoplasmic inclusion bodies) may be seen in myeloblasts and monoblasts (Fig. 8-7). More mature forms (prolymphocytes, progranulocytes, and promonocytes) are also present in the peripheral blood, especially in patients with more slowly progressive or subacute disease. In some patients a hiatus leukemicus is evident in which there are blast cells and mature forms without intermediate precursors; there

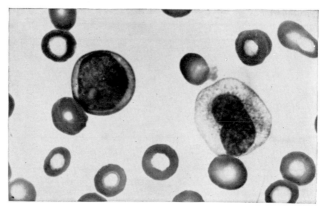

Figure 8-4. Undifferentiated blast cell and an atypical promonocyte in the peripheral blood of a patient with acute myelomonocytic leukemia.

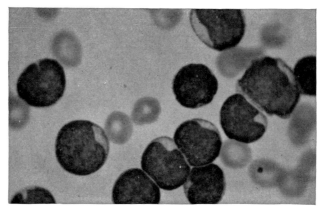

Figure 8-5. Primitive lymphosarcoma cells in the peripheral blood of a patient with acute lymphosarcoma cell leukemia (see Table 8-1).

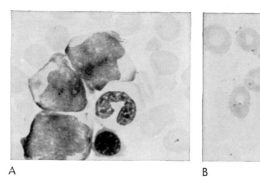

A   B

Figure 8-6. Monoblasts and promonocytes in the peripheral blood of a patient with acute monocytic leukemia. A. Monoblasts (see Table 8-1), band neutrophil, and nucleated red cell. B. Promonocytes.

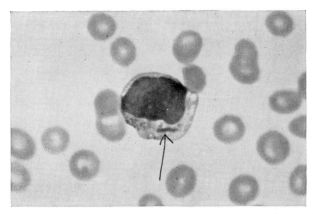

Figure 8-7. Early progranulocyte containing an Auer body in the peripheral blood of a patient with acute granulocytic leukemia.

is most often, however, a deficiency in the peripheral blood of the mature end products of the marrow cell compartment that is involved in the leukemic process. Mature neutrophils are usually decreased in patients with lymphocytic and lymphosarcoma cell leukemias, whereas most patients with acute granulocytic, myelomonocytic, and monocytic leukemias have normal numbers of circulating lymphocytes. The alkaline phosphatase content of mature granulocytes is decreased in acute granulocytic leukemia. In some patients with acute lymphocytic or lymphosarcoma cell leukemia, occasional immature granulocytes appear in the peripheral blood. They probably reflect a pathogenic mechanism similar to that which operates in a myelophthisic process (p. 241).

Thrombocytopenia, usually marked, is almost always present at the time of diagnosis. In certain patients with acute or subacute myelomonocytic leukemia, large atypical platelets are present in normal numbers; however, thrombocytosis almost excludes the diagnosis of acute leukemia arising *de novo*. Thrombocytopenia is responsible for prolonged bleeding times and positive capillary resistance tests. A variety of coagulation defects has been described in patients with acute leukemia, but no consistent pattern has been evident.

BONE MARROW. The pathognomonic finding of acute leukemia is a hyperplastic bone marrow with extensive replacement of normal elements by excess numbers of immature cells. In rapidly progressing disease the marrow contains few cells other than blasts. Marrow pictures differ among the various types of acute leukemia only insofar as the individual morphology of the blast cells differs (Fig. 8-8). Variable degrees of maturation and differentiation are seen, especially in patients with subacute myelomonocytic leukemia (Fig. 8-9); however, immature cells are always disproportionately increased. In acute lymphocytic and

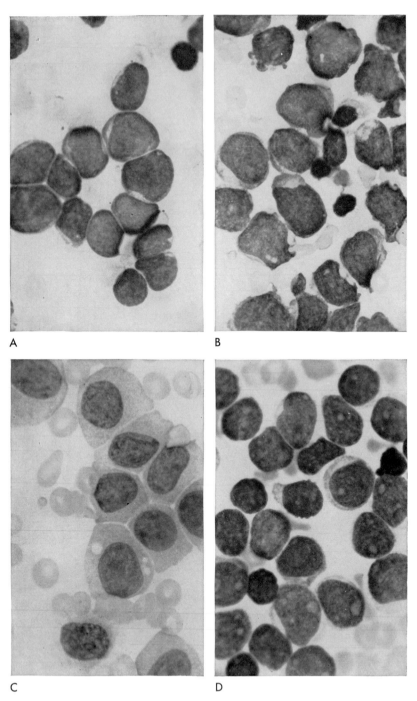

A

B

C

D

Figure 8-8. Bone marrow aspirates from patients with acute leukemia. _A._ Acute lymphocytic leukemia. _B._ Acute granulocytic leukemia. _C._ Acute monocytic leukemia. _D._ Acute lymphosarcoma cell leukemia.

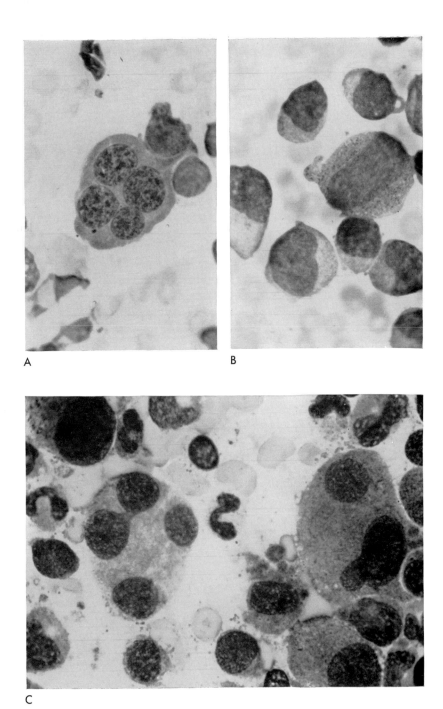

Figure 8-9. Marrow abnormalities in acute myelomonocytic leukemia. *A.* Atypical, multinucleated red cell precursor. *B.* Atypical, monocytoid granulo-cytic precursors. *C.* Atypical megakaryocytes.

349

lymphosarcoma cell leukemias normal myeloid elements (granulocytic precursors, nucleated red cells, and megakaryocytes) are decreased to absent. Erythropoiesis and thrombopoiesis are also decreased in patients with acute granulocytic and monocytic leukemias. In patients with acute myelomonocytic leukemia, atypical erythrocytic precursors and megakaryocytes may be present in normal, decreased, or increased numbers. Erythrocytic elements exhibit changes best described as "megaloblastoid" or paramegaloblastic (Fig. 8-9). In many patients with acute myelomonocytic leukemia, megakaryocytes are also abnormal with reticulated nuclear chromatin and hyperlobulated or multiple nuclei (Fig. 8-9).

OTHER LABORATORY FINDINGS. *Bone x-rays* are abnormal in many patients, especially in children (narrow transverse bands of diminished density proximal to the metaphyses of long bones are particularly common). Other bone findings include diffuse osteoporosis, osteolytic lesions, and periosteal thickening (osteosclerosis is rare); pathologic fractures are unusual. *Hyperuricemia* and *uricosuria* are common. *Serum proteins* may be abnormal, but the changes are not specific (alpha globulins are often increased in acute lymphocytic and gamma globulins in granulocytic and myelomonocytic leukemias; albumin is ordinarily decreased in all types). Hypogammaglobulinemia is a rare occurrence in acute leukemia. The *basal metabolic rate* may be elevated, but radioiodine uptake is normal. Evidence of renal insufficiency is seldom encountered, even though the kidneys are frequently involved by the leukemic process. In patients with meningeal leukemia, the *cerebrospinal fluid* contains increased protein, normal to decreased glucose, and increased numbers of cells; when films of the cellular sediment are stained with Wright's stain, these cells are identifiable as blasts (Fig. 8-10). For the most part, other laboratory findings lack specificity and reflect the nature

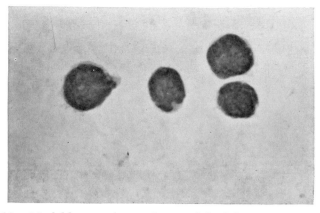

Figure 8-10. Myeloblasts in the cerebrospinal fluid from a patient with acute granulocytic leukemia and meningeal involvement (Wright's stain of cellular sediment).

and site of involvement (e.g., abnormal liver function tests). It is of interest that the serum glutamic oxaloacetic transaminase is generally normal, unless the patient develops superimposed hepatitis. The blood glucose may fall in vitro in bloods with high blast cell counts consequent to the glycolytic activity of the immature cells. Therefore the specimen must be processed promptly; the addition of fluoride as a preservative is also helpful.

DIAGNOSIS

The diagnosis of acute leukemia is suggested by the symptoms and physical findings, supported by the abnormalities in the peripheral blood, and confirmed by the bone marrow. The presence of an acute leukemia is ordinarily evident in the peripheral blood. Even if immature or abnormal cells are not seen (a most unlikely occurrence), an unexplained anemia and/or thrombocytopenia indicate the need for a marrow examination. An absolute diagnosis of acute leukemia is contingent on the bone marrow histology; in the absence of a "leukemic" marrow, such a diagnosis cannot be made.

In virtually all patients it is possible to recognize the various blast cells on the basis of their morphology. Accurate morphologic diagnosis is thus possible and should be made. This kind of characterization has been criticized and some have suggested dropping attempts to classify the acute leukemias morphologically, an approach that cannot be recommended. Admittedly, morphology is perhaps more of an art than a science; morphologic differentiation is sometimes difficult, and many morphologic variances are difficult to describe. Nonetheless, trained observers, given well-made and well-stained peripheral blood and marrow films, can with relative ease and consistent reproducibility correctly characterize the type of acute leukemia. Differentiation can usually be made with Wright-stained films alone; supravital staining or examination of living cells by phase microscopy often supplies additional information. Cells are rarely identified on the basis of single attributes. When stained with Wright's or some other polychrome stain, blast cells do not manifest consistent differences in size, position or shape of the nucleus, amount of cytoplasm, or tinctorial properties. Some of the pertinent differences in blast cell morphology are listed in Table 8-1. The presence of Auer bodies (Fig. 8-7) is particularly significant because these cytoplasmic inclusion bodies exclude the possibility of acute lymphocytic or lymphosarcoma cell leukemia. Many attempts have been made to distinguish among the various blast cells by other means (e.g., cytochemical differences). For the most part these techniques have either failed to reveal adequate specificity or are too cumbersome for routine clinical use. In view of the unequivocal differences in response to treatment, accurate morphologic diagnosis is a requisite for the selection of ap-

Table 8-1. Differences in Morphology of Leukemic Blasts (Wright's Stain)

Type of Cell	Nuclear Chromatin Pattern	Nucleoli	Nuclear Membrane	Cytoplasm
Myeloblast	Finely stippled or "ground-glass-like"	2 or more	Indistinct	1. No granules 2. Auer bodies may be present
Lymphoblast	Homogeneous with scattered small clumps	1 to 2	Relatively dense	1. Clear without granules 2. No Auer bodies 3. Perinuclear clear zone may be present
Lymphosarcoma cell	Reticulated or spongy with scattered clumps	1 to 2 (prominent with dense chromatin border)	Dense	1. Usually agranular; rarely, a few reddish granules 2. No Auer bodies 3. Perinuclear clear zone may be present
Monoblast	Fine lacework	1 to 2 (indistinct)	Indistinct	1. Often contain small reddish granules 2. Auer bodies may be present

propriate therapy, prognostication, and, most important, the evaluation of newer therapeutic agents as they become available. A diagnosis merely of acute leukemia is not acceptable. Even in those patients with very undifferentiated disease (i.e., "stem cell leukemia"), it is generally possible to make a more exact diagnosis after careful study.

Because the diagnosis of acute leukemia is predicated on the marrow findings, some mention must be made of the rare patients in whom adequate marrow specimens cannot be obtained. Failure to obtain marrow usually reflects a myeloid cavity densely packed with cells that are difficult to dislodge. Use of a larger syringe and the rapid application of negative pressure will often produce a satisfactory specimen; even a single drop in the lumen of the needle may be diagnostic. If repeated aspirations fail to yield adequate material and acute leukemia is suspected, an open marrow biopsy is indicated. In addition to fixed sections, imprints should be made and stained with Wright's stain. In most patients marrow involvement is diffuse, but focal areas of hyperplasia do occur. Myelofibrosis has even been observed in a few patients. It should be re-emphasized that a positive diagnosis cannot be made in the absence of a "leukemic" marrow. Specific treatment is never justified so long as there is doubt of the correctness of the diagnosis. Rare patients manifest certain nonspecific hematologic abnormalities (usually anemia, thrombocytopenia, and/or neutropenia) for months to several years before developing the typical findings of acute myelomonocytic or granulocytic leukemia. During this *preleukemic state* the marrow is often hypocellular without the pathognomonic abnormalities in proliferation and maturation needed to make a positive diagnosis. Only supportive therapy is indicated, pending unequivocal confirmation of the diagnosis of acute leukemia.

The symptoms and physical findings of acute leukemia may suggest a number of other diagnoses. In fact, the presenting manifestation is often that of some associated disorder such as an infection. Even the peripheral blood abnormalities are not always specific. A white count of 100,000/cu mm with 90 per cent lymphoblasts is diagnostic, but leukemoid reactions with normal or slightly elevated counts and only rare immature cells in the peripheral blood may cause some confusion. In children and adolescents infectious mononucleosis is especially troublesome (p. 323); however, the characteristic bone marrow findings of the acute leukemias eliminate all other diagnoses. Thus awareness of the possibility of acute leukemia and the indications for a marrow examination is the only requirement for the differential diagnosis.

TREATMENT AND COURSE

Acute leukemia is uniformly fatal; no patient has been cured. Untreated, the median survival is less than three months, with only rare patients (mostly adults with subacute myelomonocytic leukemia) living as long as a year. With specific therapy the median survival in children is 12 to 14 months. Prolongation of life is less evident in a group of adults; however, some patients do respond, and symptoms can be controlled in most. Several factors determine the responsiveness of an acute leukemic process to specific therapy. The type of disease is most important. Acute lymphocytic leukemia responds the best; acute granulocytic, myelomonocytic, and monocytic leukemias respond poorly, if at all. Therefore it is not surprising that the best results are seen in children under the age of 14. Because of the rarity of acute monocytic and lymphosarcoma cell leukemias, the terms childhood and adult leukemia are, for the purposes of discussion, considered to be synonymous, respectively, with acute lymphocytic leukemia and with acute granulocytic or myelomonocytic leukemia.

Specific Therapy (Systemic). Approximately 5 per cent of these patients (almost always children) exhibit spontaneous improvement. The remissions are short-lived, rarely complete, and follow a stressful situation such as an infection. They are most likely the result of enhanced endogenous corticosteroid elaboration. Before the introduction of antimetabolite therapy, no drug had been known to alter the course of acute leukemia. A number of agents have since been shown to exert a suppressive, antileukemic effect, but only a few have proved to be clinically useful. With the exception of the corticosteroids, all types of specific therapy inhibit cell growth by destroying or inactivating nucleic acids or by inhibiting their synthesis. No qualitative difference has yet been found between normal and leukemic cells. All proliferating cells require constant synthesis of purines and pyrimidines. The needs of leukemic cells are greater than those of normal cells, and it is possible to exploit these quantitative differences and selectively inhibit growth of leukemic cells. However, such agents affect normal cells as well. All too often the requirements of rapidly proliferating normal cells (e.g., blood cell precursors) do not differ significantly from those of the leukemic cells. Consequently, therapeutic and toxic effects cannot always be easily separated, and careful titration of doses is needed to prevent serious damage to normal cells.

FOLIC ACID ANTAGONISTS.   An antimetabolite is a structural analogue of a physiologically occurring metabolite that competes with normal substrate for an enzyme, thereby introducing a block in an essential biochemical pathway. The first antimetabolites used in the treatment of acute leukemia were analogues of folic acid (Fig. 8-11). Since the initial report by Farber and his associates in 1948, the therapeutic effectiveness of these substances has been clearly proved. *Methotrexate* (formerly called amethopterin) is the antifolic agent of choice because

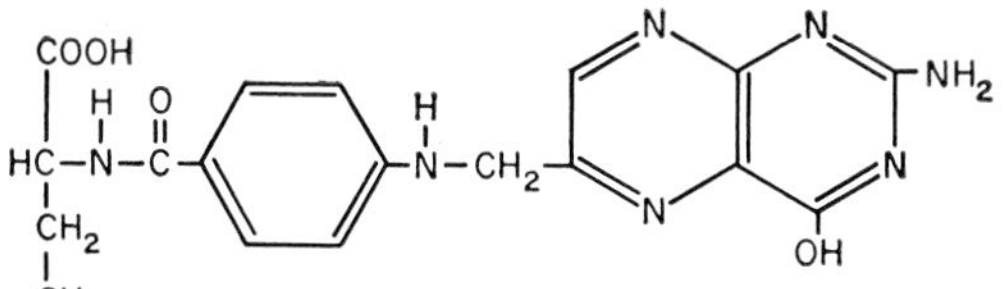

pteroylglutamic acid

FOLIC ACID

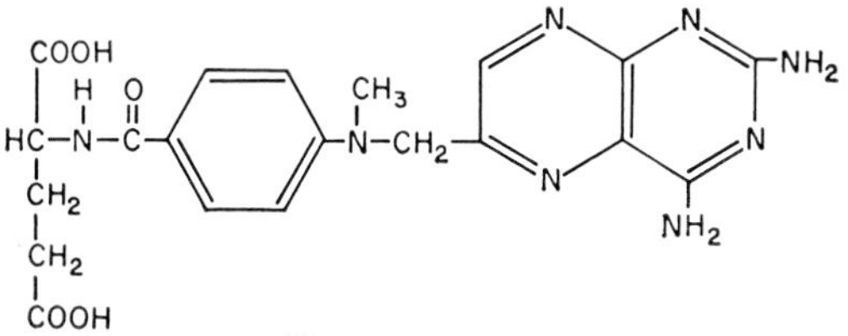

4, amino-N[10]-methyl-pteroylglutamic acid

METHOTREXATE

Figure 8-11. Structural formulas of folic acid and methotrexate.

it is somewhat less toxic and more easily controlled; however, *aminopterin* is equally effective. The folic acid antagonists act at different sites to block the conversion of folic acid to the various reduced tetrahydrofolic forms such as N5-formyltetrahydrofolic acid (folinic acid or the citrovorum factor). The metabolically active forms of folic acid play important roles in the transfer of one-carbon fragments, the basic building blocks in many biochemical reactions which include the synthesis of purines and pyrimidines. Thus the folic acid antagonists ultimately interfere with nucleic acid production (especially by affecting DNA biosynthesis) and in this manner inhibit cell proliferation.

The daily dose of methotrexate varies from 2.5 mg in a child to 5.0 mg in an adult; the dose of aminopterin is 0.5 to 1.0 mg/day. Both drugs are given orally but can be administered parenterally. There is a two- to three-week latent period before a therapeutic effect can be detected; six to eight weeks may be needed to obtain maximal benefit. Toxicity is encountered often and is frequently severe. Marrow depression and painful ulcerations of the oral mucosa are the initial toxic manifestations. Unless the dose is adjusted, marrow depression will progress to irreversible aplasia and the ulcerations will involve the entire gastrointestinal tract. Alopecia and exfoliative dermatitis are other evidences of toxicity. Toxic reactions can be lessened by the intramuscular administration of folinic acid (citrovorum factor), but the therapeutic effect will also be negated. The folic acid antagonists are excreted in the urine (about

60 per cent of a single dose is eliminated in the following 24 hours). Therefore impaired renal function will hasten the development of toxicity.

About 50 per cent of the children with acute leukemia respond favorably to treatment with a folic acid analogue; half of this number will develop complete remissions, that is, temporary eradication of all clinical and hematologic evidence of leukemia. Adults respond poorly, if at all; only 5 to 10 per cent improve, and a complete remission is very unusual. Beneficial responses are most frequent in patients in their teens or early 20's; above the age of 30, the chances of therapeutic benefit are almost nil, whereas the chances of inducing serious toxicity are great. Consequently, the age of 25 constitutes a relative contra-indication to the use of the antifolics, at least as initial therapy.

ANTIPURINES. A number of purine analogues are effective agents in the treatment of acute leukemia. 6-Mercaptopurine (6MP) was first used in 1952 and has been employed most extensively (Fig. 8-12).

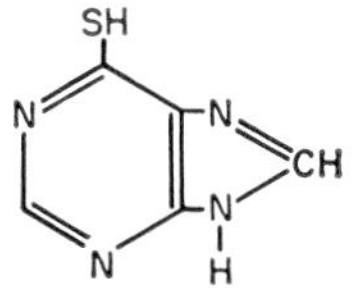

purine-6-thiol

6 MP; 6-MERCAPTOPURINE. *(Purinethol)*

Figure 8-12.   Structural formula of 6-mercaptopurine.

Related compounds such as thioguanine, thioguanasine, and 9-ethyl-6-mercaptopurine appear to be equally effective. 6MP appears to interfere with the incorporation of purines into nucleic acids by affecting the conversion of hypoxanthine to adenine. Nucleic acid synthesis is thereby impaired, and cell growth is inhibited. 6MP is given orally in a single daily dose equivalent to 2.5 mg/kg. Two to four weeks are usually required before a therapeutic effect becomes apparent; however, very high leukocyte counts may start to fall after only five to seven days. Maximal benefit may not be obtained for 8 to 10 weeks.

6MP is less toxic than the folic acid analogues. Bone marrow depression is the major manifestation of toxicity. An occasional patient will develop oral ulcerations, but these lesions ordinarily disappear, even in the face of continued therapy. Rare patients develop cholestatic jaundice; hepatic necrosis has been described in a few instances.

In children 6MP induces complete remissions in about 40 per cent and partial remissions in an additional 30 per cent. Approximately 15 per cent of the adults manifest complete and 20 per cent partial remissions; however, it is unusual for a patient over the age of 35 to develop a complete remission.

CORTICOSTEROIDS. Since first used in 1949, the corticosteroid compounds have played an important role in the treatment of acute leukemia. Their mode of action is still unknown. These agents differ from the other antileukemic drugs in not suppressing normal myelopoiesis. The recommended dose is 15 mg of prednisone or its equivalent every six hours (60 mg/day). In small children the daily dose is 2 mg/kg. The response is often dramatic; disappearance of fever, relief of symptoms, and a striking reduction in the circulating blast cell count occur within the first few days of therapy. Three or more weeks are needed to achieve maximal benefit. Toxic manifestations include, among others, peptic ulceration, fluid retention, hyperglycemia, increased susceptibility to infections, and osteoporosis.

About 90 per cent of the children with acute leukemia respond favorably to the corticosteroids; approximately 70 per cent achieve complete remissions. In contrast, good responses occur in only 20 to 25 per cent of the adults, most of whom are patients under the age of 30 with highly undifferentiated disease. In fact, adults with moderately differentiated granulocytic or myelomonocytic disease occasionally manifest accelerated activity of the leukemic process on administration of corticosteroids. Because the corticosteroids normally stimulate granulopoiesis, it is logical to anticipate such occurrences. The frequency with which the corticosteroids aggravate acute leukemia is not known. Such an effect can probably be hidden by the simultaneous administration of an antimetabolite. Aggravation in about 10 per cent of the adult patients would appear to be a conservative estimate. Massive corticosteroid therapy (i.e., 200 to 1000 mg of prednisone a day) has been successful in occasional adults who fail to respond to more conventional doses. The over-all results, however, have not been particularly gratifying. Although this mode of therapy may be of value in certain patients with far-advanced disease, the hazards (especially increased susceptibility to infections) are such that it cannot be recommended as initial treatment.

MISCELLANEOUS AGENTS. A variety of other chemotherapeutic agents has been reported to exert beneficial effects in some patients with acute leukemia. None has achieved the clinical status of the folic acid antagonists, the antipurines, or the corticosteroids. *Vincristine*, a plant alkaloid, shows promise in children. In general, there is no place for the use of alkylating drugs in the treatment of acute leukemia, for toxicity intervenes promptly. *Cyclophosphamide* (p. 405) is of value in some children and in a few adults (the latter usually with lymphosarcoma cell leukemia); however, it cannot be considered the treatment of choice with the possible exception of patients with extremely high leukocyte counts (i.e., more than 200,000/cu mm). When the leukocyte count is very high, the cytolytic effect of cyclophosphamide may cause prompt lowering of the leukocyte count and thus avert such complications as intracerebral thromboses.

Principles of Therapy. The treatment of acute leukemia is complex and must be individualized. At some time during the course of their disease, most patients receive at least three types of therapy, that is, the antifolics, the antipurines, and corticosteroids. Although theoretically advantageous, there is no convincing evidence that the simultaneous administration of two or more agents is more efficacious than their use alone. Protagonists of combination therapy point to slightly higher initial remission rates. However, patients treated sequentially with single agents are more likely to develop subsequent remissions and appear to live as long or longer. Eventually all patients become refractory to therapy, probably because of the emergence of mutant strains of cells with different metabolic pathways. Although there is no cross resistance among the different groups of antileukemic drugs, recipients of combination therapy may respond to one while becoming resistant to another. Furthermore, therapy with a single drug is easier to control. It is often difficult to separate toxic effects of multiple agents (e.g., severe leukopenia). As a result, the drug most likely to exert the best effect may be assumed erroneously to be at fault and stopped. Pending clear-cut proof of the superiority of combination therapy, it is recommended that the antileukemic drugs be given sequentially. When one has only a few rounds of ammunition and is not sure how vulnerable the enemy may be, it would seem to be the best strategy to fire each round separately.

In children the corticosteroids induce the most favorable responses (about 90 per cent), followed by 6MP (about 70 per cent) and the antifolics (about 50 per cent). The durations of the responses show an inverse relationship. They are longest in recipients of the folic acid antagonists (usually two or more months; occasionally a year or longer) and shortest after corticosteroids (average of about 10 weeks). Because the first remission is easiest to obtain, the antifolics are the treatment of choice followed by 6MP and then the corticosteroids. Corticosteroids are given initially in addition to an antimetabolite if it seems unlikely that the patient will survive long enough to obtain an antimetabolite effect (two to three weeks) or if there is a severe hemorrhagic diathesis.

In adults 6MP is the treatment of choice in patients over the age of 25. Under this age the antifolics deserve a trial. The indications for early corticosteroid therapy are the same as in children. It should be re-emphasized that the diagnosis of acute leukemia is not an indication for immediate corticosteroid therapy because of the likelihood of aggravating the disease or of producing serious side effects. If the older patient does not respond to 6MP, a trial of methotrexate may then be worthwhile. There is some evidence to suggest that smaller, less toxic doses of methotrexate are effective after prolonged 6MP therapy. Massive doses of corticosteroids deserve a trial in some patients after this approach has failed.

In general, a diagnosis of acute leukemia is an indication for treatment. The only possible exception is the adult with subacute myelomonocytic leukemia whose only manifestation is anemia. These patients respond so poorly to specific therapy that they are more likely to develop thrombocytopenia and neutropenia as a result of the treatment than to undergo significant improvement. They might best receive transfusions alone until additional manifestations become evident. In all other patients the appropriate antileukemic agent should be started as soon as the diagnosis is made. Because of the nature of the therapy to be used, the diagnosis must be unequivocal; *there is no room for doubt.* A drug should be given for three to four weeks before it can be discarded as ineffective. If the patient responds, the agent is continued in full doses until a complete remission occurs or toxicity intervenes. In the face of toxicity, dose adjustment is indicated. It is often difficult to decide when the toxic manifestations are more dangerous than the disease. It is usually necessary to accept some toxicity. In order for any degree of normal hematopoiesis to be re-established, almost all the leukemic cells must be destroyed. This point is dangerously close to irreversible marrow aplasia, and there are no good rules to prevent such occurrences. The circulating leukocyte count is not a valid indicator; therapy should be continued as long as the marrow remains hypercellular. Although every attempt should be made to prevent serious toxicity, there is no place for ultraconservatism in the treatment of acute leukemia. Unless the process is brought under control, the alternative is death. In patients receiving antifolics the development of mouth lesions is an immediate indication to reduce the dose or stop the drug. Treatment with folinic acid should be avoided insofar as possible because it will counteract the therapeutic effect. In patients receiving 6MP jaundice is an indication to stop that agent.

A partial remission can sometimes be maintained with less than full doses. When a complete remission is achieved, the question of maintenance therapy arises. In some patients continued administration of small doses of an antimetabolite (50 to 75 mg of 6MP or 2.5 mg of methotrexate every one or two days) seems to prolong the remission. However, other patients remain in complete remission for months, even though all treatment is stopped. Pending further insight into the whole problem of suppressive maintenance therapy and unless precluded by toxicity, continuous drug administration would seem to be preferable. When relapse occurs, retreatment with full doses is indicated; the chances of obtaining a second response are not good and most patients will need another drug.

Specific Therapy (Local).   There are few indications for local therapy. The commonest is the syndrome of "meningeal leukemia" which develops in about 25 per cent of the children (it is uncommon in adults). Because antimetabolites cross the blood-brain barrier poorly, central nervous system involvement can progress, even though the leukemic proliferation elsewhere is responding to specific treatment. The symptoms and findings of "meningeal leukemia" are basically those of increased intracranial pressure. The spinal fluid contains blast cells; protein is elevated and the sugar is normal to decreased. Treatment usually evokes dramatic results and consists of x-radiation to the head (about 200 to 300 r are given over a period of one to two weeks) or intrathecal methotrexate (0.25 to 0.5 mg/kg every three to five days until cells in the cerebrospinal fluid disappear and protein returns to normal). Corticosteroids may also be helpful for these compounds do cross the blood-brain barrier. Rarely, a symptomatic tumor mass requires local x-radiation.

Complications and General Supportive Measures.   Infections and hemorrhage are the major complications of acute leukemia. For infections appropriate *antibiotics* are indicated. Prophylactic antibiotics cannot be condoned, even in the severely neutropenic patient because of the danger of infection by resistant organisms. On the other hand, there is no time for delay once an infection develops. As soon as blood, urine, and sputum have been obtained for culture, broad antibiotic coverage on an empiric basis is indicated; preference should be given to bactericidal agents in greater than customary doses. After the organism(s) is identified and sensitivities are known, the drug may be changed. Because of altered host resistance and ecology consequent to earlier antibiotic therapy and corticosteroids, clinical infections are often caused by resistant staphylococci and by bacteria and fungi that normally do not cause disease. Viral infections are not increased. The feasibility of leukocyte transfusions to tide over severely neutropenic patients is currently under investigation.

Treatment of hemorrhage leaves much to be desired. Corticosteroids are given because of their "nonspecific effect on capillary integrity," but the existence of such an effect is conjectural. Transfusions, preferably with fresh platelet-rich blood, are needed in the face of severe hemorrhage. Platelet transfusions have been recommended, but limited availability, technical difficulties, and the generally short-lived results preclude their routine use.

Although relatively rare, obstructive uropathy due to uric acid crystals deserves mention because of its potential seriousness. Following cytolytic therapy or during periods of intense proliferative activity, increased nucleic acid catabolism produces hyperuricemia and hyperuricosuria (uric acid is the end point of purine catabolism). Decreased fluid intake and urine output in the presence of pre-existent renal damage bring about deposition of uric acid crystals, especially in the distal tubules. Oliguria progressing to anuria and uremia ensues. The most effective means of treating hyperuricemic renal failure is to anticipate and prevent its occurrence by maintaining an adequate urine output (3000 ml or more a day) and by keeping the urine alkaline, which, of course, is difficult. Acetazolamide (Diamox) works for a while but soon loses its effect. Osmotic diuresis with mannitol has been used with some success to increase urine flow. Once oliguria occurs, fluids must then be restricted, thus leading to further uric acid deposition. Ureteral catheterization is indicated to exclude extrarenal obstruction, but the obstruction is almost always within the renal parenchyma. Once anuria develops, there is little that can be done. Hemodialysis will lower the serum uric acid and blood urea nitrogen concentrations, but it will not affect the basic lesion. Preliminary data on the effect of allopurinol on uric acid metabolism are encouraging. This analogue of hypoxanthine inhibits the enzyme xanthine oxidase, which is responsible for the oxidation of hypoxanthine to xanthine and uric acid. The result is a decrease in uric acid production and a fall in serum and urine uric acid levels. Further observations on the role of this agent in the prevention of uric acid uropathy are indicated.

Pregnancy does not appear to exert either a beneficial or a deleterious effect on an acute leukemic process. Fetal mortality is high, and the chances of hemorrhage during delivery are increased, but there is no clear-cut indication to interrupt a pregnancy. Specific therapy is beneficial and would appear to be safe after the first trimester. Because corticosteroids cross the placental barrier, adrenal insufficiency may contribute to infant mortality in the immediate postnatal period.

Transfusions play a vital role in the treatment of acute leukemia. They are indicated as needed to maintain satisfactory erythroid values, that is, a level commensurate with adequate physiologic adjustment or a hemoglobin of 8 to 10 gm/100 ml of blood. If abnormal bleeding has caused iron deficiency, iron therapy is indicated. There is no reason to give other antianemic agents such as vitamin B_{12} or folic acid. In fact, there is some evidence that folic acid may accelerate the leukemic proliferation. Adequate *psychologic support* for the patient and his family is essential.

Response to Treatment and Prognosis. Therapeutic responsiveness is dependent on a number of factors such as the age of the patient, type of disease, and degree of differentiation; however, histology is most important. Acute lymphocytic leukemia responds best; acute granulocytic, myelomonocytic, and monocytic leukemias rarely show a good response. Since most childhood leukemia is the acute lymphocytic variety, children do better than adults; but even children do poorly if they have granulocytic or monocytic disease, and most adults who respond favorably have lymphocytic or lymphosarcoma cell leukemia. Rapidly progressing acute leukemias with primitive, undifferentiated cells respond better than more slowly proliferating processes characterized by moderate cellular differentiation. Specific antileukemic therapy and antibiotics have greatly altered the course of acute leukemia. In children the median survival has been prolonged from three months to 12 to 14 months, and about 10 per cent live longer than two years. Almost every patient with acute lymphocytic leukemia can expect one and often two or more satisfactory remissions. Less can be accomplished for the adult; even with treatment, median survival is only four to six months. In adults complete remissions are quite unusual. Above the age of 35 it is rare to observe significant restoration of normal bone marrow activity, even though the leukemic proliferation can be adequately suppressed. In contrast to the treatment of other types of malignant disease, return of marrow function is a more important goal of antileukemic therapy than is a decrease in tumor tissue.

Hemorrhage and infection are the chief causes of death. Hemorrhage is slightly more common in acute granulocytic and myelomonocytic leukemias; infection predominates in lymphocytic disease. Acute leukemia cannot be cured or even controlled for long; however, much can be accomplished. Symptoms can be eliminated, and life can be significantly prolonged, especially in children. The outlook is not bleak. It is reasonable to predict that greater understanding of the cause of acute leukemia and of the mechanism(s) responsible for the purposeless cell proliferation will permit new therapeutic approaches. Cure (or at least permanent control of the disease) does not seem to be an unattainable goal.

Chronic Granulocytic Leukemia

Chronic granulocytic leukemia accounts for approximately 25 per cent of all cases of leukemia and for about half of the chronic leukemias. Although seen occasionally in children, it is essentially a disease of middle life and occurs most often between the ages of 20 and 50; the peak incidence is in the fourth decade.

Symptoms. Weakness, ease of fatigue, a left upper quadrant mass (with or without associated pressure symptoms), pallor, and weight loss are the typical presenting manifestations. Symptoms usually develop slowly over a period of several weeks to months, but infarcts (especially in the spleen) may produce sudden, acute pain. Fever, increased sweating, and heat intolerance are rarely prominent at the time of diagnosis. Abnormal bleeding occurs late in the course. About 1 or 2 per cent of the patients complain of priapism.

Physical Findings. Splenomegaly is the most constant physical abnormality; the spleen is massively enlarged, with the lower pole extending below the level of the umbilicus in 75 per cent or more of the patients at the time of diagnosis. It is firm, smooth, and nontender, unless the site of a recent infarct. Under the latter circumstances, an associated perisplenitis may cause a splenic friction rub. Minimal to moderate hepatomegaly is present in most patients. Lymph nodes are rarely enlarged. Some patients complain of discomfort on sternal pressure, but generalized bone tenderness is unusual. Pallor and evidence of weight loss are frequent findings. Skin lesions are uncommon. Leukemic proliferation can occur in any tissue, thus giving rise to findings unique to that particular organ (e.g., the brain or spinal cord). However, significant involvement of organs other than the marrow and spleen is seldom encountered, at least early in the disease.

Laboratory Findings. PERIPHERAL BLOOD. A minimal to moderate normocytic, normochromic anemia occurs in all patients and becomes more marked as the leukemia progresses. Red cell morphology is normal. Slight polychromasia, a reticulocyte count of 2 to 5 per cent, and occasional nucleated red cells are characteristic findings in the peripheral blood. Superimposed hemolysis occurs rarely, if ever.

Leukocytosis is invariably present; as a rule, leukocyte counts range from 100,000 to 300,000/cu mm. The leukocytosis is primarily the result of a relative and absolute neutrophilia, but eosinophils and basophils are also increased. Although mature cells predominate, all stages of granulocyte development are represented, including small numbers of myeloblasts and progranulocytes (Fig. 8-13). The number of immature cells increases as the disease advances. The alkaline phosphatase content of the mature neutrophils is almost always reduced below normal.

Thrombocytosis is typical early in the course of chronic granulocytic leukemia and may persist until the terminal phase is reached. The platelets are ordinarily morphologically normal, but large and atypical forms may be seen. Atypical megakaryocytes or fragments are present in the peripheral blood of some patients.

BONE MARROW. The marrow is markedly hypercellular because of granulocytic hyperplasia; a "maturation defect" or disorderly proliferation with predominance of a single immature cell type is evident (Fig. 8-13). Early, this cell is a myelocyte or metamyelocyte, but as the disease progresses more immature forms take over. Terminally the marrow picture is generally indistinguishable from that of acute granulocytic leukemia arising *de novo* (Fig. 8-8, p. 348). At the onset megakaryocytes are present in increased numbers; as the leukemic process

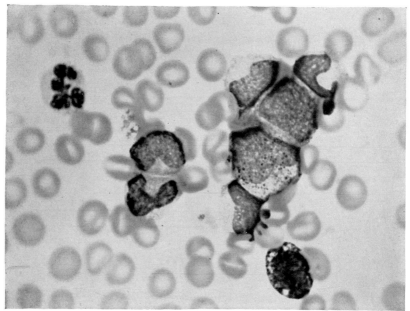

A

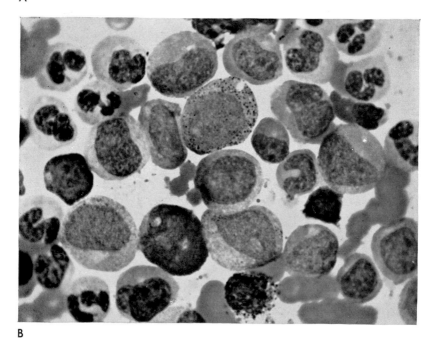

B

Figure 8-13. Hematologic findings in chronic granulocytic leukemia. *A*. Peripheral blood. *B*. Bone marrow.

advances, thrombopoiesis is eventually depressed. Erythropoiesis is al-most always decreased at the time of diagnosis. The Ph^1 chromosome can be demonstrated in the marrow cells of most, if not all, patients with chronic granulocytic leukemia (Fig. 8-14).

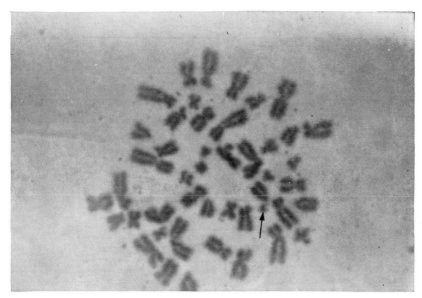

Figure 8-14. Chromosome preparation from the marrow of a patient with chronic granulocytic leukemia. Arrow points to the Ph^1 chromosome.

OTHER LABORATORY FINDINGS. Most of the other laboratory findings are nonspecific. *Hyperuricemia* is usual. The *basal metabolic rate* is frequently elevated. *Serum proteins* do not show consistent abnormalities. *Serum vitamin B$_{12}$* levels and *vitamin B$_{12}$-binding capacity* are increased. *Roentgenographic* evidence of bone involvement (lytic lesions or diffuse demineralization) is rare. Unless the specimen is processed promptly, *blood glucose* may be artifactually low because of continued glycolytic activity in vitro of the large number of leukocytes.

D I A G N O S I S

As a rule, massive splenomegaly, marked leukocytosis, and immature granulocytes in the peripheral blood point clearly to chronic granulo-cytic leukemia and the need for a marrow examination, which confirms the diagnosis. In fully developed cases it is difficult to confuse chronic granulocytic leukemia with any other disorder. It is doubtful that sub-leukemic forms exist. However, problems arise when the peripheral leukocyte count is only slightly to moderately elevated. Leukemoid reactions must then be excluded. The characteristic marrow findings, as well as other manifestations such as splenomegaly, usually permit differentiation with relative ease. Although granulocytic hyperplasia accompanies a number of disorders of varied etiology (e.g., pyogenic infections and acute blood loss), maturation is not affected and the ratio of immature to mature granulocytic precursors is normal. Agnogenic myeloid metaplasia causes the most confusion; separation of this disorder from chronic granulocytic leukemia is discussed in detail elsewhere (p. 437).

TREATMENT AND COURSE

Chronic granulocytic leukemia runs a progressive course that lasts about three years. An unequivocal diagnosis is an indication for treatment aimed at suppressing the abnormal granulocytic proliferation. It seems unlikely that the final outcome will be affected significantly if treatment is delayed, but early treatment is justified because most patients are symptomatic at the time of diagnosis or shortly thereafter. Initially, favorable responses can be obtained regularly with ionizing radiation or any of a variety of chemotherapeutic agents.

Specific Therapy (Ionizing Radiation). RADIOACTIVE PHOSPHORUS (^{32}P). This radioisotope was first used in patients with chronic granulocytic leukemia in 1936. Radioactive phosphorus is taken up by bone and granulocytic precursors where it emits beta radiation and suppresses granulopoiesis. The initial intravenous dose is 4 to 8 mc; when given orally, the dose should be about 25 per cent greater (i.e., 5 to 10 mc). Additional treatment may be needed in six to eight weeks. In the vast majority of untreated patients, radioactive phosphorus will evoke good responses. In many, all (or almost all) evidence of the disease will disappear. In others, there will be symptomatic relief, with alleviation of anemia and a decrease in the size of the spleen, even though obvious signs of the disease persist. Remissions last for several weeks to months; some patients do not require further treatment for a year or longer. Small titrated doses of radioactive phosphorus at regularly spaced intervals have been advised by some as a means of administering continuous suppressive therapy.

TOTAL BODY X-RADIATION. Spray irradiation to the whole body exerts an effect comparable to radioactive phosphorus. However, this type of therapy is time-consuming (three weeks or longer), and radioactive phosphorus or splenic radiation is preferred.

SPLENIC RADIATION. Local x-ray therapy to the enlarged spleen is an effective form of treatment. Depending on the degree and rapidity of the response, about 400 to 1200 r can be given in divided doses over a period of two to three weeks. Excellent responses similar in frequency, type, and duration to those induced by radioactive phosphorus are readily obtained in patients with early disease. When relapse occurs, another course of x-radiation to the spleen will usually bring about a second remission.

Specific Therapy (Chemotherapy). BUSULFAN (MYLERAN). This alkylating agent, a sulfonoxy ester (Fig. 8-15), was synthesized in 1953

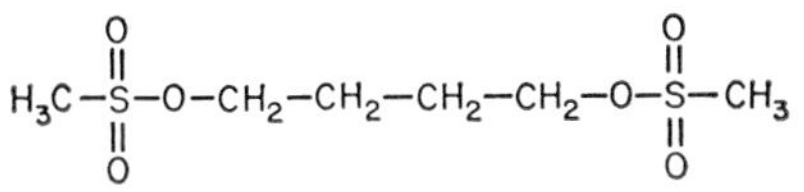

$$H_3C-\overset{\overset{O}{\|}}{\underset{\underset{O}{\|}}{S}}-O-CH_2-CH_2-CH_2-CH_2-O-\overset{\overset{O}{\|}}{\underset{\underset{O}{\|}}{S}}-CH_3$$

1, 4, dimethanesulfonoxybutane

BUSULFAN *(Myleran)*

Figure 8-15. Structural formula of busulfan (Myleran).

and is the chemotherapeutic agent of choice. It is given orally in a single daily dose equivalent to about 0.15 mg/kg. The mode of action of busulfan is similar to that of the other alkylating agents (p. 403). Although its suppressive effect is not limited to granulocytic elements, busulfan has its greatest usefulness in the treatment of chronic granulocytic leukemia. Excellent responses are observed in most patients with minimal side effects. The over-all results are at least as good as those obtained with any other form of therapy. Full doses are continued (unless signs of toxicity intervene) until the white count reaches about 10,-000/cu mm. The dose should then be stopped or reduced to one that will maintain the response without producing toxicity (e.g., 1 or 2 mg/day). The chief toxic manifestation of busulfan is bone marrow depression and pancytopenia; rarely, skin pigmentation, a picture simulating adrenal insufficiency, and pulmonary fibrosis have been ascribed to this drug. When relapse occurs, full doses of busulfan are resumed.

OTHER CHEMOTHERAPEUTIC AGENTS. A number of other drugs, including potassium arsenite (Fowler's solution), ethyl carbamate (urethane), triethylenemelamine (TEM), nitrogen mustard (HN2), desacetylmethylcolchicine (Demecolcin; Colcemide), and 6-mercaptopurine (6MP), are capable of exerting a beneficial effect in chronic granulocytic leukemia. None has proved to be superior to or less toxic than busulfan. Only 6-mercaptopurine plays a significant role, and that is in patients with an acute terminal blastic transformation. Corticosteroids will aggravate chronic granulocytic leukemia and are contraindicated.

Principles of Therapy. Radiation and busulfan are equally effective; one has not proved to be superior to the other. Therefore the type of initial treatment depends on the physician's personal experience and preference as well as such practical considerations as the availability of facilities for x-ray therapy, handling radioisotopes, and adequate follow-up. Because of the ease with which it can be given and the lack of serious or undesirable side effects, radioactive phosphorus is the preferred form of radiation. As is true for other hematologic neoplasms, continuous suppressive maintenance therapy possesses certain theoretical advantages over interval therapy and is the reason that many prefer to treat chronic granulocytic leukemia with a chemotherapeutic agent rather than with ionizing radiation. However, comparison of these treatment plans is hazardous, inasmuch as patients do develop lengthy remissions after a single injection of radioactive phosphorus, a single course of splenic x-ray, or a single course of busulfan. There is still insufficient proof, at least in patients with early disease, of the superiority of continuous therapy to warrant the close follow-up (i.e., every two to three weeks) needed to prevent the development of toxicity. Pending the acquisition of such proof, interval therapy is the simplest and least likely to be associated with serious side effects. If ionizing radiation is selected as the initial treatment, it is repeated until the patient no longer responds; chemotherapy is then indicated. If busulfan is given first, the drug may be discontinued as soon as the maximal effect is obtained. If the response is maintained, treatment need not be reinstituted until relapse occurs. If relapse occurs promptly, continuous suppressive therapy is obviously necessary. Busulfan is continued until the patient no longer responds (or until side effects necessitate its discontinuance); therapy with ionizing radiation is then indicated.

Response to Therapy. Several remissions of variable and unpredictable length can be expected. In most patients granulocyte alkaline phosphatase returns to normal; available data indicate that the Ph^1 chromosome is unaffected by treatment. In general, the first therapeutic remission is complete or almost so. Each succeeding remission is shorter and less complete until therapeutic unresponsiveness occurs. Terminally, most patients with chronic granulocytic leukemia undergo an acute blastic transformation. With the exception of the duration of the illness and the presence of a massively enlarged spleen, these patients are indistinguishable from those with acute granulocytic leukemia arising *de novo*. Ionizing radiation or busulfan are no longer of value, and these patients should be treated as for acute leukemia; 6-mercaptopurine in daily doses equal to 2.5 mg/kg is the treatment of choice, but few patients respond.

Despite the frequency and excellence of the remissions induced by specific therapy early in the course of the disease, there is little evidence that life can be significantly prolonged. Most patients live about 30 to 40 months; a few survive for shorter periods and a rare patient lives longer. There is much less variability in survival times in chronic granulocytic leukemia than in other hematologic neoplasms. Some data suggest that therapy lengthens the course by a few months, but the figures are not particularly impressive. Nevertheless, the symptomatic relief and general improvement that follow treatment clearly establish its importance. Even if death cannot be postponed, most patients can be maintained symptom-free and capable of a near normal existence until just before their demise.

Chronic Lymphocytic Leukemia

Chronic lymphocytic leukemia is a disease of late life with a peak incidence about the age of 60. It is rare under the age of 45 and most unusual before the age of 30. Chronic lymphocytic leukemia affects males two to three times as often as females. It occurs with equal frequency in all geographic locations, with the exception of Japan and other parts of Asia where it is quite uncommon. In contrast to the acute leukemias and chronic granulocytic leukemia, there is no apparent relationship between ionizing radiation and chronic lymphocytic leukemia. Chronic lymphocytic leukemia accounts for about 15 per cent of the cases of leukemia and about 30 per cent of the chronic leukemias.

Symptoms. The onset is almost always insidious. In 10 per cent or more of the patients, the diagnosis is made as an incidental finding in the absence of symptoms attributable to the leukemic process. In some patients an acute infection first calls attention to the disease. In others a hemolytic anemia is the initial manifestation. Weakness, ease of fatigue, painless lymph node enlargement, and weight loss are typical early symptoms. Skin lesions are common. Fever, heat intolerance, and increased sweating become prominent as the disease progresses. A hemorrhagic diathesis characterizes far-advanced disease. A variety of other symptoms reflects involvement of the lungs, bones, gastrointestinal or genitourinary tracts, central nervous system, and so forth.

Physical Findings. Generalized peripheral lymphadenopathy is the most characteristic physical manifestation of chronic lymphocytic leukemia. Early, the nodes are small, but in far-advanced disease they may reach massive proportions. Nodes are firm, movable, and nontender, unless involved in an infectious process. Mediastinal adenopathy may occur alone or with such lung findings as atelectasis or pleural effusion. Retroperitoneal and abdominal nodes may be evident on abdominal palpation. The spleen is almost always enlarged even at the time of diagnosis, but splenomegaly is rarely marked. Most often, the spleen extends 4 to 6 cm below the costal margin. Slight to moderate hepatomegaly is usual. Skin lesions are perhaps more common in chronic lymphocytic leukemia than in any other form of leukemia. Numerous types of lesions have been described. The incidence of herpes zoster is increased. Other physical findings depend on the site of involvement and lack diagnostic specificity.

Laboratory Findings. PERIPHERAL BLOOD. Initially, the erythroid values are normal. As the disease progresses, a normocytic, normochromic anemia develops which eventually becomes severe. Erythrocytic morphology is ordinarily normal. About 10 per cent of the patients with chronic lymphocytic leukemia manifest an overt hemolytic anemia; spherocytes are present in most of these individuals, as are increased polychromasia, circulating nucleated red cells, reticulocytosis, and abnormal erythrocyte osmotic behavior. In patients with extensive marrow involvement, erythropoiesis may be so depressed that a "normal" reticulocyte response is prevented, even though active hemolysis is present. In far-advanced disease examination of the peripheral blood reveals occasional nucleated red cells, immature granulocytes, and slight reticulocytosis, even in the absence of overt hemolysis. These findings probably reflect a myelophthisic process (p. 240).

Depending on the stage of the disease, the leukocyte count varies between 20,000 and 200,000/cu mm. Fewer than 5 per cent of the patients have white counts above 500,000. The leukocytosis is due to a relative and absolute lymphocytosis (lymphocytes make up 60 to 99 per cent of all leukocytes). Mature small lymphocytes with scant cytoplasm predominate. These cells differ from normal lymphocytes in having larger and denser clumps of nuclear chromatin and accentuation of parachromatin (Fig. 8-16). Occasional medium and large lymphocytes are

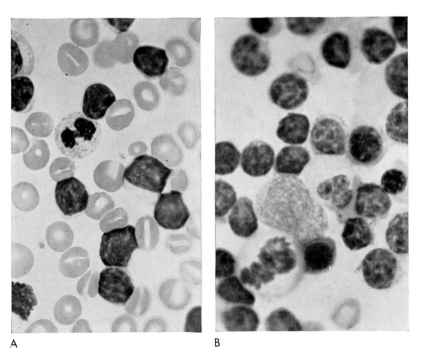

A   B

Figure 8-16. Hematologic findings in chronic lymphocytic leukemia. A. Peripheral blood. B. Bone marrow.

seen, but immature cells are infrequent. At first there is only a relative neutropenia, but as the disease progresses an absolute neutropenia develops.

Early in the course of chronic lymphocytic leukemia, platelets are not affected. As the process advances, however, thrombocytopenia occurs. Eventually it becomes marked and is associated with hemorrhagic manifestations.

BONE MARROW. Findings vary with and depend on the stage of the disease. Initially, cellularity is increased because of the increased numbers of mature small lymphocytes without associated depression of normal myelopoiesis. As the disease progresses, the overabundance of lymphocytes becomes more marked, and the number of normal marrow elements falls. To be considered diagnostic, 50 per cent or more of the cells in a cellular specimen should be lymphocytes. In far-advanced disease the marrow is extremely hypercellular and normal hemic precursors are almost completely replaced by small to medium-sized mature lymphocytes (Fig. 8-16). In patients with superimposed hypersplenism, the marrow generally reflects this complication, and there may appear to be only two types of marrow cells, that is, lymphocytes and nucleated red cells. Hypersplenic neutropenia or thrombocytopenia are also reflected by characteristic abnormalities in granulopoiesis and in megakaryocyte morphology, provided lymphocytic infiltration is not so extensive that it obscures these changes.

OTHER LABORATORY FINDINGS. About 35 per cent of the patients with chronic lymphocytic leukemia (especially those with far-advanced disease) have *hypogammaglobulinemia;* about 20 per cent have *hypergammaglobulinemia. Agammaglobulinemia* and *cryoglobulinemia* have been described but are rare findings. *X-rays* may reveal mediastinal or hilar adenopathy. Bone involvement is common (lytic lesions or diffuse demineralization predominate, but sclerosis has also been described). The *basal metabolic rate* is often elevated, but other measures of thyroid function are normal. Most patients with an acquired hemolytic anemia have positive *Coombs'* or *antiglobulin tests* (p. 97). Hemolysis may also be reflected by appropriate *pigment changes,* that is, hyperbilirubinemia of the unconjugated type with increased urinary and fecal urobilinogen. If hypersplenic neutropenia and/or thrombocytopenia is present, *leukocyte and/or platelet agglutinins* may be demonstrable. Other laboratory abnormalities lack specificity.

DIAGNOSIS

The diagnosis of a fully developed case of chronic lymphocytic leukemia presents no problem. Lymph node enlargement, splenomegaly, leukocytosis due to mature small lymphocytes, and marrow lymphocytosis in an older patient are diagnostic. Some confusion may exist in patients with early or subleukemic disease. Chronic subleukemic lympho-

cytic leukemia is unusual and most often associated with anemia, neutropenia, thrombocytopenia, and extensive marrow lymphocytic infiltration.
However, early disease may not be associated with other significant
abnormalities in the peripheral blood; other causes of lymphocytosis
must then be excluded, but differentiation is rarely difficult. The age
of the patient, morphology of the lymphocytes, and a positive heterophil agglutination test readily distinguish infectious mononucleosis from
chronic lymphocytic leukemia. The hematologic manifestations of acute
infectious lymphocytosis most closely simulate those of chronic lymphocytic leukemia, but the acute form occurs in children and the nodes
and spleen are not enlarged. Thyrotoxicosis is occasionally associated
with slight lymphocytosis, lymphadenopathy, and splenomegaly, but the
changes are rarely so marked that they suggest a diagnosis of chronic
lymphocytic leukemia. Should there be doubt about the diagnosis, follow-up observations will soon clarify the problem without depriving
the patient of the benefits of treatment or altering the final outcome.

TREATMENT AND COURSE

Although the natural course of chronic lymphocytic leukemia is progressive, it is characterized by relative benignity. Accurate survival data
are not available. Many published reports include all kinds of chronic
leukemia; even in those that separate lymphocytic from granulocytic,
few have delineated chronic lymphocytic from chronic lymphosarcoma
cell leukemia. Because the prognosis and response to therapy are somewhat poorer for the latter type, inclusion of these patients yields falsely
low survival times. Some patients with chronic lymphocytic leukemia
(especially younger patients and those with superimposed hypersplenism) exhibit rapidly progressive disease and succumb within one to
four years. More often than not, however, the disease remains stable
for several years or advances quite slowly. Chronic lymphocytic leukemia is compatible with survival for 10 to 20 years; rare patients
have been known to live as long as 35 years. Because of its variable
course, average survival times are meaningless. Available data suggest
a median survival of about six years, but about 15 per cent survive for
10 years or more. Thus the prognosis of chronic lymphocytic leukemia
is better than any other type of leukemia.

In contrast to the other hematologic neoplasms, the diagnosis of
chronic lymphocytic leukemia is *not* an indication for treatment. In fact,
injudicious suppressive therapy early in the course of the disease may
do more harm than good by injuring the marrow or by "triggering"
hypersplenism. The goal in the treatment of any type of leukemia is
control, not cure. Success depends on the establishment of a patient-
disease or host-tumor relationship favoring the patient. In many patients
with chronic lymphocytic leukemia, such a relationship exists at the

time of diagnosis and persists for several years; there is no reason to disturb it. Increased numbers of lymphocytes in the peripheral blood, marrow, and other tissues are not in themselves deleterious to the patient. If the patient is without systemic symptoms, if his erythroid values and neutrophil and platelet counts are normal, and if local tumor masses are not causing symptoms or interfering with normal function, therapy aimed at decreasing lymphocytic proliferation is not indicated. There is no proof that delaying therapy shortens survival. On the other hand, there is a very real likelihood that premature therapy will depress normal myelopoiesis and hasten the appearance of anemia, neutropenia, and/or thrombocytopenia. As soon as there is something to treat other than an elevated leukocyte count (symptoms, anemia, thrombocytopenia, neutropenia, or significant tumor masses), suppressive therapy is indicated. Control of the abnormal lymphocytic proliferation can be achieved by ionizing radiation or chemotherapy.

Ionizing Radiation. *X-radiation* to the spleen or enlarged nodes is quite effective. Patients with chronic lymphocytic leukemia are unusually sensitive to the cytotoxic effect of ionizing radiation and relatively small doses are required. Over the spleen 200 to 1200 r generally suffice. Over areas of enlarged nodes 200 to 300 r (often applied in a single treatment) may be sufficient. The indirect effect of this therapy is striking. Distant nodes melt away and lymphocytic proliferation in the marrow decreases. *Radioactive phosphorus* is also effective but must be given in much smaller doses than in chronic granulocytic leukemia (about 2 to 4 mc intravenously or 2.5 to 5 mc orally). Total body x-radiation is comparable to radioactive phosphorus. Titrated or regularly spaced therapy with radioactive phosphorus may be more effective than interval therapy.

Chemotherapy. *Chlorambucil,* an aromatic mustard introduced in 1953 (Fig. 8-17), is the agent of choice in daily doses equivalent to

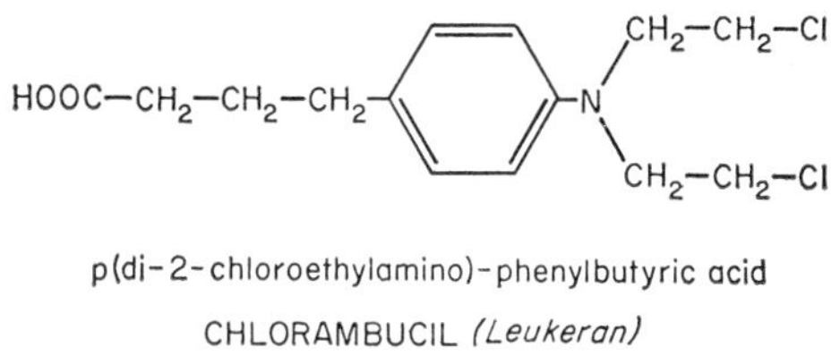

$$HOOC-CH_2-CH_2-CH_2-\underset{\underset{CH_2-CH_2-Cl}{\overset{CH_2-CH_2-Cl}{}}}{\bigcirc}-N$$

p(di-2-chloroethylamino)-phenylbutyric acid

CHLORAMBUCIL *(Leukeran)*

Figure 8-17. Structural formula of chlorambucil (Leukeran).

0.2 mg/kg. It is ordinarily well tolerated. Bone marrow depression, the major toxic manifestation, will usually necessitate a reduction of dose after four to six weeks of treatment. The drug should be continued for weeks to months with dosage adjustments as needed to avoid toxicity and to maintain (or obtain) the desired effect. Small doses of triethylenemelamine (TEM) are also effective, but this drug can no longer be recommended because of the frequency with which it produces serious marrow depression. Several other agents will suppress the abnormal lymphocytic proliferation (e.g., busulfan or nitrogen mustard), but none is superior to chlorambucil.

Other Therapeutic Measures.   *Corticosteroids* play an important role in the management of the patient with chronic lymphocytic leukemia. Although these compounds normally produce lymphocytopenia, they usually do not exert a clear-cut therapeutic effect. In fact, an unexplained increase in the circulating lymphocyte count commonly follows their administration. This seemingly paradoxical situation cannot be correlated with increased activity of the disease and often subsides even though the corticosteroids are continued. Increased susceptibility to infections is a more serious side effect. The chief indication for corticosteroids in patients with chronic lymphocytic leukemia is superimposed hypersplenism. Overt hemolysis occurs in 10 per cent or more of the patients, and the majority have occult hemolysis. Hypersplenic thrombocytopenia and/or neutropenia are also common. Hypersplenism may be correlated with increasing activity of the disease or may actually follow specific therapy, perhaps as the result of cell lysis and release of an abnormal globulin. It is treated as all other types of hypersplenism (p. 461). Corticosteroids are indicated in doses equivalent to 15 mg of prednisone every six hours; in some desperate situations massive doses (i.e., 120 mg or more of prednisone daily) may be effective when smaller doses were not. As soon as maximal improvement occurs, the dose is tapered to the smallest amount that will maintain the desired effect (usually 5 mg of prednisone two or three times daily). If the patient cannot be maintained on small doses or fails to respond, *splenectomy* should be considered. In view of the ultimate prognosis, it is desirable to avoid splenectomy if possible. On the other hand, the results are often dramatic in certain selected patients in whom hypersplenism is the major cause of disability.

Antibiotics are invaluable for the frequent infections. In some patients with hypogammaglobulinemia, exogenous *gamma globulin* has decreased the incidence of infectious complications. *Transfusions* are needed in patients with far-advanced disease to maintain satisfactory erythroid values. Fresh platelet-rich blood is often helpful in patients with abnormal bleeding.

Principles of Therapy.   The diagnosis is not an indication for therapy; significant symptoms or physical abnormalities, anemia, thrombocytopenia, neutropenia, hypersplenism, and frequent infections point to the need for treatment. Theoretically, systemic therapy (e.g., radioactive phosphorus or chlorambucil) seems preferable because chronic lymphocytic leukemia is a generalized disease. In practice, however, local x-radiation is just as effective and often better. Marrow depression is a common and serious complication of specific therapy. In contrast to the neutrophilia and thrombocytosis in patients with chronic granulocytic leukemia, granulopoiesis and thrombopoiesis are curtailed (often seriously so) in patients with chronic lymphocytic leukemia. Local irradiation of an enlarged spleen and/or enlarged lymph nodes is less likely to cause serious marrow depression than a chemotherapeutic agent or radioactive phosphorus and is frequently the treatment of choice, especially if there is significant splenomegaly or lymphadenopathy; x-radiation to the spleen is often followed by disappearance of distant tumor masses and by marrow improvement.

In patients who are no longer responsive to x-radiation or in those with marked marrow involvement and disseminated disease, chlorambucil is indicated. This agent permits long-term maintenance treatment, but proof of the superiority of continuous as opposed to interval therapy is not available. If chlorambucil evokes a complete remission, maintenance therapy (e.g., 2 mg/day) should probably be continued until toxicity intervenes or the disease reactivates. If a partial response occurs, continuous therapy is indicated as long as it does not aggravate thrombocytopenia, anemia, or neutropenia. Most patients require several types of therapy during the course of their disease.

Response to Therapy. The initial response is typically favorable, regardless of the type of therapy employed. Nodes disappear, the spleen decreases in size, and symptoms abate. The erythroid values, neutrophil count, and platelets return to normal. In patients with far-advanced disease, however, it is difficult to restore normal myelopoiesis, even if the leukemic process is suppressed. It is usual to obtain two, three, or even four remissions in patients with chronic lymphocytic leukemia. Eventually, refractoriness to all forms of treatment ensues. Therapy clearly prolongs "useful life," even though it may not materially lengthen the course. Most patients can be maintained in an asymptomatic state until shortly before death. Almost half the patients die from some cause other than their leukemia. Infection and hemorrhage are equally responsible for death in the remainder. Acute blastic transformation is a most exceptional occurrence, even in the terminal phases of chronic lymphocytic leukemia.

Chronic Lymphosarcoma Cell Leukemia

Chronic lymphosarcoma cell leukemia is rarely differentiated from chronic lymphocytic leukemia. Although their clinical manifestations are similar, they differ morphologically. Variances in length of course and responses to therapy justify the classification of these two chronic leukemias in separate categories. Because few large series have distinguished between chronic lymphocytic and chronic lymphosarcoma cell leukemias, accurate data concerning their relative incidence are not available. Chronic lymphosarcoma cell leukemia probably accounts for about 10 per cent of all kinds of leukemia and for about 20 per cent of the chronic leukemias. Clinical manifestations differ from chronic lymphocytic leukemia in the following respects:

1. Chronic lymphosarcoma cell leukemia is more likely to occur at an earlier age and usually runs a shorter course.

2. The leukocyte count is lower (usually between 20,000 to 80,000/cu mm).

3. The predominant cell in the peripheral blood and marrow is an atypical prolymphocyte. These lymphosarcoma cells resemble those in acute lymphosarcoma cell leukemia (Fig. 8-5, p. 346), but they are more mature (Fig. 8-18). Lymphosarcoma cells are usually large, with round, oval, or notched nuclei, reticulated or spongy nuclear chromatin, and a single large prominent nucleolus ringed by thick chromatin. The nucleoli are especially evident in supravitally stained films. There is a definite nuclear wall and scant to relatively abundant blue-gray opaque cytoplasm which occasionally contains a few nonspecific azurophilic granules. These cells are easily recognized by a trained observer and permit ready separation of this disease from chronic lymphocytic leukemia.

4. Fixed tissue sections (e.g., a lymph node) are identical with those from a patient with lymphosarcoma (Fig. 9-3, p. 384); similar preparations from a patient with chronic lymphocytic leukemia are identical with those in persons with lymphocytic lymphoma (Fig. 9-6, p. 387).

5. Chronic lymphosarcoma cell leukemia does not ordinarily respond to treatment quite as well as chronic lymphocytic leukemia. Relatively few patients exhibit the long fairly benign courses that characterize chronic lymphocytic leukemia.

Although the major clinical manifestations and types of therapy are similar, every effort should be made to separate chronic lymphosarcoma cell leukemia from chronic lymphocytic leukemia. Chronic lymphosarcoma cell leukemia appears to respond best when treated aggressively as lymphoma (p. 398) would be treated rather than more conservatively as recommended for chronic lymphocytic leukemia.

Other Types of Leukemia

CHRONIC MONOCYTIC LEUKEMIA

Most of the reported cases of monocytic leukemia appear to be examples of myelomonocytic disease with involvement of several cell

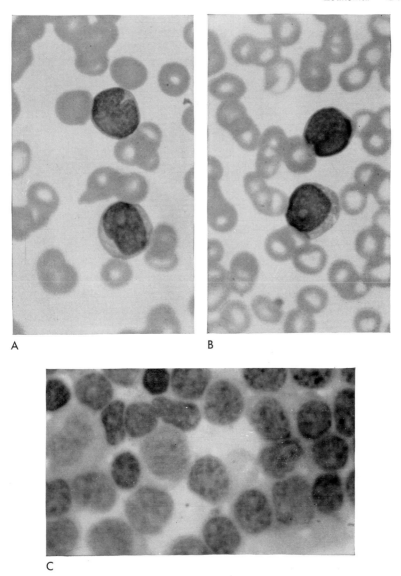

A   B

C

Figure 8-18. Hematologic findings in chronic lymphosarcoma cell leukemia. *A.* Peripheral blood film (Wright's stain). *B.* Brilliant cresyl blue peripheral blood film counterstained with Wright's stain. *C.* Bone marrow (Wright's stain).

lineages. Monocytic leukemia is rare and usually runs a subacute or acute course. Chronic monocytic leukemia of the histiomonocytic type is seldom seen. An insufficient number of patients has been studied to permit formulation of a distinct clinical picture. Leukopenia or only slight leukocytosis has been stressed. Therapeutically such patients must be considered as individual problems.

LEUKEMIC RETICULOENDOTHELIOSIS

The term leukemic reticuloendotheliosis has been used to describe disorders characterized by uncontrolled proliferation of reticulum cells in the marrow, spleen, liver, and lymph nodes. Abnormal or malignant reticulum cells have been observed in the peripheral blood. Both acute and chronic courses have been described. These proliferative disorders appear to be closely related to monocytic and myelomonocytic leukemias, especially the latter. It is preferable to classify such patients under these headings rather than to add arbitrary categories of disease.

ACUTE STEM CELL (OR HEMOCYTOBLASTIC) LEUKEMIA

An acute leukemic process involving undifferentiated blast cells is often designated "stem cell" leukemia. Because, in almost every instance, careful study will permit accurate morphologic classification, there is little justification for the retention of this category.

ERYTHREMIC MYELOSIS (DI GUGLIELMO'S DISEASE)

Uncontrolled proliferation of erythrocytic precursors as the sole proliferative abnormality is extremely rare. Only a few cases have been reported. This proliferative disorder eventually involves other marrow elements and is best classified as myelomonocytic leukemia.

EOSINOPHILIC LEUKEMIA

Eosinophilic leukemia, a rare disorder, is characterized by disorderly proliferation of eosinophilic elements. It should be noted that peripheral blood and marrow eosinophilia are not in themselves diagnostic. Abnormality in maturation is requisite for the diagnosis.

BASOPHILIC LEUKEMIA

Increased numbers of basophils are most commonly seen in patients with chronic granulocytic leukemia. However, a few patients have been described in whom abnormal proliferation of basophilic elements appears to have been the sole or at least major manifestation of the leukemic process.

MAST CELL LEUKEMIA

Mast cell leukemia, an unusual variety, is characterized by urticaria pigmentosa and excessive numbers of mast cells in the bone marrow, spleen, peripheral blood, and other tissues. Mast cell leukemia appar-

ently bears the same relationship to tissue mast cell disease that lymphosarcoma cell leukemia does to lymphosarcoma and monocytic leukemia
does to reticulum cell sarcoma.

MEGAKARYOCYTIC LEUKEMIA

The term megakaryocytic leukemia has been used by some to describe participation of megakaryocytes in a leukemic process. These
patients fall more correctly into such categories as myelomonocytic leukemia, chronic granulocytic leukemia, agnogenic myeloid metaplasia,
primary thrombocythemia, and polycythemia vera.

PLASMACYTIC LEUKEMIA

Patients with plasmacytic myeloma typically have occasional "myeloma cells" in their peripheral blood; rare patients have large numbers
and have been classified separately as plasmacytic leukemia. There is
no justification for differentiating these patients from those with the
usual type of plasmacytic myeloma (p. 411).

Lymphoma

Lymphoma is a generic term that refers to a group of diseases characterized by disorderly proliferation of lymphoid or extramedullary reticuloendothelial tissue. Several histologic types can be recognized, but similarities in clinical manifestations and therapy warrant collective consideration. Their progressive course, fatal outcome, and pathologic nature attest to the propriety of their classification as malignant neoplasms.

HISTORY

Credit for first directing attention to this group of diseases belongs to Thomas Hodgkin, who reported several patients in 1832. However, Hodgkin's article aroused little interest until Wilks brought the subject into sharper focus in 1856 and 1865 and suggested that the disorder be called Hodgkin's disease. Reference to large multinucleated cells was made by Langhans in 1872 and again by Greenfield in 1878, but these workers attached little significance to their presence. In 1898 Sternberg published a detailed description of the giant cells but concluded that the disease was a type of tuberculosis. In an erudite article published in 1902, Dorothy Reed clearly delineated Hodgkin's disease as a specific entity and accurately described its pathology, including the presence of the characteristic giant cells that now bear her name. Lymphosarcoma was recognized by Kundrat in 1893. Ewing described neoplastic proliferation of reticulum cells in 1913; this entity was named *retothelsarkom* or reticulum cell sarcoma by

Roulet in 1930. Brill and associates in 1925 and Symmers in 1927 described giant follicular lymphoma, but several years elapsed before it was recognized as a type of lymphoma. The protean manifestations of the lymphomas have been responsible for many descriptions which we now recognize as different forms of a single disease. It is of interest that mycosis fungoides (lymphomatous involvement of the skin) was described by Alibert in the early nineteenth century, a number of years before the other manifestations of lymphoma were recognized.

CLASSIFICATION

Classification of the malignant lymphomas has long been the subject of controversy. Differences in nomenclature and dispute concerning the origin and types of cells have added to the confusion. Attempts to establish rigid criteria for each subcategory serve no useful purpose. Indeed, current evidence indicates that each type may actually reflect a different host response to a similar stimulus. Transitional forms of lymphoma support this thesis, as does the evolution of giant follicular lymphoma into Hodgkin's disease or lymphosarcoma. Nevertheless, a histologic classification can usually be made and is clinically useful, especially insofar as prognosis and response to therapy are concerned. Such a classification is listed in Table 9-1. Since all lymphomas alter

Table 9-1. *Classification of the Lymphomas*

Histologic Type	Relative Frequency (%)
Hodgkin's disease	50
Lymphosarcoma	25
Reticulum cell sarcoma	10
Giant follicular lymphoma	5
Lymphocytic lymphoma	5
Unclassified	5

or destroy normal tissue architecture, differentiation must be based on cytology rather than on the more general histologic pattern of a malignant neoplasm.

Hodgkin's Disease. Hodgkin's disease is characterized by cellular heterogeneity and by complex and pleomorphic histology. Lymphocytes, neutrophils, eosinophils, plasmacytes, reticulum cells, monocytes, fibroblasts, and giant cells are present in variable numbers (Fig. 9-1). The giant Reed-Sternberg cells constitute the only cellular element that is morphologically distinct and pathognomonic of Hodgkin's disease; when studied singly, the other cells are without diagnostic features and do not differ from normal elements. Reed-Sternberg cells vary in size from 50 to 100 μ or more. Their cytoplasm is abundant, and the cell margins are frequently irregular. They contain single, multiple, or multilobed

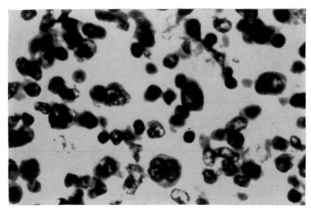

Figure 9-1. Fixed lymph node section from a patient with Hodgkin's disease (granuloma).

nuclei; very large nucleoli are typical. When imprints of involved tissue are stained with Wright's stain (a technique that permits detailed study of individual cell morphology), Reed-Sternberg cells are quite distinctive (Fig. 9-2). Variable degrees of fibrosis and necrosis complete the histologic picture.

It is generally agreed that Reed-Sternberg cells must be present before a diagnosis of Hodgkin's disease can be made. However, the other histologic components are quite variable, and Hodgkin's disease has been further divided into three subtypes:

1. Hodgkin's paragranuloma consists basically of lymphocytes and Reed-Sternberg cells. Clinically this type is earmarked by peripheral node enlargement and a relatively benign course.

2. Hodgkin's granuloma is the most common form and is distinguished by fewer lymphocytes plus plasmacytes, eosinophils, and Reed-Sternberg cells, together with necrosis and fibrosis. The clinical manifestations and course are variable. With the possible exception of the central nervous system, all tissues in the body may be involved.

3. Hodgkin's sarcoma is a highly invasive malignant process that affects all tissues and runs a rapidly progressive course. Histologically, the majority of the cells are two to three times the size of normal lymphocytes and display single nuclei and prominent nucleoli. They probably represent immature, atypical reticuloendothelial cells, that is, undifferentiated Reed-Sternberg cells.

The clinical importance of this pathologic classification is disputable. Although differences in clinical manifestations and prognoses are evident, the type and degree of clinical involvement must be determined

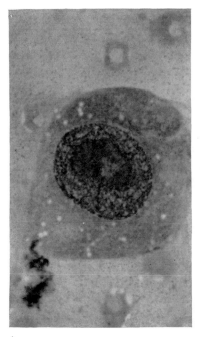

A

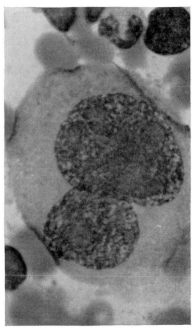

B

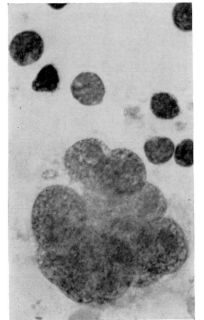

C

Figure 9-2. Reed-Sternberg cells
stained with Wright's stain. *A.*
Lymph node aspirate. *B.* Spleen
imprint. *C.* Aspirate from a skin
lesion.

for each patient and cannot be predicted from a pathologic picture. Furthermore, a relatively benign form may evolve without warning into a more malignant process, although the reverse probably never occurs. Therefore, this classification fails to permit uniformly accurate prognostication, which is difficult at best and dependent on many factors. It should also be noted that knowledge of the pathologic type of Hodgkin's disease is not requisite for the selection of appropriate therapy.

Lymphosarcoma. Lymphosarcoma is distinguished by the presence of atypical lymphocytic elements which vary in different patients from immature to relatively mature forms. In all cases, however, these cells differ from normal lymphoblasts, prolymphocytes, and lymphocytes and possess the attributes of lymphosarcoma cells (p. 376). These morphologic details are most evident in tissue imprints or node aspirates stained with Wright's stain and are often difficult to detect in fixed tissue sections (Fig. 9-3). Because of the limitations of the latter technique, confusion has been especially noticeable in the classification of lymphosarcoma, and this term has been used to include several other

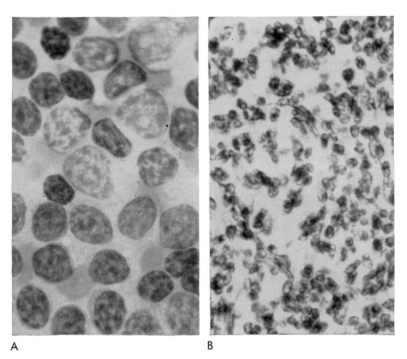

A   B

Figure 9-3. Lymphosarcoma involving a lymph node. *A.* Imprint stained with Wright's stain. *B.* Fixed tissue section stained with hematoxylin and eosin.

types of lymphoma; for example, "lymphocytic lymphosarcoma" (see lymphocytic lymphoma) and even "reticulum cell lymphosarcoma" (see reticulum cell sarcoma). Consequently, it is often difficult to be certain whether an author is referring to true lymphosarcoma (often designated "lymphoblastic lymphosarcoma") or to some other kind of lymphoma. If the same diagnostic significance is attached to the presence of lymphosarcoma cells in this disorder as to the Reed-Sternberg cells in Hodgkin's disease, this category of lymphomatous disease will be greatly clarified.

Reticulum Cell Sarcoma. This lymphoma variant is characterized by neoplastic proliferation of primitive mesenchymal or reticulum cells (Fig. 9-4). Malignant reticulum cells are specific entities closely related to monocytes or histiocytes and must be delineated from lymphocytes. They are two to four times the size of normal lymphocytes and possess relatively abundant cytoplasm and indistinct cell margins. Single nuclei are round, oval, or irregularly shaped, with finely reticulated nuclear chromatin creating the impression of lacework without points of condensation or the aggregation of nuclear chromatin so characteristic of

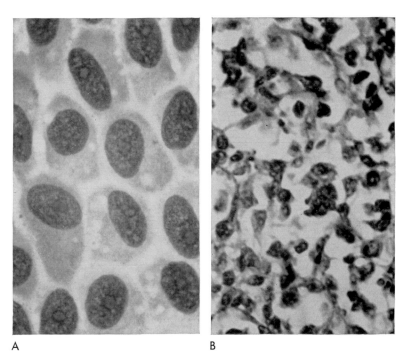

A   B

Figure 9-4. Reticulum cell sarcoma involving a lymph node. *A.* Imprint stained with Wright's stain. *B.* Fixed tissue section stained with hematoxylin and eosin.

lymphocytes. Occasionally, larger forms may be seen in which a multi-lobulated nucleus occupies most of the cell. Nucleoli are evident but are not as prominent as in Reed-Sternberg or lymphosarcoma cells. Because these tumors do not arise from cells of the lymphocytic series per se but rather from reticuloendothelial cells, the designation of lymphosarcoma, reticulum cell type is inappropriate and should be discarded. Certain lymphomas referred to by some writers as clasmatocytic and monocytic would appear to fall into this category.

Giant Follicular Lymphoma. Tightly packed masses of enlarged lymphoid follicles that fill the entire node, compress surrounding tissue, and display a tendency to fuse and destroy normal architecture characterize giant follicular lymphoma (Fig. 9-5). In fixed sections these

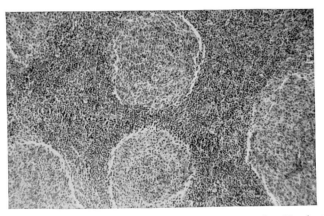

Figure 9-5. Giant follicular lymphoma in a lymph node (fixed tissue section stained with hematoxylin and eosin).

follicles are likely to "crack off"; although artifactual, this finding is of some diagnostic importance because it does not occur in simple lymphoid hyperplasia (the disorder with which giant follicular lymphoma is most likely to be confused). The centers of the follicles are filled with uniform, actively proliferating lymphocytes or their precursors. After variable periods of time, giant follicular lymphoma generally evolves into a more rapidly proliferating process such as Hodgkin's disease, lymphosarcoma, or lymphocytic leukemia. Therefore the histologic picture may be mixed and reflect two cellular patterns.

Lymphocytic Lymphoma. In lymphocytic lymphoma the proliferating cells are mature, morphologically normal lymphocytes. Although often classified as lymphocytic lymphosarcoma, it is preferable to consider this disease as a specific entity which bears the same relationship to chronic lymphocytic leukemia that lymphosarcoma does to lymphosarcoma cell leukemia (p. 376). Histologically, involved nodes are indistinguishable from those in patients with chronic lymphocytic leukemia unless a vessel is sectioned and a peripheral blood lymphocytosis is demonstrated in the leukemic node (Fig. 9-6). Giant or multinucleated cells are not seen.

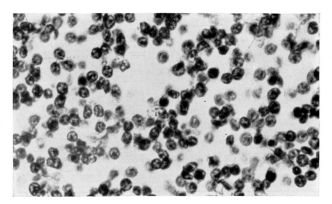

Figure 9-6. Lymphocytic lymphoma in a lymph node (fixed tissue section stained with hematoxylin and eosin).

Malignant Lymphoma, Type Unclassified. This category includes types that defy precise classification. Although relatively rare, highly malignant forms of lymphoma with undifferentiated cells do occur and must be recognized.

ETIOLOGY

The cause of the malignant lymphomas is unknown. Although histologically distinct, they may be etiologically related. Most of the mechanisms thought to participate in the pathogenesis of leukemia (p. 335) also appear applicable to the lymphomas (e.g., ionizing radiation and genetic factors). Because of the granulomatous nature of Hodgkin's disease and its resemblance to certain infectious granulomata, numerous attempts have been made to establish an infectious etiology. The possible role of the tubercle bacilli has received the attention of many investigators, but there is no convincing support that these or any other bacteria are of etiologic significance. A viral etiology has been proposed and, although not proved, remains the most promising lead. Several observations, which include, among others, the studies implicating a virus in the etiology of leukemia, the lymphoid hyperplasia that accompanies some viral infections such as infectious mononucleosis, and the demonstration of cytoplasmic inclusion bodies in certain lymphoma cells, support the tenability of such an hypothesis. Future studies along these lines may greatly clarify the pathogenesis of the lymphomas. At this time, however, they must be classified as malignant hematologic neoplasms, cause unknown.

PATHOPHYSIOLOGY

The clinical manifestations and functional disturbances attributable to the malignant lymphomas are similar for all histologic types and may be divided into three categories.

Local Proliferation with Tumefaction, Pressure Symptoms, and/or Organ Dysfunction. Lymph node enlargement and splenomegaly predominate, but in view of the widespread distribution of lymphoid and reticuloendothelial tissue, it is not surprising that the symptoms and findings are many and varied. Although frequently multicentric and eventually widely disseminated, the lymphomas are characterized, at least initially, by local tumor formation. The mechanisms determining the primary site of involvement (hence the major manifestations of the disease) are not known. One patient may have peripheral lymph node enlargement, another splenomegaly, others skin or bone lesions, and so forth. Indeed, the presence or absence of bone marrow involvement appears to constitute the chief if not the only difference between the lymphomas and certain leukemias. Leukemia and lymphoma both reflect uncontrolled proliferation of blood-forming tissues. In the leukemias the bone marrow is always involved and is responsible for most of the clinical manifestations. In the lymphomas bone marrow involvement is minimal or nil, and abnormalities in the peripheral blood and bone marrow are absent or nonspecific. However, certain patients with lymphoma do develop leukemic manifestations. Under these circumstances lymphosarcoma becomes lymphosarcoma cell leukemia (p. 375), reticulum cell sarcoma evolves into monocytic leukemia (p. 340), and lymphocytic lymphoma merges with chronic lymphocytic leukemia (p. 369). In some subjects with Hodgkin's disease, Reed-Sternberg cells are demonstrable in the marrow, and a few patients have been observed with similar cells in the peripheral blood (i.e., Reed-Sternberg cell leukemia). When a lymphomatous process becomes frankly leukemic, a diagnosis of lymphoma is no longer appropriate.

Systemic Manifestations. The nutritional and metabolic disturbances that accompany any malignant process are common in patients with lymphoma and are manifested by weakness, ease of fatigue, weight loss, fever, and increased sweating. By and large, these symptoms and findings are nonspecific and poorly explained. The heightened metabolic activity accompanying the disorderly cellular proliferation may play an important role.

Altered Cellular Function. Because many of the cells participating in a lymphomatous process are normally concerned with protein synthesis, it seems likely that certain quantitative and qualitative changes in serum proteins reflect altered cellular function. It is also reasonable to assume that cellular dysfunction may affect the production of antibodies (especially those concerned with tissue or cellular immunity), thereby explaining the increased susceptibility to certain infections as well as such immunologic defects as the commonly encountered cutaneous anergy to delayed-reacting antigens. Certain lymphoma cells can also be implicated in the production of "autoantibodies" or abnormal globulins that are responsible for the frequent occurrence of hemolysis or other types of hypersplenism in patients with lymphoma (p. 131).

CLINICAL MANIFESTATIONS

Although uncommon, the malignant lymphomas are not rare. In the United States there were 11,157 deaths, or 5.9 per 100,000 population, attributed to these disorders in 1963. Lymphoma has shown a progressive increase in incidence over the last few decades but to a lesser degree than leukemia (p. 341). It is difficult to ascertain the true frequency of each histologic type because of variability in nomenclature (some authors still use the term lymphosarcoma in a generic sense to include lymphosarcoma, lymphocytic lymphoma, and reticulum cell sarcoma). The histologic criteria for the diagnosis of Hodgkin's disease and giant follicular lymphoma are less disputable. Therefore information regarding their relative frequencies is more accurate. As shown in Table 9-1, Hodgkin's disease accounts for about half the cases. The lymphomas respect no age limits but are relatively rare under 15. In children lymphosarcoma is most common, although Hodgkin's disease does occur. Hodgkin's disease has its peak incidence in the third and fourth decades of life; lymphosarcoma occurs most often between the ages of 40 and 60. Reticulum cell sarcoma, giant follicular lymphoma, and lymphocytic lymphoma ordinarily have their onset between 50 and 70 years of age. Males are affected about twice as often as females. There are no race predilections. Although not true for other types, there is some evidence that the relatives of patients with Hodgkin's disease have a slightly greater chance of developing the disease than relatives of persons without Hodgkin's disease. At least two cases of Hodgkin's disease in identical twins have been reported. However, available data are certainly not convincing and, if heredity (or more likely environmental similarities) plays any role, it would appear to be a minor and indirect one.

Symptoms. Since the lymphomas affect all tissues, the symptoms are diverse. The onset is usually insidious but may be fulminant. In most patients the first sign of the disease is asymptomatic enlargement of cervical, axillary, and/or inguinal nodes; in a few persons the primary site of involvement is extranodal (e.g., tonsils, spleen, or gastrointestinal tract). Weight loss, ease of fatigue, weakness, fever, chills, tachycardia, and night sweats are systemic symptoms common to all types, especially in the far-advanced stages. In Hodgkin's disease fever (continuous, spiking, or intermittent) is particularly prominent and is often a major manifestation of the disease. Murchinson-Pel-Ebstein fever (recurrent or cyclic fever) occurs in less than 10 per cent of the patients, and its diagnostic importance has been overemphasized. After the ingestion of even small amounts of alcohol, about 15 per cent of the patients with Hodgkin's disease complain of the rapid onset of pain, which persists for minutes to hours at the site of active disease. This rather bizarre complaint is not limited to Hodgkin's disease and has been observed infrequently in patients with other lesions (e.g., fractures and other types of lymphoma or neoplasm). However, the association of alcohol-induced pain with Hodgkin's disease is such that it should arouse a high index of suspicion of this diagnosis. Generalized pruritus without demonstrable skin lesions occurs in 20 per cent or more of the patients with Hodgkin's disease but is much less common in the other forms of lymphoma; this symptom usually indicates widespread and deep-seated involvement.

Other symptoms lack diagnostic specificity and reflect the nature of the underlying lesion. For example, enlarged mediastinal nodes or involvement of the pulmonary parenchyma may produce cough or dyspnea; gastric lesions may mimic carcinoma of the stomach; bone lesions may cause pain, tenderness, or tumor formation; hematuria may be due to bladder infiltration; and neurologic complaints may reflect cord compression, involvement of peripheral or cranial nerves, meningeal invasion, or even lymphomatous proliferation in the cerebral cortex. Occasionally, the predominant symptoms are those of some complication such as an intercurrent infection. Because of the striking variability in manifestations of the lymphomas in different patients and in a single patient throughout the course of the disease, it serves no useful purpose to list all symptoms that have been observed or to assign relative frequencies to sites of involvement. It is more important to remember that no tissue is immune and any symptom is possible.

Physical Findings. Lymph node enlargement occurs in almost every patient with lymphoma. Any or all peripheral node-bearing areas as well as mediastinal and retroperitoneal nodes may be involved. Initially, the nodes are discrete and freely movable but may become matted and fixed as the capsules and contiguous tissues are invaded. As a rule, the overlying skin is not involved, and the nodes are seldom tender unless affected by a superimposed infection. Varying greatly in size, lymphomatous nodes are firm with a consistency best likened to hard rubber; they do not display the rocklike hardness that is characteristic of metastatic carcinoma. Splenomegaly is less common than lymphadenopathy and tends to reflect far-advanced and widespread disease; however, it occurs in about three fourths of the patients at some time during their illness. Occasionally the spleen is the primary site of involvement, especially in lymphosarcoma. Splenomegaly is most often slight to moderate, but massive enlargement can occur. Hepatomegaly is demonstrable in the majority of patients. Skin involvement is prominent in all types of lymphoma other than giant follicular; a variety of lesions may be encountered. Some patients with Hodgkin's disease exhibit a peculiar brownish pigmentation of the skin. Patients with extensive intradermal infiltration and tumor masses as the major or only manifestation of their disease are often classified separately under the heading of mycosis fungoides. Herpes zoster occurs in 10 per cent or more of patients with lymphoma.

Other physical findings reflect the site of lymphomatous proliferation and for the most part are not specific. Intrathoracic disease may be manifested by obstruction of the superior vena cava, bronchial occlusion and atelectasis, diffuse or nodular pulmonary infiltrations, or pleural effusion. If the thoracic duct is affected, the pleural fluid may be chylous, a finding highly suggestive of lymphoma. Chronic congestive heart failure or pericardial effusion is rare, even though the heart is commonly involved. Lymphomatous proliferation in the gastrointestinal tract (usually in the stomach) or enlarged retroperitoneal nodes may produce palpable abdominal masses. Ascites occurs and is often chylous, especially in giant follicular lymphoma. Jaundice develops in 10 to 15 per cent and is secondary to hepatic parenchymal involvement in 50 per cent or more of these patients; less often jaundice reflects an acquired hemolytic anemia, obstruction of bile ducts by strategically placed nodes, or serum hepatitis. Bone lesions may produce tenderness, a tumor mass, or a pathologic fracture. The commonest neurologic findings are those of cord compression (e.g., paraplegia and sensory losses) secondary to extradural tumor masses or compression fractures of involved vertebrae. Signs of meningeal involvement or of expanding intracranial lesions are rare.

Laboratory Findings. PERIPHERAL BLOOD. Early in the course of the disease, the peripheral blood is characteristically normal. Eventually, all patients develop hematologic abnormalities, but for the most part they lack specificity. A slight to moderate normocytic, normochronic anemia, the severity of which varies with the activity and extent of disease, is most common. The red blood cells show little anisocytosis or poikilocytosis and the reticulocyte count is usually normal. This kind of anemia appears to reflect a slight impairment in red cell viability consequent to a poorly defined extracorpuscular or extrinsic defect, coupled with relative bone marrow failure, that is, a marrow that is incapable of increasing erythropoiesis to a sufficient degree to maintain normal peripheral erythroid values. Rare patients with lymphoma manifest slight hypochromia, especially those with Hodgkin's disease. Although plasma iron is decreased in these individuals, their tissue iron stores are not depleted. The cause of such a hypochromic anemia is obscure, but it may be similar to that of the hypochromic anemia which occasionally accompanies chronic infection (p. 178). Occult hemolysis probably occurs to some degree in most patients. Overt hemolysis is less common, but it is certainly not an unusual occurrence. In fact, a hemolytic anemia may be a major manifestation of the disease and in some patients it even antedates other evidence of lymphoma. Such an acquired hemolytic anemia is typically manifested by spherocytes and other evidence of hemolysis in the peripheral blood (increased polychromasia, reticulocytosis, nucleated red cells, abnormal osmotic behavior, and decreased red cell survival times). Coombs' and bromelin tests are usually (but not always) positive.

In patients with active Hodgkin's disease, an elevated leukocyte count is a frequent finding. The leukocytosis (typically around 15,000 and seldom more than 25,000/cu mm) reflects a relative and absolute neutrophilia with increased numbers of band forms. An eosinophilia is encountered less often than is customarily believed to be the case. A few patients with striking eosinophilia have been described, but they are the exceptions. Even when eosinophils are increased they hardly ever account for more than 6 to 8 per cent of the leukocytes. Slight to moderate monocytosis is quite common with immature and toxic forms. The most consistent of the nonspecific leukocyte abnormalities in Hodgkin's disease is a relative and absolute lymphocytopenia, especially a small lymphocytopenia. BGN (basophilic granulation of the neutrophils) is generally quite evident. More often than not, the platelet count is increased in patients with active disease. When leukopenia and/or thrombocytopenia is present, it usually reflects the myelosuppressive effect of specific therapy or superimposed hypersplenism. Infrequently, extensive replacement of the marrow by Hodgkin's disease may cause leukopenia, thrombocytopenia, or a leukemoid reaction with slight reticulocytosis, immature granulocytes, and nucleated red cells in the peripheral blood, that is, a myelophthisic process (p. 241). In exceptional cases Reed-Sternberg cells appear in the peripheral blood (Fig. 9-7).

Leukocyte and platelet counts are ordinarily normal in the other types of lymphoma; however, one or both of these cellular elements may be depressed as the result of cytotoxic therapy or superimposed hypersplenism. A trained examiner can, as a rule, detect an occasional lymphosarcoma cell (p. 376) in the blood of a patient with lymphosarcoma, and some observers have called attention to circulating "hematogones" (a peculiar type of small lymphocyte with virtually no cytoplasm and a notched or cleft nucleus) in certain patients with giant follicular lymphoma. Thus the dividing line between leukemia and lymphoma is often indistinct. When the marrow changes become

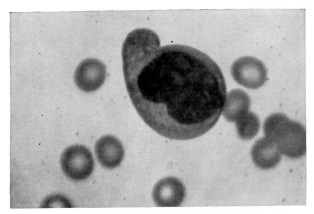

Figure 9-7. Reed-Sternberg cell in the peripheral blood of a patient with generalized Hodgkin's disease and extensive marrow involvement.

sufficiently marked to permit a diagnosis from the peripheral blood, the disorder should be classified as leukemia (see Chap. 8).

BONE MARROW. Initially, the marrow is normal in all types of lymphoma. As the disease progresses, quantitative changes are detectable, but consistent or diagnostic patterns are seldom observed. In Hodgkin's disease granulocytic and megakaryocytic hyperplasia are commonplace, and plasmacytes and eosinophilic elements are often increased, even though the circulating eosinophil count may be normal. It is unusual to observe the pathognomonic cell, that is, the Reed-Sternberg cell, in a routine marrow aspirate. Because necropsy data indicate that focal marrow lesions are common in Hodgkin's disease, serial marrow sections constitute a more rewarding approach. However, this technique does not permit retention of the morphologic detail needed to differentiate unequivocally Reed-Sternberg cells from other giant cells, most notably megakaryocytes and osteoclasts. Such delineation is relatively easy in Wright-stained marrow aspirates or imprints of biopsy specimens. The small and inconspicuous nucleoli, pachychromatic nuclei, and cytoplasmic granulation of megakaryocytes contrast strikingly with the large nucleoli, vesicular nuclear chromatin and absent or sparse granulation of Reed-Sternberg cells; osteoclasts are characterized by multiple small nuclei, each with a single small nucleolus (Fig. 9-8). In lymphosarcoma occasional lymphosarcoma cells are commonly detectable in the marrow. In giant follicular lymphoma the finding of "hematogones" has been stressed, but precise identification is difficult, and their true significance is conjectural. When present, hypersplenism is manifested by one or more of its characteristic marrow changes (p. 456).

OTHER LABORATORY FINDINGS. *Hyperuricemia* and an *elevated BMR* reflect abnormal cell proliferation. *Serum protein deviations* are common

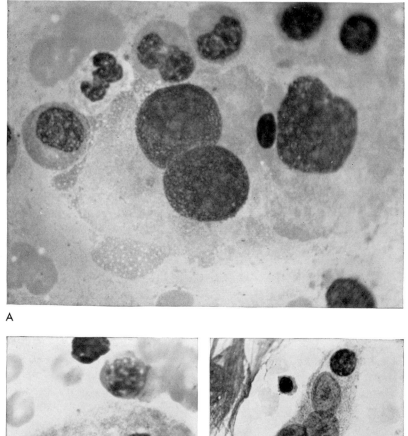

A

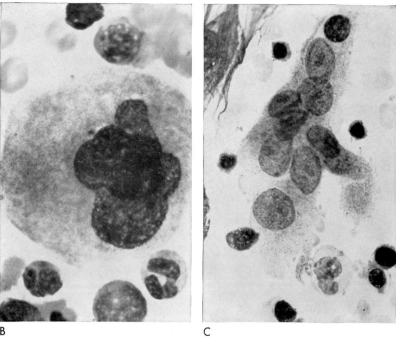

B   C

Figure 9-8. Giant cells in bone marrow aspirates (Wright's stain). *A.* Reed-
Sternberg cells. *B.* Megakaryocyte. *C.* Osteoclast.

but they lack specificity (decreased, albumin, increased globulins, or, rarely, hypogammaglobulinemia). In the presence of active disease, *tuberculin and other delayed-reacting skin tests are almost always negative.* Although most characteristic of Hodgkin's disease, patients with other lymphomas exhibit similar cutaneous anergy when their disease is generalized and symptomatic. This anergy is relative, and a sufficiently strong stimulus will elicit skin responsiveness. Thus active tuberculosis is usually associated with tuberculin positivity. Skin reactivity often returns during therapeutic remissions, particularly in patients with some form of lymphoma other than Hodgkin's disease. Other findings include varied manifestations of specific organ dysfunction (e.g., an increased serum alkaline phosphatase may be secondary to bone lesions or liver involvement; the latter may also be reflected by increased BSP retention, hyperbilirubinemia, or other evidence of hepatic dysfunction, etc.). *X-ray studies* are of great help in localizing disease. A chest film may reveal mediastinal adenopathy or parenchymal involvement, which may be diffuse or nodular. Cavitation of the lungs is most often caused by superimposed tuberculosis or a fungus infection, but it may follow necrosis of tumor tissue. Lymphoma of the gastrointestinal tract (especially the stomach) is detectable roentgenographically but cannot be distinguished from carcinoma. Intravenous pyelography occasionally reveals displacement due to retroperitoneal node enlargement. An abdominal flat plate or upper gastrointestinal tract x-ray may indicate otherwise unsuspected splenic enlargement, but careful palpation of the abdomen is normally more informative. Lymphangiography (visualization of lymph nodes following the intralymphatic injection of radiopaque substance) is a valuable technique for the demonstration of retroperitoneal node involvement. About two thirds of the bone lesions of lymphoma are mixed, osteolytic and osteoblastic; most of the remainder are osteolytic, but purely osteoblastic lesions have been described, particularly in Hodgkin's disease involving a vertebra. Compression fractures of the spine occur, but lymphoma rarely causes pathologic fractures of other bones.

DIAGNOSIS

In contrast to the importance of the findings in the peripheral blood and bone marrow in the diagnosis of leukemia (p. 351), the diagnosis of lymphoma, which by definition excludes extensive marrow involvement, is dependent on other parameters, most notably a fixed tissue section. An absolute diagnosis and differentiation between the various forms of lymphoma can be accomplished only by histologic study. In most patients a diagnosis of lymphoma is suggested by the symptoms, physical findings, and initial laboratory studies. Biopsy of an enlarged peripheral lymph node generally provides histologic confirmation. The node to be studied should be selected with careful attention to its location, size, and consistency. Whenever possible, inguinal nodes should be avoided because chronic lymphadenitis and atypical histology resulting from infections on the feet and legs are encountered frequently. Cervical, supraclavicular, or axillary nodes are preferred. Occasionally, it is necessary to biopsy more than one node before an unequivocal diagnosis can be made. In addition to routine sections, imprints of the excised node should be stained with Wright's or a similar polychrome stain. Although this technique does not permit demonstration of architectural changes, it does allow detailed study of individual cellular morphology with recognition of such abnormal elements as lymphosarcoma, metastatic carcinoma, and Reed-Sternberg cells. Similar preparations can be made from node aspirates or the cellular sediments of ascitic or pleural fluid (Fig. 9-9). The potential value of these simple

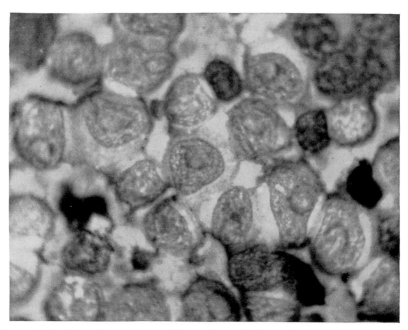

Figure 9-9. Lymphosarcoma cells in the cellular sediment of pleural fluid (Wright's stain).

diagnostic techniques has not been widely recognized; their use is strongly recommended.

When the peripheral blood is normal, it can be predicted with relative certainty that the marrow will also be normal. Even when the peripheral blood is abnormal, marrow findings are usually quantitative and lack specificity. Atypical cells (e.g., lymphosarcoma cells) may be noted, but they are not present in large enough numbers to be diagnostic unless the marrow involvement is sufficiently marked to be classified as leukemia. Under these circumstances the peripheral blood findings point clearly to a diagnosis of leukemia rather than lymphoma, thus making a marrow examination mandatory. An exception would be the demonstration of Reed-Sternberg cells in the marrow; if they can be identified with certainty, a single cell will confirm the diagnosis of Hodgkin's disease. However, Reed-Sternberg cells are rarely found in routine marrow specimens. Consequently, a bone marrow study is of little use in the diagnostic work-up of a patient with lymphoma but is of greater value in confirming the presence of superimposed hypersplenism and in evaluating the myelosuppressive effect of cytotoxic therapy.

In some patients the primary site of disease is not in the peripheral lymph nodes but in bone, liver, spleen, stomach, hilar or retroperitoneal nodes. Although tissue is harder to obtain under these circumstances, it should be emphasized that histologic proof of the diagnosis of lymphoma is still needed. When the only demonstrable involvement is mediastinal, a scalene or paratracheal node biopsy is often informative. If not, thoracotomy should be considered. In patients in whom lymphoma is suspected and abdominal or retroperitoneal involvement can be inferred by exclusion (e.g., no peripheral node enlargement or a negative chest x-ray) abdominal surgical exploration is indicated and will often clarify the picture. With the exception of certain preterminal patients, all possible attempts to obtain absolute confirmation of the diagnosis are indicated; the advantages of this diagnostic approach outweigh the risks. Because of the kind of agents used to treat lymphoma, there is no room for equivocation. When all diagnostic attempts fail or the tissue sections are only suggestive, continued observation will reveal the true nature of the disease within a short period of time without altering significantly the final outcome. Only in seriously ill patients in whom there is a very strong likelihood that lymphoma exists should consideration be given to the use of such specific therapy as x-ray or nitrogen mustard before diagnosis.

Because of the protean manifestations of the lymphomas, they mimic many diseases. Differential diagnosis is complex; all causes of lymph node enlargement, splenomegaly, fever, and so forth must be considered. Fortunately, the need for a biopsy is usually quite evident. Thus peripheral adenopathy due to lymphoma is differentiated on histologic criteria from metastatic carcinoma or sarcoidosis, even though the diagnosis might not have been clear on the basis of the clinical manifestations alone. The major problem in these cases is whether a palpable node is significantly abnormal. Several factors aid in this decision, including the size, consistency, and location of the nodes; for example, nodes in the femoral triangle, epitrochlear areas, or along the pectoral chains are less likely to be enlarged as the result of chronic lymphadenitis. Size alone is not a good criterion. Several 1- to 1.5-cm cervical nodes in an asymptomatic person assume added significance if the spleen is also palpable or if nodes of similar size are found in other areas. Each patient presents an individual problem. When any doubt exists, the suspected node should be biopsied.

Most of the diseases that simulate lymphoma have certain distinguishing characteristics of their own. Infectious mononucleosis (p. 316) deserves special mention because peripheral lymphadenopathy and splenomegaly are prominent features; however, other clinical manifestations, such as the acute onset, sore throat, and atypical lymphocytes, point to the need for additional diagnostic procedures (i.e., a heterophil agglutination test). Chronic congestive splenomegaly consequent to portal hypertension rarely causes confusion because of the evidence of cirrhosis or other findings of the primary disease. As a cause of "fever of unknown etiology," the differential diagnosis is less easy; all types of infectious and neoplastic diseases must be excluded. However, as long as the clinician thinks of lymphoma, demands histologic confirmation of the diagnosis, exhausts all attempts to establish it, and, if he fails, follows the patient closely, the diagnosis of lymphoma will not be missed and incorrect diagnoses will be few. In the presence of a disease that is obviously malignant it has been the tendency of some physicians not to require precise diagnosis. Because of the excellent responses to energetic treatment obtainable in so many patients with lymphoma, this approach cannot be sanctioned.

TREATMENT AND COURSE

Although the lymphomas run a progressive course that terminates in death, much can be accomplished by judicious treatment. In most patients symptoms can be alleviated; in many, life can be materially prolonged. Responses vary, but the principles of therapy are the same, regardless of the histologic picture. The dictum of successful management is early, energetic suppressive treatment. Inasmuch as therapy cannot effect a cure, disabling manifestations have been considered by some to be the only indication for treatment. Such a defeatist attitude is unwarranted. Treatment of disseminated disease is much less effective than treatment of localized disease. Furthermore, survival appears to be primarily dependent on the persistent pursuit of a well-planned program of specific suppressive therapy. Patients with lymphoma should be treated intensively every time there is anything to treat, provided no contraindication to treatment exists. Suppression of the proliferative process can be achieved by the application of ionizing radiation or the administration of a variety of chemotherapeutic agents.

Specific Therapy (Local Irradiation). *X-ray therapy* is the treatment of choice in all patients with lymphoma; chemotherapy serves as a valuable adjunct but does not displace x-radiation. Treatment should be directed at obvious sites of disease in an attempt to eradicate the lymphomatous process and to prevent, if possible, recurrence in the area treated. X-ray therapy was first used in the treatment of Hodgkin's disease by Pusey in 1902. Although its exact mode of action remains obscure, ionizing radiation interferes with mitosis, perhaps by inactivating some vital enzyme system; the result is an abnormality in DNA synthesis. Although suppression is most noticeable in rapidly proliferating neoplastic tissue, ionizing radiation does not discriminate between normal and abnormal cells, a fact that limits its use. All proliferating cells are affected, but some are more sensitive than others. Since hemopoietic cells possess the highest mitotic rates of any normal cells, they are the first to reflect excessive radiation.

If lymphoma cells were sensitive to levels of radiation far below those that affect normal cells, treatment would be simplified. Unfortunately, doses that exceed the tolerance of many normal tissues are needed to achieve satisfactory control over the lymphomatous process. Even larger amounts are needed to prevent local recurrence of disease. Therefore treatment must be planned carefully to inflict as little damage as possible to normal tissue. Restriction of the field and shielding of vital organs such as the kidneys and gonads minimize undesirable effects. Fractionation of the dose and interrupted therapy to allow partial recovery are also helpful, but the cumulative effect eventually precludes further treatment. Although lymphomatous tissue is generally radiosensitive, 3000 to 5000 r given over a period of three to five weeks are required to prevent local recurrence of disease. If it were possible to treat all sites of disease with doses of this magnitude, a "cure" could theoretically be achieved. However, this amount of x-radiation will cause irreparable damage to many normal tissues (the kidneys can tolerate only about 2300 r in five weeks without incurring severe to complete loss of function). Because of the widespread distribution of the tissues affected by lymphoma, it is necessary to limit treatment to a suboptimal generalized suppressive effect or to give intensive local therapy to areas of obvious involvement. The best results are obtained with the latter approach.

The diagnosis of lymphoma is an indication for therapy. Although treatment programs must be individualized, certain generalizations are justified. Specific details are the prerogative of the radiotherapist, but the general program should be a collaborative decision. The area to be treated determines the daily and total dose. A portal dose of 3000 to 3500 r given over a period of three to four weeks to a peripheral node-bearing area is well tolerated and rarely followed by recurrence locally. After 2000 r or less, local recurrence is to be expected. Disease in sites other than the peripheral node-bearing areas cannot be given sufficient irradiation to prevent local recurrence because of the limits imposed by the radiosensitivity of certain vital organs. It has been recommended by some that adjacent node areas be treated even though they do not contain detectable disease; for example, inclusion of the upper mediastinum in a patient with cervical and supraclavicular node involvement. Proponents of this approach have claimed excellent results. However, it is not known whether a lymphoma metastasizes like a carcinoma or whether the unknown stimulus persists and affects lymphoid and reticuloendothelial tissue in different sites at different times. Most students of the disease view lymphoma as a multicentric process arising in various loci at different times rather than spreading from a single focus. If this assumption is correct, there would be little to gain by treating an area of anticipated disease, unless the subsequent development of lymphoma at that site could be prevented. Doses of this magnitude cannot be administered to the chest or abdomen. Furthermore, because of exposure to normal tissues, prophylactic irradiation will seriously curtail the amount of treatment that can be applied in the future when overt disease becomes evident. Therefore it seems preferable to await locally demonstrable disease before initiating local x-ray therapy.

Marrow depression is the commonest toxic manifestation of ionizing radiation. Leukopenia precedes thrombocytopenia. Significant anemia is unusual after exposure to therapeutic x-ray; however, reticulocytopenia is often the first sign of myelosuppression. Some toxicity is acceptable because of the prognosis of the basic disease and the possible benefits to be obtained, but the undesirable side effects should be kept minimal and reversible. Irreversible marrow aplasia is too great a price to pay, even though the lymphoma is brought under control. It is necessary to balance the toxic and therapeutic effects carefully. To decide when the toxic outweigh the therapeutic requires astute clinical evaluation. In general, the white count should never be allowed to fall below 2000 or the platelets below 100,000/cu mm; but many factors must be considered, including the amount and types of prior therapy, areas being treated, rapidity of the fall, and the pretreatment counts. It is impossible to measure the marrow reserve accurately, and, even though it may be decreased, it is permissible to continue treatment as long as the peripheral neutrophil and platelet counts are maintained. If significant marrow depression develops, temporary cessation of treatment may permit sufficient recovery so that treatment can be resumed at a lower daily dose without further untoward reaction. Since hypersplenism may be manifested by leukopenia and/or thrombocytopenia, this complication must be excluded by appropriate studies (p. 460). If neutropenia or thrombocytopenia is shown to be caused by hypersplenism, continued suppressive therapy is not necessarily precluded. Anorexia, nausea, and vomiting constitute the only other immediate effects of x-ray therapy of any significant import. They are ordinarily alleviated by decreasing the daily dose or restricting the field or by some antiemetic agent. Gastrointestinal symptoms are absent or mild in patients receiving corticosteroids. It would be most exceptional, however, for radiation sickness to be so severe that it alone would warrant the risk of the undesirable side effects of corticosteroid therapy.

Giant follicular lymphoma, the most radiosensitive, is followed by Hodgkin's disease, lymphocytic lymphoma, lymphosarcoma, and reticulum cell sarcoma. Some variability is evident, however, even among patients with similar histologic pictures. The stage of the disease is also an important factor because all patients eventually become refractory to therapy, regardless of how good their initial responses might have been. Relief of symptoms and regression of tumor masses may be prompt or the maximal effect may not be realized until four to six weeks after treatment is completed. Because maximal marrow depression may not occur until after the treatment is completed, premature application of additional suppressive therapy (another course of x-ray or nitrogen mustard) can produce serious cumulative toxicity. With rare exceptions, patients should not be retreated for at least three weeks and preferably longer if there is any question of the state of marrow activity. As a rule, the faster the response, the shorter the remission. Following treatment, all patients should be re-evaluated at one- to three-month intervals. Retreatment is indicated as soon as recurrent activity of the disease becomes evident. In this regard it must be borne in mind that all symptoms and findings may not be due to lymphoma. For example, fever consequent to an intercurrent infection may be misinterpreted as active lymphoma, thus resulting in the use of cytotoxic therapy rather than the appropriate antibiotic. It can be concluded that the lymphoma is at fault only after all other causes have been excluded (e.g., tuberculosis in the case of a cavitary lesion in the lung).

Early in the course of the disease, most patients with lymphoma will respond favorably to local x-ray therapy with relief of symptoms and disappearance of tumor masses. However, it is not always possible to eradicate all clinical manifestations, especially in generalized or far-advanced disease. Under these circumstances, it is necessary to accept less than an optimal response because persistent treatment will lead to serious toxicity. X-ray therapy should be continued until an indication for chemotherapy arises. Chemotherapy, which, in effect, is a contraindication to further x-radiation, includes (1) disease that is no longer responsive to x-ray; (2) local changes that preclude additional x-radiation (e.g., skin changes, pulmonary fibrosis, or total therapy approaching the level of tolerance for such vital organs as the gastrointestinal tract or kidneys); (3) disease so generalized that it is not feasible to treat all involved areas; and (4) lesions encroaching on the spinal cord, vena cava, or trachea that may cause serious compression or occlusion due to postradiation edema (swelling is generally less marked with chemotherapy). The first two contraindications are easily recognized; it is obviously impractical as well as dangerous to continue to treat disease that shows no response or progresses under treatment. Objective findings such as skin lesions or the knowledge that further treatment may be expected to produce irreversible damage to the kidneys or other vital organs preclude additional x-ray therapy. It is more difficult to decide when the disease is too generalized to be treated with local irradiation. Methods have been devised to stage or classify the disease in an attempt to aid in this decision. However, each patient presents an individual problem, and it appears highly artificial to select treatment on this arbitrary basis. Even though disease is limited to the retroperitoneal area, prior treatment to tolerance may prevent additional x-radiation. Conversely, multiple areas may be treated successfully by localized x-ray in a previously untreated patient. If the treatment period will exceed six weeks, if the patient appears preterminal, or if some but not all of the sites of disease can be treated, it is best to employ systemic therapy. Otherwise, x-ray remains the treatment of choice. In regard to the fourth indication for systemic therapy, a chemotherapeutic agent is less likely to evoke significant edema of tumor tissue, although small fractionated doses of x-ray are equally safe.

Specific Therapy (Systemic). After it has been decided that x-ray therapy is contraindicated, one of the *alkylating agents* becomes the treatment of choice. The leukopenic and myelosuppressive effects of mustard gas were first noted in 1917 during World War I. The initial clinical trials of a nitrogen analog of sulfur mustard in the treatment of malignant disease were conducted in 1942. The therapeutic effectiveness of these compounds in the lymphomas has since been proved clearly by extensive clinical experience. Methyl *bis* (β-chloroethyl) amine hydrochloride (Fig. 9-10) or HN2 (a chemical warfare designation)

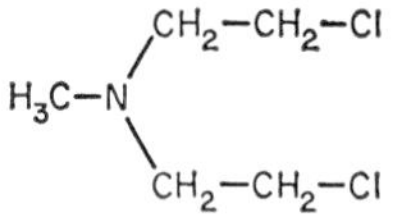

$$H_3C-N\underset{CH_2-CH_2-Cl}{\overset{CH_2-CH_2-Cl}{<}}$$

methyl-bis(β-chloroethyl) amine hydrochloride

NITROGEN MUSTARD; HN2; MECHLORETHAMINE *(Mustargen)*

Figure 9-10.   Structural formula of nitrogen mustard (HN2).

has been most widely used. In neutral or alkaline aqueous solution the tertiary amine undergoes intramolecular change with release of a chloride ion and formation of a cyclic quaternary ethylenimonium compound, which is a highly active alkylating agent that can react with many inorganic ions and organic radicals. Ionization occurs within a few minutes. In the absence of other anions, first one and then the other chloroethyl group reacts with water; the dihydroxy compound that results is chemically inactive. Therefore HN2 is unstable in aqueous solution and is inactivated shortly after its administration. However, the biologic effects of its brief period of chemical activity are much longer lasting.

The nitrogen mustards are mitotic poisons, but the exact manner by which they impede cell proliferation is not known. Although HN2 can inhibit a variety of enzyme systems, its in vivo effect appears to involve inactivation of DNA and interference with the anabolism of this vital nuclear constituent, thus rendering the cells incapable of proliferation. The proclivity of the nitrogen mustards to inhibit mitosis is similar to the biologic effect of ionizing radiation and warrants their classification as radiomimetic agents. The cytotoxic effect of these compounds is not specific; all proliferating cells are susceptible to their action.

HN2, or mechlorethamine (Mustargen), is marketed as a white crystalline solid, 10 mg to a vial. It should be diluted with sterile saline just before use and the predetermined dose injected into the tubing of a free-flowing intravenous infusion of normal saline. The usual dose is 0.4 to 0.6 mg/kg, divided into two to four daily doses; in most adults 10 mg daily for three days is an acceptable course of therapy. Immediate toxic side effects consist of a chemical thrombophlebitis (usually obviated when injected into a rapid intravenous infusion) and nausea and vomiting. The latter vary in severity but occur in most patients within one to three hours and persist for several hours. These symptoms, severest with the first injection, decrease in intensity with subsequent treatments; they are absent or markedly diminished in patients who are receiving corticosteroids. Several other drugs allay gastrointestinal symptoms, for example, chlorpromazine (25 mg four hours before the first injection and every six hours during the course of treatment) or sodium phenobarbital (0.1 gm intramuscularly at the time of the HN2 injection with repetition as needed in six hours). The delayed toxic effects of HN2 are hematologic. Because hemic precursors are the most rapidly proliferating normal cells in the body, it is reasonable to expect marrow depression after the administration of a general mitotic poison. Although a measurable decrease in circulating blood cells is usual, the myelosuppressive effect of therapeutic doses of HN2 is usually transient and reversible. Serious or permanent marrow hypoplasia is rarely encountered unless the marrow reserve has been exhausted by prior treatment or the dose is excessive. Reticulocytopenia and lymphopenia occur first and are followed by neutropenia. The maximal depression in circulating leukocytes occurs between the tenth and fourteenth days; however, the maximum fall in platelets may not be observed for 21 days. A significant decrease in the erythroid values is uncommon. After a course of HN2, recovery of bone marrow function can be expected within four to six weeks.

Symptomatic relief is often evident within a few hours, although the maximum benefit may not occur for three to four weeks. Fever may disappear after a single injection of HN2, and pruritus is often alleviated quickly. The therapeutic effect may last for days, weeks, months, or even years. As a rule, however, remissions induced by HN2 are shorter than those produced by x-radiation. Patients usually respond to subsequent courses of HN2, but it is essential that the marrow recover fully before additional treatment is given. When pleural effusion or ascites are major problems, HN2 may be injected directly into the pleural or abdominal cavities. Following removal of most but not all of the fluid, a single instillation of HN2 equivalent to 0.3 mg/kg is made. The patient is then encouraged to assume a variety of positions to ensure dilution with the remaining fluid and adequate exposure of serosal surfaces. Systemic effects such as bone marrow depression are unusual, probably because of chemical inactivation before absorption.

Contraindications to HN2 are (1) marrow depression secondary to prior treatment and (2) disease that has proved resistant to HN2. Leukopenia, thrombocytopenia, and/or anemia do not preclude the administration of HN2 when due to marrow involvement by the lymphoma or to hypersplenism; however, when cytopenia is secondary to previous cytotoxic therapy, serious and possibly fatal marrow depression may be expected if further suppressive therapy is applied. As with x-ray therapy, patients eventually become unresponsive to HN2, even though they once responded well. Continued administration of this agent may then cause serious toxicity and hasten death rather than prolong life. This state of therapeutic refractoriness usually heralds the end. If marrow function permits, some other chemotherapeutic agent may be tried; otherwise, terminal support is all that is left to offer the patient. Contrary to a once widely held view, jaundice and liver disease do not constitute contraindications to the administration of HN2.

Several hundred chemical congeners of HN2 have been synthesized and evaluated for their oncolytic effects. Most have had a low therapeutic index, and none has been shown to be superior to HN2, which remains the chemotherapeutic agent of choice for the treatment of lymphoma. Because HN2 must be given intravenously, an orally effective agent would appear to offer certain advantages. In addition to the ease of administration, such a drug would permit continuous suppressive maintenance therapy, a theoretically desirable but disputable advantage. *Triethylenemelamine* (TEM) was the first oral compound subjected to widespread use. However, the absorption of TEM is quite variable.

As a result, severe toxicity (irreversible marrow aplasia) was encountered too commonly. Since the therapeutic index of TEM is not superior to other less toxic agents, this drug should be abandoned. The absorption of *chlorambucil* (Leukeran), an aromatic mustard (p. 373), is much more uniform and its toxicity is much less, but the therapeutic effect accrues slowly. Although occasional patients with lymphoma respond to daily doses of 0.2 mg/kg, chlorambucil has found its greatest use in the treatment of chronic lymphocytic leukemia. *Cyclophosphamide* (Cytoxan) has proved to be more valuable. It is an inactive cyclic phosphamide ester of nitrogen mustard that is apparently activated intracellularly by phosphamidase (Fig. 9-11). Since malignant cells

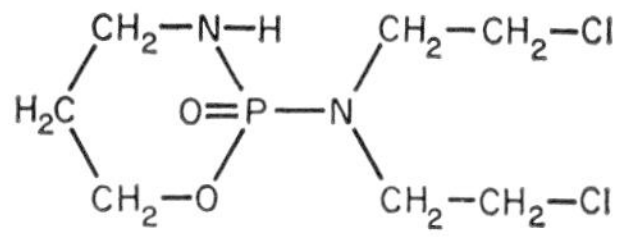

2-[bis(2-chloroethyl)amino]-1,3,2-oxazaphosphoridine,2-oxide
CYCLOPHOSPHAMIDE *(Cytoxan)*

Figure 9-11. Structural formula of cyclophosphamide (Cytoxan).

appear to contain increased phosphamidase activity, it was hoped that cyclophosphamide might have a more selective effect on malignant cells than HN2. However, experience to date indicates that it has a therapeutic spectrum quite similar to but no better than HN2 and with comparable toxicity. Therefore, intravenous cyclophosphamide offers no advantage over HN2. Oral cyclophosphamide allows continuous suppressive therapy not permitted by HN2, but the superiority of this regimen has yet to be proved and important questions concerning dosage have been asked. Certain data indicate that most, if not all, of the polyfunctional alkylating agents have comparable biologic activities and that differences in therapeutic effects and toxic manifestations reflect the dose used and the method of administration (i.e., interrupted courses versus maintenance therapy). The suggested oral dose of cyclophosphamide is 3.5 mg/kg daily until maximum tumor response is achieved or toxicity becomes evident. The drug should then be stopped or reduced to maintenance levels of 1.0 to 1.5 mg/kg/day. Leukopenia is usually the first sign of toxicity, and criteria for stopping or altering therapy are similar to those already described for x-radiation. Alopecia and hematuria occur in a significant number of patients. Hair growth is restored when the drug is stopped; hematuria can usually be prevented by maintaining a high urine output during treatment. Further evaluation is needed before the relative therapeutic effectiveness of HN2 and oral cyclophosphamide can be accurately assessed.

Although chemotherapy has much to offer the patient with lymphoma, it has not supplanted x-radiation. It is pertinent to consider the reasons for this statement, for chemotherapy is often recommended or used in the absence of a proper indication. Theoretical advantages of systemic chemotherapy include simplicity and the opportunity to exert a suppressive effect on *all* lymphoma tissue, evident and undetectable. Even though most patients with lymphoma will respond to an alkylating agent (regardless of the stage of their disease or the extent of involvement), the response is usually less complete and almost always shorter than that induced by x-ray therapy. Because these drugs are radiomimetic agents, their effects can justifiably be likened to that of total body x-radiation. Whereas 3000 r or more can be given to several restricted peripheral ports without serious side effects, a dose of 600 to 700 r to the whole body is fatal. It then follows that to obtain a local effect comparable to regional x-ray with an alkylating agent one would have to administer a lethal amount of the drug. Recurrent disease is likely after treatment with 2000 r or less; therefore recurrent disease can be expected after a standard course of treatment with HN2 or some similar compound.

Suboptimal therapy to sites of obvious disease is too great a price to pay for the speculative advantage of suppressing (also suboptimally) hidden or microscopic foci of lymphoma. For this reason x-radiation should be used until the disease reaches a stage at which a lesser therapeutic response must be accepted. Even multiple sites of disease do not always represent an indication for chemotherapy. In some previously untreated patients it is possible to irradiate virtually all peripheral node-bearing areas as well as the mediastinum and retroperitoneal area. Until absolutely necessary these patients should not be deprived of this greater tumorlytic effect. A combination of x-ray and HN2 or cyclophosphamide has been used in selected patients with excellent results, but this approach is limited because the toxic effects of these different types of therapy are cumulative. In certain acutely ill patients in whom an immediate effect is desired or in others with widely disseminated disease, HN2 may be followed by x-radiation to the remaining major sites of disease. Even in these patients, however, it is desirable to wait two or three weeks after treatment with HN2 to permit the marrow to recover at least partly. Because of the potential seriousness of the toxic effects of combined therapy, it cannot be advised as routine treatment.

Other chemotherapeutic agents have been recommended from time to time; most are quite toxic, and none has been found to be superior to HN2 or cyclophosphamide. Although an occasional patient will respond to agents such as vinblastine (Velban), a plant alkaloid, use of this or similar drugs should be restricted to patients who have become refractory to the more conventional forms of therapy and who still have an adequate marrow reserve. HN2 or cyclophosphamide will induce excellent therapeutic responses in the majority of patients in whom chemotherapy is indicated. Until a new agent is proved to be therapeutically more efficacious, with comparable or less toxicity, its use in a patient still responsive to x-ray, HN2, or cyclophosphamide is difficult to condone.

Other Types of Therapy. *Corticosteroids* do not exert a clear-cut suppressive effect on the malignant lymphomas, despite their propensity to produce lymphocytopenia. Consequently, these compounds should not be used as the sole form of treatment, even though most recipients do exhibit symptomatic relief.

Much has been written about the role of *surgery* in the management of the patient with lymphoma. Although dispute continues, there is no compelling support for the contention that lymphoma spreads from a unicentric origin. It seems more likely that the stimulus to the disorderly proliferation persists, even though the only evident focus of disease is removed surgically, and that at a later time the process will again manifest itself. Protagonists of the surgical approach cite relatively high five-year survival rates after removal of a lymphomatous lesion. However, patients with localized disease survive for equivalent periods of time after x-ray therapy. Furthermore, frequent examples of recurrent disease at a later date can be found in the apparent "five-year cures." Therefore surgery should be limited to that needed to establish the diagnosis. Available data do not justify such extensive procedures as radical neck dissections. Even though all apparent disease is removed surgically (e.g., a gastrectomy for a suspected carcinoma which turns out to be a lymphoma), the area should still be irradiated as though active disease were present.

Complications. Organ dysfunction attributable to lymphomatous proliferation generally indicates the need for cytotoxic therapy. *Spinal cord compression,* however, constitutes a specific problem and must be handled separately. Symptoms of cord involvement are usually the result of an epidural tumor mass and should be evaluated with dispatch. In addition to a careful neurologic examination, a lumbar puncture (spinal fluid protein may be markedly increased), spine x-rays, and myelograms are indicated. In the face of evidence of a compressing lesion, surgical decompression should be carried out if at all possible. In view of the fatal prognosis, some are loath to attack this problem surgically and advise instead x-ray or HN2. This approach cannot be supported. If paraplegia is to be avoided, immediate action is required. Because some patients live for several years after such an episode, any procedure that may prevent paraplegia is warranted. Although symptoms may progress slowly and in retrospect have often been present for some time, the actual complication (i.e., threatened transection of the cord) usually occurs rapidly and should be handled as an emergency. The longer a laminectomy is delayed, the less chance there is of recovering function. After decompression, x-ray therapy should be directed to the involved area. If for some reason surgery is deemed inadvisable, care must be taken so that post-treatment edema does not precipitate transverse myelitis. Such a patient should be given HN2 followed by x-ray or x-ray should be administered in titrated doses with small daily increments as tolerated.

Infections constitute a frequent and serious complication. Although patients with lymphoma can elaborate humoral antibodies in response to appropriate antigenic stimuli, they manifest definite alterations in tissue immune defense mechanisms. The incidence of tuberculosis has long been known to be increased in persons with lymphoma. The immunologic defect responsible for a negative tuberculin reaction is relative. If the stimulus is sufficiently strong, skin responsiveness can be elicited. Therefore a positive tuberculin reaction in a patient with lymphoma is presumptive evidence of active tuberculosis. Infections with fungi ordinarily of low infectivity are fairly common (e.g., moniliasis, cryptcoccosis, aspergillosis, histoplasmosis, and coccidioidomycosis). Torulosis, or infection with *Cryptococcus neoformans*, a saprophyte in nature, is of interest. Although the over-all occurrence of clinical cryptococcosis is quite low, it develops with some frequency in patients with lymphoma and must always be excluded in the presence of central nervous system symptoms or evidence of meningeal involvement. The increased incidence of herpes zoster deserves special mention. Altered immune mechanisms probably play a major role, although involvement of nerve roots by the tumor or activation of a latent virus by specific suppressive therapy may be additional factors in some patients. Occasionally herpes zoster becomes generalized and is indistinguishable from varicella. Current data indicate that the viruses of herpes zoster and varicella are probably identical and that relative immunity governs the clinical picture. Thus the individual with little or no immunity develops varicella, with partial immunity, herpes zoster, and with complete immunity, no apparent disease. Neutropenia consequent to cytotoxic therapy often contributes to an increased number of bacterial infections. Corticosteroids, which so many of these patients receive, also exert a deleterious effect on cellular reactions and immune mechanisms and lead to an enhanced susceptibility to infection.

Although an obstructive *uric acid uropathy* occurs more commonly in leukemia, it is seen occasionally in patients with lymphoma, especially after cytotoxic therapy. The most effective means of treating this complication is to prevent its occurrence (p. 361).

Hypersplenism is a common complication. A hemolytic component can be recognized in most patients with a lymphoma at some time during their disease, but it is usually occult and detectable only by careful study. In certain patients hypersplenism (hemolysis, neutropenia, and/or thrombocytopenia) constitutes an important and sometimes major manifestation of the disease. Hypersplenic activity is not directly related to activity of the disease and may antedate other evidence of lymphoma by months or even years. In fact, it is not uncommon for this complication to appear after suppressive therapy has been given, perhaps as a result of cellular destruction with release of large quantities of preformed abnormal globulins. Therapy of hypersplenism consists of corticosteroids and, in selected patients, splenectomy (p. 462). If active lymphoma is present, specific suppressive therapy is indicated. Some patients will show amelioration of hypersplenism after such treatment; however, if it continues unabated after systemic therapy, the peripheral blood cell counts may fall rapidly because marrow output will be immediately curtailed.

Pregnancy does not aggravate lymphoma, and lymphoma does not appear to affect ovulation, fertility, or the course of pregnancy adversely. Therefore interruption of pregnancy is seldom, if ever, indicated because of a diagnosis of lymphoma. It should be noted, however, that the therapeutic agents employed in the treatment of lymphoma may exert a deleterious effect on the fetus, especially during the first trimester.

A variety of *other diseases* may complicate the course of lymphoma, but they do not appear to be etiologically related and must be viewed as coincidental occurrences (e.g., a second malignancy).

General Supportive Measures. Patients with lymphoma require general support throughout all phases of their illness. Regardless of the completeness of response to specific therapy, regularly scheduled checkups are essential so that additional treatment can be given as soon as recurrent disease becomes evident. Terminally, these individuals present problems similar to those encountered in any patient with disseminated malignant disease. Supportive measures include maintenance of adequate fluid and caloric intake, relief of pain, and transfusions as needed to maintain satisfactory erythroid values (i.e., a hemoglobin of 8 to 10 gm/100 ml). Corticosteroids are invaluable when this stage of the disease is reached, and, unless specifically contraindicated, they should be given to all such patients for whatever symptomatic relief can be obtained (e.g., decrease in fever and pruritus and increase in appetite and sense of well-being). The recommended initial dose is 15 mg of prednisone (or its equivalent) every six hours (60 mg/day); as soon as the desired response is achieved, the dose should be tapered to the smallest amount capable of maintaining that effect.

Prognosis. Although all the lymphomas are progressive and ultimately fatal, there is great variability in response to therapy and duration of life, even among patients with similar histologic pictures. Thus one patient with Hodgkin's disease may live for less than a year, whereas another may survive for more than 30 years. In order of decreasing responsiveness to specific therapy are giant follicular lymphoma, Hodgkin's disease, lymphocytic lymphoma, lymphosarcoma, and reticulum cell sarcoma. The literature abounds with average or median survival times, but differences in nomenclature render interpretation of these data difficult. The median survival time for giant follicular lymphoma would appear to be about 5 years, for Hodgkin's disease, 4 years, for lymphocytic lymphoma, 3 years, for lymphosarcoma, 1.5 years, and for reticulum cell sarcoma, about 1 year. Approximate five-year survival rates are (1) giant follicular lymphoma, 50 per cent, (2) Hodgkin's disease, 30 per cent, (3) lymphocytic lymphoma, 20 per cent, (4) lymphosarcoma, 15 per cent, and (5) reticulum cell sarcoma, 10 per cent. A significant number of patients with giant follicular lymphoma or Hodgkin's disease can be expected to be alive 10 years after the diagnosis is made; the patient with lymphosarcoma or reticulum cell sarcoma who is alive at 10 years is a distinct exception.

Knowledge of the form of lymphoma permits some generalization of the expected course, but it is often difficult to distinguish at the onset of the disease between the patient who will live for years and the one who will die within a few months. Early accurate predictions are rarely possible. Even the histologic picture may be misleading because it can change without warning; for example, giant follicular lymphoma may evolve into Hodgkin's disease, lymphosarcoma, or, less often, reticulum cell sarcoma. The prognosis then becomes that of the more rapidly progressive disease. A number of attempts have been made to attach prognostic significance to certain clinical manifestations such as the presence or absence of splenomegaly at the time of diagnosis. None of these parameters has proved to be an infallible indicator of things to come. Perhaps one of the most valuable signs is early dissemination; that is, the more generalized the disease, the poorer the prognosis. However, exceptions to this rule are not hard to find. The longest survival times correlate best with a well-planned program of suppressive therapy energetically and persistently pursued, irrespective of histologic type or extent of disease. Therefore precise prognosis cannot be made at the time of diagnosis, and a more accurate prediction can usually be made after the response to initial therapy is known. Although an ultimately fatal group of diseases, guarded optimism is justified.

Plasmacytic Myeloma

Plasmacytic myeloma is a malignant neoplasm primarily involving the bone marrow. Although often referred to as multiple myeloma, there is no longer any doubt that the "myeloma cell" is an immature, atypical plasmacyte. In most patients subleukemic plasmacytic leukemia would be a more accurate designation, but myeloma is, by common usage, closely associated with this disorder. Therefore plasmacytic myeloma is recommended as an appropriate name to encompass all forms of the disease. Nonspecific terms such as multiple myeloma and myelomatosis should be discarded.

HISTORY

Plasmacytic myeloma was first recognized as a specific entity in 1845 by Watson and MacIntyre. The histology of the bone tumors in their patient was described by Dalrymple the following year. In 1847 Henry Bence Jones, the chemist, published his observations on the unique protein contained in this patient's urine. Rustizky introduced the term multiple myeloma in 1873, but there was little interest in this disease before Kahler's detailed description in 1889. In the same year Ellinger first called attention to the increased serum proteins and formation of rouleaux. In 1900 Wright concluded that the myeloma cells were identical with or closely related to plasma cells, although attempts to classify the disease into "myeloblastic" or "lymphoblastic" types continued. Electrophoretic techniques were applied to the study of plasmacytic myeloma by Longsworth in 1939; these procedures have facilitated diagnosis and contributed greatly to our understanding of the pathophysiology of this disease. More recently the discovery of a transmissible plasmacytic tumor in mice has permitted a variety of basic experimental observations.

ETIOLOGY

The cause of plasmacytic myeloma is unknown. It cannot be related to trauma, and there is no evidence that heredity or environmental similarities play a role. Certain findings, most notably cytoplasmic inclusion bodies, tend to implicate a virus, but this attractive thesis lacks experimental support. A variety of chromosome abnormalities has been observed without a consistent pattern. Once started, plasmacytic proliferation progresses relentlessly. Until the nature of the stimulus to such cell growth is clarified, plasmacytic myeloma should be classified as a malignant hematologic neoplasm, closely related to leukemia and lymphoma.

PATHOPHYSIOLOGY

The basic abnormality is the disorderly proliferation of immature, atypical plasmacytes, which vary from small differentiated forms to large anaplastic cells. There is great morphologic variability among patients; however, there is little pleomorphism in a single patient, and the myeloma cells usually maintain their morphologic characteristics throughout the course of the disease. "Typical" myeloma cells do not exist, and it serves no useful purpose to describe their widely differing morphology. Examples are shown in Figure 10-2. Two points deserve emphasis: (1) regardless of their stage of maturity, myeloma cells are always atypical, differing significantly from normal plasmacytes; (2) even though myeloma cells are abnormal plasmacytes, they always display sufficient plasmacytic characteristics to establish their relationship to this cell series.

The clinical manifestations of plasmacytic myeloma are divisible on the basis of pathogenesis into three groups.

Systemic Symptoms. Nonspecific complaints such as weight loss, fever, and weakness are attributable to the presence of a malignant neoplasm.

Altered Organ Structure and Function. As a result of uncontrolled plasmacytic growth, a variety of symptoms and findings is produced. Bone marrow involvement, with displacement of normal myeloid elements and osteolysis, usually predominates. When the lytic lesions are focal, they are responsible for bone pain, pathologic fractures, and tumor formation, especially of red marrow-containing bones such as the spine, pelvis, skull, and thoracic cage. When the proliferation is diffuse, generalized osteoporosis ensues. Bone destruction is responsible for hypercalcemia, which may in itself produce symptoms. New bone formation is almost never seen, and serum alkaline phosphatase levels are normal. Displacement of normal myeloid elements produces anemia, neutropenia, and thrombocytopenia. Thrombocytopenia contributes to a hemorrhagic diathesis; neutropenia enhances susceptibility to infections. Extramedullary lesions are less common but may cause splenomegaly, hepatomegaly, or tumor formation in such sites as the upper respiratory tract, conjunctivae, stomach, or intestine. Local symptoms are unique to the organ involved (e.g., paraplegia due to extradural cord compression by a vertebral tumor mass).

Protein Abnormalities. Normal plasmacytes elaborate immunoglobulins. Myeloma cells retain this capacity for protein synthesis, and their products are detectable in almost every patient with plasmacytic myeloma. These myeloma proteins are most likely abnormal products of abnormal cells, but the possibility that they are normal proteins produced in excess cannot be entirely excluded. They might best be termed paraproteins, pending resolution of this problem.

Normal immunoglobulin fractions consist of complex mixtures of related proteins divisible into three major groups (IgG, IgA, and IgM) on the basis of certain common immunologic, electrophoretic, chemical, and physical properties; a fourth (IgD) is present in only trace amounts. Each group contains an indeterminate number of biologically specific proteins made up of two heavy (H) and two light (L) polypeptide chains. Two kinds of light chains (type K and type L) are common to all immunoglobulins, whereas the structure of the H chains differs for each class. Although the term gamma globulins is often used interchangeably with immunoglobulins, these substances have an "extragamma" electrophoretic spread. The IgG fraction constitutes about 70 to 80 per cent of the immunoglobulins and has electrophoretic mobilities ranging from γ to α_2; it contains most of the acquired antibacterial and antiviral antibodies. The IgA group migrates as γ or β globulins and accounts for approximately 15 to 20 per cent of the immunoglobulins; these antibodies occur in relatively large amounts in bronchial secretions, tears, saliva, and so forth. Both the IgG and IgA fractions have molecular weights of about 160,000 and sedimentation constants of 7S. Normally, the IgM fraction makes up about 5 to 10 per cent of the immunoglobulins and includes such antibodies as the naturally occurring red cell isoagglutinins. These substances are macroglobulins with molecular weights of about 1,000,000 and sedimentation constants of 19 to 20S. Electrophoretically, they migrate as γ or α_2 globulins.

In most disease states associated with hyperglobulinemia (e.g., chronic infections, cirrhosis, sarcoidosis, and collagen diseases), there is a diffuse increase in all globulin fractions. In contrast, the hyperglobulinemia in patients with plasmacytic myeloma typically forms a discrete electrophoretic peak. The characteristics of the myeloma globulins vary from patient to patient but exhibit individual specificity. There is compelling experimental evidence which indicates that each patient produces his own unique paraprotein(s) and that their properties remain constant throughout the course of the disease. These observations are in accord with the hypothesis that a clone of plasmacytes is normally "selected" by an antigen, thereafter responding only to that stimulus by elaborating a specific immunoglobulin. Plasmacytic myeloma might then be envisaged as a neoplastic proliferation of a single line of cells behaving as if they were under constant antigenic stimulation but engaged in the production of proteins without known biologic specificity. However, the apparent homogeneity of myeloma proteins on paper electrophoresis has not been borne out by other techniques. Starch gel electrophoresis and ion exchange column chromatography point to heterogeneity of most myeloma globulins. Thus it would seem that a single cell must be capable of synthesizing more than one protein molecule or that several closely related clones of myeloma cells must coexist.

There are two types of myeloma paraprotein, plasma globulins and Bence Jones proteins. The plasma globulins are immunologically, physically, and chemically related to normal immunoglobulins. Most of the myeloma globulins have molecular weights of about 160,000 and sedimentation constants of 7S; about 70 per cent of these proteins are related to the IgG and 30 per cent to the IgA immunoglobulins. Occasionally, myeloma globulins are macroglobulins. These substances are immunologically related to the IgM fraction. In some patients the myeloma globulins, especially the macroglobulins, are cold-precipitable or cryoglobulins. Rarely, the 7S myeloma globulins may be pyroglobulins (i.e., heat-precipitable at 56°C). Because of displacement of normal plasmacytes by myeloma cells or perhaps to competition for metabolic precursors, normal immunoglobulins are markedly decreased.

The term Bence Jones protein refers to a group of proteins of small molecular weight (approximately 22,000). These substances possess the unique property of precipitating at 45 to 60°C and redissolving at 85°C. Bence Jones proteins are synthesized *de novo* and promptly excreted in the urine because of their small molecular weight. Consequently, they are not detectable in serum by routine electrophoresis but can be demonstrated by more sensitive immunoelectrophoretic techniques. In urine the electrophoretic mobility of Bence Jones proteins is that of a globulin, but it does not necessarily conform to that of the 7S plasma paraprotein. Bence Jones proteins display less homogeneity in individual patients than the myeloma plasma globulins. They possess immunologic determinants common to both IgG and IgA immunoglobulins. Bence Jones proteins are not degradation products of the plasma myeloma globulins, as was once widely believed. Instead they are light or L-chain subunits from which the larger plasma paraprotein molecules are constructed. When the synthesis of light and heavy chains is balanced, plasma myeloma globulins are formed; when light chains are produced in excess, Bence Jones proteins appear in the urine.

There is no longer any doubt that the myeloma cells elaborate the paraproteins. However, numerous attempts have failed to correlate morphology of the myeloma cells with specific protein properties such as electrophoretic mobility. Nearly all patients with plasmacytic myeloma manifest some protein abnormality. About 60 per cent have hyperglobulinemia; approximately 50 per cent have Bence Jones proteinuria. In some patients the paraproteins are well tolerated. In others they interfere seriously with a number of physiologic processes. The following clinical manifestations are attributable in whole or in part to protein abnormalities.

ERYTHROCYTE CLUMPING. Because of the presence of hyperglobulinemia, rouleaux are evident in stained peripheral blood films; they may interfere with blood typing and red cell counting and are responsible for an increased erythrocyte sedimentation rate. This tendency may also contribute, along with increased blood viscosity, to circulatory stasis and capillary damage.

COAGULATION DEFECTS. A bleeding tendency may result from the interaction of the myeloma proteins with certain coagulation factors, most notably factors I (fibrinogen), II (prothrombin), IV (calcium), V, and VII.

INFECTIONS. A marked deficiency of biologically effective antibodies is characteristic of plasmacytic myeloma. Recurrent infections with pyogenic bacteria are common occurrences, especially pneumonia (usually pneumococcal) and urinary tract infections. Although viral and fungal infections are less frequently encountered, the incidence of herpes zoster is increased.

COLD SENSITIVITY. When cryoglobulins are present, they may be responsible for a variety of symptoms and findings triggered by exposure to cold. These include purpura, epistaxis, urticaria, Raynaud's phenomenon, skin ulcerations, and even peripheral gangrene.

HYPERSPLENISM. Occasionally, patients with plasmacytic myeloma develop overt hypersplenism manifested by a hemolytic anemia, thrombocytopenia, and/or leukopenia (p. 448). In view of the evidence implicating abnormal globulins in the pathogenesis of "autoimmune" hypersplenism, it is surprising that this occurrence is not seen with greater frequency in a disease with such evident protein abnormalities.

RENAL FAILURE. Impaired renal function occurs in more than 50 per cent of the patients with plasmacytic myeloma. Although a number of pathogenic mechanisms may be involved (hypercalcemia, decreased renal blood flow secondary to increased blood viscosity, plasmacytic infiltration of the kidneys, or paramyloid deposition), the damaging effect of Bence Jones proteins is the most important. In a "myeloma" kidney the distal and proximal convoluted tubules become obstructed by large laminated casts of precipitated Bence Jones protein surrounded by giant cells. In addition, the tubular cells become swollen and engorged with hyaline droplets; these changes may progress to atrophy and degeneration. The damaging effect on the renal tubules appears to be the result of an interaction between certain Bence Jones proteins and the tubular epithelial cytoplasmic proteins. Eventually, the entire nephron becomes markedly distorted and nonfunctional. All modalities of renal function are affected (i.e., both tubular and glomerular). It is of interest that the blood pressure is generally normal even in the presence of marked renal insufficiency. Rarely, alterations in specific tubular functions may produce an adult Fanconi syndrome. The nephrotoxicity of some but not all Bence Jones proteins apparently reflects specific physicochemical properties.

AMYLOIDOSIS. Increased amyloid deposition or paramyloidosis occurs in about 10 per cent of the patients. The distribution and tinctorial properties of these amyloid deposits differ from those of secondary amyloidosis and are identical with those of primary amyloidosis. In fact, the primary form bears a close nosologic relationship to plasmacytic myeloma and cannot be delineated clearly from it. Amyloid is chemically and immunologically related to the immunoglobulins; available evidence indicates that the atypical or paramyloid deposits, which are not metachromatic and show little affinity for Congo red, represent insoluble complexes of myeloma paraproteins (probably the Bence Jones type) and normal tissue polysaccharides. The tongue, heart, blood vessels, gastrointestinal tract, kidneys, peripheral nerves, carpal ligaments, and joint capsules are the usual sites of paramyloid deposition.

CLINICAL MANIFESTATIONS

Plasmacytic myeloma accounts for less than 1 per cent of all types of malignant disease and about 10 per cent of all hematologic malignancies. In 1963 in the United States there were 3182 deaths, or 1.7 per 100,000 population, attributable to this disorder. It is about twice as common in men as in women. The disease usually has its onset between the ages of 40 and 70, with its peak incidence in the sixth decade of life. It is uncommon below the age of 40 and rare below the age of 30. Plasmacytic myeloma occurs in all races and geographic locations.

Symptoms. Because plasmacytic myeloma is predominantly a disease of the marrow with secondary osteolysis, it is not surprising that bone pain, typically in the back and less often in the chest or extremities, is present at the time of diagnosis in about 90 per cent of the patients.

Pain is ordinarily gradual in onset but may develop suddenly as the result of a pathologic fracture. Bone tenderness and deformity are common. The symptomatology of plasmacytic myeloma is otherwise varied. Neurologic complaints are often encountered; paraplegia caused by cord compression deserves emphasis, but peripheral neuropathies also occur. Weakness, weight loss, and fever are frequent, especially in far-advanced disease. Abnormal bleeding, most often in the form of epistaxis or purpura, is a prominent complaint. In some patients the major symptoms are the result of an acute infection or of some other complication such as uremia, hypercalcemia, or paramyloidosis. Hypercalcemia may be manifested by nausea, vomiting, apathy, polydipsia, and polyuria. Congestive heart failure, the nephrotic syndrome, joint symptoms, or a peripheral neuropathy may reflect paramyloidosis. Cryoglobulinemia may be responsible for symptoms on exposure to cold. Rarely, extramedullary tumors in the upper respiratory tract, conjunctivae, or elsewhere produce local symptoms. Sjøgren's syndrome has been observed in a number of patients.

Physical Findings. Bone tenderness and pallor are the most common physical abnormalities. Bone deformity, pathologic fractures, and tumor formation are also encountered frequently. Splenomegaly (usually slight) occurs in about 15 per cent and hepatomegaly in about 25 per cent of the patients. Lymph nodes are rarely enlarged. With the exception of petechiae and purpura, skin involvement is uncommon. Findings due to local lesions depend on their site; for example, extradural cord compression by a vertebral tumor mass may produce paraplegia or even quadriplegia if the cervical spine is involved. Extramedullary plasmacytomas have been described in almost all tissues. Paramyloidosis may bring about such diverse abnormalities as defects in cardiac conduction, congestive heart failure, macroglossia, joint findings (even joint effusion has been observed), or the carpal tunnel syndrome due to compression by amyloid deposits of the median nerve as it traverses the volar carpal tunnel.

Laboratory Findings. PERIPHERAL BLOOD. A normocytic, normochromic anemia occurs eventually in every patient and is present in the majority at the time of diagnosis. Most often it is slight to moderate (hemoglobin, 10 to 11 gm/100 ml of blood; hematocrit, 32 to 35 per cent). Severe anemia indicates some complicating factor such as uremia or hemolysis. The erythrocytes vary little in size or shape, but rouleaux are characteristic (Fig. 10-1). Increased polychromasia, slight reticulocytosis, and occasional nucleated red cells are frequent findings in the peripheral blood; these changes are more marked in the presence of overt hemolysis. The erythrocyte sedimentation rate is typically increased. A blue-gray staining background on the peripheral blood film is common and presumably reflects the dysproteinemic state.

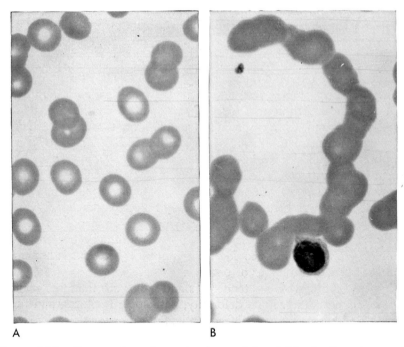

A   B

Figure 10-1. Increased rouleaux in the peripheral blood of patients with plasmacytic myeloma. *A.* Mild. *B.* Marked.

The leukocyte count is most often normal or slightly decreased. Occasionally, it is slightly elevated. It is not unusual to find a few immature granulocytes in the peripheral blood, that is, a leukemoid reaction similar to that observed in any myelophthisic process (p. 242). A slight eosinophilia is common. Although usually present in very small numbers, and therefore missed, atypical plasmacytes or myeloma cells identical to those in the marrow can be found in the peripheral blood of almost every patient; a careful search by a trained observer rarely goes unrewarded. Rare patients manifest clear-cut plasmacytic leukemia with white counts as high as 50,000/cu mm and large numbers of myeloma cells in the peripheral blood.

The platelet count is usually normal. Thrombocytopenia occurs in far-advanced disease with extensive marrow replacement. A number of coagulation defects have been described without a specific or diagnostic pattern.

BONE MARROW. The presence of atypical, immature plasmacytes in the bone marrow is pathognomonic of plasmacytic myeloma (Fig. 10-2). These cells generally make up 20 per cent or more of all nucleated cells but may represent less than 5 to almost 100 per cent of the marrow cells. They may be present diffusely, in small clumps, in syncytia, or in large sheets. Marrow involvement is usually focal rather than

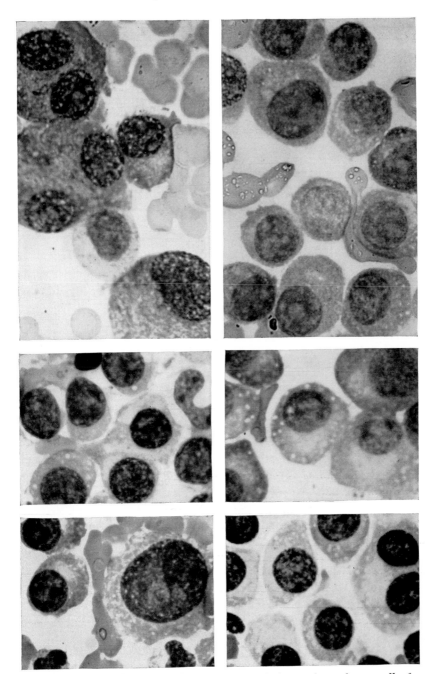

Figure 10-2. Examples of the differing morphology of myeloma cells from six patients with plasmacytic myeloma. Myeloma cells vary greatly in size. They ordinarily have large prominent nucleoli and may contain a variety of cytoplasmic inclusions, such as colorless vacuoles (Mott bodies) and eosinophilic globules (Russell bodies). Multinucleated forms are common.

diffuse. Consequently, separate specimens often differ strikingly; one may consist of nothing but myeloma cells, whereas marrow obtained from another site may be normal or almost so. Myeloma cells are most likely to be confused with osteoblasts (Fig. 10-3). Quantitative de-

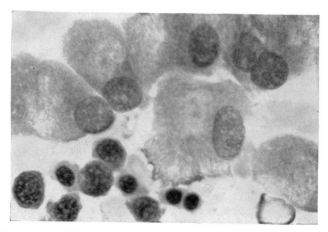

Figure 10-3. Osteoblasts showing a superficial similarity to cells of the plasmacytic series. Osteoblasts are relatively large; the nuclei contain one to two nucleoli, and the chromatin pattern is reticular, with sharp contrast between basichromatin and parachromatin. The basophilic cytoplasm is abundant and frequently contains a rounded pale area distinct from a perinuclear clear zone. These cells are present normally in the bone marrow of infants and children and may be found in adults with a variety of disorders involving bone (e.g., metastatic malignancy).

creases in normal myeloid elements constitute the only other consistent findings.

Protein Abnormalities. *Hyperglobulinemia* occurs in about 60 per cent of the patients; *serum electrophoretic abnormalities* are detectable in about 80 per cent. The characteristic pattern on paper electrophoresis is a sharp, homogeneous peak, with mobility varying from as slow as the γ globulins to as fast as the α globulins (Fig. 10-4). Although the amount may change, the electrophoretic mobility of the paraprotein ordinarily remains remarkably constant in a patient throughout the course of his disease. About 50 per cent of the patients have a peak that migrates as a γ globulin, 15 per cent in the β fraction, and 10 per cent have the "M" pattern, with mobility between the γ and β globulins. Five per cent or less have paraproteins migrating as α globulins. The remaining 20 per cent have normal serum electrophoretic patterns or exhibit minor nonspecific changes. *Bence Jones proteinuria* is detectable by the usual techniques employing heat in about half the patients with plasmacytic myeloma. It is of interest that patients with the most marked Bence Jones proteinuria usually show no hyperglobulinemia and vice versa. With electrophoretic techniques, an abnormal protein with the mobility of a globulin can be demonstrated in the urine of approximately 70 per cent. If cryoglobulins are present, a precipitate will form when serum is refrigerated and will dissolve on warming.

X-ray Findings. Bone x-rays are abnormal in about 90 per cent of the patients with plasmacytic myeloma. In approximately 25 per cent diffuse bone lysis is manifested by generalized osteoporosis. The classic lesions are "punched out" lytic areas *without* associated osteoblastic reactions. They may be sharply circumscribed or, when superimposed on diffuse bone demineralization, poorly defined. Condensed trabeculae may create a soap-bubble or honeycomb appearance. The vertebrae, skull, thoracic cage, pelvis, and proximal humeri and femora are the usual sites of involvement. Pathologic fractures are common, especially vertebral collapse. In contrast to the frequency with which they are the site of metastatic carcinoma, the vertebral pedicles are rarely involved. Soft tissue extensions are frequently observed. Evidence of new bone formation is almost never seen unless in response to specific therapy or secondary to a fracture with subsequent callus formation. Although osteoblastic reactions and even osteosclerosis of the spine have been attributed to plasmacytic myeloma, these findings are so unusual that the demonstration of new bone deposition in an untreated patient without fracture virtually excludes this diagnosis. It should be noted that one out of every ten patients exhibits no x-ray abnormalities.

Other Laboratory Findings. *Hypercalcemia,* occasionally reaching levels of 18 to 20 mg/100 ml occurs in about 30 per cent of the patients with plasmacytic myeloma. In the absence of fracture with callus formation, *serum alkaline phosphatase* is normal. *Serum phosphorus* levels are also normal unless raised by renal failure. *Serum uric acid* is often elevated. Some degree of renal insufficiency is present in more than half the patients and will be reflected by an increase in the blood urea nitrogen and other evidence of renal dysfunction. Other laboratory determinations are nonspecific.

DIAGNOSIS

Bone pain, anemia, and rouleaux constitute a triad that demands exclusion of plasmacytic myeloma. A number of findings should suggest the diagnosis, such as multiple osteolytic lesions, pathologic fractures, bone tumors, osteoporosis, hypercalcemia, uremia without hypertension, the carpal tunnel syndrome, Sjøgren's syndrome, cold sensitivity phenomena, cryoglobulinemia, pyroglobulinemia, hyperglobulinemia, Bence Jones proteinuria, or protein electrophoretic abnormalities. An unequivocal diagnosis is predicated on the demonstration of the "myeloma cell." Although protein changes are highly suggestive, they are not always

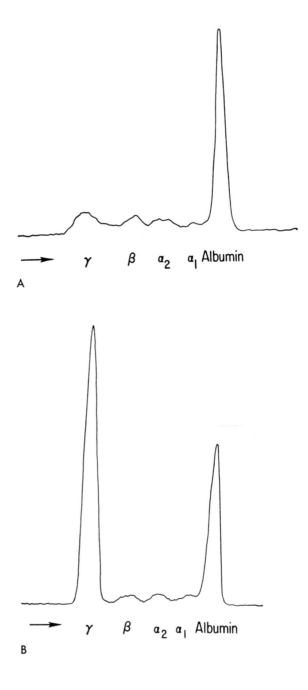

Figure 10-4. Serum electrophoretic patterns. *A.* Normal. *B.* Myeloma globulin with a γ mobility. *C.* Abnormal serum protein migrating electrophoretically as a β globulin in a patient with plasmacytic myeloma.

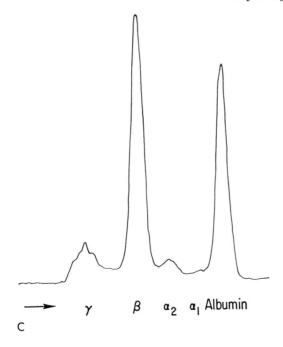

$\longrightarrow$ γ β α_2 α_1 Albumin

C

pathognomonic. Cryo- and pyroglobulins are uncommon and not restricted to plasmacytic myeloma; Bence Jones proteinuria has also been
observed in rare patients without plasmacytic myeloma; hyperglobulinemia accompanies a number of seemingly unrelated disorders such
as sarcoidosis, liver disease, and kala-azar.

Serum electrophoretic patterns are possible exceptions to the relative
nonspecificity of the other protein abnormalities. On paper electrophoresis a sharp homogeneous peak migrating as a γ, β, or even an α
globulin is virtually diagnostic of plasmacytic myeloma. A urinary protein with the electrophoretic mobility of the globulins is equally specific. Approximately 50 per cent of the patients have electrophoretic
abnormalities in blood and urine, 30 per cent in blood alone, and 20
per cent in urine alone. Therefore simultaneous electrophoresis of serum
and urine will reveal an abnormality in almost every patient. When
the serum protein peak is sharp and tall, interpretation is easy, but
when there are only minor quantitative differences, interpretation is
difficult. Furthermore, certain other disorders (e.g., primary macroglobulinemia, p. 442) may have similar electrophoretic patterns. Therefore
a positive diagnosis rests on the demonstration of myeloma cells. "Typical" electrophoretic abnormalities almost never occur without easily
demonstrable cytologic evidence of the disease.

Marrow plasmacytosis is not unique to plasmacytic myeloma and
can be found in patients with certain infections (especially chronic

granulomatous processes), cirrhosis, malignancies, collagen diseases, and hypersensitivity states. Plasmacytes usually make up less than 20 per cent of the marrow nucleated cells in these conditions and more than that number in plasmacytic myeloma, but exceptions occur. Therefore the diagnosis of plasmacytic myeloma depends on the *type* of cell. Myeloma cells are *always* immature and atypical. Because of focal marrow involvement, a negative marrow does not exclude the diagnosis. Repeated marrow examinations may be necessary; "aimed punctures" (needle aspirations of tender areas or tumor masses) are often rewarding. Inasmuch as fractures of the sternum have followed sternal punctures in patients with plasmacytic myeloma, the iliac crest is the preferred site from which to aspirate marrow. Rarely, it may be necessary to biopsy an extramedullary plasmacytoma.

When considered singly, some of the manifestations of plasmacytic myeloma mimic other diseases. For example, bone x-rays may suggest metastatic carcinoma, postmenopausal osteoporosis, or even hyperparathyroidism; hyperglobulinemia and marrow plasmacytosis occur in other disorders; and so forth. When certain findings are viewed collectively, however, precise diagnosis can generally be established with relative ease. Osteoblastic reactions, an elevated serum alkaline phosphatase, or a decreased serum phosphorus are not typical of plasmacytic myeloma; other causes of hyperglobulinemia have broad electrophoretic patterns reflecting an increase in all globulin fractions; and so forth. Knowledge of the various clinical manifestations of plasmacytic myeloma is the prime requisite for accurate diagnosis. Awareness of such a possibility will lead to the diagnostic procedures (serum and urine electrophoresis and bone marrow examination) needed to confirm or exclude the diagnosis. Occasionally, the more typical manifestations of plasmacytic myeloma may be obscured by those of some complication such as the "myeloma kidney" or paramyloidosis. Uremia may suggest primary renal disease, or paramyloidosis may be responsible for congestive heart failure, the nephrotic syndrome, or a picture simulating rheumatoid arthritis. Even in these patients, however, there is always some clue to the correct diagnosis, such as bone pain, an unexplained anemia, rouleaux, or uremia without hypertension. It is especially important to consider the possibility of plasmacytic myeloma in patients with uremia of unknown cause because several instances of acute renal failure have followed intravenous pyelography, an otherwise benign procedure. The explanation is not clear, but a number of factors such as dehydration and abdominal pressure probably act together to enhance precipitation of Bence Jones protein in the renal tubules.

TREATMENT AND COURSE

Plasmacytic myeloma runs a progressive course; most patients succumb within one to three years, although rare patients have survived for 10 years or even longer. Median survival time is about 24 months. Plasmacytic leukemia, solitary plasmacytoma, or extramedullary plasmacytoma represent differing manifestations of a single disease; there is no justification for classifying them separately. The patient with plasmacytic leukemia has a poorer prognosis than the patient with a solitary lesion, but the shorter course reflects more generalized involvement rather than a different disease.

Specific Therapy. The role of *surgery* in the treatment of a solitary plasmacytoma is disputable. There is no proof that surgical extirpation can "cure" such a patient; instead, there is every reason to believe, as in lymphoma (p. 407), that the disease will eventually recur. Even so, removal of a readily accessible extramedullary lesion is probably indicated, although they are extremely rare. Surgery plays a more important role in patients with extradural cord compression. Because of the slow suppressive effect of ionizing radiation or chemotherapy, one cannot rely on tumor lysis by these means. If paraplegia is to be prevented, prompt diagnosis and decompression are needed. The ultimate prognosis should not unduly influence the decision to operate; survival for only a year as an ambulatory patient is certainly to be preferred over permanent paraplegia.

X-radiation is a more useful form of local therapy and is indicated postoperatively in situations such as those already described. It also effectively relieves pain in most patients. Because plasmacytic myeloma is almost always a generalized disease at the time of diagnosis, x-radiation should not be employed as the sole form of suppressive therapy. Small doses (1000 to 1500 r) will usually alleviate pain; systemic therapy can then be instituted. It is best to complete palliative x-ray therapy before starting chemotherapy because their myelosuppressive effects may be cumulative.

Specific Therapy (Systemic). CYCLOPHOSPHAMIDE (CYTOXAN). This alkylating agent (p. 405) has recently been subjected to extensive clinical trial. When cyclophosphamide is given orally in relatively small doses (50 to 150 mg/day) for prolonged periods of time (three to six months or longer), approximately 45 per cent of the patients manifest some kind of objective response; an additional 25 per cent report subjective improvement. The former includes an increase in the peripheral erythroid values and a decrease in hyperglobulinemia and/or Bence Jones proteinuria (electrophoretic abnormalities may disappear completely). New bone formation (recalcification) is rare, even in patients who otherwise exhibit a favorable therapeutic response. The drug is generally well tolerated. Bone marrow depression is the major toxic manifestation. Although leukopenia occurs in most patients and may require adjustment of the dose, it is not ordinarily necessary to stop the cyclophosphamide unless the leukocyte count falls below 2000/cu mm. Even at those levels, the bone marrow should be examined before the drug is discontinued because leukopenia (or thrombocytopenia) may reflect the basic disease or hypersplenism rather than drug-induced marrow depression.

Patients improve slowly and require long-term therapy; maximal improvement may not be achieved for eight to nine months or even longer. The duration of treatment appears to be a more important factor than the total amount of drug given. In other words, large doses given in short courses seem to be less effective than small doses continued for a longer period of time. Available data indicate that the drug should be administered for a minimum of 90 days before it is discarded as useless. If the disease regresses, cyclophosphamide should be continued indefinitely until the patient either shows evidence of increasing activity of the malignant process or toxicity of sufficient severity to warrant stopping the drug.

MELPHALAN (ALKERAN). This alkylating agent has an active nitrogen mustard radical attached to the amino acid, L-phenylalanine (Fig. 10-5). It was synthesized in 1953 on the assumption that this physio-

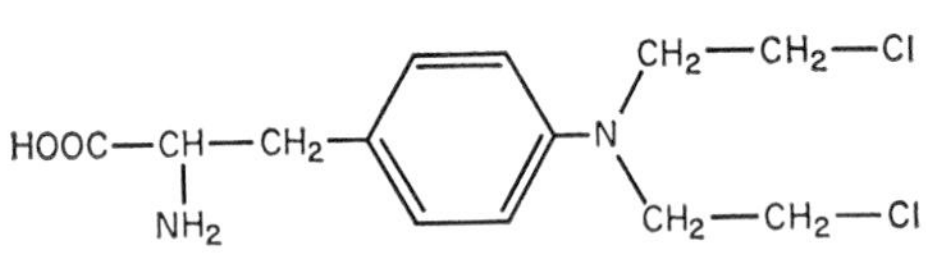

p-di(2-chloroethyl)-amino-L-phenylalanine

MELPHALAN; L-SARCOLYSIN *(Alkeran)*

Figure 10-5.   Structural formula of melphalan (Alkeran).

logically important amino acid might be selectively taken up by metabolically active tumor cells. This compound appears to exert a therapeutic effect comparable to that of cyclophosphamide. Long-term treatment is essential. Numerous dosage schedules have been suggested (e.g., large doses in short interrupted courses and small doses over a prolonged period of time). A daily dose of 2 to 3 mg continued indefinitely (unless the disease progresses or toxicity intervenes) seems to be the most effective regimen. The toxic manifestations of melphalan are similar to those of cyclophosphamide. Bone marrow depression is most common. Some recipients of large doses complain of mild nausea and vomiting, and ulcerations of the gastrointestinal tract have been observed in a few. Significant untoward reactions rarely accompany the recommended doses; however, some type of toxicity can be expected in the majority of patients treated with larger doses (e.g., 5 to 6 mg/day).

URETHANE (ETHYL CARBAMATE). This mitotic inhibitor exerts a fairly specific suppressive effect on plasmacytic proliferation, but gastrointestinal symptoms limit its usefulness. The precise mode of action of this simple compound (Fig. 10-6) is not known. When given in divided doses of 3 to 5 gm/day for periods of 8 to 12 weeks, subjective improvement occurs slowly in approximately 40 per cent and ob-

$$O=C \overset{\displaystyle NH_2}{\underset{\displaystyle OC_2H_5}{}}$$

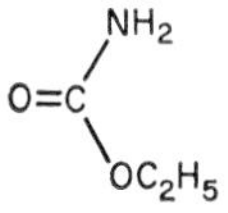

ethyl carbamate

URETHANE

Figure 10-6. Structural formula of urethane.

jective improvement in an additional 20 per cent of the patients. Gastrointestinal side effects (anorexia, nausea, and vomiting) are quite common and more often than not preclude adequate therapy. Bone marrow depression and acute hemorrhagic centrilobular hepatic necrosis are the other major toxic manifestations of urethane. Hepatic necrosis is rare but should be watched for in all patients receiving urethane. It is necessary to give 3 gm or more a day for 60 to 90 days before concluding that urethane is ineffective. If the patient improves, the drug should be continued until toxicity occurs or the disease progresses. Occasional patients improve after the drug is discontinued. Second courses of treatment are rarely of value.

OTHER CHEMOTHERAPEUTIC AGENTS. Other cytotoxic drugs have little place in the treatment of plasmacytic myeloma. Stilbamidine, triethylenemelamine (TEM), 6-mercaptopurine (6MP), and others have been used but can no longer be recommended; their toxic effects outweigh any potential advantage.

Supportive Therapy. *Corticosteroids* are of definite value in the management of patients with plasmacytic myeloma, even though they do not appear to suppress the plasmacytic proliferation significantly. They are indicated when hypersplenism is present and are quite effective in lowering blood calcium, although the exact manner by which this is accomplished is not known. Corticosteroids are also indicated in patients with uremia. Even though few respond, there is little else to offer these patients. Unless renal function can be improved, death will intervene before a suppressive agent can exert an effect. Corticosteroids also appear to modify protein production; symptoms of cryoglobulinemia and certain manifestations of paramyloidosis may respond to such treatment. The diagnosis of plasmacytic myeloma is *not* an indication for corticosteroid therapy; the deleterious side effects of these substances, especially in patients already prone to infections, must not be ignored.

At some time during the course of the disease, however, almost every patient will be an appropriate candidate, if only for terminal symptomatic support. Prednisone, 60 mg/day (or an equivalent dose of some other corticosteroid), is given until maximal benefit is achieved. The dose is then tapered to the smallest amount capable of maintaining the desired effect (e.g., a normal serum calcium).

Physiotherapy is an essential part of the over-all treatment program, as is adequate *nursing care*. With suitable braces, ambulation should be attempted. Dramatic results are often achieved, even in those patients with extensive bone destruction. Appropriate *antibiotics* are indicated for the frequent infections. Because normal immunoglobulins are decreased, treatment with exogenous *gamma globulin* may be of value in some patients with repeated infections. *Transfusions* are given as needed to maintain erythroid values commensurate with the patient's activity (i.e., a hemoglobin of 7 to 10 gm/100 ml of blood).

Principles of Therapy. Although available therapy results in only temporary control of the proliferative process, much can be accomplished for the patient's comfort. With rare exceptions, the diagnosis appears to be an indication for treatment. Local x-radiation is used as needed for relief of pain, after which the patient should be started on cyclophosphamide, melphalan, or urethane. Since cyclophosphamide and melphalan are better tolerated and because significant improvement rarely follows treatment for less than 60 to 90 days, they are the drugs of choice. The selection of one over the other is largely a matter of personal preference and experience (cyclophosphamide and melphalan appear to exert comparable therapeutic effects). When one agent proves to be ineffective or the patient becomes refractory to it, another drug can then be used. Supplemental treatment and supportive care must be individualized. Infections, renal failure (uremia), and hemorrhage are the usual causes of death.

Other Myeloproliferative and Lymphoproliferative Disorders

A precise definition is requisite for accurate diagnosis, but nature shows little respect for rigid, compartmentalized classifications of disease. As a result, it is often difficult to provide diagnostic criteria that are sufficiently discriminating to prevent inclusion of other disorders, yet broad enough to encompass all variations of the disease in question. The similarities between certain of the proliferative abnormalities of the blood-forming organs have prompted the introduction of such broad terms as myeloproliferative and lymphoproliferative syndromes. Examples of the former include polycythemia vera (p. 292), chronic granulocytic leukemia (p. 362), and myelomonocytic leukemia (p. 340); examples of the latter are the various types of malignant lymphoma (p. 380) and chronic lymphocytic leukemia (p. 369). In addition to certain common clinical manifestations, it is not unusual for one member of a group to evolve into another. Thus some patients with polycythemia vera develop granulocytic leukemia, and giant follicular lymphoma may change into Hodgkin's disease, lymphosarcoma, or chronic lymphocytic leukemia. For these reasons attempts to subdivide the myelo- and lymphoproliferative disorders into separate entities have been criticized as serving no useful purpose. However, most protagonists of this classification have based their conclusions on histologic findings alone. Although it may be impossible to differentiate histologically between acute leukemia arising *de novo* and acute leukemia developing in a patient with polycythemia vera, they can be delineated on clinical

429

grounds. Even though all bone marrow elements may participate in a proliferative process, some cell types do so to a greater or lesser degree than others, thereby creating variable and separable clinical syndromes. The fact that polycythemia vera and chronic granulocytic leukemia may terminate as an acute leukemia is not a valid reason to deny their existence.

The clinical usefulness of a classification of disease depends on its reliability in predicting patterns of presentation, the natural course, and responses to specific therapy. The concept of the myeloproliferative and lymphoproliferative syndromes has certainly clarified the relationships between these disorders. Clinically, however, it is necessary to make more exact diagnoses, for the therapy and prognosis of each disease category differ. Therefore the clinician must be cognizant of individual clinical pictures. When one type is transformed into another, the original diagnosis should be discarded but not denied; the patient is then managed exactly as if the new diagnosis had been the original manifestation of the myelo- or lymphoproliferative disorder. In view of the close relationships between several clinically distinct entities and the possibility that they may reflect different responses to a similar pathologic stimulus, it is not surprising that disease in an occasional patient will defy accurate classification. These individuals must be handled as unique problems.

Agnogenic Myeloid Metaplasia

Agnogenic (idiopathic or primary) myeloid metaplasia is a slowly progressive proliferative disease involving the pluripotential mesenchymal cells; it is characterized by extramedullary hematopoiesis, especially in the spleen, and usually by myelofibrosis or osteosclerosis. Heuck first called attention to this syndrome in 1879 when he described a patient with anemia, leukocytosis, massive splenomegaly, and generalized osteosclerosis. Its nature and relationship to chronic granulocytic leukemia remained a controversial subject for many years. Increasing awareness of the disorder gradually led to the formulation of a composite clinical and pathologic picture, and during the last two decades its separable identity has been firmly established. Case reports have appeared under a variety of names. Agnogenic myeloid metaplasia is recommended as an inclusive term to describe the condition adequately and to set it apart from extramedullary hematopoiesis secondary to some other primary disease. It is preferable to myelofibrosis or myelosclerosis (both widely used), for these histologic findings are neither limited to this disease nor requisites for the diagnosis.

ETIOLOGY

Many theories have developed with respect to the pathogenesis of agnogenic myeloid metaplasia. A once popular but unproved thesis is that of "primary" bone marrow failure with "compensatory" extramedullary hematopoiesis. However, myeloid metaplasia does not always follow myelofibrosis or bone marrow failure; hypoplastic anemia is a notable example. Furthermore, a marrow of normal or even increased cellularity is not incompatible with the diagnosis. Among factors considered to be etiologically significant are exposure to some marrow toxin such as benzene, tuberculosis, liver dysfunction, and endocrine disease, but there is no compelling support for such causal relationships. The possibility of a mesenchymal reaction to some type of marrow injury cannot be excluded, but it seems more reasonable to consider agnogenic myeloid metaplasia as a proliferative disorder in which both hematopoietic and stromal cells are involved and in which myelofibrosis and osteosclerosis are a consequence of the disease rather than a cause. Although closely related to other myeloproliferative syndromes, such as chronic granulocytic leukemia, polycythemia vera, myelomonocytic leukemia, and primary thrombocythemia, it is a distinct entity. The stimulus to the abnormal proliferation is unknown.

PATHOPHYSIOLOGY

Mesenchyme, the embryonic connective tissue, constitutes the ontogenetic anlage of the blood cells. At birth functional extramedullary hematopoiesis ceases, with the exception of lymphocytes and possibly monocytes; however, pluripotential mesenchymal cells persist throughout life in the spleen, liver, lymph nodes, and elsewhere as part of the reticuloendothelial system. These cells are normally quiescent, but their embryonic potentialities remain intact. Agnogenic myeloid metaplasia is envisaged as a proliferative disorder involving these pluripotential cells. In extramedullary sites they resume active blood formation. Stromal differentiation with fibroblastic proliferation generally predominates in the bone marrow. Although one or more cell series may be increased out of proportion to the others, creating variability in symptoms and findings, disorderly proliferation of a single hemic precursor (the pathognomonic finding of leukemia) is not seen. The bone marrow is usually hypocellular and fibrotic; occasionally osteosclerosis is present. Decreased erythropoiesis secondary to marrow hypocellularity contributes significantly to anemia, which is a major cause of disability. Deposition of excess fibrous or osseous tissue in the myeloid cavity may evoke bone pain and may be roentgenographically demonstrable. The findings in the peripheral blood are similar to those of a myelophthisic process (p. 241).

Myeloid metaplasia occurs in the spleen and, to a lesser degree, in the liver and abdominal lymph nodes. Occasionally, foci of hematopoiesis are present in other organs such as the peripheral lymph nodes, kidneys, lungs, adrenals, and gastrointestinal tract. Basic architectural patterns are distorted but rarely destroyed. In the spleen areas of developing erythrocytes and granulocytes plus megakaryocytes are present in a massively enlarged, slightly to markedly fibrosed organ, which is ordinarily without infarcts. In most cases the lymphoid follicles are preserved, and the splenic cords and sinuses remain well demarcated. Lymphocytes make up 20 to 50 per cent of all nucleated cells in the spleen. Pressure symptoms consequent to marked splenomegaly are common. Splenic enlargement can also be implicated in the pathogenesis of hypersplenism (p. 452), a rather frequent occurrence. Active hematopoiesis in other tissues may produce organ enlargement (e.g., hepatomegaly), but it is rarely responsible for significant functional derangement. Although it is tempting to attribute the striking morphology of the erythrocytes to their formation in extramedullary sites, the bizarre cells probably reflect the basic proliferative abnormality. Systemic symptoms such as weight loss and fever reflect the underlying proliferative process, as do elevated blood uric acid levels.

CLINICAL MANIFESTATIONS

Agnogenic myeloid metaplasia affects both sexes and usually has its onset in the sixth or seventh decade of life. Although uncommon, it is not rare and probably has a frequency about half that of chronic granulocytic leukemia (p. 362). Approximately 10 per cent of the patients have a prior diagnosis of polycythemia vera.

Symptoms. A long history (months to years) of slowly progressive complaints referable to anemia (e.g., weakness or ease of fatigue) or to a massively enlarged spleen is characteristic. Often the diagnosis is made in an asymptomatic person during the course of a periodic health examination. About 15 per cent of the patients complain of bone pain, which is predominantly localized. Abnormal bleeding (most often in the form of petechiae, purpura, epistaxis, or gingival bleeding) occurs in some. Fever, weight loss, and increased sweating are not prominent until the disease becomes far advanced. An occasional patient develops secondary gout.

Physical Findings. Marked to massive splenomegaly (generally below the level of the umbilicus at the time of diagnosis), minimal to moderate hepatomegaly, and pallor are the principal physical abnormalities. Splenic enlargement is a consistent finding, and hepatomegaly is present in most. Peripheral nodes are hardly ever enlarged. Bone tenderness is fairly common.

Laboratory Findings. PERIPHERAL BLOOD. Depending on the duration of the disease, there is a minimal to moderate normocytic, normochromic anemia. Increased polychromasia, occasional nucleated red cells (1 to 10/100 leukocytes), and a slight reticulocytosis (3 to 8 per cent) are characteristic; these findings are more marked in patients with superimposed hemolysis. There is appreciable anisocytosis and moderate to marked poikilocytosis; tailed, teardrop, comma, and other bizarrely shaped cells are particularly prominent (Fig. 11-1). As a rule,

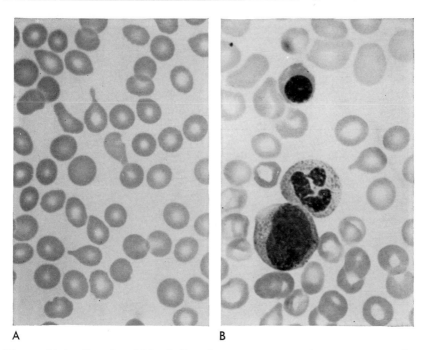

A   B

Figure 11-1.   Peripheral blood films from a patient with agnogenic myeloid metaplasia. *A.* Bizarre tailed erythrocytes. *B.* Immature granulocyte (neutrophilic myelocyte) and a nucleated red cell with atypical erythrocytes.

spherocytes are evident in those patients (about 10 per cent) who manifest overt hemolysis.

The leukocyte count may be normal or even below, but it is most often modestly elevated. A count above 50,000 is uncommon; it almost never exceeds 100,000/cu mm. The leukocytosis reflects a relative and absolute increase in granulocytic elements, neutrophils predominating. With few exceptions, small numbers of immature granulocytes (including myeloblasts and progranulocytes) are found in the peripheral blood irrespective of the circulating leukocyte count. The alkaline phosphatase content of the mature granulocytes is usually increased, but in a few patients it may be normal or even decreased.

Thrombocytosis (often quite marked) is the most common finding, although normal platelet counts are seen and occasional patients are thrombocytopenic. Large and bizarre platelets are characteristic, regardless of their numerical status. Atypical megakaryocytes are present in the peripheral blood of some patients.

Bone Marrow. The marrow is hypocellular in more than 90 per cent of the patients, but specimens of normal or even increased cellularity are not incompatible with the diagnosis. Marrow fibrosis is usual; deposition of excessive osseous tissue is much less common. Increased bone consistency or a gritty sensation may be encountered during penetration of the marrow cavity. Although members of one cell lineage may be increased out of proportion to other elements derived from the myeloid reticulum, maturation remains orderly; typical leukemic changes are not found. Because of the hypocellularity, it is frequently difficult to procure adequate specimens, and multiple sampling from different sites may be necessary. Marrow biopsy is often more informative than aspiration alone and is required to demonstrate myelofibrosis or osteosclerosis (Fig. 11-2). Large clumps and masses of platelets

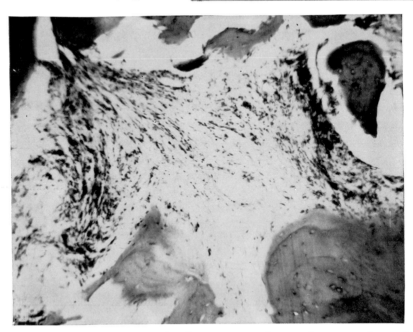

Figure 11-2. Fixed section of a bone marrow biopsy from a patient with agnogenic myeloid metaplasia showing decreased cellularity and increased fibrous tissue.

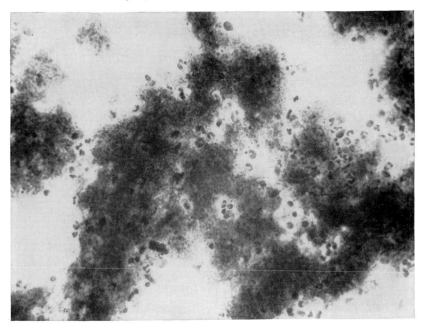

Figure 11-3. Large masses of platelets in the sternal marrow aspirate of a patient with agnogenic myeloid metaplasia; the specimen is otherwise hypocellular.

in the absence of a parallel increase in megakaryocytes and in an otherwise hypocellular specimen are quite suggestive of agnogenic myeloid metaplasia (Fig. 11-3).

SPLENIC CYTOLOGY. The cellular composition of splenic aspirates is remarkably similar to that of normal bone marrow (Fig. 11-4). Developing erythrocytes, granulocytic elements, and megakaryocytes are all present, and maturation appears orderly. Lymphocytes account for 20 to 50 per cent of all nucleated cells.

OTHER LABORATORY FINDINGS. Increased bone density is demonstrable roentgenographically in about 25 per cent of the patients. Both flat and long bones may be involved; however, the skull is rarely affected. For the most part other laboratory data are nonspecific. There may be a variety of coagulation defects without a consistent or diagnostic pattern. Serum uric acid is often elevated. Superimposed hemolysis is reflected by appropriate pigment changes, abnormal erythrocyte osmotic behavior, and a decrease in red cell survival time; the Coombs' test is usually negative. In patients who have marked thrombocytosis, serum acid phosphatase may be elevated, presumably because of the acid phosphatase contained in platelets (plasma acid phosphatase levels are normal).

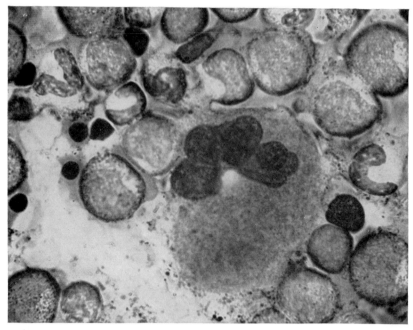

Figure 11-4. Splenic aspirate from a patient with agnogenic myeloid metaplasia, showing all normal myeloid elements (Wright's stain).

DIAGNOSIS

There is no single test or histologic finding that is pathognomonic of agnogenic myeloid metaplasia. Splenic hematopoiesis is found in other disorders (e.g., hemolytic anemias, thalassemia, some types of leukemia, and certain infections). Although osteosclerosis occurs rarely (if at all) in leukemia, myelofibrosis is demonstrable in some patients with far-advanced chronic granulocytic leukemia, the disease with which agnogenic myeloid metaplasia is most likely to be confused. Thus accurate diagnosis depends on the careful interpretation of all clinical data. In fully developed cases the clinical picture is distinctive and diagnostic. It can be differentiated with relative ease from Albers-Schönberg or marble bone disease, a rare familial disorder characterized by generalized osteopetrosis. Osteopetrosis almost always has its onset in infancy or early childhood and invariably involves the skull. Furthermore, only 25 per cent of these patients have evidence in their peripheral blood of a myelophthisic process. Chronic congestive splenomegaly, leishmaniasis (kala-azar), malaria, tuberculosis, Gaucher's disease, lymphoma, and chronic lymphocytic leukemia may be associated with massive splenomegaly but seldom cause confusion because of the evident differences in their clinical manifestations. In contrast, chronic granulocytic leukemia and agnogenic myeloid metaplasia are characterized by similarities; exclusion of leukemia is a prerequisite for the diagnosis of agnogenic myeloid metaplasia and vice versa.

Pertinent differences between agnogenic myeloid metaplasia and chronic granulocytic leukemia are listed in Table 11-1. Examination

Table 11-1. *Differential Diagnosis of Agnogenic Myeloid Metaplasia and Chronic Granulocytic Leukemia* *

	AGNOGENIC MYELOID METAPLASA	CHRONIC GRANULOCYTIC LEUKEMIA
Age	Usually over 50	20 to 50
Sex distribution	Equal	Slightly more common in males
Symptoms		
Onset	Insidious	Insidious
Duration	Months to years	Weeks to months
Type	Secondary to anemia or massive splenomegaly	Secondary to anemia or massive splenomegaly
Physical findings		
Splenomegaly	Marked	Marked
Hepatomegaly	Minimal to moderate	Minimal to moderate
Lymph nodes	Usually not enlarged	Usually not enlarged
Bone tenderness	Frequently present	Rare
Peripheral blood		
Anemia	Minimal to moderate	Minimal to moderate
Reticulocytes	3 to 8 per cent	2 to 5 per cent
Nucleated RBC	1 to 10/100 WBC	0 to 5/100 WBC
Hemolytic component	Common (often spherocytic)	Rare, if ever
Red cell morphology	Marked poikilocytosis, moderate anisocytosis	Normal
Leukocyte count	Low, normal, or modestly increased (usually below 50,-000, rarely more than 80,-000)	100,000 to 300,000 or higher
Immature granulocytes	Present	Present
Granulocyte alkaline phosphatase	Usually increased (may be normal or below)	Decreased
Platelets	Usually increased but may be normal or decreased (large and bizarre forms)	Normal to increased (decreased in far advanced disease)
Bone marrow	Usually hypocellular and fibrotic (orderly maturation); occasionally large clumps of platelets without megakaryocytic hyperplasia	Granulocytic hyperplasia (predominance of a single immature precursor)
Splenic aspirate	Active hematopoiesis with all myeloid elements present (lymphocytes 20 to 50 per cent)	Immature granulocytes predominate (lymphocytes less than 20 per cent)

* J. W. Linman: *Med Clin N Amer*, **46**:49–62, 1962. Reprinted by permission.

of marrow always provides relevant information and is mandatory in the work-up of all such patients. Since a splenic aspiration is accompanied by some risk, it is indicated only when accurate diagnoses cannot be made by any other means. In chronic granulocytic leukemia the splenic aspirate consists chiefly of granulocytic elements with a single precursor (usually myelocytes) predominating; erythrocytic precursors and megakaryocytes are either absent or rare, and lymphocytes constitute less than 20 per cent of the nucleated cells. In agnogenic myeloid metaplasia lymphocytes ordinarily make up 20 to 50 per cent of the nucleated cells and all normal myeloid elements are present. However, a clear-cut dividing line does not always exist between the splenic cytology of these two disorders. Singly, the clinical manifestations of agnogenic myeloid metaplasia are of little diagnostic value. On the other hand, when all the findings are considered together, few diagnostic problems resist solution. Occasional patients will remain an enigma, despite careful study. Close observation is then indicated; the more rapid evolution of chronic granulocytic leukemia will reveal the true diagnosis within a short period of time.

TREATMENT AND COURSE

Agnogenic myeloid metaplasia runs a progressive course, but its relative benignity in many patients deserves emphasis. Duration of life varies from less than a year to 15 years or longer. Extremely short courses are the exception rather than the rule; average survival after onset is about six years. If patients with agnogenic myeloid metaplasia live long enough, it seems likely that most will develop a picture closely simulating and in many cases indistinguishable from acute leukemia. When this change occurs, the outlook and management become those of acute leukemia (p. 353). There is no valid reason to give separate consideration to the patient with a prior diagnosis of polycythemia vera.

Treatment varies according to the major clinical manifestations and must be individualized (Table 11-2). The diagnosis is not necessarily an indication for treatment. Some patients remain asymptomatic for years and require no therapy during that time. The commonest cause of disability is progressive anemia. At first, periodic *transfusions* may suffice, but the anemia eventually becomes severer. If a hemolytic component is present (about 10 per cent of patients), *corticosteroids* are indicated and may alter transfusion requirements strikingly. The initial daily dose of 60 mg of prednisone (15 mg every six hours) or its equivalent should be tapered, as soon as maximal benefit is obtained, to the smallest amount capable of maintaining the desired effect (usually 15 mg of prednisone a day). Prolonged therapy is generally necessary and may, of course, be accompanied by such complications of

Table 11-2. *Therapy of Agnogenic Myeloid Metaplasia*

MANIFESTATION	TREATMENT
Asymptomatic	None
Anemia	1. Transfusions
	2. Corticosteroids
	(if hemolysis is present)
	3. Androgens
Splenomegaly	1. Busulfan
	2. Splenic x-radiation
Hypersplenism	1. Corticosteroids
(hemolysis and/or thrombocytopenia)	2. Splenectomy (rarely)
Thrombocytosis	^{32}p
(thromboembolism or hemorrhage)	
Systemic systems	1. Busulfan
(weakness, weight loss, fever, bone pain)	2. 6-Mercaptopurine (?)
	3. Corticosteroids (?)
	4. General supportive measures

this treatment as increased susceptibility to infections, osteoporosis, and peptic ulcer. In most patients the anemia is not basically hemolytic and will not respond to corticosteroids. *Testosterone* has been of value in some of these patients when given in massive doses (400 to 600 mg of testosterone enanthate weekly) for long periods of time. The exact mechanism responsible for this effect is not known (p. 16).

Pressure symptoms secondary to massive splenomegaly are prominent complaints in many patients. Occasionally *x-radiation to the spleen* is effective; however, the potential danger of this treatment must be borne in mind. If the spleen is the major site of hematopoiesis, intensive splenic irradiation will be deleterious. Partial shielding of the spleen may preserve areas of active hematopoiesis, but the therapeutic benefit is usually disappointing, even if serious hematopoietic depression is avoided. *Busulfan* (Myleran) would appear to be a more effective means of reducing splenic size. The recommended dose (2 to 4 mg/day for three to four weeks, followed by a maintenance dose of 2 mg two to three times a week) is less than that used for chronic granulocytic leukemia (p. 367). Even so, patients treated in this way must be observed carefully for evidence of toxicity (hematopoietic depression). *6-Mercaptopurine* (Purinethol) has been used but is less effective and more toxic than busulfan.

Splenectomy plays a limited role in the treatment of agnogenic myeloid metaplasia. Although once considered absolutely contraindicated, it is not necessarily disastrous. More often than not splenectomy is tolerated well, although the only indication for this procedure is hypersplenism (hemolysis and/or thrombocytopenia) that is unresponsive to corticosteroid therapy. Splenectomy should not be employed to relieve pressure symptoms or to prevent their future development. Technical difficulties often preclude splenectomy to relieve pressure symptoms, and if the spleen is removed early in the course of the disease, marked hepatomegaly can be expected to replace the massive splenomegaly and to be equally symptomatic. Although most patients will not, as once thought, succumb to hematopoietic failure after splenectomy, an occasional patient will. Furthermore, the operative risk is, on the whole, high. Even when clearly indicated, the hypersplenic component fails to improve in about half the patients. In addition, the development of striking thrombocytosis with thromboembolic or hemorrhagic complications is a common postoperative hazard. Therefore the decision to remove the spleen should be made only after careful consideration of all aspects of the individual case: the age of the patient, associated diseases, size of the spleen, presence of preoperative thrombocytosis, and extent of hematopoiesis in other sites. It is also highly desirable to confirm splenic red cell sequestration by the ^{51}Cr technique (p. 88) and to assess the degree of erythropoiesis in other sites by determining ^{59}Fe uptake before recommending splenectomy.

When hemorrhage or thromboembolic phenomena can be attributed to thrombocytosis (either as a primary manifestation of the disease or following splenectomy), *radioactive phosphorus* (^{32}P) is indicated. Megakaryocytes are especially sensitive to ionizing radiation; 2 to 3 mc of ^{32}P given intravenously (or 2.5 to 3.75 mc give orally) will usually lower the platelet count without depressing other aspects of hematopoiesis. ^{32}P can be repeated in six to eight weeks as needed.

Systemic symptoms (weight loss, fever, hypermetabolism, and bone pain) may respond to busulfan or, less often, to 6-mercaptopurine. If these complaints are disabling, corticosteroids may also be tried, but their side effects ordinarily outweigh the minimal subjective improvement that may be obtained. Bone pain will often respond to simple measures such as salicylates. Appropriate antibiotics are indicated for intercurrent infections. Secondary infections, bleeding, or thromboembolism are the usual causes of death.

Primary Thrombocythemia

A transient increase in the number of circulating platelets follows acute tissue necrosis (infection or trauma), bleeding, or hemolysis. Persistent thrombocytosis occurs after splenectomy and in patients with such diverse disorders as carcinoma, sarcoidosis, Cushing's syndrome, and Hodgkin's disease. Thrombocytosis is also a prominent manifestation of polycythemia vera, chronic granulocytic leukemia, and agnogenic myeloid metaplasia. Infrequently thrombocytosis occurs in the absence of any other disease to which it can be attributed; these patients have been diagnosed as primary (essential) thrombocythemia or hemorrhagic thrombocythemia. Although hemorrhage is often prominent, not all patients bleed. Therefore primary thrombocythemia is a more appropriate designation. Fewer than 100 patients have been reported, and in most the thrombocytosis appears to have reflected some other entity (e.g., polycythemia vera, agnogenic myeloid metaplasia, or the postsplenectomy state). Because of its rarity, lack of a unique histologic picture, and resemblance to other more clearly defined myeloproliferative disorders, it has been concluded by some that primary thrombocythemia does not exist as a disease *sui generis*. However, for occasional patients the clinical diagnosis of primary thrombocythemia is both appropriate and justified. The cause of the overproduction of platelets is not known. The predominant clinical manifestations of hemorrhage and/or thrombotic phenomena are directly attributable to the thrombocytosis. The excess platelets probably interfere with thromboplastin generation, but other mechanisms may also contribute to the hemorrhagic diathesis. Megakaryocytic hyperplasia is prominent, but there is no evidence of uncontrolled proliferation (i.e., "megakaryocytic leukemia").

Hemorrhage, thromboembolism, minimal to moderate splenomegaly, thrombocytosis (1 to 10 million/cu mm), and megakaryocytic hyperplasia in the marrow are the characteristic clinical manifestations. Platelets are frequently large, and megakaryocyte fragments may be found in the peripheral blood. The erythroid values are usually at the upper limits of normal but may be decreased as a result of acute or chronic hemorrhage; in the latter case the anemia will, of course, be microcytic and hypochromic. Polychromasia, reticulocytosis, nucleated red cells, and immature granulocytes have been described in the peripheral blood but probably reflect either acute hemorrhage or another diagnosis such as agnogenic myeloid metaplasia. The white count is generally normal or slightly increased. Tests of the coagulation mechanism, platelet function, and capillary integrity yield inconsistent and variable results.

Diagnosis is based on thrombocytosis in the absence of any other disorder known to be associated with this finding. When thrombocytosis and megakaryocytic hyperplasia are the only hematologic abnormalities in a patient with splenomegaly and thrombotic or hemorrhagic manifestations, the diagnosis is not difficult. When the erythroid values are slightly above normal or there is leukocytosis or anemia with immature granulocytes and nucleated red cells in the peripheral blood, exclusion of other myeloproliferative syndromes becomes a difficult task, for which careful follow-up is often needed. Too few patients have been studied to ascertain accurately the natural course of primary thrombocythemia. If death from hemorrhage or thrombosis is barred, it would appear to run a slowly progressive course similar to that of polycythemia vera. Because both hemorrhage and thrombosis can be attributed directly to the thrombocytosis, therapeutic measures are indicated to decrease platelet production and the peripheral platelet count. *Radioactive phosphorus* (2 to 3 mc intravenously or 2.5 to 3.75 mc orally) is the treatment of choice and may be repeated as needed at six- to eight-week intervals. *Total body x-radiation* or *busulfan* may be equally effective, but greater care must be taken with busulfan to prevent depression of other aspects of myelopoiesis. In view of the close relationship between the myeloproliferative disorders, it is not surprising that primary thrombocythemia has been observed to evolve into acute granulocytic leukemia. If patients with primary thrombocythemia live long enough, it is reasonable to surmise that many will develop an acute uncontrolled myeloproliferative process, as some patients with polycythemia vera (p. 306), agnogenic myeloid metaplasia, and chronic granulocytic leukemia (p. 368) seem to do.

Primary Macroglobulinemia
(Waldenström's Syndrome)

Lymphoid hyperplasia and macroglobulinemia characterize this syndrome which was first described by Waldenström in 1944. It bears certain similarities to plasmacytic myeloma, lymphoma, and chronic lymphocytic leukemia and should be classified as a hematologic neoplasm (a lymphoproliferative disorder) of unknown cause.

PATHOPHYSIOLOGY

The basic abnormality is the uncontrolled proliferation of lymphoid cells of variable morphology. In many patients these cells cannot be distinguished on morphologic criteria from normal small lymphocytes; in others they are atypical and might best be described as a cross between a lymphocyte and a plasmacyte (Fig. 11-5). The stimulus to this proliferative process is unknown. A disease has been observed in mice that is quite similar to primary macroglobulinemia in man. Lymphoid hyperplasia is responsible for lymphadenopathy, splenomegaly, and hepatomegaly, and tissue architecture is altered as in other lymphomatous processes. Lymphocytic proliferation in the marrow contributes significantly to the development of anemia.

Normally, about 5 per cent of the serum proteins are macroglobulins. These proteins (IgM immunoglobulins) have sedimentation constants of 15S or greater and molecular weights of about 1,000,000. They are approximately 10 per cent carbohydrate and appear to be polymers of polypeptide units with molecular weights similar to those of the 7S

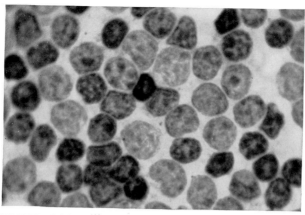

Figure 11-5. Atypical lymphocytes in the imprint of a lymph node from a patient with primary macroglobulinemia (Wright's stain).

immunoglobulins bound together by disulfide bonds. Red cell isoagglutinins, cold agglutinins, heterophil and Wassermann antibodies, and the rheumatoid factor are macroglobulins. Macroglobulinemia may occur in a variety of disorders, including plasmacytic myeloma, lymphoma, chronic lymphocytic leukemia, other malignancies, chronic infections, collagen diseases, cirrhosis, and the nephrotic syndrome. In these secondary macroglobulinemias macroglobulins generally make up only 5 to 15 per cent of the serum proteins. In primary macroglobulinemia or Waldenström's syndrome these high molecular weight globulins account for more than 15 per cent of the serum proteins.

There is abundant evidence that plasmacytes elaborate 7S myeloma globulins. The cell that synthesizes macroglobulins is less well defined, but a small lymphoid cell is the most likely suspect. The lymphoid cells in patients with primary macroglobulinemia possess endoplasmic reticulum which indicates active protein synthesis; fluorescent immunocytochemical techniques also point to these cells as the site of macroglobulin production. On paper electrophoresis these proteins usually migrate as homogeneous fractions; however, the presence of several components on ultracentrifugal analysis attests to their heterogeneity. Waldenström's macroglobulins manifest immunologic individuality but are antigenically related to one another and to normal immunoglobulins. Although the question of their "normalcy" cannot be answered with certainty, it seems most likely that these macroglobulins are anomalous products of abnormal cells with a perverted mechanism of protein synthesis.

Macroglobulins are directly responsible for many of the clinical manifestations of Waldenström's syndrome, such as increased blood viscosity, rouleau formation, a greatly increased erythrocyte sedimentation rate, hyperglobulinemia, abnormal electrophoretic patterns, cold-sensitivity phenomena (macroglobulins are often cold-precipitable), and abnormal bleeding. Although thrombocytopenia often contributes to a hemorrhagic diathesis, interference by the macroglobulins with a variety of coagulation factors is more important (e.g., the release of factor 3 by platelets). The abnormal protein undoubtedly plays a major role in the development of hypersplenism by extrinsic cellular damage (p. 453). Complexes between the macroglobulins and normal cellular proteins appear to explain a number of other findings, such as interference with glandular secretions (Sjögren's syndrome) and amyloid deposits. Bence Jones-like proteins are demonstrable in the urine of about 10 per cent of the patients, although renal failure is quite unusual. Precipitation of the macroglobulins in the central nervous system, with bleeding and perivascular lymphocytic infiltrations, is responsible for a high incidence of neurologic abnormalities. Macroglobulinemia is associated with decreased production of normal immunoglobulins, thus contributing to a high incidence of infections.

CLINICAL MANIFESTATIONS

Primary macroglobulinemia is rare. Fewer than 300 patients have been reported in the world's literature, but the wider use of electrophoretic and ultracentrifugal analyses will probably uncover many previously unrecognized cases. It also seems likely that some cases have been classified in the past as atypical lymphoma or plasmacytic myeloma. Primary macroglobulinemia most commonly affects males between the ages of 50 to 70. As a rule, the onset is insidious.

Symptoms. Weakness, ease of fatigue, dyspnea, abnormal bleeding, visual disturbances, neurologic complaints, recurrent bacterial infections, cold-sensitivity phenomena (p. 415), and weight loss are the common symptoms. In contrast to plasmacytic myeloma, bone pain is unusual. A hemorrhagic diathesis occurs in more than one half the patients, visual disturbances in one third, and neurologic abnormalities in approximately one fourth. Neurologic abnormalities may take the form of an encephalopathy, a peripheral neuropathy, or a stroke syndrome.

Physical Findings. Pallor, minimal splenomegaly, hepatomegaly, and peripheral lymphadenopathy are the most prevalent physical abnormalities. Retinal lesions (hemorrhages, exudates, and venous congestion with vascular segmentation or "sausage" formation) are frequent. Bleeding into the skin (petechiae and purpura) is common, and skin ulcerations may be present, especially over the lower legs. Diverse lesions may produce a variety of neurologic findings. Bone tenderness, deformity, or tumor formation does not ordinarily occur.

Laboratory Findings. PERIPHERAL BLOOD. A moderate to severe normocytic, normochromic anemia is present in almost every patient;

decreased erythropoiesis and a hemolytic component are the usual causes. When the hemolytic component predominates, it is reflected by polychromasia, reticulocytosis, and nucleated red cells in the peripheral blood. Rouleau formation is striking, and the erythrocyte sedimentation rate is greatly increased. Leukocyte and platelet counts are normal to decreased. A relative or slight absolute lymphocytosis is a common finding.

BONE MARROW. Lymphocytes generally make up 40 per cent or more of the marrow nucleated cells. In most cases these cells have scanty cytoplasm and resemble small mature lymphocytes (Fig. 11-6).

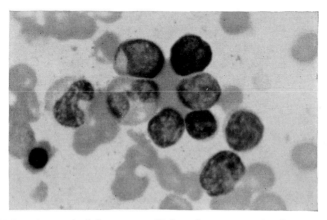

Figure 11-6. Atypical, "plasmacytoid" lymphocytes in the bone marrow aspirate of a patient with primary macroglobulinemia.

Naked nuclei are abundant and cytoplasmic shedding may be evident. Occasionally these lymphocytic elements have plasmacytoid characteristics. Mast cells are often increased, an interesting finding, for heparin has been shown to precipitate macroglobulins. Normal myeloid elements are usually decreased in number.

PROTEIN ABNORMALITIES. Hyperglobulinemia is to be expected. The Sia water test is ordinarily positive (moderate to heavy precipitate forming within 10 seconds after a drop of plasma is added to 10 ml of distilled water), as is the formol-gel test, but these tests are nonspecific reflections of the hyperglobulinemic state. The serum protein electrophoretic pattern is indistinguishable from that of plasmacytic myeloma and is characterized by a sharp peak migrating with γ or, less often, β globulin mobility. Ultracentrifugal analysis is the *sine qua non* for the diagnosis of macroglobulinemia and reveals one or more protein components with sedimentation constants of 15S or greater (usually 20S). Macroglobulins make up 15 per cent or more of the serum proteins; normal immunoglobulins are decreased. The serum protein

immunoelectrophoretic pattern is also specific for primary macroglobulinemia. Cryoglobulins are demonstrable in 10 to 15 per cent of the
patients. About 10 per cent will have Bence Jones proteinuria.

Other Laboratory Findings. Bone x-rays are most often normal
but may show diffuse osteoporosis; focal lytic lesions are almost never
seen. As a reflection of the dysproteinemic state, flocculation tests may
be abnormal in the face of otherwise normal liver function studies.
Serum uric acid may be slightly increased. Other laboratory findings
are, for the most part, nonspecific.

DIAGNOSIS

The symptoms, physical findings, and protein abnormalities (rouleau
formation, hyperglobulinemia, and abnormal electrophoretic patterns)
should suggest the diagnosis. Although these patterns also point toward
plasmacytic myeloma, histologic confirmation is unobtainable. A positive
diagnosis is based on the demonstration of macroglobulinemia by ultracentrifugal analysis in the absence of any other disease known to be
associated with this finding and in the presence of a clinical picture
and histology compatible with primary macroglobulinemia. Serum protein immunoelectrophoretic patterns are also diagnostic. Because an
ultracentrifuge is not routinely available, attempts have been made to
devise simpler and more usable diagnostic techniques such as starch
gel electrophoresis. Although macroglobulins will not migrate in starch
gel, they can be readily depolymerized into units similar in size to the
7S globulins by low molecular weight thiols. These protein subunits will
then migrate as sharp peaks similar to those of the myeloma globulins.
Therefore macroglobulins can be detected in starch gel to which 2-
mercaptoethanol has been added.

Major problems in differential diagnosis center around the exclusion
of plasmacytic myeloma, chronic lymphocytic leukemia, and certain
forms of lymphoma, especially lymphosarcoma. In some patients primary
macroglobulinemia actually appears to evolve into plasmacytic myeloma
or one of the other lymphoproliferative disorders; it should also be
noted that macroglobulinemia may occur in otherwise "typical" cases
of plasmacytic myeloma or lymphoma. These diseases are closely
related, and some patients actually have findings characteristic of more
than one disorder. Pending the development of more discriminating
tests, enough patients fail to meet the criteria for some other diagnosis
to warrant the retention of the category of primary macroglobulinemia
as a specific hematologic neoplasm. To prevent confusion, however,
the diagnosis of primary macroglobulinemia should be made only when
other diagnoses are not possible; for example, the presence of myeloma
cells demands the diagnosis of plasmacytic myeloma, even if peculiar
lymphocytes predominate in the marrow, and bone lesions are absent.

TREATMENT AND COURSE

Primary macroglobulinemia runs a chronic progressive course lasting 2 to 10 years or longer. Some patients tolerate macroglobulinemia well; others manifest a more malignant process.

Specific therapy should be directed toward suppression of the abnormal lymphocytic proliferation. A number of chemotherapeutic agents have been used with varying degrees of success. In several patients beneficial effects have been ascribed to *chlorambucil* after prolonged administration in doses similar to those used in chronic lymphocytic leukemia (p. 373), but the number treated is still small. In view of the response to long-term oral *cyclophosphamide* in patients with plasmacytic myeloma (p. 425), this agent deserves a therapeutic trial. Since many of the clinical manifestations of primary macroglobulinemia are directly attributable to the presence of the abnormal proteins, attempts have been made to attack the problem from this angle. The macroglobulin level can be reduced by repeated plasmaphereses or the administration of a low molecular weight thiol, such as penicillamine (*d,* 1-dimethylcysteine), which depolymerizes the macroglobulins. Although the effect of such therapeutic measures is transient, they are useful adjuncts in certain selected patients. Some patients respond symptomatically to *corticosteroids,* but these compounds are of greatest use in the treatment of superimposed hypersplenism. Other supportive measures include *transfusions* as needed and appropriate *antibiotics* for intercurrent infections. Hemorrhage and infection are the usual causes of death. The development of another malignant disease occurs with a greater frequency than can be attributed to chance alone.

Hypersplenism

Hypersplenism is a clinical syndrome of varied etiology characterized by peripheral blood cytopenia with normal or increased numbers of bone marrow precursors; it may involve erythrocytes, granulocytes, and/or thrombocytes. Hypersplenism arises from the overactivity or exaggeration of one or more of the spleen's functions. The spleen is often palpable, and improvement frequently follows removal of all splenic tissue. Since certain of the spleen's functions are attributable to cells common to other tissues (i.e., reticuloendothelial cells, lymphocytes, and plasmacytes), "hypersplenic" activity can persist even in the absence of the spleen. In this regard the term hypersplenism, first introduced by Chauffard in 1907, is a misnomer; however, it has gained wide acceptance in recent years and is useful when defined broadly because it emphasizes the nature of the pathogenic mechanisms involved in these hematologic syndromes.

PATHOGENESIS

In many respects the spleen still fits Galen's description as an "organ of mystery." Although certain aspects of the histology and physiology of the normal spleen remain obscure, much has been learned from the study of the effects of splenectomy and of various disturbances affecting the spleen; these observations bear directly on the pathogenesis of hypersplenism.

Anatomy. The basic structural components of the spleen are (1) a branching arterial tree, (2) a system of venous sinusoids lined with reticuloendothelial cells, (3) lymphoid elements (white pulp), (4) an intercommunicating network of finer capillaries (red pulp), and (5) a smooth muscle-reinforced capsule that penetrates the parenchyma as trabeculae. The nature of the splenic arteriovenous communications is disputable. The consensus is that the vascular system is closed with muscular sphincters in the distal venous sinusoids that control blood flow; others favor an open vascular system. Despite this controversy, there is general agreement that splenic structure permits deplasmatization of blood with sequestration and concentration of hemic cells. Thus the spleen might best be viewed as a large distensible blood filter interposed between an artery and a vein; it possesses a variable stasis compartment and abundant lymphoid and reticuloendothelial tissue.

Effects of Splenectomy. The spleen is not essential for life and can be removed with relative impunity; however, the hematologic effects of splenectomy are definite and provide insight into the functions of the normal spleen. All blood cells are affected by "hyposplenism." In otherwise normal subjects the erythroid values do not usually change. Although slight anemia and even polycythemia have been described, alterations in the peripheral erythroid values are not constant and probably reflect some underlying disease. On the other hand, certain qualitative changes in the erythrocytes are striking. Howell-Jolly bodies (p. 63) occur in 100 per cent of splenectomized individuals, and siderocytes are commonly found. Other peripheral blood manifestations of the postsplenectomy state include polychromasia, slight reticulocytosis, target cells (p. 62), and even occasional nucleated red cells. Thrombocytosis and leukocytosis are rather consistent findings after removal of the spleen. The platelet increase often develops gradually and may be quite marked. The leukocyte count is ordinarily between 10,000 and 15,000/cu mm but may be much higher, especially in the immediate postoperative period when the leukocytosis reflects a neutrophilia. Later on, the differential count is characterized by a relative (but not an absolute) neutropenia and by relative and absolute increases in large lymphocytes and monocytes. The hematologic effects of splenectomy persist indefinitely. Similar changes are demonstrable in patients with congenital absence of the spleen as well as in others who develop decreased splenic activity consequent to a disorder such as sickle cell anemia (p. 255). There is suggestive evidence that some children are more susceptible to acute infections after splenectomy, perhaps because of impaired immunologic response. Although prophylactic antibiotics have been recommended, there is little support for this approach, and the problem requires further study before a definitive answer can be reached.

Functions of the Spleen. The following functions can be attributed to the normal spleen.

HEMATOPOIESIS. The spleen is the chief erythrocytogenic organ in lower vertebrates and is an important site of hematopoiesis in human fetal development. In postnatal life the spleen does not actively produce blood cells other than lymphocytes and probably monocytes; however, splenic reticulum cells retain their embryonic potentialities and are capable of resuming active hematopoiesis in response to a variety of stimuli.

CELL REMOVAL. The unique splenic anatomy, which favors cell sequestration, and the presence of phagocytic reticuloendothelial cells support the contention that the spleen plays a major role in the removal of effete red cells as they reach the end of their finite life-span. It is not known what role, if any, the normal spleen plays in the destruction or removal of thrombocytes or leukocytes.

CELL RESERVOIR. In man the spleen normally contains about 1 to 2 per cent of the circulating red cell mass; there is no significant non-circulating erythrocyte reserve as in the spleens of certain other species. However, it has been estimated that a normal red cell spends about two days out of a normal life-span of 120 days in the stasis compartment of the spleen.

ANTIBODY PRODUCTION. The spleen contains large numbers of cells that are capable of synthesizing protein (i.e., plasmacytes and lympocytes). Consequently, it is an important site of antibody or immunoglobulin production.

CULLING AND PITTING EFFECT. The normal spleen removes defective and misshapen erythrocytes from the circulation. It has been estimated that up to 10 per cent of the red cells produced by the marrow fail to meet minimum requirements and are selectively removed by the normal spleen. The spleen is also capable of removing certain erythrocyte inclusion bodies, such as Howell-Jolly bodies and iron granules, without damaging the cell, which is returned to the circulation. The loss of this function accounts for the presence of Howell-Jolly bodies and siderocytes after splenectomy.

EFFECT ON RED CELL MEMBRANE. After splenectomy, the erythrocytes lost by normal attrition are replaced by a population of large thin cells or target cells. These cells most likely reflect the loss of a maturing or controlling effect of the spleen on the lipid content of the stroma and surface membrane of the erythrocyte, thus affecting the active metabolic processes serving to maintain the normal configuration of the cell.

IRON METABOLISM. Hemoglobin released from red cells destroyed in the spleen is catabolized, and the iron is returned to the marrow for reutilization. This function of the spleen contrasts with that of other organs (e.g., the lungs), which are incapable of returning iron to the body.

HORMONAL EFFECTS ON MYELOPOIESIS. There exists some evidence that the spleen, presumably by humoral factor elaboration, exerts an inhibitory effect on the maturation of marrow precursor cells or on the release of mature elements into the circulation. So far, however, the search for a splenic hormone or hormones with a physiologic effect on myelopoiesis has proved unrewarding.

Etiology of Hypersplenism. Exaggeration of the following functions of the spleen has been implicated in the production of hypersplenism: (1) the ability to remove and destroy aged or defective cells, (2) the ability to sequester normal cells for variable periods of time, and (3) the production of immunoglobulins. Other splenic functions are noticeable when absent or decreased (e.g., Howell-Jolly bodies and target cells following splenectomy), but clinical manifestations are not associated with their hyperfunction. The thesis that hypersplenism is due to inhibition of marrow activity by a splenic hormone was once a widely held view. Perhaps the strongest argument for the existence of a humoral hematopoietic depressant stems from the presence of atypical megakaryocytes without evidence of platelet formation in patients with idiopathic thrombocytopenic purpura. Defects in maturation are less impressive in the granulocytic and erythrocytic series, but they are nonetheless typically demonstrable. However, numerous attempts to isolate a splenic hormone(s) have yielded negative or inconclusive results, whereas other theories of the causation of hypersplenism have acquired compelling experimental and clinical support. Therefore the role of a hormonal factor(s) in the production of hypersplenism, although not excludable with absolute certainty, must be viewed as conjectural.

Based on the pathogenic mechanism involved, the hypersplenic syndromes may be separated into three categories.

Removal of Defective or Injured Cells by a Normal Spleen. Certain types of erythrocyte are more susceptible to splenic sequestration and destruction than others. For example, spherocytes, deformed or fragmented erythrocytes, and cells that have been injured by certain antibodies or metallic cations are selectively retained by the spleen. After a sufficiently long sojourn in the spleen, the surface membrane of an erythrocyte is changed in some manner so that the cell attracts destruction by splenic phagocytes. Hereditary spherocytosis is an excellent example of this form of hypersplenism. Because of an inborn cellular defect, red cells from patients with hereditary spherocytosis are unable to maintain a normal shape and become spherocytic (p. 101). These spherocytes disappear quickly when transfused into a normal recipient, but they possess a nearly normal life-span when transfused into a splenectomized recipient. Thus a normal spleen is apparently behaving in an essentially normal manner toward a group of abnormal erythrocytes. Excessive splenic sequestration of damaged or defective cells is demonstrable by several techniques. When such cells are tagged with ^{51}Cr, their increased localization in the spleen can be detected by external surface counting. Comparison of body and venous hematocrits will also reveal abnormal trapping of red cells in the spleen, but this is a more cumbersome and less reliable technique. Methods permitting study of the role of splenic hypersequestration in the production of thrombocytopenia and leukopenia are just becoming available; however, it may be logically inferred from existent data that a similar pathogenic mechanism is operative in certain cases of hypersplenic thrombocytopenia and leukopenia.

INCREASED REMOVAL OF NORMAL CELLS BY AN ENLARGED SPLEEN. Greatly enlarged spleens contain an expanded vascular bed and stasis compartment which can assume major clinical significance. An enlarged spleen may be likened to a hypertrophied, sequestering, and phagocytic organ in which increased numbers of red cells are exposed to the metabolic stress of normal splenic stasis, a damaging effect that is similar to enzymatic depletion in vitro. Sequestered cells undergo rather rapid injury (perhaps as the result of separation from glucose and the source of energy needed to maintain their integrity); repeated short periods of splenic stasis appear to result in cumulative cell damage which eventually becomes irreversible. Therefore splenic sequestration is an important conditioning factor affecting cell survival. The increased stasis compartment in an enlarged spleen can be demonstrated by the administration of ^{51}Cr-tagged erythrocytes; uptake of the isotope by the spleen is initially high and remains so for an hour or more after injection because of slow mixing of "splenic" and circulating cells. This form of hypersplenism (i.e., the "big spleen" syndrome) has also been studied experimentally. Repeated intraperitoneal injections of methyl cellulose in normal rats induce infiltration with phagocytic monocytes in the spleen, liver, kidneys, and other tissues, together with splenomegaly, anemia, reticulocytosis, leukopenia, thrombocytopenia, and myeloid hyperplasia. Splenectomized recipients manifest similar histologic lesions in other tissues, but these animals do not develop hematologic abnormalities. Clinical counterparts of these experimental observations include patients with Banti's syndrome (portal hypertension with chronic congestive splenomegaly and hypersplenism), Gaucher's disease, and agnogenic myeloid metaplasia of the spleen. Red cells from these patients have shortened in vivo life-spans but survive normally in normal recipients. Although other factors (e.g., abnormal cells or abnormal splenic activity) may contribute in some cases, there is rather compelling support for the contention that massively enlarged spleens can remove increased numbers of normal cells primarily by quantitative changes. The role of splenomegaly in the production of hypersplenic thrombocytopenia and leukopenia is less clear; however, these hemic cells are probably affected in a similar manner.

IMMUNOLOGIC REACTIONS. Strong experimental and clinical evidence implicates antigen-antibody responses in the pathogenesis of certain hypersplenic syndromes. The elaboration of abnormal globulins capable of affecting one or more types of blood cell may be primary (idiopathic) or secondary (associated with a collagen disease, certain viral infections, or proliferative disorders involving antibody- or protein-producing cells such as chronic lymphocytic leukemia, lymphoma, or plasmacytic myeloma). In these "autoimmune" disorders the nature of the stimulus (or antigen) that evokes the formation of the immunoglobulin directed against autologous cells is not known. These disorders do not appear to reflect the usual type of immunologic response (i.e., a specific antigen stimulating the production of a specific antibody that is capable of reacting with and destroying the foreign substance). It seems more likely that they are manifestations of the proliferation of a clone or clones of antibody-producing cells whose product or products fortuitously exhibit an affinity for one or more hemic cells. Blocking or incomplete red cell antibodies are demonstrable in certain patients with acquired hemolytic anemia (p. 96) and platelet agglutinins can be identified by in vitro and in vivo techniques in many patients with idiopathic thrombocytopenia purpura (p. 490). Recent studies indicate that leukoagglutinins play a role in the pathogenesis of certain types of hypersplenic neutropenias (p. 332). Since the spleen contains large numbers of antibody-producing cells, it is rational to assume that this organ plays an important (but not necessarily an essential) role in the production of immunologic hypersplenism.

Many questions remain unanswered. Enhanced splenic sequestration of cells, an expanded stasis compartment, or abnormal immunoglobulins are not always demonstrable even in the presence of clear-cut clinical hypersplenism. In addition, the possible role of marrow inhibition by a hypothetical splenic hormone or perhaps by circulating immunoglobulins cannot be eliminated. It should also be emphasized that few hypersplenic syndromes are the result of a single pathogenic mechanism; for example, the passage of abnormal cells such as spherocytes through a normal spleen will lead to "work hypertrophy," an expanded vascular bed (or stasis compartment), and the promotion of a vicious cycle. A similar sequence occurs in the immunologic forms of hypersplenism in addition to the important role of the spleen in the elaboration of the abnormal globulins that injure the cells and render them more susceptible to splenic destruction. It is apparent that the causes of hypersplenism are multiple and varied; its pathogenesis, more often than not, is complex. An etiologic classification of the hypersplenic syndromes is given in Table 12-1.

Table 12-1. Etiologic Classification of Hypersplenism

I. *Cell Defects (Intrinsic)*

A. Erythrocytes
1. Hereditary spherocytosis (p. 100)
2. Hereditary elliptocytosis (p. 121)
3. Other hereditary hemolytic anemias (p. 112)
4. Paroxysmal nocturnal hemoglobinuria (p. 150)
5. Vitamin B_{12} or folic acid deficiencies (p. 186)

B. Granulocytes
1. None known

C. Platelets
1. None known

II. *Cell Defects (Extrinsic)*

A. Erythrocytes
1. Iso- and autoantibodies (see below)
2. Physical damage (e.g., heat, p. 147)
3. Chemical damage (e.g., heavy metals, snake venoms, and drugs, p. 147)
4. Parasites (e.g., malaria, p. 149)
5. Bacterial infections (e.g., cholera and gas gangrene, p. 149)
6. Hyperlipemic hemolysis—Zieve's syndrome (p. 148)

B. Granulocytes
1. Iso- and autoantibodies (see below)

C. Platelets
1. Iso- and autoantibodies (see below)

III. *Splenomegaly* *
1. Banti's syndrome (p. 457)
2. Agnogenic myeloid metaplasia (p. 430)
3. Infectious splenomegaly (e.g., tuberculosis and syphilis, p. 458)
4. Sarcoidosis (p. 460)
5. Gaucher's disease (p. 458)

454

IV. *Immunologic*
 1. Autoantibodies (primary)
    a. Idiopathic acquired hemolytic anemia (p. 131)
    b. Idiopathic thrombocytopenic purpura (p. 491)
    c. Hypersplenic neutropenia (p. 328)
 2. Autoantibodies (secondary) *
    a. Chronic lymphocytic leukemia (p. 369)
    b. Lymphoma (p. 380)
    c. Plasmacytic myeloma (p. 411)
    d. Primary macroglobulinemia (p. 442)
    e. Disseminated carcinoma and other neoplasms (p. 460)
    f. Systemic lupus erythematosus and other collagen disorders (p. 460)
    g. Viral infections (e.g., infectious mononucleosis, p. 316)
    h. Drug-induced (pp. 147, 328, and 499)
 3. Isoantibodies
    a. Transfusion reactions (p. 532)
    b. Erythroblastosis fetalis (p. 123)
    c. Neonatal neutropenia (p. 329)
    d. Neonatal thrombocytopenia (p. 489)

V. *Miscellaneous (Cause Unknown)*
 1. Felty's syndrome (p. 459)
 2. Hereditary hemoglobinopathies (p. 246)
 3. Thrombotic thrombocytopenic purpura (p. 501)

* May affect erythrocytes, granulocytes, platelets, all three, or any combination.

PATHOPHYSIOLOGY

Although the pathogenesis differs, the pathophysiology of the hypersplenic syndromes is similar, regardless of cause. Despite the pathogenic importance of the spleen, its histologic picture is nonspecific. The spleen usually reveals only congestion and reticuloendothelial hyperplasia; erythrophagocytosis, myeloid metaplasia, and hemosiderosis may also be evident. The major clinical manifestations of hypersplenism reflect a deficiency in the peripheral blood of one or more hemic cells; that is, anemia, neutropenia, and/or thrombocytopenia, which evoke, respectively, the symptoms and findings of anemia, an enhanced susceptibility to infection, a hemorrhagic diathesis, or various combinations. The peripheral blood cytopenia, operating through normal homeostatic controls, such as the humoral erythropoietic regulatory mechanism (p. 13), stimulates myeloid activity and produces a hypercellular marrow. The attempt on the part of the marrow to correct the peripheral cytopenia will, depending on the cell involved, be reflected in the circulating blood by polychromasia, reticulocytosis, and nucleated red cells or occasional immature granulocytes. In many cases qualitative marrow changes are also demonstrable, especially in the megakaryocytes, which often exhibit sharp cytoplasmic borders without evidence of platelet formation. Comparable "maturation arrests" in granulopoiesis or erythropoiesis with preponderance of a single precursor and a paucity of more mature cells are often noticeable but are usually less apparent than the changes in the megakaryocytes. In contrast to a leukemic marrow, maturation is orderly up to a point but does not appear to proceed beyond that stage. These marrow findings have been interpreted as evidence of marrow inhibition; however, these "maturation arrests" may be more apparent than real, for the changes may reflect premature release of more mature cells into the circulation. It is also possible that a circulating antibody may exert a direct effect on the marrow in patients with immunologic hypersplenism, thus affecting both cell production and destruction.

Other clinical manifestations depend on the type of cell that is involved and on the nature of the underlying process. Incomplete erythrocyte antibodies, positive Coombs' or bromelin tests, leukoagglutinins, or platelet agglutinins are often demonstrable in patients with immunologic hypersplenism. Hemolysis will evoke typical pigment changes (unconjugated bilirubinemia with increased fecal and urinary urobilinogen). In some patients the major manifestations are those of the basic disease (e.g., a patient with lymphoma and a superimposed acquired hemolytic anemia). Since hypersplenism more often than not is secondary to some other primary disease, the clinical manifestations as a rule are diverse. Only the hematologic findings are constant, and even they often depend on the nature of the basic disease. For example, a patient with chronic lymphocytic leukemia may not respond in the usual manner because of marrow involvement by the leukemic process.

CLINICAL MANIFESTATIONS

Because of the many different causes of hypersplenism, the true incidence of this hematologic syndrome cannot be ascertained. It is associated with a variety of diseases more often than is generally appreciated. The characteristic clinical manifestations of hypersplenism are (1) splenomegaly, (2) a hemolytic anemia, neutropenia, and/or thrombocytopenia, and (3) a cellular marrow with or without a "maturation arrest." Splenomegaly is to be expected, but it is not invariably found, especially in such disorders as idiopathic thrombocytopenic purpura, splenic neutropenia, and splenic pancytopenia. Hypersplenism can exist, therefore, in the absence of gross splenic enlargement. Most of the hypersplenic syndromes are primary hematologic disorders and are discussed in detail in other chapters (see Table 12-1). Several non-hematologic diseases may be complicated by superimposed hypersplenism and are considered below.

Chronic Congestive Splenomegaly with Hypersplenism (Banti's Syndrome)

In 1898 Banti described a type of "splenic anemia" characterized by splenomegaly, anemia, leukopenia, hemorrhage, and progressive hepatic dysfunction. He concluded that the basic abnormality lay in the spleen and the eponym, "Banti's disease," gained popular usage. It is now evident, however, that this disorder is not a clinical entity in itself but is instead hypersplenism accompanying chronic congestive splenomegaly consequent to portal hypertension from any of a variety of causes. The term Banti's disease is no longer applicable and should be dropped; Banti's syndrome or, more appropriately, chronic congestive splenomegaly with hypersplenism is preferred. In about 75 per cent of the patients, portal hypertension is secondary to intrahepatic obstruction resulting from cirrhosis (e.g., Laennec's, postnecrotic, and schistosomiasis). Extrahepatic obstruction, secondary to thrombosis of the splenic or portal veins or obstruction due to other causes (e.g., an adjacent tumor), is seen less often. Splenomegaly, which may be massive, is always present. Although hypersplenism does not invariably accompany chronic congestive splenomegaly, the diagnosis of hypersplenism secondary to chronic congestive splenomegaly is untenable in the absence of splenomegaly. Evidence of hepatic dysfunction and bleeding esophageal varices usually dominate and color the clinical picture.

Laboratory findings include anemia, thrombocytopenia, and/or leukopenia. The anemia is typically normocytic, normochromic but may reflect iron deficiency due to chronic blood loss (microcytic, hypochromic) or liver disease (macrocytic, normochromic). In contrast to most hypersplenic anemias, evidence of hemolysis is minimal and, in the absence of recent hemorrhage, the reticulocyte count is ordinarily normal or only slightly increased. The leukopenia also differs from the usual hypersplenic syndromes and reflects a parallel decrease in all cell types with a normal differential count. The bone marrow reveals the characteristic findings of hypersplenism, but the picture may be influenced by hepatic dysfunction, iron deficiency, and so forth. This form of hypersplenism appears to be an example of the "big spleen" syndrome. Abnormal antibodies are not demonstrable, and these patients do not as a rule respond to corticosteroids. Death is most often caused by hepatic failure or bleeding from esophageal varices; however, hypersplenic manifestations are occasionally severe and warrant specific therapy. These hematologic abnormalities generally show a satisfactory response to removal of the spleen, but splenectomy cannot be recommended routinely because it does not alter the course of the basic disease and most of these patients are poor operative risks. If the superimposed hypersplenism is so severe that it necessitates splenectomy, some type of vascular shunt should probably be performed at the same time.

Gaucher's Disease

This rare familial disorder of cerebroside metabolism was first described by Gaucher in 1882. It affects all age groups and is characterized by an insidious onset, a protracted course, splenomegaly (often massive), hepatomegaly, pingueculae (brown wedge-shaped conjuctival thickenings at the lateral scleral margins), brownish skin pigmentation, skeletal defects, and hematologic abnormalities. Hematologic abnormalities occur in 80 per cent or more of the patients and consist of anemia, neutropenia, and/or thrombocytopenia in the presence of normal or increased numbers of marrow precursors. The hypersplenism of Gaucher's disease is apparently secondary to massive splenic enlargement. The diagnosis is based on the demonstration of the characteristic "foam" cells (atypical histiocytes loaded with cerebrosides) in the bone marrow, spleen, or liver (Fig. 12-1). Prompt and sustained hematologic improvement has followed splenectomy in patients with clear-cut hypersplenism.

Infectious Splenomegaly

A variety of infectious diseases may be associated with splenomegaly [e.g., tuberculosis, syphilis, and leishmaniasis (kala-azar)]. Although superimposed hypersplenic manifestations (anemia, neutropenia, and/or

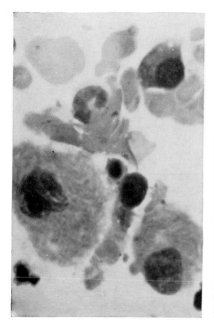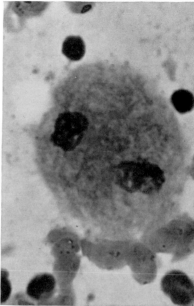

Figure 12-1. Gaucher cells in a bone marrow aspirate (Wright's stain). These large cells possess one to several round, oval, or irregularly shaped nuclei. The abundant, blue-gray cytoplasm has a fibrillar appearance.

thrombocytopenia) are not common, they have been observed. The pathogenesis is somewhat obscure. In certain patients the hematologic abnormalities probably reflect "big spleen" syndromes, and these patients usually respond to splenectomy. In other infectious diseases (e.g., infectious mononucleosis and infectious hepatitis) available data indicate that an abnormal globulin is at fault. In some cases both factors probably contribute to the development of hypersplenism.

Felty's Syndrome

This rare clinical syndrome is characterized by chronic rheumatoid arthritis, splenomegaly, hepatomegaly, adenopathy, anemia, and leukopenia. Leukopenia is due specifically to a relative and absolute neutropenia (there is a relative but not an absolute increase in lymphocytes and monocytes). The marrow typically reveals granulocytic hyperplasia with a "maturation arrest" at the myelocyte-metamyelocyte level. The cause of the hypersplenism is obscure. In view of the evident protein abnormalities in rheumatoid arthritis (i.e., the presence of the rheumatoid factor), it seems most likely that it represents an immunoneutropenia. Some (but certainly not all) patients respond to corticosteroids; splenectomy appears to be more beneficial and is indicated in patients with profound neutropenia and frequent infections.

Sarcoidosis

Splenomegaly occurs in about 25 per cent of patients with sarcoidosis. A few manifest thrombocytopenia, anemia, and/or neutropenia on the basis of superimposed hypersplenism. The cause is not known. Since this disorder is associated with hypergammaglobulinemia, an autoimmune mechanism seems likely.

Nonhematologic Neoplasms

Although hypersplenism occurs much more often in patients with lymphoma, chronic lymphocytic leukemia, and plasmacytic myeloma, rare patients with nonhematologic neoplasms (e.g., disseminated carcinoma and certain ovarian tumors) develop overt and often severe hypersplenism. The explanation is not apparent. Metastatic carcinoma almost never produces splenic enlargement, and even microscopic metastases are uncommon (less than 5 per cent of patients who die of nonhematologic malignancies have splenic metastases).

Systemic Lupus Erythematosus

A hemolytic anemia (usually spherocytic), neutropenia, and/or thrombocytopenia are common findings in patients with systemic lupus erythematosus. There is abundant evidence favoring the concept that this disease is an autoimmune process, and protein abnormalities are evident [e.g., the L.E. cell phenomenon (p. 313)]. In many (but not all) of these patients the demonstration of incomplete erythrocyte antibodies, platelet agglutinins, and/or leukocyte agglutinins supports the thesis that the hypersplenism associated with systemic lupus erythematosus (and less often with other types of "collagen" disease such as scleroderma and polyarteritis nodosa) is immunologic.

DIAGNOSIS

The diagnosis of hypersplenism is based on hematologic criteria (i.e., cytopenia in the peripheral blood in the presence of normal or, more often, increased numbers of marrow precursors). Although the marrow frequently reveals a "maturation arrest," the disorderly proliferation characteristic of leukemia (p. 337) does not occur. Splenomegaly and improvement following splenectomy have been mentioned as additional diagnostic requirements; however, the spleen is not always palpably enlarged and, with certain rare exceptions (e.g., hereditary spherocytosis), splenectomy is not always curative. Therefore the diagnosis of hypersplenism is contingent on the careful study of the peripheral blood and bone marrow and on an awareness of the many and varied clinical abnormalities that may be associated with this hematologic syndrome.

In most cases it is relatively easy to recognize the presence of hypersplenism; the diagnosis of the primary disease is much more difficult. Peripheral blood abnormalities (e.g., spherocytes, increased polychromasia, reticulocytosis, and nucleated red cells) often call attention to the possibility of a hemolytic anemia. Osmotic fragility measurements, the Coombs' or bromelin tests, unconjugated bilirubinemia with increased urine urobilinogen, and red cell survival data are other laboratory procedures that afford relevant information in the diagnosis of hypersplenic anemia or hemolytic disease (p. 85). The demonstration of platelet or leukocyte agglutinins may aid in the diagnosis of hypersplenic thrombocytopenia or leukopenia. The problem is complicated when involvement of the marrow by the primary disease prevents the usual peripheral blood and marrow responses. If erythropoietic tissue is severely curtailed as the result of infiltration with leukemic lymphocytes, a hemolytic anemia may not be accompanied by a clear-cut reticulocytosis or significant myeloid erythrocytic hyperplasia. Other defects that impair hematopoiesis such as the recent application of cytotoxic therapy are also capable of drastically altering the expected hematologic findings or response.

Several specialized diagnostic procedures have been devised to aid in the recognition of certain types of hypersplenism. It has been claimed that an increase in circulating cell count(s) after the injection of epinephrine reflects the release of cells from the spleen and is indicative of excessive cell sequestration therein. Although the Adrenalin test was once widely used to diagnose hypersplenism and predict response to splenectomy, the results are variable and often inconclusive. Furthermore, the observation of identical findings in normal and splenectomized subjects has seriously challenged the reliability and significance of this test, and it can no longer be recommended. Radioisotopic techniques have proved to be much more valuable; for example, splenic sequestration of red cells can be demonstrated by external surface counting after the injection of ^{51}Cr-tagged erythrocytes. A prompt high initial uptake of labeled cells by the spleen and slow mixing are indicative of an increase in the spleen's vascular bed and stasis compartment. However, with the exception of their use in predicting response to splenectomy, most of these specialized, complex techniques are investigative rather than clinical tools. Details of the diagnosis of the many diseases that may be accompanied by hypersplenism are discussed elsewhere (see Table 12-1).

TREATMENT AND COURSE

The course, response to treatment, and prognosis of the hypersplenic syndromes differ widely and depend on the nature of the underlying disease process. Therefore it serves no useful purpose to discuss these aspects of hypersplenism without knowledge of its cause. The forms of, indications for, and results of therapy are considered separately for each of the disorders that may be complicated by hypersplenism (see Table 12-1); however, certain principles of management are the same for all types of hypersplenism. In general, there are three therapeutic approaches to the problem.

Treatment of the Basic Disease. Depending on the cause of the hypersplenism, eradication of the basic disorder may eliminate the hematologic abnormality; for example, the hypersplenism caused by malaria will respond to antimalarial therapy, a drug-induced immunoneutropenia or thrombocytopenia can be "cured" merely by discontinuing the offending agent, and so forth. Occasionally specific suppressive therapy for a disorder such as lymphoma is followed by a decrease in hypersplenic activity. In many of these cases, however, the hypersplenism must be attacked directly in addition to the treatment of the primary disease.

Corticosteroids. These compounds are invaluable in the treatment of hypersplenism. With only a few exceptions, such as hereditary spherocytosis and the other intrinsic cell defects (Table 12-1), corticosteroids are indicated in most patients with hypersplenic disease. The immunologic types of hypersplenism show the best response, but because more than one factor may be operating in the production of hypersplenism, few patients should be denied the benefits of corticosteroid therapy. Thus patients with agnogenic myeloid metaplasia of the spleen and hypersplenism may respond, even though most cases appear to be examples of the "big spleen" syndrome. The response to corticosteroids in specific disorders is variable and is considered elsewhere (Table 12-1).

Splenectomy. Much has been written on the role of splenectomy in the management of hypersplenism. Before the advent of corticosteroid therapy, there was little else to offer these patients. Many patients show dramatic improvement after removal of the spleen, but splenectomy is by no means always effective in alleviating the symptoms and findings of hypersplenism. Splenectomy is uniformly effective only if the spleen is primarily at fault because of a normal function (e.g., hereditary spherocytosis). Sometimes splenectomy serves a dual function by eliminating a major site of antibody production in addition to the organ that is a primary (but not the only) site of removal of injured or damaged cells.

Recurrences of hypersplenic activity have, in some cases, been related to the presence of accessory spleens. However, their importance appears to have been overrated. Depending on the type of hypersplenism, splenectomy failures are not surprising because the procedure certainly does not eliminate all antibody-producing or phagocytic cells.

Even so, the possibility of an accessory spleen should be considered in patients with recurrent or persistent hypersplenic postoperative activity, especially if the hypersplenism was dependent on an essentially normal splenic function (e.g., removal of spherocytes). The incidence of accessory spleens is about 20 to 30 per cent. They are most often found in the splenic hilum or pedicle, the gastrosplenic or gastrocolic ligaments, or the mesentery of the small intestine. Detailed considerations of the indications for and the role of splenectomy in the various disorders that may be accompanied by hypersplenism are contained in the discussions of the individual diseases (Table 12-1).

Hemorrhagic Disorders

The blood possesses the ability to clot. Without this attribute, breaks in the continuity of a vessel would lead to exsanguination. On the other hand, improper intravascular clotting (thrombosis) causes serious and often fatal consequences. The prevention of hemorrhage and the maintenance of the blood's fluidity involve the complex interaction of a number of plasma factors. In addition, platelets and the status of the vascular endothelium figure importantly in hemostasis. Knowledge pertaining to the functions of platelets and the manner by which blood clots is requisite for a discussion of the clinical syndromes characterized by bleeding.

PHYSIOLOGY OF HEMOSTASIS

Normally, the blood is contained within a closed system of vessels. Breaks in major vessels occur as the result of trauma or some pathologic process involving the vascular wall. Because capillaries consist of a single layer of endothelial cells, defects are spontaneous as well. To prevent blood loss, the vascular defect must be sealed (large breaks with a fibrin clot, minor ones with a plug of platelets). Thus hemostasis (prevention of bleeding) is contingent on coagulation and the presence of adequate numbers of normal platelets. However, other factors also help to arrest the flow of blood. Under normal conditions extravascular, vascular, and intravascular factors operate together to bring about prompt and effective hemostasis.

Vascular Factors. The escape of blood from a vascular defect is temporarily controlled (at least partly) by extravascular tissues (e.g., skin and muscle) consequent to their normal tone and the pressure exerted on the bleeding vessel by blood that has already entered the tissues. Local vasoconstriction also plays an essential role early in hemostasis. Therefore the size, type, and location of an injured vessel are of great importance, as are the subject's age and the presence or absence of vascular disease. For example, the contractility of a small normal vessel greatly exceeds that of a larger diseased one.

Platelets. The major biologic activities of the blood platelets (p. 34) have to do with hemostasis. These functions are divisible into four categories.

ADHESIVENESS AND AGGREGATION. Platelets adhere readily to a variety of surfaces (e.g., glass, damaged blood vessels, and connective tissue fibers) as well as to one another. Recent observations indicate that this property, which may be the result of electrostatic forces, can be likened to phagocytosis in which the size of the particle determines the final response (i.e., platelets ingest small particles; they adhere to large surfaces). Platelets attach to the edges of a damaged blood vessel within seconds after injury occurs. Additional platelets quickly join those adherent to the vascular endothelium and an aggregate or plug is formed. Aggregation of platelets is enhanced in vitro by a variety of substances; in vivo, adenosine diphosphate (ADP) appears to play a major role. Platelet aggregation is a key event in hemostasis. At first the plug of platelets is permeable to blood; however, it rapidly becomes impermeable in a process known as *viscous metamorphosis.*

Viscous metamorphosis is initiated by thrombin (probably produced by the extrinsic thromboplastin system—see later) acting with fibrinogen present in the periplatelet atmosphere or adsorbed to the platelet's surface; divalent ions (calcium and magnesium) also contribute to this process. It is accompanied by platelet degranulation and the release of serotonin, ADP (this nucleotide enhances further aggregation), inorganic phosphate, platelet factor 3 (phospholipids that participate in the formation of a fibrin clot), free amino acids, potassium, acid phosphatase, and other constituents. Adherent platelets then contract consequent to the presence of thrombosthenin, a contractile protein bearing certain similarities to muscle actomyosin.

The end result of viscous metamorphosis is an impermeable, hemostatic plug which may completely seal breaks in small vessels. Larger defects in larger vessels require, in addition, the formation of a fibrin clot; even in these situations, however, the platelet plug or white thrombus serves as a nidus around which fibrin is deposited. Although a platelet aggregate appears to be "fused" into an amorphous mass during viscous metamorphosis, electron microscopy reveals preservation of platelet membranes. Thus the platelets are only tightly adherent and are not actually fused.

COAGULATION. Platelets contain a variety of substances that participate in blood coagulation. Four of these platelet factors have been assigned Arabic numerals to distinguish them from the plasma coagulation factors, which are designated by Roman numerals. Platelet factor 1 is adsorbed factor V (see later). Platelet factor 2 accelerates the conversion of fibrinogen to fibrin. Platelet factor 3 is a lipoprotein (a mixture of phospholipids) that participates in the intrinsic thromboplastin system (see later); this substance is generally thought to be associated with a platelet's granules, although some evidence suggests that it may be provided by a lipoprotein in the surface membrane. Platelet factor 4 is a protein or high molecular weight polypeptide that can directly neutralize heparin; it appears to be a physiologically significant intracellular component. Other plasma coagulation factors found in or on platelets include factors II, VII, VIII, IX, X, XI, and XII (Table 13-1); most, if not all, of these materials appear to exist in the periplatelet plasma environment or are adsorbed to the platelets' surfaces.

CLOT RETRACTION. The initial fibrin clot consists of a loose network that does not function as a firm plug for a vascular break until it contracts and exudes serum. Clot retraction depends on the presence of intact, viable (metabolically active) platelets. Since it requires the expenditure of energy in the form of adenosine triphosphate (ATP), glucose must be available; calcium also participates in this process. Clot retraction apparently reflects contraction of platelet pseudopods attached to fibrin strands and is probably brought about by the contractile protein, thrombosthenin.

VASCULAR INTEGRITY. Capillary fragility is increased in thrombocytopenic states, and there is rather convincing evidence that platelets contribute directly to the integrity of vascular walls. However, the manner by which this beneficial effect on the vascular endothelium is mediated remains to be clarified. Certain observations indicate that it does not require the presence of viable platelets.

Coagulation. The lifesaving property of shed blood to clot has fascinated man for centuries. Despite the intensive research endeavors of numerous investigators, many important questions have yet to be answered; however, much has been learned. Some understanding of the coagulation mechanism is essential if the problem of the bleeding patient is to be approached in a logical, rational manner.

HISTORY. In the mid-seventeenth century, Malpighi demonstrated the basic structure of a clot to be a white fibrous material separable from the blood cells. It was not until 1892, however, that Alexander Schmidt pointed out the origin of this material; he concluded that fibrin arose from a soluble precursor, fibrinogen, consequent to the action of a "fibrin ferment," which was subsequently designated thrombin.

It was further recognized that thrombin was not normally present in the blood but was formed from an inactive precursor (prothrombin) following the addition of particles of tissue (thromboplastin). Around this same time the importance of calcium in the clotting process was pointed out. These observations led Morawitz in 1905 to propound a theory of coagulation that has withstood investigation and remains the framework about which the modern concept of coagulation has evolved.

The classic theory of Morawitz is as follows: (1) phase 1 consisted of the formation of thrombin from prothrombin by thromboplastin in the presence of calcium; thromboplastin was believed to originate in platelets and other tissue cells; (2) phase 2 involved the conversion of fibrinogen to fibrin by thrombin. Little new information was added to this scheme until the last two or three decades, when, in rapid succession, a number of additional coagulation factors were described. Research activity in this area continues at a rapid pace, and the final words have not been written. Current concepts undoubtedly will require revision in the future. Nonetheless, the physician must have available a scheme of coagulation that will permit him to make accurate diagnoses and recommend appropriate treatment.

NOMENCLATURE. Even when reduced to its simplest form, the coagulation mechanism remains a complicated subject. Confusion has arisen and the inherent complexity of the clotting process has been enhanced by the development of a variable nomenclature. Recently a uniform terminology has been devised and is being widely adopted. These terms, together with their descriptive names, are listed in Table 13-1. The use

Table 13-1. *Plasma Coagulation Factors*

FACTOR	DESCRIPTIVE NAME
I	Fibrinogen
II	Prothrombin
III	Tissue thromboplastin
IV	Calcium
V	Proaccelerin
*	
VII	Proconvertin
VIII	Antihemophilic factor (AHF)
IX	Plasma thromboplastin component (PTC)
X	Stuart factor
XI	Plasma thromboplastin antecedent (PTA)
XII	Hageman factor
XIII	Fibrinase or fibrin-stabilizing factor

* There is no recognized factor VI. This numeral was at one time used as a designation for activated factor V.

of Roman numerals to designate the different plasma-clotting factors is strongly advised as a necessary step to facilitate communication in this field.

Physiology of Clotting.   The modern theory of blood coagulation envisages clotting as a dynamic process in which positive forces aimed at the production of a fibrin clot are opposed by a variety of negative forces. The coagulation mechanism consists of a series of reactions culminating in the enzymatic conversion of soluble fibrinogen into insoluble fibrin; it is depicted schematically in Figure 13-1 and can be divided into three phases: (1) phase 1 is concerned with the generation of thromboplastin and its activation, (2) phase 2 involves the formation of thrombin from its inactive precursor, prothrombin, and (3) during phase 3 fibrinogen is converted to fibrin. Normally, each of the coagulation factors is present in greater amounts than are needed for clotting to take place.

Phase 1.   Although a number of factors are known to participate in the first phase of coagulation, their modes of action and the order in which they participate are obscure. For purposes of testing, it is appropriate to divide this phase into the intrinsic and extrinsic thromboplastin systems. Initially, thromboplastin was believed to arise solely from platelets and other tissue cells. However, it soon became evident that plasma from which all tissue juices are excluded and from which all blood cells are removed still clots. Consequently, tissue thromboplastin is not required for coagulation to take place in vitro. Conversely, plasma thromboplastin can be replaced in vitro by tissue thromboplastin. Therefore tests that employ tissue (or extrinsic) thromboplastin as a reagent (e.g., a one-stage prothrombin time) are normal in disorders involving the generation of plasma (or intrinsic) thromboplastin. In vivo the relationship between plasma and tissue thromboplastins is disputable and the subject of much conjecture. Both are apparently necessary for normal hemostasis, since one cannot make up for a deficiency of the other; for example, the extrinsic thromboplastin system cannot substitute for the impaired generation of plasma thromboplastin consequent to a deficiency of factors VIII, IX, or XI, and an intact intrinsic system does not prevent abnormal bleeding in persons who are deficient in factor VII (factor VII appears to participate in the activation of tissue but not of plasma thromboplastin). As shown in Figure 13-1, factors X and V are concerned with the activation of both thromboplastins. The relationship between the intrinsic and extrinsic prothrombin activators (or prothrombinases) is problematic. Some workers contend that they are identical; others believe they are different. In any event, the active forms of both plasma and tissue thromboplastin appear to be essential participants in the conversion of prothrombin to thrombin.

Plasma coagulation factors VIII and V are not found in serum; factors VII, IX, X, XI, and XII are present both in plasma and serum. Factors VII, IX, and X are adsorbed by aluminum hydroxide or barium

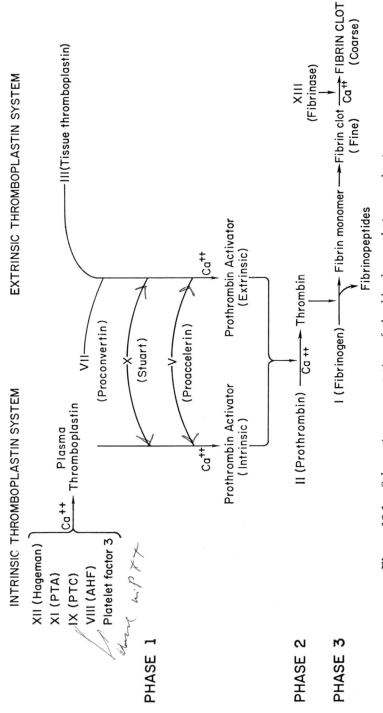

INTRINSIC THROMBOPLASTIN SYSTEM

EXTRINSIC THROMBOPLASTIN SYSTEM

III (Tissue thromboplastin)

XII (Hageman)
XI (PTA)
IX (PTC)
VIII (AHF)
Platelet factor 3

$\xrightarrow{Ca^{++}}$ Plasma Thromboplastin

VII (Proconvertin)

X (Stuart)

V (Proaccelerin)

Prothrombin Activator (Intrinsic)

Ca^{++}

Prothrombin Activator (Extrinsic)

Ca^{++}

PHASE 1

II (Prothrombin) $\xrightarrow{Ca^{++}}$ Thrombin

PHASE 2

I (Fibrinogen) → Fibrin monomer → Fibrin clot (Fine) $\xrightarrow{Ca^{++}}$ FIBRIN CLOT (Coarse)

Fibrinopeptides

XIII (Fibrinase)

PHASE 3

Figure 13-1. Schematic representation of the blood coagulation mechanism.

469

sulfate; factors V, VIII, XI, and XII are not. The factors removed by adsorbents are also those whose production requires vitamin K and a functioning liver. Factors VIII and V are labile on storage; the others are stable. In addition to these seven plasma factors and tissue thromboplastin (factor III), platelet factor 3 (a lipoprotein) participates in phase 1 of clotting. Although platelets are essential for the generation of plasma thromboplastin, only a few (probably about 30,000/cu mm) furnish enough phospholipid to permit normal coagulation. Calcium appears to be required in all steps concerned with the generation and activation of thromboplastin (Fig. 13-1).

The intrinsic thromboplastin system of phase 1 is the most time-consuming part of the coagulation process, as evidenced by a normal in vitro coagulation time at 37°C of three to four minutes and a normal one-stage prothrombin time of about 12 seconds. Because the latter test utilizes exogenous tissue thromboplastin and bypasses the formation of plasma thromboplastin, it follows that tissue thromboplastin activation, thrombin production, and fibrinogen conversion occupy but a few seconds, whereas the generation of plasma thromboplastin requires several minutes.

Coagulation involves a series of enzymatic reactions. The plasma factors are present normally as inactive precursors and must be activated by an appropriate agent. Factors VIII and V are consumed during the clotting process; factors VII, IX, X, XI, and XII are not. These observations suggest that factors VIII and V may be substrates acted on enzymatically by the others. It should be emphasized that the precise steps in phase 1 of the coagulation mechanism have not yet been worked out. Current evidence suggests (but does not prove) that the following sequence may operate.

In vitro factor XII is activated by contact with some foreign surface such as glass; activated factor XII then appears to initiate clotting. The action of this factor in vivo is not known (patients who have a deficiency of factor XII do not ordinarily bleed, even though they have greatly prolonged in vitro coagulation times); however, it may be presumed to act in some way to start the clotting process. Activated factor XII probably functions enzymatically to convert factor XI to its active form, which in turn activates factor IX. Activated factor IX, together with platelet factor 3 and in the presence of calcium, then appears to act on factor VIII to form a clot-promoting substance which has been designated plasma thromboplastin (Fig. 13-1). Factor VII is probably activated by tissue thromboplastin or factor III.

The manner by which factors X and V affect (or more likely activate) plasma (intrinsic) and tissue (extrinsic) thromboplastin is unclear. It has been proposed that the active form of factor VII activates factor X, which then reacts with plasma thromboplastin to activate factor V. Activated factor V (accelerin) would, according to this scheme, be the end product of phase 1 and as such would be synonymous with prothrombin activator or prothrombinase. Despite the attractiveness of this thesis, it lacks proof.

There is some evidence that a small amount of thrombin formed by the extrinsic thromboplastin system acts in an autocatalytic fashion to bring about the formation of large amounts of prothrombin activator (presumably by way of the intrinsic thromboplastin system). Intrinsic prothrombin activator is probably responsible for the conversion of sufficient quantities of prothrombin to thrombin to permit the deposition of a fibrin clot.

Many intricacies of phase 1 of the coagulation mechanism remain to be clarified. Pending answers to these problems, it is nonetheless essential for the physician, who is confronted by a bleeding patient, to be cognizant of the factors participating in this aspect of clotting and of their differing properties to assess accurately the results of laboratory procedures. Although precise details of its formation are lacking, the end product of phase 1, that is, a potent prothrombin activator (or activators), has been established beyond reasonable doubt.

Phase 2. The second phase of coagulation deals with the conversion of factor II or prothrombin (the inactive precursor of thrombin) to thrombin. Prothrombin is a glycoprotein with a molecular weight of about 68,000 and containing 18 different amino acids. The formation of prothrombin in the liver is contingent on the availability of vitamin K. The normal concentration of prothrombin is approximately 12 mg/100 ml of plasma. Inasmuch as prothrombin is utilized in the clotting process, it is not found in serum. Normally, however, the plasma prothrombin concentration is far greater than that needed to form a fibrin clot in vitro; consequently, some prothrombin remains in serum for a short time after coagulation has occurred and is the basis for the prothrombin consumption test (see later). Prothrombin is adsorbed by aluminum hydroxide or barium sulfate. It is stable on storage and withstands heat without much loss of activity.

The formation of thrombin from prothrombin is not clearly understood; in addition to prothrombin activator(s) (Fig. 13-1), calcium is an essential participant. The molecular weight of thrombin is about half that of prothrombin, and their amino acid compositions are similar. Available data favor the concept that thrombin is formed as a consequence of the proteolytic breakdown or degradation of the prothrombin molecule. There is convincing evidence that derivatives of prothrombin possess thrombin activity. The conversion of prothrombin to thrombin is an autocatalytic reaction.

Phase 3. The final phase in blood coagulation is concerned with the transformation of the soluble protein, factor I or fibrinogen, into an insoluble fibrin meshwork or clot. Thrombin acts as a proteolytic enzyme. Fibrinogen is one of the plasma proteins and is present normally in a concentration of 250 to 400 mg/100 ml of plasma. Its molecular weight is about 340,000, and 19 different amino acids have been identified in the fibrinogen molecule. This protein is relatively stable in storage, but it denatures irreversibly on heating. Fibrinogen is consumed during coagulation and is not present in serum.

The first step in the conversion of fibrinogen to fibrin involves the splitting off by proteolysis of two types of soluble fibrinopeptide, leaving a fibrin monomer (Fig. 13-1). The fibrin monomers then undergo polymerization with end-to-end and side-to-side alignment of the fibrils, thus forming coarser fibrin strands. The result of such polymerization is the production of a fine fibrin clot that is soluble in urea. The next step consists of the formation of a coarse fibrin clot that is insoluble in urea; this reaction appears to reflect disulfide bond formation and is brought about by the action of factor XIII (fibrinase or the fibrin stabilizing factor) in the presence of calcium ions. The fibrin clot constitutes the visible end point of the coagulation mechanism. However, it is not an adequate seal for a disrupted vessel until clot retraction occurs. This process, which requires the presence of viable platelets, brings about the exudation of serum and the formation of an effective vascular plug. During clot retraction thrombin is expressed and accumulates in the serum, where it acts on additional prothrombin and so favors further clot formation. Other factors affecting clot retraction include, among others, the concentration of fibrinogen which determines the size of the clot and the level of the peripheral erythroid values (the higher the erythroid values, the larger the clot; the lower the erythroid values, the greater the concentration of serum to be extruded and the smaller the clot). Normally, clot retraction begins about 30 minutes after coagulation has taken place and is good within one to three hours.

Anticoagulants. There is still a great deal to be learned about the interacting mechanisms that maintain the blood's fluidity intravascularly, cause shed blood to clot, and stop the coagulation process once it has started. It is apparent that negative forces or inhibitory factors play important roles; otherwise, once started, intravascular coagulation would continue unabated with disastrous results. The subject of the naturally occurring anticoagulants rivals that of the coagulation mechanism in its over-all complexity; however, even less is known about the coagulation inhibitors. There appear to be anticoagulants for every factor and reaction concerned with clotting. For example, a variety of antithrombins have been described, one of the more potent of which seems to be fibrin itself. Still poorly understood is the physiologic significance of heparin. This mucopolysaccharide, which is a normal body constituent, is formed by mast cells and basophils (p. 29); it possesses a strong negative electrical charge and displays potent anticoagulant properties. Although heparin is primarily an antithrombin, it also inhibits most, if not all, other phases of the coagulation process. This substance probably plays an important physiologic role as a natural inhibitor of the clotting process and appears to cause abnormal bleeding in rare patients.

Fibrinolysis. In addition to a variety of anticoagulants, there is also a mechanism for the dissolution of a fibrin clot. This fibrinolytic system has been the subject of much research in recent years and is still under intensive study. Normal blood contains profibrinolysin (plasminogen), a substance that appears to be formed by eosinophils (p. 28). Following activation to fibrinolysin (plasmin), it is capable of hydrolyzing the internal peptide bonds of fibrin as well as certain other structurally similar proteins. The mechanism by which profibrinolysin is transformed to an active enzyme is unclear. In vitro profibrinolysin can be activated by a variety of substances, including tissue extracts, urokinase, and bacterial filtrates such as streptokinase. Profibrinolysin can also be activated by fibrinolysin. The presence of activator and inhibitor substances seems likely, and the majority opinion contends that kinases activate a plasmatic substance, which in turn converts profibrinolysin (plasminogen) to fibrinolysin (plasmin). Epsilon-aminocaproic acid (a structural analogue of lysine) interferes with the activation of profibrinolysin and with the proteolytic effects of fibrinolysin. The fibrinolytic system probably contributes to normal hemostasis by bringing about the removal of clots, which, at best, are only temporary hemostatic barriers.

INTERACTION OF HEMOSTATIC FACTORS. After a break in a blood vessel, the various hemostatic factors act jointly to occlude the defect and prevent the loss of blood. Local vasoconstriction and pressure on the injured vessel by the surrounding tissues and by blood that has already entered the tissues exert an immediate hemostatic effect. Within seconds platelets adhere to the damaged endothelium, and additional platelets participate quickly in the formation of a platelet aggregate or plug. These platelets undergo viscous metamorphosis to release, among other substances, platelet factor 3 and serotonin. Consequent to viscous metamorphosis, the platelet aggregate becomes an impermeable plug, which may in itself be capable of sealing minor breaks in small vessels. If not, the coagulation mechanism is activated. Coagulation soon ceases as a result of the action of the inhibitory factors that keep the blood fluid. Clot retraction follows, and an effective seal for the vascular defect results. Permanent hemostasis is achieved by the formation of new tissue. Concomitant with the healing process, the fibrin clot disappears, probably as the direct result of the fibrinolytic system. Thus hemostasis is dependent on a delicately balanced equilibrium that involves a number of highly complex physiologic processes.

PATHOPHYSIOLOGY OF THE HEMORRHAGIC DISORDERS

Abnormalities of any of the normal hemostatic mechanisms can cause bleeding. Therefore a hemorrhagic disorder may reflect (1) vascular disease or increased capillary pressure, (2) quantitative or qualitative platelet defects, or (3) impaired coagulation. Impaired coagulation may reflect a deficiency of one or more of the positive factors that contribute to clotting or the overactivity of one of the inhibitory substances that keep the blood fluid. For clinical purposes it is convenient to separate the hemorrhagic diseases into vascular, platelet, and coagulation disorders (Table 13-2).

Table 13-2. *Classification of the Hemorrhagic Disorders*

I. *Vascular Disorders*
   A. Focal abnormalities
      1. Injury
      2. Emboli
      3. Hereditary hemorrhagic telangiectasia
   B. Generalized disease
      1. Scurvy
      2. Defective connective tissue (e.g., Marfan's syndrome, hypercorticosteroidism, and purpura senilis)
      3. Vascular (allergic) purpura
      4. von Willebrand's disease

II. *Platelet Disorders*
   A. Quantitative
      1. Thrombocytopenia
      2. Thrombocythemia
   B. Qualitative
      1. Thrombopathy
      2. Thrombasthenia

III. *Coagulation Disorders*
   A. Phase 1
      1. Intrinsic thromboplastin system
         a. Factor VIII deficiencies
         b. Factor IX deficiencies
         c. Factor XI deficiency
         d. Factor XII deficiency
      2. Factor VII deficiencies
      3. Factor X deficiencies
      4. Factor V deficiencies
   B. Phase 2
      1. Factor II deficiencies (hypoprothrombinemia)
   C. Phase 3
      1. Factor I deficiencies (hypofibrinogenemia)
   D. Intravascular coagulation syndrome and fibrinolysis
   E. Circulating anticoagulants
   F. Dysproteinemias

Regardless of the nature of the basic abnormality, the clinical manifestations (i.e., a hemorrhagic diathesis) are remarkably similar. Because of differing etiologies and treatments, however, it is essential to make precise diagnoses. Differentiation is usually dependent on laboratory documentation. Unfortunately, the complexity of the hemostatic mechanisms precludes simple laboratory evaluation. Furthermore, confusion is heightened by the need to use the same visible end point in many tests (i.e., the conversion of fibrinogen to fibrin). Techniques providing the most specific and direct information are, for the most part, complicated procedures that yield *accurate* data only in the hands of a specially trained technician working in a coagulation laboratory. With the exception of some of the larger medical centers, these measurements are not available for the routine evaluation of a bleeding patient. Furthermore, the results are likely to be misleading and inaccurate unless the technique is in constant use (the incidence of most coagulation disorders is quite low). Consequently, it is pertinent to consider the simpler and more universally available laboratory procedures and the nature of the information they furnish before discussing the pathophysiologic manifestations of the hemorrhagic disorders.

General Tests of Hemostasis. Many laboratory tests have been designed to assess the integrity of the coagulation mechanism and the other factors contributing to hemostasis. Since some reflect several different abnormalities, it is necessary to rely on a group of tests rather than a single one. On the basis of "six simple tests," it is possible to determine in most bleeding patients the nature of the abnormality or at least the phase of coagulation in which the defect is located; this information then permits a rational selection of the additional laboratory procedures needed to establish the diagnosis. These screening tests, which are available in all medical facilities, include (1) whole blood coagulation time, (2) clot retraction, (3) a bleeding time, (4) platelet count, (5) capillary resistance or fragility test, and (6) one-stage prothrombin time. Singly, these measurements are nonspecific and difficult to interpret; when they are considered collectively, important diagnostic information accrues. It should be noted that this group of tests ordinarily will not uncover minor hemostatic abnormalities. In other words, they are not suitable to predict bleeding (e.g., preoperative detection of potential bleeders). On the other hand, few, if any, bleeding patients fail to exhibit appropriate abnormalities. Consequently, this "battery" of tests constitutes the first step in the work-up of all persons with a hemorrhagic diathesis.

COAGULATION TIME. The time required in vitro for a specimen of whole blood to form a solid clot in the absence of tissue factors is designated a coagulation or clotting time. Several minor modifications have been proposed and change slightly the normal values. In most laboratories a normal coagulation time at room temperature is between 6 and 12 minutes. This technically simple test reflects abnormalities in the intrinsic thromboplastin system of phase 1 (Fig. 13-1). This phase, which is concerned with the generation of plasma thromboplastin is the most time-consuming portion of the clotting mechanism; consequently, a delay in this process grossly alters the coagulation time. The coagulation time is normal in the face of abnormalities in the extrinsic thromboplastin system (e.g., factor VII deficiency) because of the activity of the intrinsic system. However, it is prolonged in the presence of certain circulating anticoagulants as well as in persons with hypofibrinogenemia. On the other hand, it is not a valid indicator of deficiencies of factors X, V, or II. Because of the speed with which plasma thromboplastin is activated and prothrombin is converted to thrombin (i.e., a few seconds), even gross defects that markedly prolong the prothrombin time fail to lengthen the coagulation time significantly. Although a coagulation time is a clinically useful test, its relative insensitivity must be borne in mind. This rather crude measure of a sensitive, complicated process may be normal, even in the face of clear-cut disturbances in coagulation.

Clot Retraction. Blood is incubated at 37°C in a water bath and permitted to clot. The tube is then allowed to stand for an hour, after which the degree of clot retraction is determined. A clot normally retracts 50 to 60 per cent of its original volume within one to three hours. A commonly used modification involves the evaluation of retraction at 2 and 24 hours in tubes maintained at room temperature. Defective clot retraction indicates thrombocytopenia or qualitative platelet dysfunction.

Bleeding Time. This test evaluates hemostasis in small wounds. A small incision is made, usually in the lobe of the ear, and bleeding is timed. Bleeding normally ceases within five minutes due to vascular factors and the hemostatic effects of platelets; the coagulation mechanism does not participate in this process, even though it may eventually be necessary for permanent hemostasis. Therefore prolongation of the bleeding time reflects vascular abnormalities and/or platelet defects (quantitative or qualitative). Other factors, such as the thickness of the skin, the superficiality of the vessels, and the environmental temperature, contribute to the length of the bleeding time and must be considered in the interpretation of the test. Slight prolongation of the bleeding time may or may not be indicative of disease.

Platelet Count. Techniques for quantifying platelets are described elsewhere (p. 46).

Capillary Fragility Test. This test is designed to assess the ability of small vessels to withstand increased pressure. Therefore it reflects vascular integrity and/or the quantitative and qualitative status of the platelets. Attempts to quantify the results of this procedure precisely are to be discouraged. Although clinically useful, it is a crude measure of vascular and platelet diseases and should be interpreted as such. Otherwise, it is more likely to confuse than to clarify. A sphygmomanometer is placed on an arm and inflated to 100 mm Hg or to a pressure midway between systolic and diastolic blood pressures; the pressure should never exceed 100. The cuff should not be allowed to remain in place longer than five minutes and should be removed sooner if petechiae appear promptly. The results are interpreted in the light of the speed with which petechiae develop, the number of petechiae induced, and other factors such as the superficiality of the vessels (or the thickness of the skin). Interpretations based solely on the number of petechiae developing in a predetermined area in a given period of time are useless, for there is no way to predict where the petechiae will occur. It is more appropriate to rate the test as negative (none or only a rare lesion developing after five minutes) or slightly, moderately, or markedly positive.

PROTHROMBIN TIME (ONE-STAGE). In brief, this test involves the addition of exogenous tissue thromboplastin and calcium to citrated or oxalated plasma; the time required for a visible fibrin clot to form in this mixture is known as the prothrombin time. Depending on certain modifications in technique, a normal one-stage prothrombin time varies from 12 to 20 seconds. In all in vitro tests, tissue thromboplastin substitutes completely for plasma thromboplastin. Therefore the one-stage prothrombin time reflects the activities of factors VII, X, V, and II (Fig. 13-1); it does not assess the generation of plasma thromboplastin. In the face of significant hypofibrinogenemia, the one-stage prothrombin time is also prolonged because its end point is a visible clot.

Special Tests of Hemostasis. Although the tests already described are simple, they provide, for the most part, fairly general information. Thus more complicated procedures yielding more directly informative data are needed to pinpoint the precise cause of a bleeding disorder. Numerous techniques are available for this purpose. The following are examples of the types of test currently in use and the nature of the information they afford.

THROMBOPLASTIN GENERATION TEST. When the general screening tests point to an abnormality in the formation of intrinsic prothrombin activator (Fig. 13-1), a thromboplastin generation test provides relevant data. There are three ingredients: platelets, adsorbed plasma, and serum. This mixture, which contains all the clotting factors but prothrombin (Table 13-3), is incubated with calcium at 37°C. At regular intervals (usually every minute) an aliquot is removed and added with calcium to a specimen of normal plasma; the time required for the substrate plasma to clot is then measured. Such clotting times reflect the amount

Table 13-3. *Some Properties of the Plasma Coagulation Factors*

Factor	Present in Aged (Stored) Plasma	Present in Serum (Fate during Clotting)	Adsorbed by $Al(OH)_3$ or $BaSO_4$
XII	Yes	Yes	No
XI	Yes	Yes	No
IX	Yes	Yes	Yes
VIII	No	No	No
VII	Yes	Yes	Yes
X	Yes	Yes	Yes
V	No	No	No
II	Yes	No	Yes
I	Yes	No	No

of intrinsic prothrombin activator generated in the reaction mixture; successive determinations indicate the rate of generation. The thromboplastin generation test is primarily useful in the detection of deficiencies of those plasma factors concerned with the generation of plasma thromboplastin and of platelet factor 3 (Fig. 13-1). In addition, it reflects inadequacies of factors V and X; however, these deficiencies also cause a prolonged one-stage prothrombin time and can, by this means, be differentiated with ease. If normal platelets are used in the reaction mixture, the thromboplastin generation test may be normal in the face of a factor V deficiency because of the factor V adsorbed to the platelet's surface.

By utilizing the different properties of the various coagulation factors (Table 13-3), it is possible to determine which one is deficient. For example, a mixture of normal platelets, normal serum, and the patient's adsorbed plasma will display impaired thromboplastin generation only if the patient has a deficiency of factor VIII or V. These factors are not present in serum and are not removed by adsorbents such as aluminum hydroxide; therefore their only source in the reaction mixture is the patient's adsorbed plasma (a normal prothrombin time excludes factor V deficiency and vice versa). By varying the sources of the reaction materials, the deficient factor in the intrinsic thromboplastin system can be pinpointed. Disadvantages of the thromboplastin generation test are (1) the preparation of test materials is time-consuming, (2) the technique is difficult and requires considerable skill, and (3) it is not sufficiently sensitive to detect all mild coagulation factor deficiencies.

Prothrombin Consumption Test. During coagulation in vitro, all the available prothrombin is eventually converted to thrombin. If the generation of plasma thromboplastin is impaired (Fig. 13-1), a considerable amount of prothrombin remains in the serum after clotting has taken place. The prothrombin consumption test assesses the coagulant activity of serum at a specified interval (generally one hour) after coagulation; since serum contains no fibrinogen or factor V, these materials must be supplied. Actually, the test reflects the activities of factors VII and X as well as residual prothrombin. Normally, less than 20 per cent of the original "prothrombin" activity, as measured by the one-stage technique, remains one hour after clotting has taken place. The prothrombin consumption test reveals defects similar to those uncovered by the thromboplastin generation test, (i.e., abnormal plasma thromboplastin formation). However, it does not permit precise identification of the deficient coagulation factor; it is also less sensitive than the thromboplastin generation test. Even so, it is simple and often provides valuable information.

PROTHROMBIN TIME (MODIFIED). A one-stage prothrombin time measures the combined activities of factors VII, X, V, and II (prothrombin). When this test is abnormal, it is possible to find out which factor is deficient by combining various reagents containing some but not all of the clotting factors with the test plasma. For example, the addition of normal adsorbed plasma will correct a prolonged one-stage prothrombin time due to factor V deficiency but not if it is an inadequacy of factor II, VII, or X (the latter are adsorbed by agents such as aluminum hydroxide or barium sulfate, whereas factor V is not). Even better is the use of plasmas from patients who are known to lack an individual factor. By using a little ingenuity and designing a variety of coagulation mixtures, few deficiencies will escape detection.

QUANTIFICATION OF PLASMA COAGULATION FACTOR ACTIVITY. Techniques exist for the quantitative analysis of the plasma coagulation factors. Some are relatively easy (e.g., measurement of plasma fibrinogen concentration); however, most are complicated and technically difficult. With few exceptions, accurate measurements are obtainable only in special laboratories carrying out research in blood coagulation.

OTHER SPECIAL TESTS. A list of the many different tests available for assessing the various hemostatic mechanisms is beyond the scope of this text. Several up-to-date books describe these procedures in detail. Certain of these techniques measure similar phases of clotting and often appear to have been recommended by a particular author for obscure personal reasons. As a result, confusion in this field has been increased and compounded. It is fortunate for the clinician that most bleeding patients can be diagnosed by simpler parameters. When more complicated techniques are required to make a positive diagnosis, they are considered in the discussions of specific hemorrhagic disorders.

Manifestations of Hemorrhagic Disorders. The clinical manifestations of the different hemorrhagic diseases are often similar. Vascular and platelet abnormalities are more likely to cause petechiae (pinpoint hemorrhages from capillary loops) and mucosal bleeding (e.g., gingival hemorrhage and menorrhagia), whereas coagulation abnormalities are generally reflected by more profuse bleeding (ecchymoses, bleeding into the joints, melena, hematuria, and excessive hemorrhage following trauma). More often than not, however, precise differentiation is contingent on laboratory documentation. Thus it is more informative to consider the pathophysiologic manifestations insofar as they are reflected by certain tests, especially the battery of tests just listed (i.e., coagulation time, clot retraction, bleeding time, platelet count, capillary resistance test, and one-stage prothrombin time). It should be re-emphasized that these screening tests must be interpreted collectively and that they lack the sensitivity needed to detect minor defects. On the other hand, few bleeding patients fail to exhibit a significant abnormality or group of abnormalities. The characteristic findings in the different types of hemorrhagic disorders are shown in Table 13-4. With the foregoing discussion as background material, it is now appropriate to consider the clinical manifestations, diagnosis, and treatment of the hemorrhagic disorders and syndromes listed in Table 13-2.

Vascular Disorders

INJURY

The commonest vascular lesion responsible for bleeding and the most frequently encountered cause of hemorrhage is injury consequent to trauma or damage by some pathologic process. If the vessel is large enough or the injury sufficiently severe, bleeding ensues, regardless of the activities of the hemostatic mechanisms. Factitial or self-induced (psychogenic) purpura falls into this category, as do the purpuric lesions caused by increased capillary pressure secondary to severe bouts of coughing or vomiting, mechanical obstruction, prolonged standing or sitting, and so forth. In the latter situations the vessels are normal but are unable to withstand the increased intravascular pressure. Several infectious processes produce localized damage to capillary walls and are manifested by purpura (e.g., scarlet fever, smallpox, diphtheria, measles, and certain rickettsial infections). With the exception of a positive capillary fragility test in a few patients with capillary damage secondary to some infection, all tests of the hemostatic mechanisms are normal. As a rule, the cause of the abnormal bleeding is quite apparent. Treatment consists of local measures to arrest the flow of blood and therapy of the underlying cause (e.g., an infection or a psychogenic disturbance).

EMBOLI

Vascular occlusion by a thrombus causes local hemorrhage (probably caused by hypoxic damage to the vascular endothelium) which surrounds

Table 13-4. Laboratory Manifestations of the Hemorrhagic Disorders

Type of Disorder	Coagulation Time	Bleeding Time	Clot Retraction	Platelet Count	Capillary Fragility	Prothrombin Time (One-Stage)
Vascular	N	N or ↑	N	N	N or ↑	N
Thrombocytopenia	N	↑	↓	↓	↑	N
Thrombopathy	N	N or ↑	N	N	N	N
Thrombasthenia	N	N or ↑	↓	N	N	N
Coagulation Factor Deficiencies						
1. Intrinsic Thromboplastin System (VIII, IX, XI, and XII)	↑	N	N	N	N	N
2. Factor VII	N	N	N	N	N	↑
3. Factor X	N or ↑	N	N	N	N	↑
4. Factor V	N or ↑	N	N	N	N	↑
5. Factor II	N	N	N	N	N	↑
6. Factor I	↑	N	N	N	N	N or ↑
Circulating anticoagulant	↑	N	N	N	N	N or ↑

N = Normal
↑ = Increased
↓ = Decreased

or infiltrates the ischemic area. The size and location of the occluded vessel determine the nature and severity of the clinical manifestations. Blockage of a large vessel in the lung evokes severe consequences with chest pain and hemoptysis; capillary embolization is reflected by petechiae and splinter hemorrhages. Septic emboli accompany a variety of infections, most notably subacute bacterial endocarditis and meningococcemia. Tumor emboli also produce focal hemorrhagic lesions in certain patients with carcinomatosis. Bleeding is not the primary problem in these situations, even though hemorrhagic phenomena may be a prominent feature. The nature of the underlying disease is ordinarily evident. All tests of the hemostatic mechanisms (including capillary fragility) are normal. These conditions rarely masquerade as primary hemorrhagic disorders.

H E R E D I T A R Y   H E M O R R H A G I C   T E L A N G I E C T A S I A

Rendu (1896), Osler (1901), and Weber (1907) published the first clear descriptions of this inheritable vascular abnormality. It is still designated on occasion by their names. Hereditary hemorrhagic telangiectasia is transmitted as a simple autosomal dominant and occurs in both sexes. Affected vessels are thinned and dilated. Veins are involved to a greater degree than is the arterial side of the circulation, but visible capillary and arteriolar dilations occur and may lead to the development of arteriovenous fistulae or aneurysms, especially in the lungs.

The vascular lesions vary in appearance. Macular and nodular types are most common. The macular lesions are bright red, flat, and pinpoint in size; the nodular lesions are larger (up to 5 to 10 mm), raised, and bright red or more characteristically violaceous. Less common lesions are reminiscent of the spider telangiectasia of liver disease or pregnancy (these are seen most often in older patients and may not appear for several years after the development of other vascular abnormalities). The lesions of hereditary hemorrhagic telangiectasia usually blanch on pressure and are demonstrable predominantly in the skin and mucous membranes; however, they also affect other organs such as the lungs, spleen, liver, kidneys, and brain. They may bleed spontaneously or because of trauma. The lack of adequate muscle in the involved vessel prevents vasoconstriction and potentiates blood loss.

Hereditary hemorrhagic telangiectasia generally has its clinical onset somewhere between the second and third decades of life. The characteristic symptom is hemorrhage, particularly expistaxis, melena, hemoptysis, and hematuria. Most patients complain of overt bleeding or the manifestations of an acute hemorrhagic anemia (p. 67), but some seek medical assistance because of an iron deficiency anemia (p. 172) consequent to chronic blood loss. The pertinent physical findings are the typical telangiectatic lesions which may occur anywhere but are most likely to be located on the fingers, ears, lips, toes, trunk, and nasal or oral mucosa. Sometimes they can be demonstrated endoscopically in the esophagus, stomach, or rectum. In an occasional family the location of the telangiectasia appears to be genetically determined. Laboratory abnormalities consist of the hematologic manifestations of an acute hemorrhagic anemia or those of an iron deficiency anemia. All tests of the hemostatic mechanisms are normal.

The diagnosis of hereditary hemorrhagic telangiectasia is based on the demonstration of the characteristic vascular lesions and a positive family history. Although a positive family history is most helpful, it is not essential because the disease has its onset at different ages. This bleeding disorder also varies greatly in severity, and mild involvement may be easily missed. The lesions of hereditary hemorrhagic telangiectasia must be differentiated from spider angiomas in patients with cirrhosis or in pregnant women and from the commonly observed cherry angiomas. The spider angiomas affect the upper part of the body, and their small pulsating centers, fiery red color, erythematous halos, and peripheral branches ordinarily permit easy identification. Furthermore, evidence of the basic underlying disease (e.g., the stigmata of cirrhosis) provides valuable clues. Cherry angiomas are bright red, well circumscribed, and usually round; as a rule, they are raised and blanch little with pressure. These overgrowths of dilated vessels occur most often on the trunk and rarely affect the face. After puberty they are very common and increase in number with advancing age. Angiokeratoma corporis diffusum universale rarely causes confusion because of its distinctive features (the lesions of this rare syndrome are characteristically found over the lower trunk; they are keratotic and do not bleed).

The course of hereditary hemorrhagic telangiectasia is ordinarily progressive with advancing age. Thus bleeding can be expected to worsen as the years go by. In general, episodes of hemorrhage occur with unpredictable frequency and severity. In a small but significant number of patients, a pulmonary arteriovenous aneurysm may cause arterial hypoxemia and a secondary erythrocytosis (p. 294).

Treatment consists primarily of local measures designed to stop the bleeding. Epistaxis is a particularly difficult and commonly encountered problem. Septal dermoplasty has recently been successful in some patients. Estrogens have been claimed to be therapeutically efficacious, but it is the current consensus that they do little, if any, good. Most patients require iron; bleeding may be so profuse that both parenteral and oral iron are needed to maintain positive balance. Since hereditary hemorrhagic telangiectasia is passed on as a mendelian dominant, genetic counseling is appropriate.

SCURVY

A deficiency of vitamin C (ascorbic acid) has long been known to cause bleeding under the periosteum, into the muscle and skin, and from the mucous membranes. This hemorrhagic tendency presumably reflects increased capillary permeability (vitamin C is necessary for the formation of the intercellular or cement substance of the vascular wall). Although once a common cause of abnormal bleeding, scurvy is now rarely encountered. The other manifestations of this deficiency state permit its easy recognition. With the exception of a positive capillary fragility test, other hemostatic tests are normal. The treatment is administration of vitamin C.

DEFECTIVE CONNECTIVE TISSUE

Consequent to ineffective vascular support because of connective tissue atrophy or other inadequacy, capillary bleeding may follow minor trauma. Examples of this type of vascular disorder include Marfan's syndrome, the Ehler-Danlos syndrome, hidrotic ectodermal dysplasia, hypercorticosteroidism (endogenous and exogenous), purpura senilis in older persons, and purpura cachectica in patients with chronic wasting diseases. With the exception of capillary fragility tests, which, as a rule, are positive, other evidence of a hemostatic defect is lacking.

VASCULAR "ALLERGIC" PURPURA

This category of hemorrhagic disorders is probably a heterogeneous group rather than a single entity. Bleeding appears to be a manifestation of increased capillary permeability. Synonyms include nonthrombocytopenic purpura, anaphylactoid purpura, and Henoch-Schönlein's purpura (Schönlein first described joint manifestations and Henoch emphasized the gastrointestinal components). Although the pathogenesis remains obscure, available data favor an immune reaction involving small blood vessels. This "allergic" angiitis is characterized by a marked perivascular infiltration consisting of neutrophils, eosinophils, lymphocytes, and macrophages. A variety of antigens, including bacteria (especially beta hemolytic streptococci), drugs, and foods, have been implicated. More often than not, the inciting agent cannot be identified with certainty. It is conjectural whether the angiitis reflects a specific antibody against the vascular endothelium or a nonspecific side effect of an antigen-antibody reaction. The suggestion has recently been advanced (with some experimental support) that vascular purpura may be an auto-immune disease.

Allergic purpura affects all ages and both sexes but is more common in children, adolescents, and young adults. Because of widespread involvement, the clinical picture is distinguished by striking variability.

The onset may be insidious or explosive. Manifestations are divisible into the following major categories.

Skin. Purpuric lesions are characteristic. Most hemorrhagic areas are large; occasionally they are raised and tender. They are commonest over the lower extremities and buttocks, and less often the arms, trunk, and face are involved. Petechiae are uncommon, thus serving to distinguish nonthrombocytopenic from thrombocytopenic purpura. In some patients the initial lesions are urticarial.

Gastrointestinal. Cramping abdominal pain, diarrhea, and melena are the usual symptoms. Occasionally this disorder may simulate (or even cause) intussusception, especially in young children.

Joints. Pain in the joints with or without swelling and tenderness is typical. Often, the pain shifts from one joint to another, and the wrists, knees, and ankles are most frequently involved. Joint swelling is generally periarticular, although effusion may occur.

Renal. Hematuria (microscopic or gross), proteinuria, renal insufficiency, and hypertension are frequent manifestations of renal involvement. This aspect of "allergic" purpura is the most serious, for impaired renal function may persist after all other evidence of the disease has subsided.

Other. Less often the central nervous system or heart may be involved. A few patients complain of epistaxis but other hemorrhagic manifestations are rare.

As a rule, the diagnosis is suggested by the clinical picture. Thrombocytopenic purpura is excluded by a normal platelet count, and the capillary fragility test may or may not be positive. All other tests of the hemostatic mechanisms (platelet function and coagulation) are normal. With the exception of a slight neutrophilia in some patients, there are no other laboratory abnormalities.

In general, the course of vascular (allergic) purpura is benign and self-limited. A single episode rarely lasts longer than a few weeks, but some patients have periodic recurrences. When the offending agent is known and contact with it can be eliminated, the patient ordinarily improves. In a few cases renal insufficiency persists and eventually leads to the patient's death; however, fatal cases are quite unusual. Numerous types of treatment have been tried, but none has been shown to be consistently effective. Corticosteroids are warranted in severely ill patients, but the results leave much to be desired.

Two other disorders appear to be closely related to vascular or allergic purpura. They are the Gardner-Diamond syndrome or autoerythrocyte sensitization and DNA hypersensitivity. In the Gardner-Diamond syndrome painful ecchymoses appear spontaneously or follow trauma; it is commonest in women, especially those with emotional problems, and appears to reflect sensitivity to the stroma of the patient's own erythrocytes. DNA hypersensitivity is clinically similar to auto-erythrocyte sensitization. Hematoxylin bodies have been noted in skin lesions like those observed in patients with systemic lupus erythematosus. Available data are in accord with the thesis that this unusual disorder reflects sensitivity to the patient's own deoxyribonucleic acid.

VON WILLEBRAND'S DISEASE

In 1931 von Willebrand first described this hemorrhagic diathesis in a group of people living in the Åland Islands. Abnormal bleeding begins in childhood; epistaxis, gingival bleeding, melena, hematuria, and menorrhagia are common, whereas purpura (i.e., petechiae and ecchymoses) and bleeding deep within the tissues (e.g., hemarthroses) are rare. It affects both sexes and is inherited as a simple autosomal dominant. The synonyms, pseudohemophilia and vascular hemophilia, are misleading terms and should be abandoned.

Confusion about the pathogenesis of this syndrome persists. It seems likely that a number of hemorrhagic disorders caused by various vascular and/or platelet abnormalities have been classified under this heading. In fact, recent studies of the islanders initially described by von Willebrand indicate the presence in this group of more than one bleeding abnormality. A prolonged bleeding time is characteristic; in addition, about half the patients have a positive capillary fragility test. As a rule, tests of the coagulation mechanism are fairly normal despite the fact that factor VIII activity is usually decreased. Platelets are present in normal numbers and do not appear to be morphologically abnormal; however, recent studies suggest that they fail to aggregate normally in vivo. Also some evidence favors the concept that a plasma factor needed for the maintenance of vascular integrity is lacking.

At the present time, this category of hemorrhagic disorders remains unclear. Current data indicate that it is probably an inherited abnormality of capillaries (the absence of bleeding from large vessels suggests that they are not affected). In addition, platelet dysfunction (i.e., impaired aggregation) and factor VIII deficiency appear to be components of the disease in its full expression. The precise contribution of each of these abnormalities remains to be defined. It has been suggested that the deficiency of factor VIII may reflect depletion consequent to widespread capillary defects and superficial bleeding rather than a primary manifestation of the hemorrhagic diathesis.

Pending clarification of its pathogenesis, there is no objection to the continued use of the eponym, von Willebrand's disease. However, only patients with a prolonged bleeding time and factor VIII deficiency should be classified under this heading; the diagnostic role of tests of platelet aggregation must await further study. Thus the diagnosis is based on the clinical picture, a positive family history with bleeding affecting both sexes, a prolonged bleeding time, and a deficiency of factor VIII.

Treatment consists of local measures to control bleeding plus transfusions as needed. Transfusions are quite effective for short periods of time; for obscure reasons increases in factor VIII levels persist longer after transfusions than in patients with classical hemophilia. Because the gene causing von Willebrand's disease acts as a mendelian dominant, genetic counseling is in order.

Platelet Disorders

THROMBOCYTOPENIA

A decreased number of platelets in the peripheral blood may reflect increased destruction and/or decreased production. It is possible to classify the thrombocytopenias (Table 13-5) in a manner analogous to the etiologic classifications of the anemias (Table 3-2, p. 56) and the neutropenias (Table 7-3, p. 328). The thrombocytopenias caused by increased loss are characterized by normal or increased numbers of megakaryocytes in the bone marrow; those that reflect decreased production are accompanied by a decreased number of megakaryocytes.

Table 13-5. *Classification of the Thrombocytopenias*

I. *Increased Loss* (Normal or ↑ # megs in BM)
   A. Hypersplenic thrombocytopenia (No intrinsic platelet defect)
      1. Isoimmune
      2. Autoimmune
         a. Primary (idiopathic thrombocytopenic purpura)
         b. Secondary
      3. Drug-induced immunothrombocytopenia
      4. Big spleen syndrome
   B. Massive blood transfusion
   C. Thrombotic thrombocytopenic purpura
   D. Increased utilization

II. *Decreased Production*
   A. Deficiencies—vitamin B_{12} and folic acid (p. 186)
   B. Diversion of growth potential—granulocytic leukemia (p. 338)
   C. Destruction or depression—hypoplastic anemias (p. 222)
   D. Displacement—myelophthisic anemias (p. 240), chronic lymphocytic leukemia (p. 369), plasmacytic myeloma (p. 411), and primary macroglobulinemia (p. 442)

Pathophysiology of Thrombocytopenia. Regardless of cause, the pathophysiologic manifestations of thrombocytopenia are similar. Platelets are primarily concerned with hemostasis, and a platelet deficiency causes a hemorrhagic diathesis. As a rule, significant bleeding does not occur unless the circulating platelet count falls below 50,000/cu mm. Although platelets contribute to blood clotting, small numbers suffice for this purpose. About 30,000 platelets/cu mm of blood appear adequate to provide enough platelet factor 3 to permit normal coagulation in vitro. Therefore, routine tests of the coagulation mechanism (e.g., the whole blood coagulation time) are normal in most thrombocytopenic patients.

For the most part the bleeding phenomena attributable to thrombocytopenia reflect (1) the loss of platelet thrombi or plugs needed to seal breaks in small vessels, (2) abnormal clot retraction, and (3) impaired vascular integrity. Abnormal bleeding from large vessels is not characteristic of thrombocytopenia, and hemarthroses and soft tissue hematomas are rarely the result of quantitative platelet deficiencies. On the other hand, purpuric lesions (petechiae and ecchymoses) are typical of thrombocytopenia; in fact, these hemorrhagic disorders are usually designated thrombocytopenic purpuras. Petechiae (pinpoint bleeding from the arterial end of a capillary loop) are typical. They may be generalized but are most prominent over dependent areas (e.g., the lower legs) or over sites subjected to pressure or constriction. Other common hemorrhagic manifestations of thrombocytopenia are epistaxis, gingival bleeding, menorrhagia, melena, and hematuria.

The laboratory findings are rather clear-cut. A decrease in the platelet count is, of course, the *sine qua non* for the diagnosis of thrombocytopenia. Other abnormalities include a prolonged bleeding time, impaired clot retraction, a positive capillary fragility test, and a shortened serum prothrombin time.

Although the manifestations of all thrombocytopenias are similar, other aspects of the clinical picture (as well as the treatment) vary with the nature of the primary disease. Therefore it is appropriate to consider certain of the disorders characterized by thrombocytopenia separately.

Hypersplenic Thrombocytopenias

Hypersplenism, its cause and pathophysiology, are discussed in detail elsewhere (Chap. 12, p. 448). Thrombocytopenia is a common manifestation of certain types of hypersplenism. In many cases the decrease in platelets is associated with a hemolytic anemia and/or neutropenia. However, thrombocytopenia may be the sole, or at least the predominant, manifestation. No intrinsic defects are known to affect the survival of platelets adversely (Table 12-1, p. 454). Extrinsic damage, probably caused by platelet antibodies, and increased destruction consequent to greatly enlarged spleens do produce hypersplenic thrombocytopenia.

ISOIMMUNE THROMBOCYTOPENIA

Erythroblastosis fetalis is an isoimmune disorder affecting red cells (p. 123). Occasionally, neonatal neutropenia can be attributed to a fetal-maternal leukocyte incompatibility (p. 329). Recent studies indicate that platelets also possess antigenic specificity. It is not surprising, therefore, that a few infants have been observed in whom maternal antibodies (presumably elaborated in response to fetal platelets of a different antigenic makeup entering the maternal circulation) have been implicated in the pathogenesis of thrombocytopenia. Such antibodies are probably responsible for thrombocytopenia in some patients with erythroblastosis fetalis. This category must be distinguished from the other causes of thrombocytopenia in the newborn. The presence of normal or increased numbers of megakaryocytes eliminates such possibilities as congenital hypoplastic thrombocytopenia. In the absence of disease in the mother (e.g., idiopathic thrombocytopenic purpura or drug-induced thrombocytopenia), it can be assumed that the platelet deficiency reflects a maternal-fetal incompatibility. Bleeding is self-limited and ceases within a few days to weeks. However, available data point to a fairly high mortality rate. Exchange transfusions to rid the infant of the antibodies have been advocated if the bleeding is severe.

AUTOIMMUNE THROMBOCYTOPENIAS

The autoimmune thrombocytopenias can be divided into two categories: (1) primary or idiopathic thrombocytopenic purpura (this disorder is commonly referred to by the abbreviation ITP) and (2) secondary. The secondary autoimmune thrombocytopenias are associated with three groups of primary disorders.

1. Hematologic neoplasms such as lymphoma, chronic lymphocytic leukemia, plasmacytic myeloma, and primary macroglobulinemia.
2. Collagen diseases, particularly systemic lupus erythematosus.
3. Certain infections (e.g., rubella and other exanthemata, visceral tuberculosis with involvement of the spleen, and infectious mononucleosis).

The diagnosis of ITP is contingent on the exclusion of all causes of a secondary autoimmune thrombocytopenia. The relative incidence of idiopathic and secondary autoimmune thrombocytopenias is not known. Although most series point to a predominance of idiopathic thrombocytopenic purpura, it must be borne in mind that close follow-up eventually reveals many of these patients to be examples of secondary disease.

The autoimmune thrombocytopenias would appear to be caused by autoantibodies. Although the subject of platelet antibodies is in its infancy, the existence of humoral factors possessing the attributes of immunoglobulins and the capabilities of bringing about the destruction of platelets cannot be denied. Much of the discussion pertaining to erythrocyte autoantibodies (p. 133) probably applies as well to antibodies directed against platelets. Plasmas from some patients with ITP have been shown to evoke a prompt thrombocytopenia in normal recipients. In addition, about 70 per cent of the children born to mothers with idiopathic thrombocytopenic purpura manifest thrombocytopenia at birth which clears over the ensuing few days to weeks. Furthermore, it is possible to demonstrate in vitro the presence of platelet agglutinins in many patients with chronic ITP (50 per cent or more of some series). These observations, together with the demonstration of a greatly accelerated rate of removal of transfused platelets in patients with ITP, provide convincing support for the thesis that a circulating factor (presumably a platelet antibody) plays a major role in the pathogenesis of these thrombocytopenic states. However, technical problems concerned with the demonstration of immunoglobulins with antiplatelet activity have impeded acquisition of knowledge concerning these substances (none of the tests available for the study of platelet antibodies is wholly satisfactory). It should be noted that some investigators, who have been unable to detect antiplatelet factors or autoantibodies, dispute the significance of immune mechanisms in the causation of these thrombocytopenias. Further studies and more reliable techniques are needed to resolve this problem.

The possible role of a capillary defect in the causation of these bleeding disorders also remains to be clarified. Increased capillary fragility, the severity of which does not always go hand-in-hand with the platelet count, is evident in patients with this form of thrombocytopenia. Furthermore, comparable degrees of thrombocytopenia secondary to marrow hypoplasia are frequently not accompanied by spontaneous capillary hemorrhage (capillary hemorrhages are characteristic of the autoimmune thrombocytopenias). It has been suggested, with some experimental support, that the abnormal protein contributing to the premature destruction of platelets also adversely affects the capillary endothelium. Another poorly explained observation is the atypical appearance of the megakaryocytes in most of these patients. If thrombocytopenia reflected only accelerated platelet destruction by a circulating antibody, evidence of increased thrombopoiesis in the marrow would be expected. Although megakaryocytes are usually overabundant, they are often abnormal and have sharply demarcated cytoplasmic margins and little or no evidence of platelet budding. There are at least two alternative explanations for these findings. The megakaryocytes may be producing platelets so rapidly that evidence of their formation is not obtainable (this explanation seems unlikely, especially in view of the abundant cytoplasm of many of these cells). More feasible is the possibility that an abnormal protein (i.e., a platelet antibody) affects megakaryocytes as well as platelets. Because platelets are composed of megakaryocytic cytoplasm, it is logical to surmise that these cellular particles and the parent cells may be equally susceptible to damage by a platelet antibody. In this regard, erythrocyte antibodies have been shown to affect nucleated red cell precursors in the marrow. Thus the autoimmune thrombocytopenias may reflect an element of decreased production as well as accelerated destruction.

At the present time the premise that these thrombocytopenias are due to the presence of a circulating factor (probably an autoantibody) seems justified. This substance appears to injure or condition circulating platelets so that they are removed and destroyed prematurely; it also appears to affect megakaryocytes, thus interfering with platelet formation. In ITP the stimulus to the formation of such antiplatelet factors is unknown; in the secondary autoimmune thrombocytopenias the abnormal protein is probably a reflection of benign or malignant proliferation of cells capable of synthesizing immunoglobulins. Most likely the spleen plays an important role in these disorders as a major source of antibodies and as an organ that serves to remove "sensitized" or damaged platelets.

Idiopathic Thrombocytopenic Purpura. ITP can be divided into two subcategories, acute and chronic. Acute ITP has a sudden onset and usually subsides or terminates fatally within three to four months. Chronic ITP ordinarily has an insidious onset and may persist for months to years. Certain variations suggest that these two kinds of ITP reflect different pathogenic mechanisms. For example, platelet agglutinins, which are demonstrable in 50 per cent or more of the patients with chronic ITP, are rarely found in the acute form.

CLINICAL MANIFESTATIONS. ITP affects all ages and both sexes. However, it is more common in children and young adults (less than 10 per cent of the patients are over the age of 40 years and about two thirds are under 20) and is more frequent in females than in males (this sex predilection is especially evident after puberty). ITP may appear with dramatic suddenness or it may develop gradually. In children it is particularly likely to have an explosive onset and often follows an acute infection. The clinical pictures reflect both the severity of the thrombocytopenia and the site of bleeding; consequently, there is considerable variation among patients.

Symptoms. The symptomatology of ITP consists of overt bleeding or of manifestations ascribable to hemorrhage. Purpura is the most consistent complaint. Epistaxis, gingival bleeding, menorrhagia, hematuria, and melena are the usual forms. However, no organ is immune, and the manifestations are varied and often bizarre (e.g., bleeding into the central nervous system). If blood loss has been severe, the patient may complain of the symptoms caused by an acute hemorrhagic anemia (p. 67); occasionally, chronic blood loss may be responsible for the development of an iron deficiency anemia (p. 172).

Physical Findings. Purpura (petechiae and ecchymoses) occurs in almost every patient. Petechiae are characteristic; these small hemorrhagic lesions affect the skin and mucous membranes and are not associated with swelling or evidence of inflammation. They are most numerous over dependent areas (e.g., the legs) and at sites of pressure; in the face of severe thrombocytopenia, they may be generalized. Other physical findings are directly attributable to hemorrhage and vary with the organ involved and the severity of the bleeding. Hemarthroses are distinctly unusual; soft tissue hematomas are rare. Splenomegaly is *not* a characteristic finding. Although the tip of the spleen may be palpable in a few patients (perhaps 10 per cent or less), the presence of an enlarged spleen is so unusual that it suggests another diagnosis (e.g., a secondary autoimmune thrombocytopenia). Lymph nodes are not enlarged; neither is the liver. Bone tenderness is not found. In patients with acute bleeding, tachycardia, hypotension, and pallor (manifestations of an acute hemorrhagic anemia) may be prominent.

Laboratory Findings. The laboratory manifestations of ITP include a low platelet count, a prolonged bleeding time, impaired clot retraction, a positive capillary fragility test, a shortened serum prothrombin time, and the presence of normal or increased numbers of megakaryocytes in the bone marrow. The megakaryocytes are often abnormal (rounded with sharply demarcated borders and little or no evidence of platelet budding, Fig. 13-2). The coagulation time is typically normal, as is the one-stage prothrombin time. Other hematologic abnormalities are attributable to an acute hemorrhagic anemia (p. 69) or to an iron deficiency anemia (p. 174). Reticulocytosis, circulating nucleated red cells, and marrow erythrocytic hyperplasia are usually manifestations of recent acute hemorrhage; however, a minor hemolytic component is often demonstrable and may contribute to these findings. The leukocyte count may be increased (a reflection of acute hemorrhage, p. 70), normal, or slightly decreased. When neutropenia is present, it probably reflects an immunoneutropenia and may be accompanied by the appropriate marrow changes of hypersplenism (p. 456). The relationship between an autoimmune hemolytic anemia, thrombocytopenia, and neutropenia is discussed elsewhere (p. 135). A few patients exhibit peripheral blood and/or marrow eosinophilia. The significance of these findings is obscure; attempts to attach prognostic significance to an overabundance of eosinophils in the marrow have not been particularly convincing. Skin lesions of all kinds are often associated with an eosino-

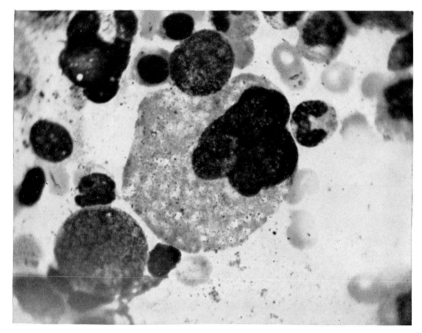

Figure 13-2. Megakaryocyte with sharply demarcated cell margins and no evidence of platelet formation in the bone marrow aspirate of a patient with idiopathic thrombocytopenic purpura.

philia (p. 315); consequently, eosinophilia in patients with ITP may be caused by bleeding into the skin. Some patients have an elevated serum acid phosphatase, a probable reflection of increased platelet destruction (platelets contain this enzyme in relative abundance). Other laboratory findings are nonspecific, with the exception of platelet agglutinins which can be found in the majority of patients with chronic ITP (they are rarely demonstrable in persons with acute disease).

DIAGNOSIS. The diagnosis of ITP is contingent on (1) the demonstration of thrombocytopenia in the presence of normal or increased numbers of megakaryocytes in the bone marrow and (2) the exclusion of all disorders known to produce thrombocytopenia by accelerating platelet destruction (Table 13-5). The history and physical examination usually suggest thrombocytopenia; the absence of splenic, hepatic, and/or node enlargement points to ITP. Examination of the peripheral blood readily confirms the presence of thrombocytopenia. The next step, a marrow examination, is mandatory in the work-up of all thrombocytopenic patients to exclude those thrombocytopenias caused by decreased platelet production (e.g., acute leukemia and hypoplastic anemia). The demonstration of platelet agglutinins supports the diagnosis of an immunothrombocytopenia; however, it does not provide proof of such a diagnosis, and a negative test does not eliminate this possibility. Having confirmed the existence of a hypersplenic thrombocytopenia, a diagnosis of *idiopathic* thrombocytopenic purpura is justified only after all secondary thrombocytopenias have been excluded. Thus the diagnosis of ITP is in effect one of exclusion. Even those patients who appear to fall clearly into the category of idiopathic thrombocytopenic purpura deserve close follow-up. Many will subsequently develop overt manifestations of some other primary disease (e.g., systemic lupus erythematosus or lymphoma). Therefore the diagnosis of ITP is, at best, a presumptive one.

TREATMENT AND COURSE. ITP is characterized by remissions and relapses. Thus it is difficult to define a typical or average course. Improvement is to be expected, but recurrences are common. In children the disease is more likely to be self-limited and to subside spontaneously. On the other hand, ITP often runs a protracted course in adults and generally requires specific therapy. Often, the dividing line between acute and chronic ITP is indistinct and arbitrary. Average or median survival data are meaningless because of variations among patients in severity, the tendency to undergo spontaneous remission, the type of therapy employed, and the response to treatment. Central nervous system bleeding is the commonest cause of death. Corticosteroids and splenectomy are the cornerstones of therapy. Because of differences in the response or course of childhood and adult forms of ITP, it is desirable to consider them separately.

Idiopathic Thrombocytopenic Purpura in Adults. The diagnosis of ITP is not necessarily an indication for treatment. In persons with few, if any, hemorrhagic manifestations and a platelet count greater than 50,000/cu mm, observation may be all that is needed. In more severely thrombocytopenic patients and those with overt bleeding, corticosteroids are indicated. In adolescents or young adults with disease of short duration, it has been advocated that they be observed for one to two weeks before starting corticosteroids to see whether a spontaneous remission will occur. However, the risks of serious bleeding (e.g., intracranial hemorrhage) ordinarily outweigh those associated with the administration of corticosteroids. Consequently, all adults who are actively bleeding and have no specific contraindication to such treatment deserve an immediate trial of corticosteroids.

Prednisone in a dose of 15 mg every six hours (60 mg/day) or an equivalent amount of some comparable compound will evoke a beneficial response in most patients. In about half the platelet count returns to normal or near normal, and all abnormal bleeding ceases. Improvement often occurs with dramatic suddenness (i.e., within 24 to 48 hours). Among the remaining patients many will manifest a suboptimal platelet response, but most will exhibit improvement in capillary integrity and lessening of their hemorrhagic manifestations, even though their platelet counts fail to show a significant increase. If a patient does not show improvement within a few days and hemorrhage is deemed to be life-threatening, massive corticosteroid therapy may be worthwhile (prednisone in doses of 400 mg or more a day has been effective in a few cases). The mechanism(s) by which corticosteroids exert their therapeutic effect are obscure. Possible explanations include (1) a decrease in antibody synthesis, (2) interference with an antigen-antibody reaction, and (3) a poorly defined beneficial effect on the capillary endothelium.

If the patient responds optimally to corticosteroids (i.e., all hemorrhagic phenomena cease and a normal platelet count is restored), the dose should be tapered and, if possible, stopped. About 30 per cent of these individuals develop sustained remissions following corticosteroids. These persons, who have usually had their disease for less than four months, require no further treatment, although they should be followed closely, for the likelihood is great that bleeding will recur at some time in the future. In most of the patients who respond well to large doses of corticosteroids (especially those who have had purpura for four months or longer before treatment), thrombocytopenia and bleeding recur as the dose is being tapered or after treatment is stopped. These patients are potential candidates for splenectomy, as are those who respond suboptimally or not at all (an adequate trial of corticosteroids appears to be 14 to 21 days). It is most unusual for a partial response (e.g., decreased capillary fragility) to be maintained as the dose of prednisone is reduced or after it has been discontinued. Because the majority of these individuals respond favorably to splenectomy, there is less justification for long-term corticosteroid therapy in patients with ITP than in persons with a primary acquired autoimmune hemolytic anemia (p. 141). Thus maintenance corticosteroid therapy is best reserved for those patients who do not respond to splenectomy or in whom some other disease precludes surgery or increases the operative risk.

The value of splenectomy in the management of patients with ITP has been known for half a century. Characteristically, the platelet count increases rapidly (often within the first 24 to 48 hours). In some patients high counts are reached in 7 to 10 days and are followed by a gradual return to more normal levels. In about 80 per cent of adolescents and adults with ITP, the platelet count returns to normal and all bleeding ceases after splenectomy. Under these circumstances corticosteroids should be tapered and discontinued as soon as possible. At some time in the future, certain of these patients will develop recurrent disease. Available data do not permit a precise appraisal of the incidence of relapse after a remission has been induced by splenectomy, but it would not appear to be particularly common. Those patients who do not respond to splenectomy and those who improve suboptimally but continue to have bleeding of sufficient severity to warrant therapy are candidates for long-term treatment with corticosteroids (the lowest dose that will maintain the desired effect—preferably 15 mg of prednisone a day or less).

Some dispute continues in regard to the role of splenectomy in the treatment of ITP. Those who are opposed to this therapeutic approach cite such disadvantages as a high rate of relapse, exacerbation of latent lupus erythematosus, and the possibility that splenectomized persons might be more susceptible to infections. None of these criticisms militates strongly against splenectomy. Admittedly, some patients fail to respond or relapse after an initial period of improvement; however, most manifest a sustained remission. Failure in the minority (about one out of five) is not a valid reason to deny the majority a completely effective form of treatment. Although it has been suggested that splenectomy enhances the development of systemic lupus erythematosus, a causal relationship has not been proved. It seems likely that most of the patients who develop systemic lupus erythematosus after splenectomy actually have an immunothrombocytopenia as the first manifestation of their collagen disease. There is little support for the contention that splenectomized individuals are more prone to develop acute infections (p. 449). The bulk of available evidence indicates that splenectomy plays an essential role in the treatment of ITP. Thus every patient who fails to develop a sustained remission with corticosteroid therapy and who continues to have a moderate to severe hemorrhagic diathesis is a potential candidate for surgery.

Before the availability of corticosteroids, it was often necessary to resort to splenectomy on an emergency basis in an attempt to control severe hemorrhage. Under these circumstances the mortality rate was quite high. Now it is rarely, if ever, necessary to perform an emergency splenectomy; with few exceptions, all patients should be pretreated with corticosteroids before surgery. Even those persons who show no increase in their platelet counts with prednisone may manifest decreased capillary fragility, thus making the surgeon's task much easier. If a patient relapses as corticosteroids are being tapered or after they have been stopped, he should be restarted on full doses and maximal control over the hemorrhagic process attained before operation.

Iron is indicated in those patients who have bled chronically and have become iron deficient. Whole blood transfusions should be used as needed for the management of an acute hemorrhagic anemia (p. 71). Platelet transfusions are of limited value in the majority of patients with ITP (one of the characteristic manifestations of this disorder is a markedly shortened platelet survival time). Since transfused platelets are generally destroyed promptly, they accomplish little. Nevertheless, when available, platelet transfusions are warranted in certain patients with life-threatening hemorrhage and may tide the patient over until the hypersplenic process can be brought under control. Platelet substitutes exert no effect because bleeding reflects too few viable platelets, not decreased platelet factor 3 activity. A few patients have responded to cytotoxic drugs (p. 145), but further observations are needed before conclusions can be reached.

Idiopathic Thrombocytopenic Purpura in Children. Treatment of acute ITP in children differs insofar as the indications for splenectomy are concerned. Most of these patients have an acute self-limited course that subsides spontaneously within a few days or weeks (serious bleeding generally lasts for only a few days). About 80 per cent of children with acute ITP undergo spontaneous remissions. Therefore it is desirable to avoid splenectomy if at all possible. Unless bleeding is life-threatening and uncontrollable, these patients should be observed for four to six months before they are subjected to splenectomy. Even in those persons with severe hemorrhage who fail to respond to other forms of therapy, it is preferable to wait one to two weeks before removing the spleen. Corticosteroids and transfusions play important roles in the management of the child with acute ITP; the indications for their use are essentially those applicable to the adult. The majority can be supported until remission occurs. Since few of these patients have demonstrable platelet agglutinins, the use of platelet transfusions is on a firmer footing. About 20 per cent of children with ITP exhibit a chronic course (i.e., thrombocytopenia will persist for four to six months or longer). In these cases the indications for splenectomy are similar to those in the adult (significant bleeding and/or a platelet count below 50,000/cu mm in a patient who fails to develop a sustained remission with corticosteroids).

Secondary Autoimmune Thrombocytopenia. Hypersplenic thrombocytopenia accompanies a variety of primary diseases, including hematologic neoplasms, collagen disorders, and certain infections. Presumably these thrombocytopenic states have an immune pathogenesis. Such an assumption is based largely on observations of the role of autoantibodies in the pathogenesis of the secondary acquired autoimmune hemolytic anemias (p. 453) and the frequency with which hypersplenic thrombocytopenia accompanies these hemolytic states. Because of the limitations of available techniques, it has not been possible to document this thesis. However, it seems likely that these thrombocytopenias reflect the presence of an abnormal globulin directed against platelets. The discussion pertaining to the pathogenesis of the secondary acquired autoimmune hemolytic anemias (p. 133) is applicable to the probable role of such factors in the causation of the secondary autoimmune thrombocytopenias.

Clinical Manifestations. The age and sex distributions of the secondary autoimmune thrombocytopenias are those of the primary diseases. Thus this form of thrombocytopenia affects males and females of all ages. For example, infections are more common in children, systemic lupus erythematosus in adolescent or young adult females, and hematologic neoplasms in older males. The clinical picture is determined by the nature of the underlying disease with the superimposed manifestations of thrombocytopenia. Occasionally, the symptoms and physical findings are those of idiopathic thrombocytopenic purpura. More often, however, the predominant symptoms and physical abnormalities are attributable to the primary disease [e.g., lymphoma (p. 389), chronic lymphocytic leukemia (p. 369), infectious mononucleosis (p. 320), and systemic lupus erythematosus].

The laboratory findings consist of thrombocytopenia, a prolonged bleeding time, impaired clot retraction, a positive capillary fragility test, and a shortened serum prothrombin time. Platelet agglutinins may or may not be demonstrable. Provided the marrow has not been affected by the primary disorder, megakaryocytes are present in normal to increased numbers; they are usually atypical without evidence of platelet formation. If the basic disease involves the marrow (e.g., chronic lymphocytic leukemia), megakaryocytes may be decreased; however, they often display the morphologic abnormalities of hypersplenism and may be present in disproportionately greater numbers than are other normal myeloid elements. The coagulation time and other tests of the clotting mechanism are normal unless they reflect the underlying disease [e.g., a prolonged coagulation time in a patient with systemic lupus erythematosus who has a circulating anticoagulant (p. 516)]. Most patients have an associated hemolytic anemia and/or hypersplenic neutropenia. In some, however, thrombocytopenia is the sole (or at least the major) hypersplenic manifestation. Other laboratory abnormalities are those of the primary disorder [e.g., a positive LE cell test (p. 313), the peripheral blood and marrow findings of chronic lymphocytic leukemia (p. 370), or plasmacytic myeloma (p. 417)].

DIAGNOSIS. The diagnosis of a secondary autoimmune thrombocytopenia is based on the demonstration of (1) hypersplenic thrombocytopenia (an inadequate number of platelets in the peripheral blood in the face of normal or increased numbers of megakaryocytes in the bone marrow) and (2) a disorder known to be associated with such a thrombocytopenia. Therefore the diagnosis is largely based on association rather than on the positive demonstration of a platelet autoantibody. For this reason the diagnostic criteria are those of the primary disease; they are discussed in the sections dealing with these disorders (see Table 12-1, p. 454).

TREATMENT AND COURSE. The course of a secondary autoimmune thrombocytopenia is contingent on the underlying disease. For example, patients with thrombocytopenia secondary to infectious mononucleosis recover; those with a lymphoproliferative disorder succumb to their hematologic malignancy. Treatment consists of those measures indicated for the primary disease plus the therapeutic regimen outlined for idiopathic thrombocytopenic purpura. Most of the special problems encountered in the treatment of the secondary autoimmune hemolytic anemias (p. 146) apply to the management of patients with secondary autoimmune thrombocytopenia. Corticosteroids are indicated in all patients, provided a specific contraindication to their use does not exist; most will respond, at least suboptimally. The role of splenectomy is less clear. If the underlying disorder is benign and self-limited (e.g., infectious mononucleosis), splenectomy is not indicated. In general, it is desirable to avoid splenectomy if possible in those patients with progressive diseases such as leukemia or lymphoma. However, splenectomy deserves serious consideration in certain patients who have uncontrollable and life-threatening bleeding as the major manifestation of their disease. Dramatic improvement has been observed.

DRUG-INDUCED IMMUNOTHROMBOCYTOPENIA

Many drugs are capable of producing thrombocytopenia; most cause megakaryocytic hypoplasia and a decrease in platelet production (i.e., a hypoplastic anemia). However, some induce antibody formation and bring about an immunothrombocytopenia. The best and most thoroughly studied examples are the thrombocytopenias caused by quinidine and the sedative Sedormid (allylisopropylacetyl carbamide). These drugs appear to act as haptenes or incomplete antigens. They may combine with platelets to stimulate the formation of an antibody, which will then react with the drug-platelet complex to bring about platelet destruction. An alternative thesis contends that a drug-plasma factor complex evokes antibody elaboration and that platelet destruction is a nonspecific side effect of an antigen-antibody reaction. It is also possible that such an antibody might coat the platelets and render them susceptible to damage on subsequent contact with the drug. Whatever the pathogenic mechanism, both the drug and antibody are required to affect platelets in vivo and in vitro.

The clinical manifestations of a drug-induced immunothrombocytopenia are all attributable to a decreased platelet count (i.e., a hemorrhagic diathesis). The laboratory findings reflect thrombocytopenia; the marrow contains normal or increased numbers of megakaryocytes. The history is particularly important. The story is that of prior (or prolonged) drug exposure; even in susceptible persons, thrombocytopenia will not follow the initial contact, since antibody formation will not have taken place.

Proof of a drug-induced immunothrombocytopenia can be obtained by in vivo and in vitro testing. The administration of even a small amount of the offending drug to a patient who has recently recovered from such an immunothrombocytopenia will bring about a prompt (within minutes or hours) fall in the circulating platelet count. This diagnostic maneuver is obviously not without hazard and should be avoided if possible. In vitro tests consist of the demonstration of platelet clumping in the patient's platelet-rich plasma after the addition of the drug (in markedly thrombocytopenic patients normal donor platelets will be needed). In the presence of complement platelet lysis follows the clumping. Antibodies have been shown to persist for as long as six months after a thrombocytopenic episode, but the test described is usually positive only in the acute phase of a drug-induced immuno-thrombocytopenia. Treatment consists of removing the responsible drug and avoiding future contact with it. Patients who are sensitive to quinidine may react to structurally similar compounds such as quinine. There is no place for splenectomy in the management of this type of thrombo-cytopenia. Improvement occurs promptly after the drug is stopped; there is no convincing evidence that corticosteroids hasten recovery.

BIG SPLEEN SYNDROMES

As discussed in Chapter 12 (p. 448), hypersplenism is sometimes caused by simple enlargement of the spleen. Examples of this type of increased blood cell destruction include agnogenic myeloid metaplasia (p. 430), Gaucher's disease (p. 458), and Banti's syndrome, that is, portal hypertension with chronic congestive splenomegaly (p. 457). A hemolytic anemia is the dominant hypersplenic manifestation in these situations and has been most extensively studied. However, many of these patients are also thrombocytopenic and/or neutropenic, presumably because of a similar pathogenesis. The diagnosis is based on the demonstration of thrombocytopenia in the face of normal or increased numbers of megakaryocytes in the marrow of a patient with massive splenomegaly. These entities and their treatment are discussed in other chapters.

Massive Blood Transfusion

Patients who lose large quantities of blood and require numerous blood transfusions over a short period of time (about 7500 ml or 15 units/hour) become thrombocytopenic and may develop a generalized hemorrhagic diathesis. The explanation for such occurrences appears to be loss of circulating platelets consequent to hemorrhage and re-plenishment with bank blood containing few, if any, viable platelets. Because there is no marrow platelet reserve (p. 33), the remaining platelets are diluted; thrombocytopenia ensues. It may also reflect a mixture of incompatible platelet types.

Thrombotic Thrombocytopenic Purpura

Thrombotic thrombocytopenic purpura is a rare syndrome characterized clinically by thrombocytopenia, a hemolytic anemia, and changing
neurologic signs and symptoms; pathologically, it is distinguished by
hyaline thrombi in small blood vessels. The vascular lesions involve all
organs with a special predilection for the brain, kidneys, heart, pancreas,
and adrenals. Histologically, there are masses of hyaline material beneath
the endothelium of capillaries and between the endothelium and muscu-
lature of arterioles. Other features include endothelial proliferation
in the absence of hyaline deposits and cylindrical and globular aneurysms
of small arteries. The hyaline material was once thought to be masses
of platelets. This possibility has been eliminated, and recent studies
indicate that it is fibrin or some other derivative of fibrinogen.

The cause of thrombotic thrombocytopenic purpura is not known.
Current data favor the concept that it is an autoimmune disorder primarily affecting small blood vessels. Neither erythrocyte nor platelet
antibodies are demonstrable. The thrombocytopenia may be caused by
intravascular clotting with platelets being utilized during the coagulation process or injured so that they are removed prematurely by normal
destructive mechanisms (e.g., the spleen). The hemolytic anemia most
likely reflects trauma to red cells consequent to the vascular defects,
thus leading to erythrocyte cytoclasis with impaired viability of the red
cell fragments (the presence of schistocytes in the peripheral blood
supports such a pathogenesis).

Thrombotic thrombocytopenic purpura affects all ages, although it is
commonest in the third and fourth decades of life. There is no sex or
race predilection. The clinical features include (1) those symptoms and
physical abnormalities that characterize any thrombocytopenic state (p.
488), as well as those attributable to an acute hemolytic anemia (p.
85), and (2) those symptoms and physical findings relating to the
damage done to specific organs by vascular lesions. Central nervous
system signs and symptoms include irritability, confusion, delirium, convulsions, motor paralysis, and sensory changes; spinal cord and peripheral nerve lesions have also been observed. Neurologic findings are
typically fleeting and variable. Most patients are febrile.

Laboratory abnormalities include thrombocytopenia and an anemia
distinguished by the presence of schistocytes in the peripheral blood
(Fig. 13-3) and, on occasion, by spherocytes. Reticulocytosis and circulating nucleated red cells reflect the hemolytic process. The bone
marrow reveals erythrocytic hyperplasia and normal to increased numbers of megakaryocytes. Hematuria is common. Other laboratory findings
include the pigment changes of hemolysis (p. 86) and the manifestations of thrombocytopenia (a prolonged bleeding time, impaired clot

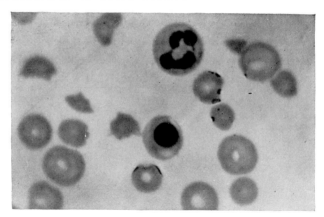

Figure 13-3. Schistocytes or red cell fragments in the peripheral blood of a patient with thrombotic thrombocytopenic purpura.

retraction, and a positive capillary fragility test). The Coombs' test is typically negative as are tests for platelet agglutinins.

In most of the reported cases (about 150), the diagnosis was made postmortem. However, an awareness of this entity permits a presumptive diagnosis in the face of a characteristic clinical picture (thrombocytopenia, a hemolytic anemia with numerous poikilocytes or red cell fragments in the peripheral blood, and bizarre, variable neurologic manifestations). In a few cases the diagnosis has been proved antemortem by the demonstration of typical vascular lesions in fixed sections of bone marrow or lymph nodes (Fig. 13-4).

The course of thrombotic thrombocytopenic purpura is usually progressive and terminates fatally within a few days or weeks. Occasionally the disorder runs a chronic course in which remissions and relapses

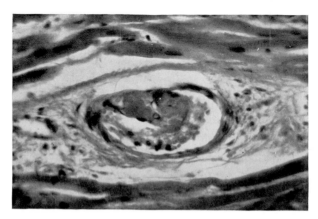

Figure 13-4. Typical vascular lesion of thrombotic thrombocytopenic purpura (fixed section of myocardium).

occur over a period of months to years. Renal insufficiency may be a prominent feature.

Treatment of this syndrome leaves much to be desired. Splenectomy has produced variable results. Corticosteroids have been more effective, especially when given in massive doses. Benefit has been observed in a few patients treated with anticoagulants on a long-term basis. The rationale for this treatment is the prevention of intravascular clotting and the deposition of the hyaline material. Further evaluation of this therapeutic approach is indicated.

Increased Utilization

A few children have been observed to have thrombocytopenia in association with large congenital hemangiomas. This hemorrhagic disorder apparently reflects sequestration of platelets within the vascular lesion with resultant peripheral thrombocytopenia. Following regression or eradication of the hemangioma, normal platelet counts are restored. Thrombocytopenia caused by increased utilization is also a feature of the intravascular coagulation syndrome (p. 516).

Decreased Production

The majority of the thrombocytopenic states reflect decreased production rather than increased destruction. These thrombocytopenias are characterized by decreased numbers of megakaryocytes in the bone marrow (vitamin B_{12} and folic acid deficiency anemias are exceptions). They can be separated into several groups based on their differing etiologies (Table 13-5). As a rule, other aspects of myelopoiesis are also affected (i.e., anemia and neutropenia generally accompany the thrombocytopenia). Rare patients have been observed with congenital or hereditary hypoplastic thrombocytopenia. However, most of the diseases associated with these secondary thrombocytopenias are acquired; their clinical manifestations, diagnosis, treatment, and course are discussed elsewhere (see Table 13-5).

THROMBOCYTHEMIA

Thrombocytopenia is manifested clinically by abnormal bleeding; thrombocythemia is often associated with intravascular thrombosis. Paradoxically, a platelet excess may also cause abnormal bleeding. Thus patients with polycythemia vera (p. 298), primary thrombocythemia (p. 440), and agnogenic myeloid metaplasia (p. 430) often exhibit a hemorrhagic diathesis. The mechanism(s) of such bleeding is obscure. Excess platelets have been shown to interfere with thromboplastin generation. An alternative explanation is intravascular clotting with depletion of plasma factors I, II, V, and VIII. In addition, hemorrhagic infarcts secondary to platelet thrombi may contribute to bleeding from mucosal surfaces.

QUALITATIVE PLATELET DISORDERS

Several hemorrhagic syndromes have been attributed to defective platelet function. Numerous terms have been proposed, and, in general, this category of bleeding disorders is distinguished by confusion often bordering on chaos. A logical classification involves division into the thrombopathies (or thrombocytopathies) and thrombasthenia. The thrombopathies are the result of deficient platelet factor 3 activity; thrombasthenia is characterized by impaired clot retraction. The platelet count is normal in all the qualitative platelet disorders.

Thrombopathies. Patients whose platelets contain deficient amounts of factor 3 are classified under the heading of *deficit thrombopathy*. When the platelets contain normal amounts of factor 3, but release of this phospholipid is impaired or faulty, the designation *functional thrombopathy* is appropriate. Functional thrombopathy is more common than the deficit thrombopathy. Both congenital and acquired thrombopathies have been observed. Congenital deficit thrombopathy is uncommon. Most bleeding disorders caused by a deficiency of platelet factor 3 are secondary to some other primary disease (usually liver disease or uremia). On the other hand, congenital functional thrombopathies are not rare and may, in fact, be one of the commonest of the minor bleeding disorders. Less often, a functional thrombopathy is secondary to a dysproteinemic state or accompanies systemic lupus erythematosus with a circulating anticoagulant. Patients with one of the thrombopathies usually bleed (often profusely) after trauma or a surgical procedure; relatively few complain of spontaneous hemorrhage.

As a rule, the thrombopathies can be recognized only by certain direct and indirect tests of platelet function. The platelet count is normal, and the platelets rarely display morphologic abnormalities. Most of the usual tests of the hemostatic mechanisms are normal, although the bleeding time may be prolonged in some patients and capillary fragility may be increased. The whole blood coagulation time, prothrombin time, and clot retraction are normal. However, the prothrombin consumption test is abnormal, as is the thromboplastin generation test when the patient contributes the platelet fraction of the reaction mixture. A simple modification of the prothrombin consumption test yields information of great diagnostic significance. An abnormal prothrombin consumption test will be corrected by the addition of a platelet substitute such as Inosithin (a phospholipid derived from soybeans) if the abnormality reflects a thrombopathy or thrombocytopenia (thrombocytopenia is readily excluded by a normal platelet count). An abnormal prothrombin consumption test will not be affected by the soybean derivative if the defect reflects a deficiency of one of the plasma coagulation factors. If the thrombopathy is due to faulty release of platelet factor 3 (the commoner type), activity of this factor will be restored to normal after the platelets are disrupted by suspension in distilled water or exposure to ultrasonic oscillation. Transfusions of viable platelets will correct the bleeding tendency in the thrombopathies; all too soon, however, platelet antibodies will develop and negate the therapeutic effect of subsequent transfusions.

Thrombasthenia. This qualitative platelet disorder is characterized by a normal platelet count and normal platelet factor 3 activity; however, clot retraction is abnormal. It is often referred to by the eponym, Glanzmann's thrombasthenia. Platelet spreading and adhesiveness are absent or impaired, and the bleeding time is ordinarily prolonged. In peripheral blood films the platelets are isolated and fail to clump. Platelets often appear morphologically abnormal, especially when examined with the electron microscope. The platelets of some of these patients have a decreased content of adenosine triphosphate (ATP); it has been suggested (but not proved) that this finding may reflect impaired glycolysis consequent to some enzymatic deficiency. Thrombasthenia can be recognized by the finding of impaired clot retraction in the face of a normal platelet count.

Combined Qualitative Platelet Disorders. This category of bleeding syndromes includes those patients who have been observed to have various combinations of thrombopathy and thrombasthenia with and without certain plasma coagulation factor deficiencies. These patients emphasize dramatically the existent voids in our knowledge of platelet disorders. Much remains to be learned. However, it can be predicted with reasonable certainty that the acquisition of new techniques will elucidate many of the intricacies of the qualitative platelet disorders, thereby permitting easier recognition and more effective treatment.

Coagulation Disorders

Each of the plasma coagulation factors (Table 13-1) contributes in an essential manner to the clotting process. Therefore a deficiency of any of these substances will impair coagulation and cause abnormal bleeding. The only exception to this rule appears to be calcium. Although calcium plays a vital role in coagulation, hypocalcemia cannot be implicated in the pathogenesis of a hemorrhagic disorder; to affect coagulation in vivo, profound hypocalcemia is required (levels well below those that produce other serious and life-threatening clinical manifestations). The diagnosis of a coagulation disorder is contingent on the recognition in the laboratory of an abnormality in the coagulation mechanism. Tests that reflect quantitative or qualitative platelet disorders and vascular defects are normal (bleeding time, clot retraction, platelet count, and capillary resistance test). The hemorrhagic diathesis is usually severe and generally involves large vessels in contrast to the bleeding from small vessels so characteristic of the vascular and platelet hemorrhagic diseases. The clinical pictures of the coagulation disorders are often similar, but their laboratory manifestations and treatment differ. They are all rare. Plasma coagulation factor deficiencies may be congenital or acquired.

FACTOR VIII DEFICIENCIES

Hemophilia. Synonyms for this hereditary hemorrhagic disorder include classical hemophilia and hemophilia A. This bleeding disorder was recognized centuries ago. It was first described clearly by Otto in 1803, and Hopff introduced the term hemophilia in 1828. Although its mode of inheritance was recognized early, it was not until 1937 that hemophilia was shown to be the result of a deficiency of a previously undescribed plasma factor needed for blood to clot. Originally, patients with factor IX deficiency were included in this category; with the recognition of this coagulation factor in 1952, it became evident that the clinical manifestations of congenital deficiencies of factor VIII and IX are identical. Hemophilia is the commonest heritable coagulation disorder (about 80 per cent of these bleeding diatheses are due to a hemophilia); however, it is a rare disease. It has been estimated that there are approximately 20,000 persons with hemophilia in the United States (an incidence of about 5 per 100,000 population). Hemophilia is found most often in persons from northern Europe and their descendents.

PATHOGENESIS. Hemophilia is transmitted as a sex-linked recessive mendelian trait. With few exceptions, the disease occurs only in hemizygous males who have acquired the defective gene on the X chromosome obtained from their mothers. In general, a heterozygous female does not bleed (apparently the unaffected X chromosome dominates the abnormal gene and prevents its expression); however, half of her sons and half of her daughters will acquire the mutant gene (the sons manifest abnormal bleeding, whereas the daughters are asymptomatic carriers). The sons of a hemophiliac male are entirely normal (they acquire their X chromosome from their mother), but *all* his daughters possess the hemophilia gene.

Until recently, hemophilia had not been observed in a female, and it was generally assumed that homozygosity was lethal *in utero*. The discovery of hemophilia in dogs dispelled this concept, for it became possible to breed homozygous females; these animals have classical hemophilia indistinguishable from the disease occurring in their male siblings. Thus half of the female offspring of a heterozygous female and a hemizygous male should have a bleeding disorder, and the rest should be carriers. A few authentic examples of hemophilia in human females have now been found. The scarcity of this occurrence undoubtedly reflects the improbability of a chance mating between a hemophiliac male and a carrier female. The development of more sensitive techniques has permitted the demonstration of less than normal factor VIII activity in some asymptomatic carriers; however, the demonstration of hemophilia in one of her male children remains the only sure way to recognize a female carrier. About 30 per cent of patients with hemophilia have a negative family history. These sporadic cases presumably reflect mutations.

The coagulation abnormality of hemophilia is decreased factor VIII activity. It is assumed by most that synthesis of this coagulation factor is governed by a gene on the X chromosome and that hemophilia reflects inadequate formation; however, this theory does not possess unequivocal proof. Some studies point to the existence of an inhibitor, and it has been proposed that such a factor may have pathogenic significance (it should be noted that the end result would be the same, i.e., inadequate factor VIII activity).

Because factor VIII plays an essential role in the first phase of coagulation (Fig. 13-1), a deficiency impairs clotting and causes a hemorrhagic diathesis. The severity of the hemorrhagic manifestations is contingent on the magnitude of the deficiency; the deficiency varies greatly among patients and appears to be a function of the particular gene, for factor VIII activity is similar in all the affected members of a family. Patients with classical hemophilia and a severe bleeding disorder have virtually no detectable factor VIII (less than 1 per cent of normal); in these persons the coagulation abnormality is readily detectable. Patients with levels of factor VIII between 1 to 5 per cent of normal have moderate disease. Relatively insensitive tests such as the whole blood coagulation time and prothrombin consumption test are usually normal in these individuals; the thromboplastin generation test is abnormal. When factor VIII levels are greater than 5 per cent, the disease is mild and requires extremely sensitive techniques for its detection (e.g., direct factor VIII assay). As a rule, spontaneous bleeding does not occur unless factor VIII is less than 10 per cent of normal; however, abnormal bleeding may follow trauma or surgery in persons with higher levels. Recognition of the disease in these persons is a difficult task.

CLINICAL MANIFESTATIONS. Hemophilia is characterized by a lifelong tendency to bleed. In typical cases bleeding is manifested shortly after birth (often at the time of circumcision) or in early childhood. The history is usually one of profound and persistent hemorrhage occurring spontaneously or after a surgical procedure or other trauma. Trauma is likely to be so trivial as to go unnoticed; therefore, unexplained hematomas are common. Since bleeding may affect any organ and occurs from every orifice and into every body cavity, the symptoms are highly variable. The most frequently encountered hemorrhagic manifestations include hemarthroses; hematuria; epistaxis; hematemesis; melena; retroperitoneal, retropharyngeal, and laryngeal hemorrhage; and intracranial bleeding. Petechiae are rare, as is pulmonary hemorrhage. Bleeding into joints is particularly bothersome because it often eventuates in permanent deformity and disability. *Physical findings* depend on the site of bleeding; for obvious reasons, they are diverse.

Laboratory findings consist of (1) evidence of the coagulation defect and (2) manifestations of abnormal bleeding, which are nonspecific and consist of the hematologic abnormalities accompanying an acute hemorrhagic anemia (p. 69) or, if bleeding has been persistent and iron stores have been depleted, those of an iron deficiency anemia (p. 174). Manifestations of the coagulation defect include a prolonged whole blood coagulation time, reduced prothrombin consumption, an abnormal thromboplastin generation test, and a quantitative decrease in factor VIII activity. In almost every patient who is actively bleeding consequent to low levels of factor VIII, the whole blood coagulation time is increased (30 to 60 minutes or longer). It should be emphasized, however, that this relatively insensitive test will not detect the presence of mild hemophilia, and a normal coagulation time in a nonbleeding patient *does not exclude hemophilia*. On the other hand, a normal coagulation time in a person with an overt hemorrhagic diathesis tends to eliminate hemophilia. Other tests are normal [e.g., platelet count, bleeding time, clot retraction, capillary fragility, and prothrombin time; tissue thromboplastin substitutes for plasma thromboplastin in the performance of a one-stage prothrombin time (p. 468)].

The presence of a normal bleeding time in a person with hemophilia deserves comment. When properly performed, a bleeding time assesses vascular integrity and platelet status (quantitative and qualitative); it does not reflect abnormalities of the coagulation mechanism. Vascular and platelet factors ordinarily control bleeding from small wounds, even if the blood is almost incoagulable. However, a word of caution is indicated. Although the actual bleeding time may be normal, hemorrhage may recur at a later time after subsidence of local vasoconstriction. Serious bleeding has been encountered under these circumstances.

DIAGNOSIS. The diagnosis of hemophilia in an actively bleeding patient is based on the exclusion of all other hemorrhagic disorders and on the demonstration of deficient factor VIII activity. A characteristic mode of inheritance often provides valuable information (disease occurring in brothers and maternal male cousins and uncles but not in females or paternal relatives), It should be borne in mind, however, that factor IX deficiency is inherited in an identical fashion.

A prolonged coagulation time (the prothrombin consumption test is also abnormal) and a normal prothrombin time point to an abnormality in the intrinsic thromboplastin system of phase 1 of coagulation (see Fig. 13-1 and Table 13-4). Separation of factor VIII deficiency from inadequacies of IX, XI, and XII requires more sophisticated techniques. The thromboplastin generation test provides valuable information. If the deficient factor is VIII, coagulation will be retarded when the patient's adsorbed plasma is added to normal serum and normal platelets; this combination will be normal if the inadequacy involves factor IX, XI, or XII (these factors are present in normal serum, see Table 13-3). Coagulation in a mixture made up of normal adsorbed plasma, the patient's serum, and normal platelets will be abnormal if the patient has factor IX deficiency and normal in the face of factor VIII, XI, or XII inadequacy (these factors are present in normal adsorbed plasma). If both mixtures are normal but coagulation is retarded when normal platelets are added to the patient's serum and adsorbed plasma, the deficiency involves factor XI or XII. As a rule, these two disorders can be separated on clinical grounds (patients with factor XI deficiency bleed; those with factor XII have few, if any, clinical manifestations).

The diagnosis of mild or moderate hemophilia is much more difficult. However, the recognition of these states is essential, especially in the evaluation of patients for surgery. In this regard the importance of a detailed history cannot be overemphasized. A clear-cut history of a hemorrhagic diathesis carries a great deal of weight, even though laboratory documentation cannot be obtained. To diagnose mild or moderate deficiencies of factor VIII, sensitive techniques are needed. The thromboplastin generation test will detect factor VIII levels that are less than 10 per cent of normal. When the concentration of factor VIII is greater, it must be quantified directly (normal values exhibit a wide range, varying from 50 to 200 per cent of the average). Thus a whole blood coagulation time and a prothrombin consumption test will uncover almost all patients with severe disease. In mild or moderate cases both tests may be normal; in many of these patients, the thromboplastin generation test will establish the diagnosis. However, there remain a few individuals with very mild disease in whom assay of factor VIII is required for a positive diagnosis. The coexistence of factor VIII deficiency and a prolonged bleeding time points to von Willebrand's disease; unlike classical hemophilia, this bleeding disorder occurs equally in both sexes.

TREATMENT AND COURSE. In general, hemophilia is a serious disease with a poor prognosis. Patients with mild disease have minimal difficulty, and some are capable of leading an essentially normal life with little or no shortening of life-span. However, about half the persons with this coagulation disorder die during the first five years of life, and relatively few live beyond the age of 40 years. Because of the trauma to which children are exposed, childhood is a particularly dangerous time. Bleeding is often episodic, but the once widely held concept that the hemorrhagic diathesis improves with advancing age is probably not valid. It seems more likely that most older hemophiliacs have always had mild disease.

Treatment of hemophilia consists of those local measures needed to staunch the flow of blood and to restore clotting to normal. Local measures depend on the site of bleeding and include pressure and hemostatic agents such as thrombin preparations (Russell's viper venom also has powerful thromboplastinlike activity and will coagulate factor VIII deficient blood). Although the application of pressure and coagulants usually helps, effective hemostasis requires the formation of a clot. Factor VIII is needed for this purpose.

Factor VIII should be administered intravenously in the form of fresh whole blood or plasma. Whole blood may be needed in persons with an acute hemorrhagic anemia, but in most cases plasma is preferable. Serum contains no factor VIII. Because this factor is labile on storage, even at 4°C, either fresh plasma or freshly frozen or lyophilized plasma must be used. Factor VIII activity remains unchanged for years in lyophilized plasma; it does deteriorate slowly in frozen plasma (at very low temperatures, e.g., −30°C, there is little deterioration). Factor VIII has been concentrated from human plasma; however, these materials are in short supply. Concentrates of animal origin are available, but immunization to the foreign protein is a formidable problem seriously limiting their use. Recent observations on a cryoprecipitated fraction of plasma indicate that this easily obtainable material is rich in factor VIII and may have considerable therapeutic potentiality.

The goal of replacement therapy is to elevate the blood factor VIII activity and control the abnormal bleeding. Spontaneous bleeding ordinarily ceases when the factor VIII level is about 15 per cent of normal; however, control of traumatic bleeding requires higher levels (hemorrhage is unlikely when factor VIII levels are 20 to 30 per cent of the normal average). As a rule, 20 to 30 ml of plasma/kg of body weight are required as an initial dose to achieve a factor VIII level of 20 to 30 per cent. It is important that the priming dose be large enough to overcome the need for equilibration between the intravascular and extravascular compartments. Once equilibration has been achieved, 3 to 6 ml of plasma/kg of body weight every 6 to 8 hours usually suffice to maintain satisfactory hemostasis. Some patients require more, whereas others are controlled with less. Thus each patient is an individual problem. In addition to the management of bleeding episodes, all patients require plasma before a surgical procedure. When surgery cannot be avoided, the level of factor VIII should be raised to 30 per cent or more before operation and maintained at this level for 10 to 14 days postoperatively. It is always better to give too much rather than too little.

Patients who receive large amounts of blood or plasma run a definite risk of acquiring serum hepatitis (p. 535). In addition, a few persons develop circulating anticoagulants that negate the benefit of subsequent therapy. It is probable that most of these anticoagulants are antibodies. Fortunately, these occurrences are rare.

Other aspects of treatment include the needs of the patient and his family for psychologic support. Although undue exertion or exposure to trauma should be avoided, it is important that the individual with hemophilia not be made an invalid. The physician must be well versed in the scientific aspects of this disorder; however, successful treatment is also predicated on the art of medicine. Since hemophilia is a heritable disorder, genetic counseling is indicated.

von Willebrand's Disease. This hereditary coagulation disorder includes as one of its manifestations decreased factor VIII activity. It is discussed in the section dealing with vascular disorders (p. 486).

FACTOR IX DEFICIENCIES

Congenital. This hereditary coagulation disorder was first recognized in 1952. Synonyms include PTC (plasma thromboplastin component) deficiency, Christmas disease (after the surname of the second patient shown to have a factor IX deficiency), and hemophilia B. It is transmitted by asymptomatic female carriers as a sex-linked recessive; active disease affects hemizygous males. In addition to an identical mode of inheritance, the clinical manifestations of this hemorrhagic disease mimic exactly those of hemophilia A or factor VIII deficiency. Both mild and serious forms have been observed; in general, however, bleeding appears to be milder than in patients with classical hemophilia. Factor IX deficiency can be distinguished from factor VIII deficiency only by the thromboplastin generation test or direct coagulation factor assay. In addition, plasma from a patient with factor IX deficiency will correct the clotting defect in the plasma of a patient with classical hemophilia and vice versa. The relative frequencies of factor IX deficiency and classic hemophilia vary considerably in different parts of the world; classic hemophilia is 2 to 10 times more common than factor IX deficiency. The principles of therapy for these two bleeding disorders are the same. However, factor IX is present in serum and stable on storage; therefore, stored blood or plasma is fully effective.

Acquired. The formation of factor IX depends on the presence of vitamin K and adequate hepatic function. Consequently, production is retarded in recipients of one of the coumarin congeners. These antico-agulants resemble vitamin K and presumably compete successfully with it for an essential enzyme functioning in the synthesis of factors II, VII, IX, and X. Some patients with liver disease also have an acquired deficiency of factor IX.

FACTOR XI DEFICIENCY

This rare coagulation disorder is transmitted as an autosomal domi-nant with variable expressivity. It affects both males and females. As a rule, bleeding is less severe than that of classical hemophilia or factor IX deficiency. The routine laboratory manifestations of factor XI or PTA (plasma thromboplastin antecedent) deficiency are similar to those of hemophilia and Christmas disease. Factor XI is present in both serum and adsorbed plasma; thus factor XI inadequacy can be detected by a thromboplastin generation test (the coagulation abnor-mality is corrected by normal serum as well as normal plasma). Treat-ment is similar to that outlined for factor VIII or IX deficiencies; stored plasma or serum is effective, although some data suggest that factor XI is not so stable on storage as factor IX.

FACTOR XII DEFICIENCY

A deficiency of factor XII (Hageman trait) is responsible for the unique combination of a prolonged whole blood coagulation time in glass tubes without significant clinical abnormalities. The affected per-son generally does not bleed even after surgery or trauma. Prothrombin consumption is markedly decreased, and the thromboplastin generation test is abnormal (the latter is corrected by normal serum as well as normal adsorbed plasma; see Table 13-3). The laboratory manifestations of factor XI and factor XII deficiencies are similar; however, these dis-orders can be separated on clinical grounds. Patients with factor XI deficiency bleed spontaneously or as a result of trauma; those with fac-tor XII deficiency ordinarily do not. Factor XII deficiency is rare and appears to reflect homozygosity for an autosomal recessive gene. The explanation for the absence of hemorrhagic manifestations in persons with factor XII deficiency is obscure.

FACTOR VII DEFICIENCIES

Congenital. Less than 100 cases of this hereditary coagulation dis-order have been reported. A hemorrhagic diathesis is usually mani-fested in the first or second decade of life. When factor VII activity is less than 10 per cent of normal, serious bleeding ensues. Overt bleeding affects both sexes and appears to reflect homozygosity for an autosomal recessive character (heterozygotes have decreased factor VII activity without abnormal bleeding). Factor VII participates in the activation of tissue thromboplastin (Fig. 13-1); therefore a deficiency causes prolongation of the one-stage prothrombin time. Tests of the intrinsic thromboplastin system (clotting time, prothrombin consumption, and thromboplastin generation) are ordinarily normal. The differing modes of action and properties of factors VII, II, V, and X permit separation of disorders due to their deficiency (see Fig. 13-1 and Table 13-3). Treatment consists of the administration of factor VII in the form of whole blood, plasma (stored plasma is effective), serum, or a plasma concentrate. Vitamin K is without effect in the congenital disease.

Acquired. The synthesis of factor VII requires vitamin K and a functioning liver. Consequently, levels of this coagulation factor are depressed by anticoagulants of the coumarin or indanedione types as well as by liver disease and vitamin K deficiency. Vitamin K deficiency accompanies biliary obstruction (bile is needed for vitamin K absorption) and certain gastrointestinal disorders characterized by impaired absorption (e.g., the sprue syndromes). With the exception of hepatic disease, each of these disorders responds to parenteral vitamin K by an increase in factor VII activity. Factor VII levels are low in newborn infants and, with a deficiency of factor II, contribute to the production of hemorrhagic disease of the newborn (see later).

FACTOR X DEFICIENCIES

Congenital. Factor X participates in both the intrinsic and extrinsic thromboplastin systems (Fig. 13-1); therefore a deficiency of this factor is reflected by a prolonged prothrombin time as well as by an abnormal thromboplastin generation test. Because the one-stage prothrombin time of serum is long when factor X is in short supply (factor X participates in the activation of exogenous tissue thromboplastin), prothrombin consumption appears to be normal. This rare disorder is probably transmitted as an autosomal recessive trait; it affects both sexes. The heterozygous state is not accompanied by abnormal bleeding, and the homozygote ordinarily has mild hemorrhagic manifestations. Factor X deficiency is most likely to resemble factor V deficiency; however, the different properties of these factors (Table 13-3) permit a positive diagnosis.

Acquired. An acquired deficiency of factor X is found in the same conditions as those causing an acquired deficiency of factor VII.

FACTOR V DEFICIENCIES

Congenital. This coagulation disorder was originally designated parahemophilia. It is extremely rare; little is known about its mode of inheritance, but it is probably an autosomal recessive trait. Tests of both the intrinsic and extrinsic systems are abnormal. Factor V deficiency can be distinguished from factor X deficiency because of the different properties of these factors (factor V is labile and is used in clotting; factor X is stable and is present in serum). Therapy consists of blood or plasma. Vitamin K is not required for the synthesis of factor V and exerts no therapeutic effect.

Acquired. Factor V activity has been found to be decreased in a variety of disorders associated with intravascular clotting (p. 516) or fibrinolysis (p. 473). It may also be decreased in patients with acute leukemia or liver disease and is regularly depressed in the presence of acute inflammatory disease, especially scarlet fever.

FACTOR II DEFICIENCIES

Congenital. Congenital factor II deficiency or hypoprothrombinemia is extremely rare. Bleeding is generally severe. The prothrombin time is prolonged; however, the coagulation time is ordinarily normal (p. 476). The properties of factor II (Table 13-3) differ from those of factors V, X, and VII (other plasma factors, the deficiencies of which cause an abnormal prothrombin time) and can be used to make the diagnosis. Vitamin K is without therapeutic effect, but, provided liver dysfunction can be excluded, the response to parenteral vitamin K may be diagnostically significant; that is, lack of response points to a congenital deficiency.

Acquired. The formation of prothrombin requires vitamin K and a functioning liver. Vitamin K deficiency generally reflects impaired absorption or defective utilization. It is rarely the result of nutritional inadequacy unless the limited intake of food is coupled with large doses of oral antibiotics. Most foods contain significant amounts of this vitamin; furthermore, large quantities are normally synthesized by bacteria in the gastrointestinal tract and are readily absorbed as long as bile is available. An acquired hypoprothrombinemia usually accompanies liver dysfunction, obstructive jaundice, or gastrointestinal disorders affecting absorption; it is also caused by anticoagulants of the coumarin or indanedione types. These hypoprothrombinemic states respond to vitamin K given parenterally, provided liver function is adequate. Acquired hypoprothrombinemia is associated with deficiencies of the other coagulation factors that require vitamin K and a functioning liver (i.e., factors VII, X, and IX) for their synthesis.

Hemorrhagic disease of the newborn deserves special mention. This self-limited, but sometimes fatal, bleeding disorder is caused by deficiencies of those coagulation factors whose synthesis is contingent on the availability of vitamin K (factors II, VII, IX, and X). Levels of these factors are subnormal at birth and fall even lower during the first few days of life. Hemorrhage is severer in premature infants. The prophylactic administration of vitamin K to all infants has virtually eliminated hemorrhagic disorder of the newborn. However, a word of caution is indicated. Because vitamin K is an oxidation-reduction mediator, it is capable of evoking oxidative hemolysis (p. 115). Massive doses may cause hemolysis in normal recipients; smaller doses may exert a deleterious effect when coupled with such factors as prematurity, hypoglycemia, functional immaturity of the liver, or hereditary glucose-6-phosphate dehydrogenase deficiency (p. 112). If hemolysis in a newborn is severe and hyperbilirubinemia is sufficiently marked, it may lead to kernicterus and death (p. 127). Small doses of vitamin K are ample to treat and prevent hemorrhagic disease of the newborn. There is never any justification to exceed a dose of 5 mg; as prophylaxis, 1 mg is quite adequate. Because serious reactions have followed intravenous vitamin K, it should not be given by this route.

FACTOR I DEFICIENCIES

Because fibrinogen is the immediate precursor of a fibrin clot, a deficiency of this substance seriously impairs the coagulation process. Fibrinogen levels can be quantified with ease (normally, the concentration of fibrinogen is about 250 to 400 mg/100 ml of plasma). Hypofibrinogenemia is reflected by a prolonged whole blood coagulation time; when the concentration of fibrinogen falls below 50 mg/100 ml of plasma, the one-stage prothrombin time is also lengthened. If the prothrombin time is normal, the usual tests may suggest an abnormality in the generation of plasma thromboplastin. However, the addition of a small amount of tissue thromboplastin used in the performance of a one-stage prothrombin time quickly resolves the problem (the blood will clot if the deficiency involves the intrinsic thromboplastin system but will remain fluid in the presence of hypofibrinogenemia).

Congenital. Fewer than 50 patients have been reported with congenital hypo- or afibrinogenemia. It affects both sexes, is generally present at birth, and is characterized by significant hemorrhagic manifestations, although bleeding appears to be less severe than in most hemophiliacs. This coagulation disorder is probably inherited as an autosomal recessive character. As already noted, severe fibrinogen deficiency is distinguished by the absence of clotting in all the tests employing the formation of a fibrin clot as the end point. Treatment consists of the administration of fibrinogen in the form of whole blood, plasma, or fibrinogen concentrates. Fibrinogen levels must be raised to about 60 mg/100 ml of plasma to achieve effective hemostasis. Some patients appear to have developed antibodies to the infused fibrinogen.

Acquired. Acquired hypofibrinogenemia may be secondary to liver disease, the intravascular coagulation syndrome, or an active fibrinolytic mechanism. Bleeding is usually acute and quite severe. Fibrinolysis and the intravascular coagulation syndrome are also associated with the depletion of other coagulant substances.

INTRAVASCULAR COAGULATION SYNDROME AND FIBRINOLYSIS

Intravascular coagulation is often referred to as the defibrination syndrome; however, this term fails to emphasize the depletion of other factors concerned with hemostasis. Factors II, V, VIII, and platelets are also consumed during clotting and are depleted by intravascular coagulation. Thus this hemorrhagic disorder is characterized by numerous laboratory abnormalities. However, a fibrinogen deficiency generally dominates the picture. This syndrome accompanies a variety of disorders, particularly certain obstetric complications such as abruptio placentae, retention of a dead fetus, and amniotic fluid embolism. Presumably intravascular coagulation is caused by the liberation of large quantities of thromboplastic materials into the circulation.

Most cases of intravascular coagulation are complicated by or associated with active fibrinolysis. It is noteworthy, however, that fibrinolysis can occur without preceding intravascular coagulation. A fibrinolytic mechanism may be activated in response to (1) severe stress or trauma (e.g., extensive burns or surgery, especially operations on the lungs, uterus, pancreas, or breasts), (2) obstetric emergencies such as those described, (3) the presence of certain malignant disorders, most notably carcinoma of the prostate, and (4) a variety of other disorders including leukemia, polycythemia vera, liver disease, and hemolytic transfusion reactions. Because an active fibrinolytic mechanism eventually depletes supplies of fibrinogen as well as platelets and factors II, V, and VIII, it may be difficult to distinguish fibrinolysis from certain other hemorrhagic disorders, especially the intravascular coagulation syndrome. As a rule, clot dissolution can be observed, particularly if the patient is actively bleeding because of fibrinolysis. However, lysis may occur so promptly that evidence of clotting may not be seen. Differentiation between fibrinolysis and intravascular coagulation requires astute clinical judgment. Treatment differs considerably. Heparin should be given if the problem is one of intravascular coagulation; epsilon-aminocaproic acid (p. 473) may be indicated if the bleeding is caused by fibrinolysis. Since the latter agent may aggravate intravascular coagulation, there is little room for diagnostic equivocation.

CIRCULATING ANTICOAGULANTS

Anticoagulants occasionally appear in the circulation in sufficient amounts to cause a hemorrhagic diathesis. These substances, which may interfere with any phase of coagulation, have been observed most often in association with a collagen disease such as systemic lupus erythematosus and in patients with macroglobulinemia. However, they have also been known to follow parturition and multiple transfusions and have been demonstrated in a variety of other situations (e.g., hemophilia, acute leukemia, chronic nephritis, and liver disease) as well as in otherwise normal persons.

In general, the laboratory manifestations of a bleeding disorder consequent to a circulating anticoagulant(s) are variable and hard to explain on the basis of any other known hemorrhagic disorder. The ability of the patient's plasma to interfere with the coagulation process in normal blood establishes the presence of an anticoagulant. Treatment is difficult and largely ineffective. Very rarely, bleeding is due to a heparinlike anticoagulant; protamine sulfate or toluidine blue may then be of value.

DYSPROTEINEMIAS

Bleeding may accompany any of the disorders characterized by protein abnormalities; for example, plasmacytic myeloma (p. 411) and primary macroglobulinemia (p. 442). The pathogenesis of the hemorrhagic diathesis is variable. In some cases platelet function is impaired, particularly the release of factor 3, when they become coated with the abnormal protein. In other patients the abnormal globulins appear to react with and inactivate certain of the coagulation factors and may interfere with the conversion of fibrinogen to fibrin. Purpura is particularly common in patients with cryoglobulinemia (p. 415).

Blood Groups and Transfusions

Transfusion of blood from one human being into another is a rational form of replacement therapy of proved clinical value. Most of the problems that plagued early transfusion attempts have been solved, and blood is now widely available in abundant amounts.

HISTORY

References to the feasibility and desirability of blood transfusions appear in the writings of the ancient Greek and Egyptian civilizations. The first recorded attempt to use blood therapeutically involved Pope Innocent VIII in 1492; it seems likely, however, that in this instance blood was given orally and not injected. Following the announcement in 1616 of Harvey's discovery of the circulation of the blood, several important events set the stage for the first transfusion. In 1656 Sir Christopher Wren, the famous English architect, gave beer and wine intravenously to dogs and made them "extremely drunk," thus proving that materials given by this route were carried to all parts of the body. Influenced by Wren's experiments, Lower, also an Englishman, successfully transfused blood from one dog into another in 1665. Two years later, Denys, a Frenchman, gave the first transfusion (lamb's blood) to a human recipient. His fourth attempt at transfusion (this time with the blood of a calf and unfortunately the second such transfusion the patient had received) was followed by a fatal hemolytic reaction. Denys was subsequently tried for manslaughter. Although he was exonerated, transfusions were banned in Paris, London, and Rome, and no progress was recorded for 150 years. Interest in transfusion therapy was revived in 1818 after Blundell, an English obstetrician, successfully carried out the first man-to-man transfusion. The use of blood transfusions increased, but frequent serious and often fatal reactions prevented widespread adoption of this form of therapy. In two articles published in 1900 and 1901, Landsteiner reported his epochal discovery of the ABO blood group system. For some strange reason this vital information, on which safe transfusion therapy is based, was not used clinically until 1911. The other major blood grouping (the Rh system) was discovered by Landsteiner and Wiener in 1940. Citrate was shown to be an effective nontoxic anticoagulant in 1914. Several advances, such as the addition of dextrose to the anticoagulant solution, followed thus prolonging significantly in vitro cell survival. The first blood bank was established in Chicago by Fantus in 1937. The use of blood transfusions increased dramatically during World War II, after which modern blood banks became commonplace.

Blood Groups

RED CELL ANTIGENS AND ANTIBODIES

Erythrocytes contain a variety of genetically determined antigens (blood group factors) which give them their serologic identity or type and permit them to be agglutinated by specific antisera. These antigens, which are also demonstrable on nucleated red cells, are complex mucopolysaccharides. They appear early in fetal life and persist unchanged with only rare exceptions (a few patients with leukemia have lost their A blood group factor and some with lower intestinal disease—usually carcinoma—have been known to acquire a B-like antigen). Although the normal function of the erythrocyte antigens is unknown, they provide a biologic label that is important in certain genetic, anthropologic, and medicolegal work. Thirteen well-defined blood group systems have been described (Table 14-1) plus a number of "public" (present in virtually all individuals) and "private" (present in only rare families) groupings. A single system may involve one or several antigens or blood group factors. An infinite number of combinations is possible, and it seems likely that a person's precise blood type is as individually specific as are his fingerprints. The clinical significance of the red cell blood group factors revolves around their antigenic properties and their ability to react with the antibodies so produced. There are two types of erythrocyte antibody or isoagglutinin, spontaneous or *naturally occurring* and acquired or *immune.*

Naturally occurring antibodies are present without prior exposure

Table 14-1. *Major Blood Group Systems*

	Date of Discovery
ABO	1900–1902
MNSs	1927
P	1927
Rh	1940
Lutheran	1945
Kell	1946
Lewis	1946
Duffy	1950
Kidd	1951
Diego	1955
Sutter	1958
Auberger	1961
Xg	1962

to a specific antigen. Most of these antibodies are macroglobulins, with molecular weights of about 1,000,000 and sedimentation constants of 19S; they do not pass the placental barrier, or they do so to a very limited extent. These antibodies are most active in the cold, at 4 or 20°C; however, some are also active at 37°C, most notably anti-A and anti-B. With the aid of complement, naturally occurring red cell antibodies bring about rapid intravascular lysis of erythrocytes in vivo. Most naturally occurring antibodies are complete (polyvalent) and saline agglutinating; that is, they attach to more than one cell at a time and bring about visible clumping in saline.

Immune erythrocyte antibodies are produced in response to an appropriate antigenic stimulus such as exposure to "foreign" red cells consequent to transfusions or pregnancies (variable numbers of fetal red cells enter the maternal circulation in all pregnancies). For the most part, immune antibodies are 7S gamma globulins with molecular weights of about 160,000. They pass the placental barrier freely and are reactive at 37°C. Immune antibodies are typically incomplete or univalent. Because they attach to only one cell at a time, visible agglutination does not occur in a saline medium; however, such cells will conglutinate or stick together when suspended in a medium of high molecular weight such as serum, plasma, or 20 to 30 per cent bovine albumin. Cells coated with an incomplete antibody will also conglutinate in Coombs' reagent (antihuman globulin rabbit sera) and will therefore give a positive direct Coombs' test. Because an incomplete antibody prevents red cells from being agglutinated by a complete antibody, the term blocking antibodies has been used to describe these immunoglobulins. In contrast to the prompt intravascular lysis brought about by complete or naturally occurring red cell antibodies, incomplete or immune antibodies render the erythrocytes susceptible to sequestration and destruction by reticuloendothelial cells, especially in the spleen and liver. Red cell antibodies serve no known useful purpose and cause no harm unless they come in contact with cells possessing appropriate antigens.

ABO System. This blood group system divides all persons into four types based on the presence or absence of the erythrocyte antigens A and B (Table 14-2). These blood group factors are inherited as mendelian dominants and are under the control of allelic genes. Conversion of the cell's basic mucoid to H substance is controlled by a gene termed X; the allele x is an amorph without effect. Rare individuals whose genotypes are xx have no ABO type (the so-called "Bombay" blood); all others have their H substances affected by genes A, B, and O. The A and B genes are responsible for the conversion of most (but not all) of the cell's H substance to A or B antigens; the O gene is an amorph, and cells from such individuals possess the greatest amount of H substance. There are four phenotypes and six genotypes (Table 14-2). A antigens can be subdivided into A_1 and A_2; about 80 per cent of the persons with blood types A or AB fall into A_1 or A_1B groups, and 20 per cent into A_2 or A_2B groups (the A_2 antigen reacts less strongly with anti-A sera than the A_1 blood group factor). Antigens similar to the red cell blood group factors are present in all tissue cells. About 80 per cent of the individuals are known as "secretors" and have H substances in their saliva, gastric and pancreatic secretions, semen, and so forth. In addition, those secretors with A and/or B erythrocyte antigens will also have variable amounts of water-soluble A and/or B antigens in their secretions.

The most important feature of the ABO blood group system is the presence of naturally occurring, reciprocal isoagglutinins (Table 14-2); the basis for their production is obscure. Anti-H (anti-O) antibodies are demonstrable in individuals with "Bombay" blood but have been observed in only a few A_1, A_1B, and B subjects; these antibodies are usually active only in the cold and are rarely responsible for disease. In the presence of complement, naturally occurring anti-A and anti-B antibodies are hemolytic. These antibodies, which react both at low temperatures and at 37°C, are responsible for most hemolytic transfusion reactions. They are saline agglutinating antibodies and do not freely cross the placental barrier. Immune anti-A and anti-B antibodies occur as the result of prior transfusions, pregnancies, or even nonspecific stimuli, such as the administration of bacterial antitoxins or horse serum. These immune antibodies may cause subsequent transfusion reactions; because they readily cross the placental barrier, they are also capable of producing hemolytic disease of the newborn even in primiparae. Although ABO incompatibility causes about two thirds of the cases of erythroblastosis fetalis, ABO hemolytic disease is usually

Table 14-2. ABO Blood Group System

PHENOTYPE (BLOOD TYPE)	GENOTYPE		ERYTHROCYTE ANTIGENS	NATURALLY OCCURRING ERYTHROCYTE ANTIBODIES	APPROXIMATE FREQUENCY (UNITED STATES-CAUCASIAN)
A	AA;	AO	A	Anti-B	40%
B	BB;	BO	B	Anti-A	10%
AB	AB		A and B	Neither anti-A nor anti-B	5%
O	OO		Neither A nor B (H substance)	Anti-A and Anti-B	45%

mild and few infants require treatment. It has been suggested that ABO incompatibility may be a cause of infertility (i.e., incompatibility between sperm and cervical secretions). Attempts to relate ABO blood type and a variety of other diseases have failed to provide unequivocal evidence of such associations.

Rh System. This complex blood group system involves six erythrocyte antigens or blood group factors and ranks second only to the ABO system in clinical significance. Since the original observations on this system involved the agglutination of human erythrocytes by serum from rabbits that had been previously injected with red cells from rhesus monkeys, the terms Rh positive and Rh negative were introduced. It soon became evident that several antigens belonged to this blood group system, and three pairs of alternate blood group factors with varying degrees of antigenicity are now recognized. Much confusion has existed insofar as nomenclature is concerned (Table 14-3); the terminology of

Table 14-3. *The Rh Blood Group Factors*

BRITISH TERMINOLOGY	WIENER TERMINOLOGY
C	rh'
D	Rh_0
E	rh''
c	hr'
d	Hr_0
e	hr''

Fisher and Race (British) has won the widest acceptance because of its simplicity.

About 85 per cent of all persons possess $D(Rh_0)$, which is the most clinically important Rh blood group factor. These individuals are usually classified as "Rh positive," whereas the remaining 15 per cent without this antigen are said to be "Rh negative." However, $D(Rh_0)$ positive or negative are more appropriate terms. Several weak variants of $D(Rh_0)$ have been recognized and are designated D^u antigens; inasmuch as cells possessing these antigens do not react with the usual anti-$D(Rh_0)$ testing sera, they may be erroneously typed as $D(Rh_0)$ negative. The Rh blood group factors are inherited as mendelian autosomal dominants, although the precise genetics of this blood group system have not been worked out. Available data indicate that their production is controlled by a single pair of genes. A multiplicity of phenotypes and genotypes is possible.

For practical purposes, all antibodies against the Rh blood group factors result from immunization; only rare examples of naturally occurring Rh antibodies have been described. Immune antibodies are produced in response to incompatible transfusions or pregnancies (fetal cells entering the maternal circulation by placental hemorrhage). $D(Rh_0)$

is the strongest antigen; a single transfusion of $D(Rh_o)$ positive blood will evoke the formation of anti-$D(Rh_o)$ in at least 50 per cent of the $D(Rh_o)$ negative recipients. $D(Rh_o)$ is followed, in descending order of antigenic potency, by $c(hr')$, $E(rh'')$, C (rh'), $e(hr'')$, and $d(Hr_o)$. Antibodies have been demonstrated against all the Rh blood group factors with the exception of $d(Hr_o)$. Most Rh antibodies are of the incomplete type. They are capable of causing hemolytic transfusion reactions and hemolytic disease of the newborn in individuals sensitized by prior transfusions or pregnancies. Most instances of severe erythroblastosis fetalis are caused by Rh antibodies (p. 123). Although only one third of the cases of hemolytic disease of the newborn result from Rh incompatibility, most of these infants require therapy.

Other Blood Group Systems. The other blood group systems (Table 14-1) are of little clinical importance. Their significance is basically dependent on the relative frequency of the antigens as well as their antigenic potency. Naturally occurring antibodies are quite rare and, when present, usually react only at low temperatures. With the exception of the A, B, and $D(Rh_o)$ antigens, most erythrocyte blood group factors are weakly antigenic or, if strongly antigenic, occur with very low frequency. Therefore the chances of immunization are slight, and blood groups other than the ABO and Rh systems need be considered only when transfusion reactions or erythroblastosis fetalis cannot be explained on the basis of ABO or Rh incompatibility. It should be noted, however, that most of the other blood group systems have, in a few cases, been implicated in the pathogenesis of transfusion reactions and erythroblastosis fetalis. These other blood groups do serve as important biologic labels in certain genetic and medicolegal studies (e.g., determination of parentage). The gene controlling the Xg blood group system is carried on the sex chromosome. All other blood group factors appear to be inherited as autosomal mendelian dominants; no clear-cut recessive character has yet been described.

LEUKOCYTE AND PLATELET ANTIGENS AND ANTIBODIES

Leukocytes and platelets also possess a complicated system of antigens. Leukocytes appear to have the same ABO, MN, P, and possibly $D(Rh_o)$ antigens as red cells plus many more. Platelets have ABO antigens in addition to several other poorly elucidated factors. Technical problems have prevented precise identification of all leukocyte and platelet antigens, which are obviously complex. Leukocyte and platelet antibodies are demonstrable in many multiparous women and in recipients of multiple transfusions. These antibodies can be implicated in the pathogenesis of certain transfusion reactions (p. 531) as well as in some instances of neonatal neutropenia (p. 329) and thrombocytopenia (p. 489).

Transfusions

It is difficult for the modern physician to envisage the practice of medicine without ready access to abundant amounts of fresh blood. Approximately 10,000,000 transfusions are given each year in the United States alone. The widespread availability of blood has saved many lives and permitted numerous dramatic accomplishments such as open heart surgery. However, the ease with which blood can now be obtained has also created problems; all too often blood is given without clear-cut indications or due consideration of the risks involved. A transfusion is not always an innocuous procedure. Consequently, all who utilize this form of replacement therapy must be fully aware of its hazards and benefits, as well as the indications for its use.

INDICATIONS

One cannot set forth guidelines for transfusion therapy applicable to all cases, but certain principles deserve emphasis. A transfusion is indicated only when anticipated benefits clearly exceed the associated risks. Blood is not a tonic or stimulant; it will not promote wound healing or suppress an infection, and its oxygen-carrying capacity is rarely, if ever, a limiting factor in surgery. A transfusion serves only to augment total blood volume, to enhance the oxygen-carrying capacity of the blood, and as a source of normal plasma constituents such as coagulation factors. The effect on blood volume is immediate, but readjustment to pretreatment levels occurs rapidly in normovolemic recipients. The effect on the erythroid values is longer lasting. Unless damaged by storage or attacked by specific antibodies, some transfused red cells will survive in the recipient for as long as 100 to 120 days. After storage for three weeks, only 70 per cent of the erythrocytes are viable; however, 90 per cent or more will survive storage for periods up to 14 days. In a normal-sized adult one unit (500 ml) of whole blood will, in general, increase the circulating hemoglobin 1.5 gm/100 ml, the venous hematocrit 4 per cent, and the erythrocyte count 400,-000/cu mm. Stored, bank blood does not contain significant numbers of leukocytes or platelets that will survive in the recipient. With special equipment and precautions, platelets can be procured in large numbers and transfused; however, the development of platelet antibodies in the recipient has prevented platelet transfusions from becoming uniformly effective, routine procedures. A number of problems remain to be solved before the feasibility and practicality of leukocyte transfusions can be ascertained.

The three basic indications for a blood transfusion are (1) to increase blood volume when hypovolemia threatens the integrity of the circulatory system, (2) to increase the oxygen-carrying capacity of the blood to prevent serious tissue hypoxia, and (3) to supply deficient plasma factors in patients with certain coagulation abnormalities. Efficient physiologic compensatory mechanisms serve to maintain an adequate cardiac output and oxygen supply to vital organs in the face of a reduction in blood volume or circulating hemoglobin. Therefore blood transfusions are needed in patients with acute hemorrhagic anemia only when shock is present or imminent. Shock resulting from causes other than acute hemorrhage is better treated with plasma or other volume expanders. The concept of "chronic shock" in a debilitated person is a myth; it does not exist.

An anemia is not in itself an indication for a blood transfusion. Each patient presents his own problem; however, several rules apply.

1. Asymptomatic patients should never be transfused solely to restore normal erythroid values. A hemoglobin of 9 to 10 gm/100 ml of blood will not cause significant symptoms or altered organ function; with the exception of patients who are actively bleeding, there is no need to fear serious untoward effects until the hemoglobin falls below 7.0 to 7.5 gm/100 ml.

2. Patients with an anemia for which there is specific therapy (e.g., pernicious or iron deficiency anemia) should never be transfused unless their erythroid values are extremely low and the delay needed to augment the oxygen-carrying capacity of the blood by increased erythropoiesis would endanger their lives.

3. Few valid indications exist for a single transfusion; if one transfusion will suffice, the chances are excellent that the patient could have done just as well without it. However, a single transfusion is occasionally justified to restore circulatory stability in a patient who has bled acutely but in whom there is little likelihood that hemorrhage will recur.

4. Each patient's needs must be considered carefully before the decision to transfuse is reached. If the patient is bedridden for other reasons, a lower hemoglobin level than would be tolerated by a more active person may be quite satisfactory.

The role of blood and plasma transfusions in the management of patients with coagulation defects is considered elsewhere (p. 510). Other unique uses for blood include exchange transfusions, which play such an important part in the treatment of infants with erythroblastosis fetalis (p. 130). Whole blood is also a requisite for the establishment of extracorporeal circulation for open heart surgery and dialysis with an artificial kidney.

TECHNIQUE

Technical details concerned with donor selection and with the procurement, storage, and processing of whole blood and its fractions are beyond the scope of this book. Modern blood bank techniques have contributed importantly to the safety of transfusion therapy. The following points deserve emphasis.

Sterility. Blood must be obtained in sterile containers (preferably single-use, disposable equipment) under aseptic conditions. It should be refrigerated promptly and not removed until just before its use. Once opened or entered for any reason, blood should be used as soon as possible and always within three hours.

Anticoagulation. ACD (acid-citrate-dextrose) solution is the anticoagulant of choice (125 ml/500 ml of blood). National Institutes of Health Formula B is most widely used; it consists of trisodium citrate, 1.32 gm, citric acid, 0.48 gm, dextrose, 1.47 gm, and distilled water to make 100 ml. The presence of dextrose prolongs cell survival. Citrate intoxication is not a problem, unless hepatic or renal clearance of citrate is impaired or the blood is given extremely fast. Heparin is an effective anticoagulant if the blood is to be used at once; however, heparinized blood deteriorates rapidly and cannot be stored. Chelating agents such as EDTA [ethylene diamine tetra-acetic acid (Versene or Sequestrene)] are effective but not clearly superior to ACD solution.

Storage. Aged blood possesses several disadvantages, and most blood banks consider blood stored for more than 21 days unsuitable for use. After storage for three weeks, 30 per cent of the erythrocytes fail to survive in the recipient. Furthermore, potassium leaves the cells and enters the plasma, in which it may reach levels that are toxic in patients with renal insufficiency or marked oliguria. In addition, certain coagulation factors are labile and deteriorate with storage. The chance of gross bacterial contamination is also greater in aged blood (bacteria that multiply at refrigerator temperatures grow slowly and rarely reach concentrations capable of producing disease in less than 14 days).

Typing and Cross Matching. The ABO type of donor and recipient must be ascertained with care on the basis of both cell antigens and serum antibodies. Confirmation of ABO blood type by serum antibody determinations aids in the detection of subjects with weak variants of these blood group factors. The only exceptions are infants under the age of four to six months, in whom circulating antibodies are largely derived from the mother (endogenous production of anti-A and anti-B antibodies does not appear until several months after birth). Potent anti-A testing sera known to react with both A_1 and A_2 cells should be used. Donors and recipients must also be grouped within the Rh system, but testing with anti-D(Rh_o) sera will suffice. All D(Rh_o) negative donors must be further tested for the presence of D^u antigens by using the indirect antiglobulin (Coombs') test and sera known to detect these D(Rh_o) variants. D^u positive blood should be given only to D(Rh_o) positive recipients. There is no need to test the recipient for D^u antigens. To be classified as Rh negative blood, some transfusion centers recommend that donor cells also be negative for C(rh′) and E(rh″) antigens; however, it is difficult to justify this additional testing procedure because C(rh′) is a weak antigen and E(rh″) occurs in less than 0.5 per cent of D(Rh$_o$) negative individuals. Ordinarily, other blood group factors are not specifically tested for because of their low antigenicity and the absence of naturally occurring reciprocal isoantibodies (p. 524).

Donor blood of the same ABO and Rh type as the recipient must also pass certain in vitro compatibility tests before transfusion. The major cross match involves the behavior of donor cells in recipient serum; the minor cross match, recipient cells and donor serum. The minor cross match is less important than the major because of prompt dilution of donor antibodies in the recipient. On the other hand, potent antibodies in the recipient readily cause destruction of donor cells and a hemolytic reaction ensues. In addition to these procedures, donor cells and recipient serum should be matched in a high-protein medium, and a Coombs' indirect antiglobulin test should be done to exclude the presence of incomplete antibodies in the recipient. It is also desirable to test the recipient's own cells and serum to exclude false positives consequent to autoagglutination or increased rouleaux. If all matching tests indicate compatibility, it can be safely assumed that the cells will survive in the recipient.

In general, blood of the same ABO and Rh type as the recipient should always be administered. Because of dilution of donor antibody in the recipient, subjects with group O blood whose cells contain neither A nor B antigens are often referred to as "universal donors." Persons with type AB are called "universal recipients," for they lack naturally occurring anti-A and anti-B antibodies. In some group O bloods, however, very high titers of isoagglutinins may cause a hemolytic reaction by destroying recipient cells. In urgent situations in which it is necessary to give blood with a different ABO type than that of the recipient, the titer of donor antibodies should be determined and, if greater than 1:100, water-soluble group A or B specific substances should be added. Although these materials will adsorb and effectively lower the titer of naturally occurring (but not immune) anti-A or anti-B antibodies, they are potentially antigenic and may incite antibody formation in the recipient. D(Rh$_o$) negative persons should not be given D(Rh$_o$) positive blood because of the very real danger of sensitization. This rule must never be violated in girls or in women of childbearing age; in males and elderly females, it may be permissible in certain emergency situations. There is no reason to fear the administration of D(Rh$_o$) negative blood to a D(Rh$_o$) positive recipient because of the very low antigenicity of d(Hr$_o$).

Administration.   Before starting a transfusion, it must be established with certainty that the blood is intended for that particular patient and that suitable in vitro compatibility tests have been performed. Single-use, disposal equipment is preferred, and a filter will eliminate the possibility of injecting unwanted particulate matter. A blood transfusion is preferably given intravenously. There is little, if any, justification for infusion into an artery. Under certain circumstances, blood may be given intraperitoneally (a technique sometimes used in children) or directly into the bone marrow cavity (e.g., intrasternally). With the exception of patients who are actively bleeding, blood should be infused simply by gravity. The first 50 to 100 ml should be given slowly over a period of 15 to 30 minutes. If no untoward reaction occurs, the rate of flow may be increased to 10 to 20 ml/minute. In most cases one unit of blood should be infused over a period of about 90 minutes; slower rates serve no useful purpose, unless there is a real danger of circulatory overload. It is safer to give chronically anemic patients no more than one transfusion per day. In acutely bleeding patients it may be necessary to give the first one or two units of blood at rates approximating 100 ml/minute. Under these circumstances it is necessary to supplement gravity in order to obtain a faster flow. Care is then needed to prevent the injection of air; a manual pump inserted in the line below the filter chamber will eliminate such a risk. The bleeding patient should be given whole blood. Packed red cells (a concentrated suspension of erythrocytes prepared by removing most of the plasma and anticoagulant solution) will lessen the likelihood of circulatory overload in chronically anemic patients; the packed cell volume or hematocrit of such preparations should be about 70 per cent.

Patients receiving blood must be observed closely for possible reactions. Their temperatures should be recorded before the transfusion is begun and at 15-minute intervals until completed; the temperature should then be recorded every 30 minutes for the next four hours. If the patient becomes febrile while the transfusion is in progress, the blood should be stopped at once and the cause of the fever sought. If a hemolytic reaction or gross bacterial contamination can be excluded, or if the fever can be shown to be unrelated to the blood, the transfusion may be restarted. If doubt remains, it is better to discard the remaining blood and transfuse with another unit than run the risk of a potentially serious reaction. In the event of a transfusion reaction, the blood remaining in the bottle should be saved, for it will permit repeat typing and compatibility tests. After a suspected reaction it is important also to save all urine so that it can be examined for the presence of hemoglobin.

COMPLICATIONS

About 5 per cent of the recipients of a blood transfusion exhibit some type of untoward effect. Many transfusion reactions can be prevented or at least minimized by appropriate attention to technical details. Others are still unavoidable, but their incidence can be reduced sharply by strict adherence to criteria governing the use of transfusions. When properly indicated, the benefits of transfusions far outweigh the risk of undesirable side effects. However, it has been estimated that as many as 50 per cent of the reactions follow transfusions for which there was no valid, clear-cut indication. Reactions occurring under these circumstances can never be justified. Fortunately, most complications are relatively mild, but some are fatal. Available data suggest a mortality of about one death in 5000 transfusions; however, this figure is most likely too high. It is difficult to obtain accurate figures because of a natural reluctance to publicize errors as well as a tendency to blame transfusions for death due to other causes. Types of transfusion reactions are listed in Table 14-4.

Table 14-4. *Types of Transfusion Reactions*

Febrile
    Leukocyte antibodies
    Platelet antibodies
    Pyrogens
    Plasma sensitivity
Allergic
Hemolytic (incompatible transfusion)
Transmission of disease
    Serum hepatitis
    Malaria
    Syphilis
    Other (e.g., brucellosis)
Gross bacterial contamination
Cardiac overload
Citrate intoxication
Potassium intoxication
Abnormal bleeding
    Incompatible transfusion
    Massive transfusion
Isosensitization
Transfusion hemosiderosis
Miscellaneous
    Thrombophlebitis
    Air embolism
    Injection of foreign material

Febrile Reactions. "Simple" febrile reactions occur in about 3 per cent of all recipients of blood and make up about 60 per cent of all transfusion complications. These reactions were once thought to be caused by *pyrogens* (bacterial products) in the bottles, tubing, or anticoagulant solutions. The advent of single-use equipment and aseptic techniques in the preparation of solutions has virtually eliminated pyrogens. However, the over-all incidence of febrile reactions remains essentially unchanged, and other factors obviously play more important roles. *Leukocyte antibodies* consequent to prior transfusions or pregnancies (i.e., production of antibodies directed against "incompatible" leukocytes) are a common cause of febrile transfusion reactions and may be responsible for as many as 80 per cent of these occurrences. It seems likely that *platelet antibodies* also play a role in the pathogenesis of some febrile reactions. *Plasma transfusion reactions* (fever resulting from sensitivity to homologous plasma) have been described but are quite rare; leukocyte and/or platelet antibodies appear to have been responsible for many of the reactions so categorized.

The manifestations of a febrile transfusion reaction include flushing, chilliness (less often frank chills), headache, apprehension, nausea, and fever (101 to 103°F). Symptoms are rarely immediate, and fever is typically manifested near the end of a transfusion or shortly thereafter (i.e., within one to four hours after the blood is started). Fever usually persists for four to eight hours and is responsive, as are the other symptoms, to salicylates. Such febrile reactions are not accompanied by evidence of hemolysis or other laboratory abnormalities. Most of these reactions are mild, and slight fever may be missed if serial temperatures are not obtained. However, severe febrile reactions occur and may be sufficiently stressful to be life-threatening in certain acutely ill patients. Treatment consists of stopping the blood if the transfusion has not been completed, warming the patient, and giving salicylates as needed to control symptoms and fever. Prevention of febrile reactions in patients known to be sensitive to leukocytes, platelets, or plasma revolves around the use of sterile equipment and solutions and of leukocyte or platelet-free blood or washed red cells resuspended in saline. Simple febrile reactions must be differentiated from hemolytic reactions and from those resulting from bacterial contamination.

Allergic Reactions. Urticaria is the commonest allergic reaction to blood, but angioneurotic edema, asthma, and even anaphylactic shock have been observed. Allergic manifestations are demonstrable in about 2 per cent of recipients and make up nearly 40 per cent of all untoward responses to transfusions. There are two types of allergic reaction. The first is immediate and is caused by antibodies in the recipient reacting with antigens contained in the transfused blood; this type occurs much more frequently in atopic individuals than in those without evidence of allergic disease. The second kind of reaction is delayed and reflects passive sensitization; that is, antibodies in donor blood to which the recipient may react days or even weeks later on contact with the appropriate antigen (antibodies persist in blood for several weeks at room temperature and for longer periods in the refrigerator).

Most allergic reactions are relatively innocuous and occur after the transfusion has been completed. As a rule, it is not necessary to stop a transfusion even if they do appear before all blood has been given. The majority of these reactions respond well to antihistamines; occasionally, severe manifestations require epinephrine. A past history of allergic responses to transfusions or a strong allergic background are indications for prophylactic antihistamine therapy, but there is no real justification for its routine administration. The incidence of allergic reactions can be reduced by careful selection of donors and by drawing blood in a fasting state in order to avoid the presence of potent food allergens.

Hemolytic Reactions. The exact incidence of this type of transfusion reaction is unknown. Fortunately they are quite rare and appear to make up only about 0.1 per cent of all transfusion complications. Hemolytic reactions are due to the administration of incompatible blood. They are almost always caused by human error and are largely preventable by adequate knowledge of blood groups and red cell antibodies and by careful attention to all details of the techniques of typing, cross matching, and the administration of blood. Most hemolytic reactions involve the ABO system and reflect the destruction of donor cells by the recipient's naturally occurring antibodies. Occasionally such reactions are caused by antibodies against other blood group factors or antigens, especially anti-D(Rh_o); for the most part these antibodies are of the immune type and reflect sensitization by prior transfusions or pregnancies. Much less often hemolytic reactions are caused by destruction of recipient cells by very high titers of donor antibodies.

The mechanisms of red cell destruction by isoantibodies are complex and not entirely understood. Naturally occurring or saline agglutinating antibodies such as anti-A and anti-B cause prompt intravascular lysis of erythrocytes. Immune or albumin agglutinating antibodies such as those of the Rh system bring about the premature removal from the circulation of affected erythrocytes which are then destroyed extravascularly by reticuloendothelial cells. Intravascular lysis is manifested by hemoglobinemia and hemoglobinuria, whereas destruction by the reticuloendothelial system (unless hemolysis is massive) is more likely to be associated with hyperbilirubinemia, with little or no free hemoglobin in the plasma or urine. Free or extracorpuscular hemoglobin in the circulating blood combines with haptoglobin (an α_2 globulin) and is cleared rapidly by the reticuloendothelial system. Normal haptoglobin levels can bind about 100 mg of hemoglobin/100 ml of plasma. Because of its high molecular weight, the hemoglobin-haptoglobin complex is not excreted in the urine. Hemoglobinuria does not occur until available haptoglobin is saturated and the free plasma hemoglobin exceeds the renal threshold of 25 mg/100 ml. After sudden intravascular hemolysis, free hemoglobin complexes with haptoglobin until this protein is saturated; a small amount of the remainder combines with albumin to form methemalbumin, and the rest is excreted by the kidneys.

The manifestations of an incompatible transfusion are variable and depend on (1) the amount of blood given, (2) the speed with which the blood is administered, (3) the potency of the donor cell antigen, (4) the titer of antibody in the recipient, and (5) the character of the responsible antibody. Thus 60 per cent or more of A cells may be destroyed within two to three minutes in a group B recipient. On the other hand, the administration of $D(Rh_o)$ positive cells to a recipient with anti-$D(Rh_o)$ immune-type antibody may not evoke untoward manifestations for 30 to 60 minutes or longer. Therefore the symptoms of a hemolytic reaction may occur after only 2 to 10 ml have been given, or they may be delayed for an hour or more. Other factors include the capacity of the reticuloendothelial system which, if overloaded, may prolong the "useful life" of an erythrocyte, even though the cell is coated with univalent or blocking antibody and already marked for destruction. Normally, the reticuloendothelial system can handle the catabolic products of 300 to 400 ml of red cells a day. Depletion of antibody will also lengthen the time that incompatible cells will survive in a recipient.

An incompatible transfusion evokes a dramatic chain of events that is usually evident within a few minutes after the mismatched blood has been started. Early manifestations include marked apprehension, tachycardia, tachypnea, pain in the back and chest, nausea, vomiting, chills, fever (103 to 105°F), hypotension, and shock. Occasionally a hemorrhagic diathesis may reflect such a reaction and in anesthetized patients may be the only sign of an incompatible transfusion. Such abnormal bleeding is associated with hypofibrinogenemia, hypoprothrombinemia, and thrombocytopenia and is presumably the result of intravascular coagulation initiated by the thromboplastic activity of hemolyzed red cells (p. 516). Hemoglobinemia and hemoglobinuria are present only during the first 12 hours or less; methemalbumin may still be detectable 24 hours after an incompatible transfusion. Hyperbilirubinemia and jaundice usually appear within 3 to 24 hours and persist for several days.

The immediate effects of a mismatched transfusion usually subside within 24 hours. Some patients show no sequelae, whereas others during the ensuing two to three days manifest acute renal failure with oliguria, anuria, and progressive uremia (lower nephron nephrosis). This phase may last for two to three weeks and often terminates in death; however, recovery does occur and will be heralded by diuresis. The precise cause of the acute renal failure is not known. Experimental data indicate that it does not result solely from hemoglobinemia or hyperbilirubinemia. Shock or profound hypotension is probably the most important factor, but other mechanisms, including decreased renal output and mechanical obstruction secondary to precipitated hemoglobin in the renal tubules, also appear to operate.

The diagnosis of a hemolytic transfusion reaction is dependent on the demonstration of increased cell destruction and of donor-recipient incompatibility. Prompt examination of the blood and urine will often achieve the first objective. Inspection of the plasma may confirm the presence of hemoglobinemia (the plasma will appear pink if the free plasma hemoglobin level exceeds 20 mg per cent and red when it reaches 100 mg per cent). It should be re-emphasized that hemoglobinemia is transient, and hemoglobinuria may be evident only in the first specimen of urine after the suspected incompatible transfusion. Careful study of the donor blood and pretransfusion specimen of the recipient's blood will almost always reveal evidence of gross incompatibility.

Management depends on the phase of the hemolytic reaction. The blood should, of course, be stopped at the first suspicion of an incompatible transfusion and the unused blood saved for testing. Initial therapeutic measures are those designed to support the patient and to combat hypotension and shock. Early and adequate fluid intake should be maintained. Because renal shutdown does not occur immediately, fluids need not and indeed should not be restricted too soon. The time to alter the fluid intake is after oliguria becomes evident. If the transfusion that caused the hemolytic reaction was indicated, the same need persists after a hemolytic reaction, and a compatible transfusion should be given as soon as possible. Fresh blood supplemented with fibrinogen is indicated in the patient who exhibits a hemorrhagic diathesis. Opinion is divided on the value of alkali in the treatment of a hemolytic reaction, but it cannot be advised routinely. Some physicians do give an agent such as sodium bicarbonate to all patients in the hope of preventing the precipitation of acid hematin in the renal tubules. However, renal ischemia appears to be the primary lesion. Furthermore, if renal function is not normal, even large quantities of sodium bicarbonate will fail to alkalinize the urine. It is more important to maintain a good urine output, if necessary with osmotic diuretics such as mannitol. Once renal insufficiency is manifested, the treatment is that of acute renal failure, regardless of cause, and consists of such measures as fluid restriction and maintenance of caloric intake. Dialysis (peritoneal or extracorporeal with an artificial kidney) has been used successfully in a few patients.

Prognosis of a hemolytic reaction depends on several factors. The amount of blood received is most important; serious reactions rarely, if ever, follow a transfusion of less than 200 ml. If the hemolytic reaction is recognized early, the prognosis is invariably good, unless there are complications such as bleeding, trauma, or surgery. Recipients of large amounts of incompatible blood do poorly, and the mortality rate in patients who develop renal failure may be as high as 30 to 50 per cent.

Transmission of Disease. *Serum hepatitis* remains a real and still unavoidable risk in every recipient of whole blood, plasma, or such blood fractions as human thrombin or fibrinogen. Careful screening of donors has reduced but not eliminated this risk. Although the exact incidence is not known, 1 to 3 per cent of the population appear to be asymptomatic carriers of the virus. Most of these individuals fail to exhibit abnormalities in liver function tests, and there is no foolproof way to detect the presence of the virus or to eliminate or inactivate the infectious agent in fresh blood. Even minute amounts of infected blood can cause disease. The incubation period varies between 30 and 180 days. Since vulnerability to hepatitis increases with the number of transfusions given, it is difficult to determine its true incidence. Icteric hepatitis occurs in less than 1 per cent; however, mild anicteric disease probably affects as many as 2 per cent. Over the age of 40, serum hepatitis, a serious complication, has a mortality rate of about 20 per cent. Human gamma globulin in a dose equivalent to 0.15 ml/kg given one week after the transfusion and repeated a month later is the only available means of modifying the disease. With this approach, the incidence of icteric (and severer) serum hepatitis can be significantly reduced; however, limited availability of gamma globulin precludes its routine use. It is hoped that such developments as the rubeola vaccine, improved methods for the procurement of gamma globulin (plasmapheresis), and more careful and thoughtful use of transfusions (thus reducing the number given) will decrease the need for gamma globulin and make more available for prophylactic use in recipients of blood, at least in older patients.

Syphilis can be transmitted by blood but does not constitute a real problem, for the spirochetes do not survive longer than 72 hours at refrigerator temperatures. *Malaria* is a bigger threat because the parasites remain viable for days to weeks at temperatures of 4 to 6°C. In certain geographic locations transmission of malaria by blood transfusion poses a real threat because the absence of symptoms (even for long periods) does not necessarily ensure lack of infectivity. A variety of other infections (e.g., *brucellosis*) has been transmitted via blood transfusions, but modern blood bank techniques and donor requirements have virtually eliminated them.

Gross Bacterial Contamination. When blood is collected in sterile containers under aseptic conditions and refrigerated promptly and continuously, there is little possibility of contamination with the common bacterial pathogens. However, certain gram-negative saphrophytic bacilli (e.g., Achromobacters and Pseudomonads) multiply at temperatures of 4 to 8°C and resist the normal bacteriostatic effect of blood.

These organisms constitute a grave threat. Although they lack the ability to multiply in the host, they can cause serious disease and even death as the result of a potent endotoxin produced outside the body. After a short latent period (30 minutes or so), manifestations in recipients of as little as 50 ml of infected blood include a shaking chill, fever, pain in the abdomen, back, and chest, nausea, vomiting, hypotension, and shock. If the patient survives the initial episode, signs of acute renal failure usually become evident one or two days later. This kind of reaction can be distinguished from an incompatible transfusion by the absence of hemolysis (hemoglobinemia or hemoglobinuria) and by the demonstration of large numbers of organisms (typically gram-negative rods) in direct smears of the donor blood. Treatment includes measures to combat shock (e.g., pressor agents) and to maintain fluid and electrolyte balance. Unless one can be absolutely sure of the identity of the responsible organism, antibiotics are indicated empirically on the outside chance that the blood was infected with an agent other than a gram-negative saprophyte. The role of corticosteroids is conjectural. Although modern blood bank methods make gross bacterial contamination an unlikely complication, any break in technique (e.g., removing the blood from the refrigerator well in advance of its use or not using the blood immediately once the bottle has been entered) invites bacterial contamination and its serious sequelae. Since bacteria proliferate logarithmically, they may reach sufficient numbers to cause difficulty if a transfusion is given very slowly over a period of six to eight hours.

Cardiac Overload.   With the exception of the hypovolemia that follows acute hemorrhage, all patients in whom transfusions are indicated can be expected to have essentially normal blood volumes. In patients with underlying heart disease, hypervolemia subsequent to blood transfusions (usually too many given too rapidly) may precipitate acute congestive failure. The acute pulmonary edema so produced may actually necessitate phlebotomies. In patients whose functional cardiac reserve is known to be impaired, cardiac overload should be anticipated. Under these circumstances packed red cells should be used instead of whole blood; the cells should be given slowly and, if possible, not more than one unit a day.

Citrate Intoxication.   Normal plasma citrate levels are about 1 mg/100 ml; levels above 50 mg/100 ml are undesirable and higher levels may be associated with such findings as muscle twitching, electrocardiographic abnormalities (e.g., a prolonged QT interval), and hypotension. These manifestations are due basically to hypocalcemia, although some direct effect is attributable to the citrate per se. There is no evidence that citrate intoxication can produce a hemorrhagic diathesis. Citrate is cleared rapidly, and normal values are restored within 60 minutes, even after rapid infusion of blood. A plasma citrate level of 50 mg/100 ml corresponds to an infusion rate equivalent to about 100 ml of whole blood in ACD solution per minute. Consequently, some defect in plasma clearance is needed for citrate intoxication to occur unless the blood is given extremely fast. Liver disease, anuria (about one fifth of injected citrate is excreted by the kidneys), and hypothermia impair citrate clearance. Citrate intoxication is rarely encountered clinically. Treatment consists of intravenous calcium chloride or gluconate. Calcium need not be given routinely unless the infusion rate exceeds 1000 ml/20 minutes (under these circumstances each 1000 ml of blood should be covered with 10 ml of a 10 per cent solution of calcium chloride or gluconate).

Aged Blood (Potassium Intoxication). When blood is stored, potassium leaves the erythrocytes and the plasma concentration rises (levels may reach 40 mEq/liter after storage for 28 days). Although harmless in most patients, excess potassium may cause trouble in certain recipients with anuria or severe renal insufficiency, especially if they are given large quantities of aged blood. Lactic acid, ammonia, and inorganic phosphate also accumulate in stored blood, but the amounts are insignificant.

Abnormal Bleeding. Patients with acute hemorrhage who require multiple transfusions over a short period of time [e.g., 7500 ml (15 units)/hour] often manifest a generalized hemorrhagic diathesis. The bleeding may reflect several causes but is basically the result of thrombocytopenia consequent to loss of platelets by hemorrhage and replacement with blood containing nonviable platelets. Bank blood collected in the usual way does not contain viable platelets. When collected in special equipment, platelets can be transfused and will survive in the recipient. Even under these circumstances, however, recipients of prior transfusions readily develop platelet antibodies that destroy donor platelets.

Sensitization. Recipients of ABO incompatible blood develop hemolytic reactions; recipients of blood that is incompatible for one of the other blood group systems may be sensitized, with the "foreign" erythrocyte antigen evoking the production of immune antibodies against that blood group factor. Such antibodies may then cause hemolytic reactions with subsequent transfusions or, if the patient is a girl or woman, may play a role in the production of hemolytic disease of the newborn.

Transfusion Hemosiderosis. Approximately 250 mg of elemental iron are contained in each unit of whole blood. In recipients who are not bleeding, iron administered in this fashion is deposited largely in reticuloendothelial cells (in primary hemochromatosis parenchymal cells are more likely to be affected). After a variable number of transfusions (usually 100 or more), excess iron begins to appear in parenchymal cells, and such patients develop skin pigmentation, hepatosplenomegaly with evidence of hepatic dysfunction, cardiac conduction defects, hyper-glycemia, and so forth. When fully developed, transfusion hemosiderosis may present a clinical picture that is indistinguishable from that of pri-mary or idiopathic hemochromatosis.

Miscellaneous Reactions. Other transfusion complications include *thrombophlebitis* in patients given multiple transfusions, *air embolism* in recipients of blood given rapidly under pressure, and the *injection of foreign material* (e.g., small pieces of glass or bits of skin). These un-wanted effects can be prevented by proper attention to the technique of blood administration.

Bibliography

***Chapter 1.* The Blood Cells. General Considerations**

1. Albritton, E. C.: *Standard Values in Blood.* Philadelphia: W. B. Saunders Company, 1952, 199 p.
2. Arnason, B. G., Jankovic, B. D., and Waksman, B. H.: A survey of the thymus and its relation to lymphocytes and immune reactions. *Blood* **20**:617–28, 1962.
3. Bessis, M.: *Cytology of the Blood and Blood-Forming Organs.* New York: Grune and Stratton, 1956, 629 p.
4. Braunsteiner, H.: Mast cells and basophilic leukocytes. In *The Physiology and Pathology of the Leukocytes,* Braunsteiner, H., and Zucker-Franklin, D., Eds. New York: Grune and Stratton, 1962, pp. 46–62.
5. Braunsteiner, H., and Zucker-Franklin, D.: The lymphocytes. In *The Physiology and Pathology of the Leukocytes,* Braunsteiner, H., and Zucker-Franklin, D., Eds. New York: Grune and Stratton, 1962, pp. 63–90.
6. Braunsteiner, H., and Zucker-Franklin, D.: Plasma cells. In *The Physiology and Pathology of the Leukocytes,* Braunsteiner, H., and Zucker-Franklin, D., Eds. New York: Grune and Stratton, 1962, pp. 114–29.
7. Brecher, G., von Foerster, H., and Cronkite, E. P.: Production, differentiation and lifespan of leukocytes. In *The Physiology and Pathology of the Leukocytes,* Braunsteiner, H., and Zucker-Franklin, D., Eds. New York: Grune and Stratton, 1962, pp. 170–95.
8. Brücher, H.: The monocytes. In *The Physiology and Pathology of the Leukocytes,* Braunsteiner, H., and Zucker-Franklin, D., Eds. New York: Grune and Stratton, 1962, pp. 91–113.
9. Cartwright, G. E., Athens, J. W., and Wintrobe, M. M.: The kinetics of granulopoiesis in normal man. *Blood* **24**:780–803, 1964.

10. Craddock, C. G., Jr., Perry, S., Ventzke, L. E., and Lawrence, J. S.: Evaluation of marrow granulocytic reserves in normal and disease states. *Blood* **15**:840–55, 1960.

11. Cronkite, E. P., and Fliedner, T. M.: Granulocytopoiesis. *New Eng J Med* **270**:1347–52; 1403–8, 1964.

12. Dittrich, H.: Physiology of neutrophils. In *The Physiology and Pathology of the Leukocytes*, Braunsteiner, H., and Zucker-Franklin, D., Eds. New York: Grune and Stratton, 1962, pp. 130–51.

13. Gordon, A. S.: Endocrine influences upon the formed elements of blood and blood-forming organs. *Recent Progr Hormone Res* **10**:339–94, 1954.

14. Gordon, A. S.: Hemopoietine. *Physiol Rev* **39**:1–40, 1959.

15. Gross, R.: The eosinophils. In *The Physiology and Pathology of the Leukocytes*, Braunsteiner, H., and Zucker-Franklin, D., Eds. New York: Grune and Stratton, 1962, pp. 1–45.

16. Harris, J. W.: *The Red Cell. Production, Metabolism, Destruction: Normal and Abnormal.* Cambridge, Mass.: Harvard University Press, 1963, pp. 3–12.

17. Jacobson, L. O., and Doyle, M., Eds.: *Erythropoiesis.* New York: Grune and Stratton, 1962, 399 p.

18. Kosenow, W.: Nuclear appendages in leukocytes and the sex pattern of chromosomes. In *The Physiology and Pathology of the Leukocytes*, Braunsteiner, H., and Zucker-Franklin, D., Eds. New York: Grune and Stratton, 1962, pp. 196–214.

19. Linman, J. W., and Bethell, F. H.: *Factors Controlling Erythropoiesis.* Springfield, Ill.: Charles C Thomas, 1960, 208 p.

20. Linman, J. W., and Pierre, R. V.: Studies on thrombopoiesis. III. Thrombocytosis-promoting effects of "thrombocythemic" and "polycythemic" plasmas. *J Lab Clin Med* **62**:374–84, 1963.

21. Little, J. R., Brecher, G., Bradley, T. R., and Rose, S.: Determinations of lymphocyte turnover by continuous infusion of H³ thymidine. *Blood* **19**:236–42, 1962.

22. Marcus, A. J., and Zucker, M. B.: *The Physiology of Blood Platelets. Recent Biochemical, Morphologic and Clinical Research.* New York: Grune and Stratton, 1965, 162 p.

23. O'Neill, B., and Firkin, B.: Platelet survival studies in coagulation disorders, thrombocythemia and conditions associated with arteriosclerosis. *J Lab Clin Med* **64**:188–201, 1964.

24. Riley, J. F.: Pharmacology and functions of mast cells. *Pharmacol Rev* **7**:267–77, 1955.

25. Schettini, F., Berni Canani, M., Di Francesco, L., and Rea, F.: Studies on the enzymes of blood platelets from healthy and thrombopathic children. *Acta Haemat* (Basel) **27**:237–45, 1962.

26. Stohlman, F., Jr.: Erythropoiesis. *New Eng J Med* **267**:342–48; 392–99, 1962.

27. Troup, S. B., and Lüscher, E. F.: Hemostasis and platelet metabolism. *Amer J Med* **33**:161–65, 1962.

28. Varsa, E. E., Dornfest, B. S., LoBue, J., Handler, E. S., and Gordon, A. S.: Mechanisms of leukocyte production and release. III. Factors influencing leukocyte release from isolated perfused legs of rats with chloroleukemia. *J Lab Clin Med* **64**:934–41, 1964.

29. Zamboni, L., and Pease, D. C.: The vascular bed of red bone marrow. *J Ultrastruct Res* **5**:65–85, 1961.

Chapter 2. Examination of the Blood and Blood-Forming Organs

30. Berman, L.: A review of methods for aspiration and biopsy of bone marrow. *Amer J Clin Path* **23**:385–402, 1953.

31. Bethell, F. H., and Meyers, M. C.: *Clinical Laboratory Diagnosis and Essentials of Hematology.* Ann Arbor: Cushing-Malloy, Inc., 5th Ed., 1961, 128 p.

32. Cartwright, G. E.: *Diagnostic Laboratory Hematology.* New York: Grune and Stratton, 3rd Ed., 1963, 352 p.

33. Miale, J. B.: *Laboratory Medicine—Hematology.* St. Louis: C. V. Mosby Company, 2nd Ed., 1962, 918 p.

34. Osgood, E. E., and Seaman, A. J.: The cellular composition of normal bone marrow obtained by sternal puncture. *Physiol Rev* **24**:46–69, 1944.

Chapter 3. Anemia. Classification and General Considerations

35. Blumgart, H. L., and Altschule, M. D.: Clinical significance of cardiac and respiratory adjustments in chronic anemia. *Blood* **3**:329–48, 1948.

36. Case, R. B., Berglund, E., and Sarnoff, S. J.: Ventricular function. VII. Changes in coronary resistance and ventricular function resulting from acutely induced anemia and the effect thereon of coronary stenosis. *Amer J Med* **18**:397–405, 1955.

37. Crosby, W. H.: Siderocytes and the spleen. *Blood* **12**:165–70, 1957.

38. Crosby, W. H., and Akeroyd, J. H.: The limit of hemoglobin synthesis in hereditary hemolytic anemia. Its relation to the excretion of bile pigment. *Amer J Med* **13**:273–83, 1952.

39. Douglas, A. S., and Dacie, J. V.: The incidence and significance of iron-containing granules in human erythrocytes and their precursors. *J Clin Path* **6**:307–13, 1953.

40. Gunton, R. W., and Paul, W.: Blood volume in congestive heart failure. *J Clin Invest* **34**:879–86, 1955.

41. Prentice, T. C., Berlin, N. I., Hyde, G. M., Parsons, R. J., Lawrence, J. H., and Port, S.: Total red cell volume, plasma volume, and sodium space in congestive heart failure. *J Clin Invest* **30**:1471–82, 1951.

42. Rodman, T., Close, H. P., and Purcell, M. K.: The oxyhemoglobin dissociation curve in anemia. *Ann Intern Med* **52**:295–309, 1960.

43. Sproule, B. J., Mitchell, J. H., and Miller, W. F.: Cardiopulmonary physiological responses to heavy exercise in patients with anemia. *J Clin Invest* **39**:378–88, 1960.

Chapter 4. Anemias Caused by Blood Loss
Acute Hemorrhagic Anemia

44. Coleman, D. H., Stevens, A. R., Jr., Dodge, H. T., and Finch, C. A.: Rate of blood regeneration after blood loss. *Arch Intern Med* (Chicago) **92**:341–49, 1953.

45. Ebert, R. V., Stead, E. A., Jr., and Gibson, J. G., II.: Response of normal subjects to acute blood loss. With special reference to the mechanism of restoration of blood volume. *Arch Intern Med* (Chicago) **68**:578–90, 1941.

46. Gregersen, M. I., and Rawson, R. A.: Blood volume. *Physiol Rev* **39**:307–42, 1959.

47. Linman, J. W.: Factors controlling hemopoiesis: thrombopoietic and leukopoietic effects of "anemic" plasma. *J Lab Clin Med* **59**:262–74, 1962.

48. Mollison, P. L.: *Blood Transfusion in Clinical Medicine*. Oxford: Blackwell Scientific Publications, 3rd Ed., 1961, pp. 87–111.

48a. Moore, F. D.: The effects of hemorrhage on body composition. *New Eng J Med* **273**:567–77, 1965.

Hemolytic Anemias

49. Allen, F. H., Jr., and Diamond, L. K.: Erythroblastosis fetalis. *New Eng J Med* **257**:659–68; 705–12; 761–72, 1957.

50. Berlin, N. I., Waldmann, T. A., and Weissman, S. M.: Life span of red blood cell. *Physiol Rev* **39**:577–616, 1959.

51. Beutler, E.: The hemolytic effect of primaquine and related compounds: a review. *Blood* **14**:103–39, 1959.

52. Bowman, H. S., and Procopio, F.: Hereditary non-spherocytic hemolytic anemia of the pyruvate-kinase deficient type. *Ann Intern Med* **58**:567–91, 1963.

53. Brody, J. I., and Finch, S. C.: Serum factors of acquired hemolytic anemia in leukemia and lymphoma. *J Clin Invest* **40**:181–87, 1961.

54. Burnet, M.: Auto-immune disease. I. Modern immunological concepts. II. Pathology of the immune response. *Brit Med J* **2**:645–50; 720–25, 1959.

55. Crosby, W. H.: Paroxysmal nocturnal hemoglobinuria. Relation of the clinical manifestations to underlying pathogenic mechanisms. *Blood* **8**:769–812, 1953.

56. Dacie, J. V.: The auto-immune hemolytic anaemias. *Amer J Med* **18**:810–21, 1955.

57. Dacie, J. V.: *The Haemolytic Anaemias Congenital and Acquired. Part I—The Congenital Anaemias.* New York: Grune and Stratton, 1960, pp. 1–339.

58. Dacie, J. V.: *The Haemolytic Anaemias Congenital and Acquired. Part II—The Autoimmune Haemolytic Anaemias.* New York: Grune and Stratton, 1962, pp. 341–718.

59. Dameshek, W., and Schwartz, R.: Hemolytic mechanisms. *Ann NY Acad Sci* **77**:589–614, 1959.

60. Dausett, J., and Colombani, J.: The serology and the prognosis of 128 cases of autoimmune hemolytic anemia. *Blood* **14**:1280–1301, 1959.

61. Davidson, R. J.: Exertional haemoglobinuria: a report on three cases with studies on the haemolytic mechanism. *J Clin Path* **17**:536–40, 1964.

62. DeGruchy, G. C., Loder, P. B., and Hennessy, I. V.: Haemolysis and glycolytic metabolism in hereditary elliptocytosis. *Brit J Haemat* **8**:168–79, 1962.

63. Dunn, I., Ibsen, K. H., Coe, E. L., Schneider, A. S., and Weinstein, I. M.: Erythrocyte carbohydrate metabolism in hereditary spherocytosis. *J Clin Invest* **42**:1535–41, 1963.

64. Emerson, C. P., Jr., Shen, S. C., Ham, T. H., Fleming, E. M., and Castle, W. B.: Studies on the destruction of red blood cells. IX. Quantitative methods for determining the osmotic and mechanical fragility of red cells in the peripheral blood and splenic pulp; the mechanism of increased hemolysis in hereditary spherocytosis (congenital hemolytic jaundice) as related to the functions of the spleen. *Arch Intern Med* (Chicago) **97**:1–38, 1956.

65. Evans, R. S., and Weiser, R. S.: The serology of autoimmune hemolytic disease. *Arch Intern Med* (Chicago) **100**:371–99, 1957.

66. Gaither, J. C.: Paroxysmal hemoglobinuria. A successful imposter. *New Eng J Med* **265**:421–30, 1961.

67. Harris, J. W.: *The Red Cell. Production, Metabolism, Destruction: Normal and Abnormal.* Cambridge: Harvard University Press, 1963, pp. 233–309.

67a. Hartmann, R. C., and Jenkins, D. E., Jr.: Paroxysmal nocturnal hemoglobinuria: current concepts of certain pathophysiologic features. *Blood* **25**:850–65, 1965.

68. Jacob, H. S., and Jandl, J. H.: Effects of sulfhydryl inhibition on red blood cells. II. Studies *in vivo. J Clin Invest* **41**:1514–23, 1962.

69. Jacob, H. S., and Jandl, J. H.: Increased cell membrane permeability in the pathogenesis of hereditary spherocytosis. *J Clin Invest* **43**:1704–20, 1964.

70. Jandl, J. H.: The Heinz body hemolytic anemias. *Ann Intern Med* **58**:702–9, 1963.

70a. Jandl, J. H.: Leaky red cells. *Blood* **26**:367–82, 1965.

71. Jandl, J. H., Jacob, H. S., and Daland, G. A.: Hypersplenism due to infection. A study of five cases manifesting hemolytic anemia. *New Eng J Med* **264**:1063–71, 1961.

72. Kellermeyer, R. W., Tarlov, A. R., Brewer, G. J., Carson, P. E., and

Alving, A. S.: Hemolytic effect of therapeutic drugs. Clinical considerations of the primaquine-type hemolysis. *JAMA* **180**:388–94, 1962.

73. Kessel, L.: Acute transient hyperlipemia due to hepatopancreatic damage in chronic alcoholics (Zieve's syndrome). *Amer J Med* **32**:747–57, 1962.

74. Klatskin, G.: Bile pigment metabolism. *Ann Rev Med* **12**:211–50, 1961.

75. Leddy, J. P., Trabold, N. C., Vaughan, J. H., and Swisher, S. N.: The unitary nature of "complete" and "incomplete" pathologic cold hemagglutinins. *Blood* **19**:379–98, 1962.

76. Lester, R., and Schmid, R.: Bilirubin metabolism. *New Eng J Med* **270**:779–86, 1964.

77. Loder, P. B., and DeGruchy, G. C.: Red-cell enzymes and co-enzymes in non-spherocytic congenital haemolytic anemias. *Brit J Haemat* **11**:21–31, 1965.

78. MacKinney, A. A., Jr., Morton, N. E., Kosower, N. S., and Schilling, R. F.: Ascertaining genetic carriers of hereditary spherocytosis by statistical analysis of multiple laboratory tests. *J Clin Invest* **41**:554–67, 1962.

79. Marsh, G. W.: Intravascular haemolytic anaemia after aortic-valve replacement. *Lancet* **2**:986–88, 1964.

80. Mollison, P. L.: *Blood Transfusions in Clinical Medicine*. Oxford: Blackwell Scientific Publications, 3rd Ed., 1961, pp. 596–675.

81. Morton, N. E., MacKinney, A. A., Kosower, N., Schilling, R. F., and Gray, M. P.: Genetics of spherocytosis. *Amer J Hum Genet* **14**:170–84, 1962.

82. Motulsky, A. G., Singer, K., Crosby, W. H., and Smith, V.: The life span of the elliptocyte. Hereditary elliptocytosis and its relationship to other familial hemolytic diseases. *Blood* **9**:57–72, 1954.

83. Murphy, J. R.: Erythrocyte metabolism. II. Glucose metabolism and pathways. *J Lab Clin Med* **55**:286–302, 1960.

84. Osgood, E. E.: Antiglobulin-positive hemolytic anemias. *Arch Intern Med* (Chicago) **107**:313–23, 1961.

85. Oski, F. A., Nathan, D. G., Sidel, V. W., and Diamond, L. K.: Extreme hemolysis and red-cell distortion in erythrocyte pyruvate kinase deficiency. I. Morphology, erythrokinetics and family enzyme studies. *New Eng J Med* **270**:1023–30, 1964.

86. Porter, I. H., Boyer, S. H., Watson-Williams, E. J., Adam, A., Szeinberg, A., and Siniscalco, M.: Variation of glucose-6-phosphate dehydrogenase in different populations. *Lancet* **1**:895–99, 1964.

87. Prankerd, T. A. J.: *The Red Cell. An Account of Its Chemical Physiology and Pathology*. Oxford: Blackwell Scientific Publications, 1961, 184 p.

88. Ramot, B., Bauminger, S., Brok, F., Gafni, D., and Shwartz, J.: Characterization of glucose-6-phosphate dehydrogenase in Jewish mutants. *J Lab Clin Med* **64**:895–904, 1964.

89. Rappaport, H., and Crosby, W. H.: Auto-immune hemolytic anemia. II. Morphologic observations and clinicopathologic correlations. *Amer J Path* **33**:429–49, 1957.

90. Roberts, F.: Haemolytic disease of the new-born. *Brit Med Bull* **15**:119–22, 1959.

91. Schneider, A. S., Valentine, W. N., Hattori, M., and Heins, H. L., Jr.: Hereditary hemolytic anemia with triosephosphate isomerase deficiency. *New Eng J Med* **272**:229–35, 1965.

92. Schwartz, R., and Dameshek, W.: The treatment of autoimmune hemolytic anemia with 6-mercaptopurine and thioguanine. *Blood* **19**:483–500, 1962.

92a. Sears, D. A., and Crosby, W. H.: Intravascular hemolysis due to intracardiac prosthetic devices. Diurnal variations related to activity. *Amer J Med* **39**:341–54, 1965.

93. Sears, D. A., Weed, R. I., and Swisher, S. N.: Differences in the mechanism of *in vitro* immune hemolysis related to antibody specificity. *J Clin Invest* **43**:975–85, 1964.

94. Shapiro, C. M., Josephson, A. M., Rozengvaig, S., and Kauffman, A.: Hereditary spherocytosis in the neonatal period. Diagnosis, incidence, and treatment. *J Pediat* **50**:308–14, 1957.

95. Sigler, A. T., Forman, E. N., Zinkham, W. H., and Neill, C. A.: Severe intravascular hemolysis following surgical repair of endocardial cushion defects. *Amer J Med* **35**:467–80, 1963.

96. Stohlman, F., Jr.: The use of FE⁵⁹ and CR⁵¹ for estimating red cell production and destruction: an interpretive review. *Blood* **18**:236–50, 1961.

97. Szeinberg, A., and Marks, P. A.: Substances stimulating glucose catabolism by the oxidative reactions of the pentose phosphate pathway in human erythrocytes. *J Clin Invest* **40**:914–24, 1961.

98. Tanaka, K. R., Valentine, W. N., and Miwa, S.: Pyruvate kinase (PK) deficiency hereditary nonspherocytic hemolytic anemia. *Blood* **19**:267–95, 1962.

99. Tarlov, A. R., Brewer, G. J., Carson, P. E., and Alving, A. S.: Primaquine sensitivity. Glucose-6-phosphate dehydrogenase deficiency: an inborn error of metabolism of medical and biological significance. *Arch Intern Med* (Chicago) **109**:209–34, 1962.

100. Wasserman, L. R., Stats, D., Schwartz, L., and Fudenberg, H.: Symptomatic and hemopathic hemolytic anemia. *Amer J Med* **18**:961–89, 1955.

101. Watson, D.: Bilirubin metabolism in disease. *Aust Ann Med* **12**:53–69, 1963.

102. Weiss, H. J.: Hereditary elliptocytosis with hemolytic anemia. *Amer J Med* **35**:455–66, 1963.

103. Young, L. E.: Hereditary spherocytosis. *Amer J Med* **18**:486–97, 1955.

104. Young, L. E., Miller, G., and Swisher, S. N.: Treatment of hemolytic disorders. *J Chronic Dis* **6**:307–23, 1957.

Chapter 5. Anemias Caused by Impaired Production
ENDOCRINE AND NUTRITIONAL DEFICIENCIES

105. Axelrod, A. R., and Berman, L.: The bone marrow in hyperthyroidism and hypothyroidism. *Blood* **6**:436–53, 1951.
106. Cartwright, G. E.: Dietary factors concerned in erythropoiesis. *Blood* **2**:111–53; 256–98, 1947.
107. Cox, E. V., Meynell, M. J., Cooke, W. T., and Gaddie, R.: Scurvy and anaemia. *Amer J Med* **32**:240–50, 1962.
108. Daughaday, W. H., Williams, R. H., and Dalano, G. A.: The effects of endocrinopathies on the blood. *Blood* **3**:1342–66, 1948.
109. Goldberg, A.: The anaemia of scurvy. *Quart J Med* **32**:51–64, 1963.
110. Gordon, A. S.: Endocrine influences upon the formed elements of blood and blood-forming organs. *Recent Progr Hormone Res* **10**:339–94, 1954.
111. Leavell, B. S., Thorup, O. A., and McClellan, J. E.: Observations on the anemia in myxedema. *Trans Amer Clin Climat Ass* **68**:137–45, 1956.
112. Schubert, W. K., and Lahey, M. E.: Copper and protein depletion complicating hypoferric anemia of infancy. *Pediatrics* **24**:710–33, 1959.
113. Tudhope, G. R., and Wilson, G. M.: Anaemia in hypothyroidism. Incidence, pathogenesis, and response to treatment. *Quart J Med* **29**:513–37, 1960.
114. Tudhope, G. R., and Wilson, G. M.: Deficiency of vitamin B_{12} in hypothyroidism. *Lancet* **1**:703–6, 1962.
115. Wintrobe, M. M., Cartwright, G. E., and Gubler, C. J.: Studies on the function and metabolism of copper. *J Nutr* **50**:395–419, 1953.

IRON DEFICIENCY ANEMIA

116. Badenoch, J., Evans, J. R., and Richards, W. C. D.: The stomach in hypochromic anaemia. *Brit J Haemat* **3**:175–85, 1957.
117. Bessis, M. C., and Breton-Gorius, J.: Iron metabolism in the bone marrow as seen by electron microscopy: a critical review. *Blood* **19**:635–63, 1962.
118. Beutler, E.: Clinical evaluation of iron stores. *New Eng J Med* **256**:692–97, 1957.
119. Beutler, E., Fairbanks, V. F., and Fahey, J. L.: *Clinical Disorders of Iron Metabolism*. New York: Grune and Stratton, 1963, 267 p.
120. Beutler, E., Robson, M. J., and Buttenwieser, E.: A comparison of the plasma iron, iron-binding capacity, sternal marrow iron and other methods in the clinical evaluation of iron stores. *Ann Intern Med* **48**:60–82, 1958.
121. Bothwell, T. H., and Finch, C. A.: *Iron Metabolism*. Boston: Little, Brown and Company, 1962, 440 p.
122. Brown, E. B., Jr., Dubach, R., and Moore, C. V.: Studies in iron transportation and metabolism. XI. Critical analysis of mucosal block by large

doses of inorganic iron in human subjects. *J Lab Clin Med* **52**:335–55, 1958.

123. Brown, E. B., and Rother, M. L.: Studies of the mechanism of iron absorption. I. Iron uptake by the normal rat. *J Lab Clin Med* **62**:357–73, 1963.

124. Brown, E. B., and Rother, M. L.: Studies of the mechanism of iron absorption. II. Influence of iron deficiency and other conditions on iron uptake by rats. *J Lab Clin Med* **62**:804–16, 1963.

125. Callender, S. T.: Iron absorption. *Brit Med Bull* **15**:5–7, 1959.

126. Cann, H. M., and Verhulst, H. L.: Accidental poisoning in young children—the hazards of iron medication. *Amer J Dis Child* **99**:688–91, 1960.

127. Chodos, R. B., Ross, J. F., Apt, L., Pollycove, M., and Halkett, J. A. E.: The absorption of radioiron labeled foods and iron salts in normal and iron-deficient subjects and in idiopathic hemochromatosis. *J Clin Invest* **36**:314–26, 1957.

128. Coleman, D. H., Stevens, A. R., Jr., and Finch, C. A.: The treatment of iron deficiency anemia. *Blood* **10**:567–81, 1955.

129. Crosby, W. H.: The control of iron balance by the intestinal mucosa. *Blood* **22**:441–49, 1963.

130. Demulder, R.: Iron. Metabolism, biochemistry, and clinical pathological physiology—review of recent literature. *Arch Intern Med* (Chicago) **102**:254–301, 1958.

131. Drabkin, D. L.: Metabolism of the hemin chromoproteins. *Physiol Rev* **31**:345–431, 1951.

132. Erslev, A. J., Lear, A. A., and Castle, W. B.: Pyridoxine-responsive anemia. *New Eng J Med* **262**:1209–14, 1960.

133. Finch, S. C., and Finch, C. A.: Idiopathic hemochromatosis, an iron storage disease. A. Iron metabolism in hemochromatosis. *Medicine* (Balt) **34**:381–430, 1955.

134. Gale, E., Torrance, J., and Bothwell, T.: The quantitative estimation of total iron stores in human bone marrow. *J Clin Invest* **42**:1076–82, 1963.

135. Granick, S.: Iron metabolism. *Bull NY Acad Med* **30**:80–105, 1954.

136. Harris, J. W.: *The Red Cell. Production, Metabolism, Destruction: Normal and Abnormal.* Cambridge: Harvard University Press, 1963, pp. 31–64.

137. Henderson, F., Vietti, T. J., and Brown, E. B.: Desferrioxamine in the treatment of acute toxic reaction to ferrous gluconate. *JAMA* **186**:1139–42, 1963.

138. Hobbs, J. R.: Iron deficiency anemia after partial gastrectomy. *Gut* **2**:141–49, 1961.

139. Jandl, J. H., and Katz, J. H.: The plasma-to-cell cycle of transferrin. *J Clin Invest* **42**:314–26, 1963.

140. Josephs, H. W.: Iron metabolism and the hypochromic anemia of infancy. *Medicine* (Balt) **32**:125–213, 1953.

141. Josephs, H. W.: Absorption of iron as a problem in human physiology. A critical review. *Blood* **13**:1–54, 1958.

142. Lichtman, H. C., and Feldman, F.: *In vitro* pyrrole and porphyrin synthesis in lead poisoning and iron deficiency. *J Clin Invest* **42**:830–39, 1963.

143. Mendel, G. A.: Iron metabolism and etiology of iron-storage diseases. *JAMA* **189**:45–53, 1964.

144. Moeschlin, S., and Schnider, V.: Treatment of primary and secondary hemochromatosis and acute iron poisoning with a new, potent iron-eliminating agent (desferrioxamine-B). *New Eng J Med* **269**:57–66, 1963.

145. Moore, C. V.: The importance of nutritional factors in the pathogenesis of iron deficiency anemia. *Scand J Clin Lab Invest* **9**:292–304, 1957.

146. Moore, C. V., and Dubach, R.: Metabolism and requirements of iron in the human. *JAMA* **162**:197–204, 1956.

147. Muir, A. R.: The molecular structure of isolated and intracellular ferritin. *Quart J Exp Physiol* **45**:192–201, 1960.

148. Pletcher, W. D., Brody, G. L., and Meyers, M. C.: Hemochromatosis following prolonged iron therapy in a patient with hereditary nonspherocytic hemolytic anemia. *Amer J Med Sci* **246**:27–34, 1963.

149. Pollycove, M., and Mortimer, R.: The quantitative determination of iron kinetics and hemoglobin synthesis in human subjects. *J Clin Invest* **40**:753–82, 1961.

150. Raab, S. O., Haut, A., Cartwright, G. E., and Wintrobe, M. M.: Pyridoxine-responsive anemia. *Blood* **18**:285–302, 1961.

151. Ramsay, W. N. M.: Plasma iron. *Advances Clin Chem* **1**:1–39, 1958.

152. Robinson, J. C., Blumberg, B. S., Pierce, J. E., Cooper, A. J., and Hames, C. G.: Studies on inherited variants of blood proteins. II. Familial segregation of transferrin $B_{1-2}B_2$. *J Lab Clin Med* **62**:762–65, 1963.

153. Schulman, I.: Iron requirements in infancy. *JAMA* **175**:118–23, 1961.

154. Schulz, J., and Smith, N. J.: A quantitative study of the absorption of food iron in infants and children. *Amer J Dis Child* **95**:109–19, 1958.

155. Schwartz, H. C., Goudsmit, R., Hill, R. L., Cartwright, G. E., and Wintrobe, M. M.: The biosynthesis of hemoglobin from iron protoporphyrin and globin. *J Clin Invest* **40**:188–95, 1961.

156. Shoden, A., and Sturgeon, P.: On the formation of haemosiderin and its relation to ferritin. II. A radioisotopic study. *Brit J Haemat* **9**:513–22, 1963.

157. Sturgeon, P.: Iron metabolism. A review with special consideration of iron requirements during normal infancy. *Pediatrics* **18**:267–98, 1956.

158. Verloop, M. C., Bierenga, M., and Diezeraad-Njoo, A.: Primary or essential sideroachrestic anaemias. Pathogenesis and therapy. *Acta Haemat* (Basel) **27**:129–45, 1962.

159. Wallerstein, R. O., and Mettier, S. R., Eds.: *Iron in Clinical Medicine.* Berkeley: University of California Press, 1958, 283 p.

MEGALOBLASTIC ANEMIAS

160. Barker, H. A.: Structure and function of cobamide coenzymes. *Fed Proc* **20**:956–61, 1961.

161. Beck, W. S.: The metabolic functions of vitamin B_{12}. *New Eng J Med* **266**:708–14; 765–71; 814–17, 1962.

162. Bingham, J.: The macrocytosis of hepatic disease. I. Thin macrocytosis. *Blood* **14**:694–707, 1959.

163. Brody, E. A., Estren, S., and Wasserman, L. R.: Treatment of pernicious anemia by oral administration of vitamin B_{12} without added intrinsic factor. *New Eng J Med* **260**:361–67, 1959.

164. Buchanan, J. M.: The function of vitamin B_{12} and folic acid coenzymes in mammalian cells. *Medicine* (Balt) **43**:697–709, 1964.

165. Callender, S. T., and Denborough, M. A.: A family study of pernicious anaemia. *Brit J Haemat* **3**:88–106, 1957.

166. Callender, S. T., Retief, F. P., and Witts, L. J.: The augmented histamine test with special reference to achlorhydria. *Gut* **1**:326–36, 1960.

167. Castle, W. B.: Present status of the etiology of pernicious anemia. *Ann Intern Med* **34**:1093–1106, 1951.

168. Castle, W. B.: Development of knowledge concerning the gastric intrinsic factor and its relation to pernicious anemia. *New Eng J Med* **249**:603–14, 1953.

169. Castle, W. B.: Factors involved in the absorption of vitamin B_{12}. *Gastroenterology* **37**:377–84, 1959.

170. Chanarin, I., Dacie, J. V., and Mollin, D. L.: Folic-acid deficiency in haemolytic anaemia. *Brit J Haemat* **5**:245–56, 1959.

171. Chanarin, I., MacGibbon, B. M., O'Sullivan, W. J., and Mollin, D. L.: Folic-acid deficiency in pregnancy. The pathogenesis of megaloblastic anaemia of pregnancy. *Lancet* **2**:634–39, 1959.

172. Chazan, J. A., and Mistilis, S. P.: The pathophysiology of scurvy. *Amer J Med* **34**:350–58, 1963.

173. Cooper, B. A., and Castle, W. B.: Sequential mechanisms in the enhanced absorption of vitamin B_{12} by intrinsic factor in the rat. *J Clin Invest* **39**:199–214, 1960.

174. Doniach, D., Roitt, I. M., and Taylor, K. B.: Autoimmune phenomena in pernicious anemia. *Brit Med J* **1**:1374–79, 1963.

175. Fallon, H. J., Lotz, M., and Smith, L. H., Jr.: Congenital orotic aciduria: demonstration of an enzyme defect in leukocytes and comparison with drug-induced orotic aciduria. *Blood* **20**:700–9, 1962.

176. Finch, C. A., Coleman, D. H., Motulsky, A. G., Donohue, D. M., and Reiff, R. H.: Erythrokinetics in pernicious anemia. *Blood* **11**:807–20, 1956.

177. Flexner, J. M., and Hartmann, R. C.: Megaloblastic anemia associated with anticonvulsant drugs. *Amer J Med* **28**:386–96, 1960.

178. Gardner, F. H.: Tropical sprue. *New Eng J Med* **258**:791–96; 835–42, 1958.

179. Gatenby, P. B. B., and Lillie, E. W.: Clinical analysis of 100 cases of severe megaloblastic anaemia of pregnancy. *Brit Med J* **2**:1111–14, 1960.

180. Girdwood, R. H.: The megaloblastic anaemias. Their investigation and classification. *Quart J Med* **25**:87–119, 1956.

181. Girdwood, R. H.: The role of folic acid in the blood disorders. *Brit Med Bull* **15**:14–18, 1959.

182. Glass, G. B. J., and Boyd, L. J.: Differentiation of macrocytic anemias and diagnosis of pernicious anemia and sprue in remission by accelerated measurement of hepatic uptake of radioactive $Co^{60}B_{12}$. *Ann Intern Med* **47**:274–92, 1957.

183. Goldhamer, S. M., Bethell, F. H., Isaacs, R., and Sturgis, C. C.: The occurrence and treatment of neurologic changes in pernicious anemia. *JAMA* **103**:1663–67, 1934.

184. Gräsbeck, R.: Physiology and pathology of vitamin B_{12} absorption, distribution, and excretion. *Advances Clin Chem* **3**:299–366, 1960.

185. Hamilton, H. E., Sheets, R. F., and DeGowin, E. L.: Studies with in-agglutinable erythrocyte counts. VII. Further investigation of the hemolytic mechanism in untreated pernicious anemia and the demonstration of a hemolytic property in the plasma. *J Lab Clin Med* **51**:942–55, 1958.

186. Hansen, H. A., and Weinfeld, A.: Metabolic effects and diagnostic value of small doses of folic acid and B_{12} in megaloblastic anemias. *Acta Med Scand* **172**:427–43, 1962.

187. Harris, J. W.: *The Red Cell. Production, Metabolism, Destruction: Normal and Abnormal.* Cambridge: Harvard University Press, 1963, pp. 146–94.

188. Hawkins, C. F., and Meynell, M. J.: Macrocytosis and macrocytic anaemia caused by anticonvulsant drugs. *Quart J Med* **27**:45–63, 1958.

189. Herbert, V.: *The Megaloblastic Anemias.* New York: Grune and Stratton, 1959, 162 p.

190. Herbert, V.: Current concepts in therapy: megaloblastic anemia. *New Eng J Med* **268**:201–3; 368–71, 1963.

191. Herbert, V., and Castle, W. B.: Intrinsic factor. *New Eng J Med* **270**:1181–85, 1964.

192. Huguley, C. M., Jr., Bain, J. A., Rivers, S. L., and Scoggins, R. B.: Refractory megaloblastic anemia associated with excretion of orotic acid. *Blood* **14**:615–34, 1959.

192a. Jeffries, G. H., and Sleisenger, M. H.: Studies of parietal cell antibody in pernicious anemia. *J Clin Invest* **44**:2021–28, 1965.

193. Johns, D. G., Sperti, S., and Burgen, A. S. V.: The metabolism of tritiated folic acid in man. *J Clin Invest* **40**:1684–95, 1961.

194. Klipstein, F. A.: Subnormal serum folate and macrocytosis associated with anticonvulsant drug therapy. *Blood* **23**:68–86, 1964.

195. Lambert, H. P., Prankerd, T. A. J., and Smellie, J. M.: Pernicious anaemia in childhood. A report of two cases in one family and their relationship to the aetiology of pernicious anaemia. *Quart J Med* **30**:71–90, 1961.

196. Leiken, S. L.: Pernicious anemia in childhood. *Pediatrics* **25**:91–100, 1960.

197. Lowenstein, L., Pick, C., and Philpott, N.: Megaloblastic anemia of pregnancy and the puerperium. *Amer J Obstet Gynec* **70**:1309–37, 1955.

198. Luhby, A. L., Cooperman, J. M., and Teller, D. N.: Urinary excretion of formiminoglutamic acid. Application in diagnosis of clinical folic acid deficiency. *Amer J Clin Nutr* **7**:397–406, 1959.

199. MacLean, L. D., and Sundberg, R. D.: Incidence of megaloblastic anemia after total gastrectomy. *New Eng J Med* **254**:885–93, 1956.

200. McIntyre, O. R., Sullivan, L. W., Jeffries, G. H., and Silver, R. H.: Pernicious anemia in childhood. *New Eng J Med* **272**:981–86, 1965.

201. McIntyre, P. A., Hahn, R., Conley, C. L., and Glass, B.: Genetic factors in predisposition to pernicious anemia. *Bull Hopkins Hosp* **104**:309–42, 1959.

202. McIntyre, P. A., Hahn, R., Masters, J. M., and Krevans, J. R.: Treatment of pernicious anemia with orally administered cyanocobalamin (vitamin B_{12}). *Arch Intern Med* (Chicago) **106**:280–92, 1960.

203. Mollin, D. L.: Radioactive vitamin B_{12} in the study of blood diseases. *Brit Med Bull* **15**:8–13, 1959.

204. Mollin, D. L.: The megaloblastic anemias. *Ann Rev Med* **11**:333–52, 1960.

205. Nieweg, H. O., Faber, J. G., deVries, J. A., and Stenfert Kroese, W. F.: The relationship of vitamin B_{12} and folic acid in megaloblastic anemias. *J Lab Clin Med* **44**:118–32, 1954.

206. O'Brien, J. S.: The role of the folate coenzymes in cellular division. A review. *Cancer Res* **22**:267–81, 1962.

207. Reisner, E. H., Jr.: The nature and significance of megaloblastic blood formation. *Blood* **13**:313–38, 1958.

208. Richmond, J., and Davidson, S.: Subacute combined degeneration of the spinal cord in non-Addisonian megaloblastic anaemia. *Quart J Med* **27**:517–31, 1958.

209. Scudamore, H. H., Thompson, J. H., Jr., and Owen, C. A., Jr.: Absorption of Co^{60}-labeled vitamin B_{12} in man and uptake by parasites, including *Diphyllobothrium latum*. *J Lab Clin Med* **57**:240–46, 1961.

210. Sheehy, T. W., and Berman, A.: The anemia of cirrhosis. *J Lab Clin Med* **56**:72–82, 1960.

211. Sheehy, T. W., Santini, R., Jr., Guerra, R., Angel, R., and Plough, I. C.: Tritiated folic acid as a diagnostic aid in folic acid deficiency. *J Lab Clin Med* **61**:650–59, 1963.

212. Smith, A. D. M.: Megaloblastic madness. *Brit Med J* **2**:1840–45, 1960.

213. Taylor, K. B., Roitt, I. M., Doniach, D., Couchman, K. G., and Shapland, C.: Autoimmune phenomena in pernicious anaemia: gastric antibodies. *Brit Med J* **2**:1347–52, 1962.

214. Victor, M., and Lear, A. A.: Subacute combined degeneration of the spinal cord. Current concepts of the disease process. Value of serum vitamin B_{12} determinations in clarifying some of the common clinical problems. *Amer J Med* **20**:896–911, 1956.

215. Waife, S. O., Jansen, C. J., Jr., Crabtree, R. E., Grinnan, E. L., and Fouts, R. J.: Oral vitamin B_{12} without intrinsic factor in the treatment of pernicious anemia *Ann Intern Med* **58**:810–17, 1963.

216. Weissbach, H., and Dickerman, H.: Biochemical role of vitamin B_{12}. *Physiol Rev* **45**:80–97, 1965.

217. Wells, R.: Nutritional vitamin B_{12} deficiency. *J Trop Med Hyg* **61**:81–92, 1958.

218. Will, J. J., Mueller, J. F., Brodine, C., Kiely, C. E., Friedman, B., Hawkins, V. R., Dutra, J., and Vilter, R. W.: Folic acid and vitamin B_{12} in pernicious anemia. Studies on patients treated with these substances over a ten-year period. *J Lab Clin Med* **53**:22–38, 1959.

219. Williams, A. W., Coghill, N. F., and Edwards, F.: The gastric mucosa in pernicious anaemia: biopsy studies. *Brit J Haemat* **4**:457–64, 1958.

220. Wilson, T. H.: Intestinal absorption of vitamin B_{12}. *Physiologist* **6**:11–26, 1963.

221. Wintrobe, M. M.: The search for an experimental counterpart of pernicious anemia. *Arch Intern Med* (Chicago) **100**:862–69, 1957.

222. Zamcheck, N., Grable, E., Ley, A., and Norman, L.: Occurrence of gastric cancer among patients with pernicious anemia at the Boston City Hospital. *New Eng J Med* **252**:1103–10, 1955.

Hypoplastic Anemias

223. Dawson, J. P.: Congenital pancytopenia associated with multiple congenital anomalies (Fanconi type). Review of the literature and report of a twenty-year-old female with a ten-year follow-up and apparently good response to splenectomy. *Pediatrics* **15**:325–33, 1955.

224. Diamond, L. K., Allen, D. M., and Magill, F. B.: Congenital (erythroid) hypoplastic anemia. A 25-year study. *Amer J Dis Child* **102**:403–15, 1961.

225. Ferrebee, J. W., and Thomas, E. D.: Transplantation of marrow in man. *Arch Intern Med* (Chicago) **106**:523–31, 1960.

226. Havard, C. W. H., and Scott, R. B.: Thymic tumour and erythroblastic aplasia. Report of three cases and a review of the syndrome. *Brit J Haemat* **6**:178–90, 1960.

227. Heaton, L. D., Crosby, W. H., and Cohen, A.: Splenectomy in the treatment of hypoplasia of the bone marrow with a report of twelve cases. *Ann Surg* **146**:637–60, 1957.

228. Hughes, D. W.: Acquired aplastic anaemia in childhood: a review of 22 cases. *Med J Aust* **2**:251–59, 1962.

229. Jacobs, E. M., Hutter, R. V. P., Pool, J. L., and Ley, A. B.: Benign thymoma and selective erythroid aplasia of the bone marrow. *Cancer* **12**:47–57, 1959.

230. Kumar, S., and Saraya, A. K.: Experimental production of bone marrow aplasia by immunologic means. *Acta Haemat* (Basel) **27**:306–20, 1962.

231. Mathé, G.: Application of hematopoietic cell grafts to the treatment of leukemias and allied diseases. A critical review. *Blood* **16**:1073–88, 1960.

232. Mohler, D. N., and Leavell, B. S.: Aplastic anemia: an analysis of 50 cases. *Ann Intern Med* **49**:326–62, 1958.

233. Osgood, E. E.: Drug induced hypoplastic anemias and related syndromes. *Ann Intern Med* **39**:1173–88, 1953.

234. Roland, A. S.: The syndrome of benign thymoma and primary aregenerative anemia. An analysis of forty-three cases. *Amer J Med Sci* **247**:719–31, 1964.

235. Rubin, D., Weisberger, A. S., Botti, R. E., and Storaasli, J. P.: Changes in iron metabolism in early chloramphenicol toxicity. *J Clin Invest* **37**:1286–92, 1958.

236. Saidi, P., Wallerstein, R. O., and Aggeler, P. M.: Effect of chloramphenicol on erythropoiesis. *J Lab Clin Med* **57**:247–56, 1961.

237. Schmid, J. R., Kiely, J. M., Harrison, E. G., Jr., Bayrd, E. D., and Pease, G. L.: Thymoma associated with pure red-cell agenesis. *Cancer* **18**:216–30, 1965.

238. Scott, J. L., Cartwright, G. E., and Wintrobe, M. M.: Acquired aplastic anemia: an analysis of thirty-nine cases and review of the pertinent literature. *Medicine* (Balt) **38**:119–72, 1959.

239. Shahidi, N. T., and Diamond, L. K.: Testosterone-induced remission in aplastic anemia of both acquired and congenital types. Further observations in 24 cases. *New Eng J Med* **264**:953–67, 1961.

240. Smith, C. H.: Hypoplastic and aplastic anemias of infancy and childhood: with a consideration of the syndrome of nonhemolytic anemia of the newborn. *J Pediat* **43**:457–82, 1953.

MYELOPHTHISIC ANEMIAS

241. Crocker, A. C., and Farber, S.: Niemann-Pick disease: a review of eighteen patients. *Medicine* (Balt) **37**:1–95, 1958.

242. Hyman, G. A.: A comparison of bone-marrow aspiration and skeletal roentgenograms in the diagnosis of metastatic carcinoma. *Cancer* **8**:576–81, 1955.

243. Jonsson, U., and Rundles, R. W.: Tumor metastases in bone marrow. *Blood* **6**:16–25, 1951.

244. Medoff, A. S., and Bayrd, E. D.: Gaucher's disease in 29 cases: hematologic complications and effect of splenectomy. *Ann Intern Med* **40**:481–92, 1954.

245. Pillers, E. M. K., Marks, J., and Mitchell, J. S.: The bone marrow in malignant disease. *Brit J Cancer* **10**:458–71, 1956.

246. Pisciotta, A. V.: Clinical and pathologic effects of space-occupying lesions of the bone marrow. *Amer J Clin Path* **20**:915–33, 1950.

247. Welsh, J. F., and MacKinney, C. C.: Experience with aspiration biopsies of the bone marrow in the diagnosis and prognosis of carcinoma of the prostate gland. *Amer J Clin Path* **41**:509–12, 1964.

Hereditary Hemoglobinopathies

248. Allison, A. C.: Genetic factors in resistance to malaria. *Ann NY Acad Sci* **91**:710–29, 1961.

249. Bannerman, R. M.: *Thalassemia. A Survey of Some Aspects.* New York: Grune and Stratton, 1961, 138 p.

250. Beaven, G. H., Ellis, M. J., and White, J. C.: Studies on human foetal haemoglobin. III. The hereditary haemoglobinopathies and thalassaemias. *Brit J Haemat* **7**:169–86, 1961.

251. Charache, S., and Conley, C. L.: Rate of sickling of red cells during deoxygenation of blood from persons with various sickling disorders. *Blood* **24**:25–48, 1964.

252. Chernoff, A. I.: The human hemoglobins in health and disease. *New Eng J Med* **253**:322–31; 365–74; 416–23, 1955.

253. Chernoff, A. I.: The hemoglobin D syndromes. *Blood* **13**:116–27, 1958.

254. Chernoff, A. I.: The distribution of the thalassemia gene: a historical review. *Blood* **14**:899–912, 1959.

255. Conley, C. L., Weatherall, D. J., Richardson, S. N., Shepard, M. K., and Charache, S.: Hereditary persistence of fetal hemoglobin: a study of 79 affected persons in 15 Negro families in Baltimore. *Blood* **21**:261–81, 1963.

256. Curtis, E. M.: Pregnancy in sickle cell anemia, sickle cell-hemoglobin C disease, and variants thereof. *Amer J Obstet Gynec* **77**:1312–23, 1959.

257. Dacie, J. V.: *The Hemolytic Anemias. Part 1. The Congenital Anemias.* New York: Grune and Stratton, 1960, pp. 200–330.

258. Diggs, L. W.: Sickle cell crises. *Amer J Clin Path* **44**:1–19, 1965.

259. Dittman, W. A., Haut, A., Wintrobe, M. M., and Cartwright, G. E.: Hemoglobin H associated with an uncommon variant of thalassemia trait. *Blood* **16**:975–83, 1960.

260. Gabuzda, T. G., Nathan, D. G., and Gardner, F. H.: Thalassemia trait. *New Eng J Med* **270**:1212–17, 1964.

261. Gerald, P. S.: Genetic determination of hemoglobin structure. *Medicine* (Balt) **43**:747–57, 1964.

262. Golding, J. S. R., MacIver, J. E., and Went, L. N.: The bone changes in sickle cell anaemia and its genetic variants. *J Bone Joint Surg* (Brit) **41-B**:711–18, 1959.

263. Goodman, G., von Sallmann, L., and Holland, M. G.: Ocular manifestations of sickle-cell disease. *Arch Ophthal* (Chicago) **58**:655–82, 1957.

264. Greer, M., and Schotland, D.: Abnormal hemoglobin as a cause of neurologic disease. *Neurology* (Minneap) **12**:114–23, 1962.

265. Harris, J. W.: *The Red Cell. Production, Metabolism, Destruction: Normal and Abnormal.* Cambridge: Harvard University Press, 1963, pp. 65–105.

266. Heller, P.: The molecular basis of the pathogenicity of abnormal hemoglobins. Some recent developments. (Analytical review.) *Blood* **25**:110–25, 1965.

267. Hill, R. J., Konigsberg, W., Guidotti, G., and Craig, L. C.: The structure of human hemoglobin. I. The separation of the α and β chains and their amino acid composition. *J Biol Chem* **237**:1549–54, 1962.

268. Ingram, V. M.: *The Hemoglobins in Genetics and Evolution.* New York: Columbia University Press, 1963, 165 p.

269. Itano, H. A., Bergren, W. R., and Sturgeon, P.: The abnormal human hemoglobins. *Medicine* (Balt) **35**:121–59, 1956.

270. Jensen, W. N.: The hemoglobinopathies. *DM* **1961**:3–39, Feb.

271. Kekwick, R. A., and Lehmann, H.: Sedimentation characteristics of the γ-chain haemoglobin (haemoglobin "Bart's"). *Nature* **187**:158, 1960.

272. Malamos, B., Belcher, E. H., Gyftaki, E., and Binopoulos, D.: Simultaneous radioactive tracer studies of erythropoiesis and red-cell destruction in thalassaemia. *Brit J Haemat* **7**:411–29, 1961.

273. McCormick, W. F.: Abnormal hemoglobins. II. The pathology of sickle cell trait. *Amer J Med Sci* **241**:329–35, 1961.

274. McCurdy, P. R.: Erythrokinetics in abnormal hemoglobin syndromes. *Blood* **20**:686–99, 1962.

275. Motulsky, A. G.: Controller genes in synthesis of human haemoglobin. *Nature* **194**:607–9, 1962.

276. Nance, W. E.: Genetic control of hemoglobin synthesis. Thalassemia and related disorders may be explained by known properties of regions of genetic duplication. *Science* **141**:123–30, 1963.

277. Neel, J. V.: Human hemoglobin types. Their epidemiologic implications. *New Eng J Med* **256**:161–71, 1957.

278. Perillie, P. E., and Epstein, F. H.: Sickling phenomenon produced by hypertonic solutions: a possible explanation for the hyposthenuria of sicklemia. *J Clin Invest* **42**:570–80, 1963.

279. Pierce, L. E., and Rath, C. E.: Evidence for folic acid deficiency in the genesis of anemic sickle cell crisis. *Blood* **20**:19–32, 1962.

280. River, G. L., Robbins, A. B., and Schwartz, S. O.: S-C hemoglobin: a clinical study. *Blood* **18**:385–416, 1961.

281. Schlitt, L. E., and Keitel, H. G.: Renal manifestations of sickle cell disease: a review. *Amer J Med Sci* **239**:773–78, 1960.

282. Schweet, R. S.: Studies on hemoglobin synthesis. *Medicine* (Balt) **43**:731–45, 1964.

283. Smith, C. H., Erlandson, M. E., Stern, G., and Schulman, I.: The role of splenectomy in the management of thalassemia. *Blood* **15**:197–211, 1960.

284. Smith, E. W., and Krevans, J. R.: Clinical manifestations of hemoglobin C disorders. *Bull Hopkins Hosp* **104**:17–43, 1959.

285. Sturgeon, P., and Finch, C. A.: Erythrokinetics in Cooley's anemia. *Blood* **12**:64–73, 1957.

286. The thalassemia syndromes. Biochemical, genetic and clinical considerations. *Amer J Med* **36**:919–35, 1964.

287. Vavra, J. D., Mayer, V. K., and Moore, C. V.: *In vitro* heme synthesis by human blood: abnormal heme synthesis in thalassemia major. *J Lab Clin Med* **63**:736–53, 1964.

288. Weatherall, D. J.: Abnormal haemoglobins in the neonatal period and their relationship to thalassemia. *Brit J Haemat* **9**:265–77, 1963.

289. Zuelzer, W. W., Robinson, A. R., and Booker, C. R.: Reciprocal relationship of hemoglobins A_2 and F in beta chain thalassemias, a key to the genetic control of hemoglobin F. *Blood* **17**:393–408, 1961.

SECONDARY ANEMIAS OF UNKNOWN CAUSE

290. Bingham, J.: The macrocytosis of hepatic disease. I. Thin macrocytosis. *Blood* **14**:694–707, 1959.

291. Cartwright, G. E., and Wintrobe, M. M.: The anemia of infection. XVII. A review. *Advances Int Med* **5**:165–226, 1952.

292. Cawein, M. J., Hagedorn, A. B., and Owen, C. A., Jr.: Anemia of hepatic disease studied with radiochromium. *Gastroenterology* **38**:324–31, 1960.

293. Freireich, E. J., Ross, J. F., Bayles, T. B., Emerson, C. P., and Finch, S. C.: Radioactive iron metabolism and erythrocyte survival studies of the mechanism of the anemia associated with rheumatoid arthritis. *J Clin Invest* **36**:1043–58, 1957.

294. Gallagher, N. I., McCarthy, J. M., and Lange, R. D.: Observations on erythropoietic-stimulating factor (ESF) in the plasma of uremic and non-uremic anemic patients. *Ann Intern Med* **52**:1201–12, 1960.

295. Kimber, C., Deller, D. J., Ibbotson, R. N., and Lander, H.: The mechanism of anemia in chronic liver disease. *Quart J Med* **34**:33–61, 1965.

296. Kurtides, E. S., Rambach, W. A., Alt, H. L., and Del Greco, F.: Effect of hemodialysis on erythrokinetics in anemia of uremia. *J Lab Clin Med* **63**:469–79, 1964.

297. Loge, J. P., Lange, R. D., and Moore, C. V.: Characterization of the anemia associated with chronic renal insufficiency. *Amer J Med* **24**:4–18, 1958.

298. Miller, A., Chodos, R. B., Emerson, C. P., and Ross, J. F.: Studies of the anemia and iron metabolism in cancer. *J Clin Invest* **35**:1248–62, 1956.

299. Naets, J. P., and Heuse, A. F.: Measurement of erythropoietic stimulating factor in anemic patients with or without renal disease. *J Lab Clin Med* **60**:365–74, 1962.

300. Parsons, W. B., Jr., Cooper, T., and Scheifley, C. H.: Anemia in bacterial endocarditis. *JAMA* **153**:14–16, 1953.

Chapter 6. Polycythemia

301. Abraham, J. P., Ulutin, O. N., Johnson, S. A., and Caldwell, M. J.: A study of the defects in the blood coagulation mechanisms in polycythemia vera. *Amer J Clin Path* **36**:7–15, 1961.

302. Bodansky, O.: Methemoglobinemia and methemoglobin-producing compounds. *Pharmacol Rev* **3**:144–96, 1951.

303. Burwell, C. S., Robin, E. D., Whaley, R. D., and Bickelmann, A. G.: Extreme obesity associated with alveolar hypoventilation—a Pickwickian syndrome. *Amer J Med* **21**:811–18, 1956.

304. Calabresi, P., and Meyer, O. O.: Polycythemia vera. I. Clinical and laboratory manifestations. II. Course and therapy. *Ann Intern Med* **50**:1182–1216, 1959.

305. Dameshek, W.: Physiopathology and course of polycythemia vera as related to therapy. *JAMA* **142**:790–97, 1950.

306. Damon, A., and Holub, A.: Host factors in polycythemia vera. *Ann Intern Med* **49**:43–60, 1958.

307. Donati, R. M., McCarthy, J. M., Lange, R. D., and Gallagher, N. I.: Erythrocythemia and neoplastic tumors. *Ann Intern Med* **58**:47–55, 1963.

308. Escobar, M. A., and Trobaugh, F. E., Jr.: Erythrocythemia. *Med Clin N Amer* **42**:253–76, 1962.

309. Finch, C. A.: Methemoglobinemia and sulfhemoglobinemia. *New Eng J Med* **239**:470–78, 1948.

310. Forssell, J.: Nephrogenous polycythaemia. *Acta Med Scand* **161**:169–79, 1958.

311. Garrett, M.: Polycythaemia vera. *Irish J Med Sci* **413**:224–36, 1960.

312. Goll, K. H.: Über die pathogenese der polycythämia vera. *Folia Haemat* (Leipzig) **77**:1–25, 1960.

313. Harrop, G. A., Jr.: Polycythemia. *Medicine* (Balt) **7**:291–344, 1928.

314. Haynal, E., and Gráf, F.: The rôle of the hypophyseal-hypothalamic system in the pathogenesis of erythraemia and symptomatic polycythaemias. *Acta Med Scand* **139**:61–77, 1950.

315. Hertko, E. J.: Polycythemia (erythrocytosis) associated with uterine fibroids and apparent surgical cure. *Amer J Med* **34**:288–93, 1963.

316. Huff, R. L., Hennessy, T. G., Austin, R. E., Garcia, J. F., Roberts, B. M.,

and Lawrence, J. H.: Plasma and red cell iron turnover in normal subjects and in patients having various hematopoietic disorders. *J Clin Invest* 29:1041–52, 1950.

317. Hurtado, A.: Some clinical aspects of life at high altitudes. *Ann Intern Med* 53:247–58, 1960.

318. Jaworski, Z. F., and Hirte, W. E.: Polycythemia (erythrocytosis) and non-neoplastic renal disease. Report of a case and review of the literature. *Canad Med Ass J* 84: 1421–27, 1961.

319. Kiely, J. M., Stroebel, C. F., Hanlon, D. G., and Owen, C. A., Jr.: Clinical value of plasma-iron turnover rate in diagnosis and management of polycythemia. *J Nucl Med* 2:1–7, 1961.

320. Killmann, S., and Cronkite, E. P.: Treatment of polycythemia vera with myleran. *Amer J Med Sci* 241:218–24, 1961.

321. Lawrence, J. H.: *Polycythemia: Physiology, Diagnosis and Treatment Based on 303 Cases.* New York: Grune and Stratton, 1955, 136 p.

322. Lawrence, J. H., and Berlin, N. I.: Relative polycythemia—the polycythemia of stress. *Yale J Biol Med* 24:498–505, 1952.

323. Ledlie, E. M.: The incidence of leukaemia in patients with polycythaemia vera treated by ^{32}P. *Clin Radiol* 11:130–33, 1960.

324. Linman, J. W., and Bethell, F. H.: *Factors Controlling Erythropoiesis.* Springfield, Ill.: Charles C Thomas, 1960, 208 p.

325. Linman, J. W., and Pierre, R. V.: Studies on thrombopoiesis. III. Thrombocytosis-promoting effects of "thrombocythemic" and "polycythemic" plasmas. *J Lab Clin Med* 62:374–84, 1963.

326. Lynch, E. C.: Uric acid metabolism in proliferative diseases of the marrow. *Arch Intern Med* (Chicago) 109:639–53, 1962.

327. Mack, I., and Snider, G. L.: Respiratory insufficiency and chronic cor pulmonale. *Circulation* 13:419–47, 1956.

328. Masouredis, S. P., and Lawrence, J. H.: The problem of leukemia in polycythemia vera. *Amer J Med Sci* 233:268–74, 1957.

329. Merino, C. F.: Studies on blood formation and destruction in the polycythemia of high altitude. *Blood* 5:1–31, 1950.

330. Mitus, W. J., Mednicoff, I. B., and Dameshek, W.: Alkaline phosphatase of mature neutrophils in various "polycythemias." *New Eng J Med* 260:1131–33, 1959.

330a. Modan, B., and Lilienfeld, A. M.: Polycythemia vera and leukemia— the role of radiation treatment. A study of 1222 patients. *Medicine* (Balt) 44:305–44, 1965.

330b. Osgood, E. E.: Polycythemia vera: age relationships and survival. *Blood* 26:243–56, 1965.

331. Pike, G. M.: Polycythemia vera. *New Eng J Med* 258:1250–55; 1297–1300, 1958.

332. Reinhard, E. H., and Hahneman, B.: The treatment of polycythemia vera. *J Chronic Dis* 6:332–46, 1957.

333. Reynafarje, C.: The influence of high altitude on erythropoietic activity. In *Brookhaven Symposia in Biology, Homeostatic Mechanisms,* 1958, pp. 132–46.

334. Rigby, P. G., and Leavell, B. S.: Polycythemia vera. A review of fifty cases with emphasis on the risk of surgery. *Arch Intern Med* (Chicago) **106**:622–27, 1960.

335. Schwartz, S. O., and Ehrlich, L.: The relationship of polycythemia vera to leukemia; a critical review. *Acta Haemat* (Basel) **4**:129–47, 1950.

336. Shaw, D. B., and Simpson, T.: Polycythaemia in emphysema. *Quart J Med* **30**:135–52, 1961.

337. Starr, G. F., Stroebel, C. F., Jr., and Kearns, T. P.: Polycythemia with papilledema and infratentorial vascular tumors. *Ann Intern Med* **48**:978–86, 1958.

338. Stroebel, C. F., and Fowler, W. S.: Secondary polycythemia. *Med Clin N Amer* **40**:1061–76, 1956.

339. Szur, L., Lewis, S. M., and Goolden, A. W. G.: Polycythaemia vera and its treatment with radioactive phosphorus. A review of 90 cases. *Quart J Med* **28**:397–424, 1959.

340. Talbott, J. H.: Gout and blood dyscrasias. *Medicine* (Balt) **38**:173–205, 1959.

341. Valentine, W. N., Beck, W. S., Follette, J. H., Mills, H., and Lawrence, J. S.: Biochemical studies in chronic myelocytic leukemia, polycythemia vera and other idiopathic myeloproliferative disorders. *Blood* **7**:959–77, 1952.

342. Waldmann, T. A., Levin, E. H., and Baldwin, M.: The association of polycythemia with a cerebellar hemangioblastoma. *Amer J Med* **31**:318–24, 1961.

343. Wasserman, L. R., and Bassen, F.: Polycythemia. *J Mount Sinai Hosp NY* **26**:1–49, 1959.

344. Wasserman, L. R., and Gilbert, H. S.: Surgery in polycythemia vera. *New Eng J Med* **269**:1226–30, 1963.

345. Ways, P., Huff, J. W., Kosmaler, C. H., and Young, L. E.: Polycythemia and histologically proven renal disease. *Arch Intern Med* (Chicago) **107**:154–62, 1961.

346. Wiseman, B. K., Rohn, R. J., Bouroncle, B. A., and Myers, W. G.: The treatment of polycythemia vera with radioactive phosphorus. *Ann Intern Med* **34**:311–30, 1951.

347. Yu, T. F., Weissmann, B., Sharney, L., Kupper, S., and Gutman, A. B.: On the biosynthesis of uric acid from glycine-N^{15} in primary and secondary polycythemia. *Amer J Med* **21**:901–17, 1956.

Chapter 7. Leukocyte Responses

348. Athens, J. W., Raab, S. O., Haab, O. P., Mauer, A. M., Ashenbrucker, H., Cartwright, G. E., and Wintrobe, M. M.: Leukokinetic studies. III. The distribution of granulocytes in the blood of normal subjects. *J Clin Invest* **40**:159–64, 1961.

349. Becker, F. T., Coventry, W. D., and Tuura, J. L.: Recurrent oral and cutaneous infections associated with cyclic neutropenia. *Arch Derm* (Chicago) **80**:731–41, 1959.

350. Bender, C. E.: Interpretation of hematologic and serologic findings in the diagnosis of infectious mononucleosis. *Ann Intern Med* **49**:852–65, 1958.

351. Bernstein, A.: Infectious mononucleosis. *Medicine* (Balt) **19**:85–159, 1940.

352. Bernstein, T. C., and Wolff, H. G.: Involvement of the nervous system in infectious mononucleosis. *Ann Intern Med* **33**:1120–38, 1950.

353. Brittingham, T. E., and Chaplin, H., Jr.: The antigenicity of normal and leukemic human leukocytes. *Blood* **17**:139–65, 1961.

354. Calabresi, P., Edwards, E. A., and Schilling, R. F.: Fluorescent antiglobulin studies in leukopenic and related disorders. *J Clin Invest* **38**:2091–2100, 1959.

355. Craddock, C. G., Jr., Perry, S., and Lawrence, J. S.: The dynamics of leukopenia and leukocytosis. *Ann Intern Med* **52**:281–94, 1960.

356. Custer, R. P., and Smith, E. B.: The pathology of infectious mononucleosis. *Blood* **3**:830–57, 1948.

357. Daland, G. A., Gottlieb, L., Wallerstein, R. O., and Castle, W. B.: Hematologic observations in bacterial endocarditis. Especially the prevalence of histiocytes and the elevation and variation of the white cell count in blood from the ear lobe. *J Lab Clin Med* **48**:827–45, 1956.

358. Davidsohn, I., and Lee, C. L.: The laboratory in the diagnosis of infectious mononucleosis. With additional notes on epidemiology, etiology and pathogenesis. *Med Clin N Amer* **46**:225–44, 1962.

359. Davidsohn, I., and Lee, C. L.: Serologic diagnosis of infectious mononucleosis. A comparative study of five tests. *Amer J Clin Path* **41**:115–25, 1964.

360. Davidsohn, I., Stern, K., and Kashiwagi, C.: The differential test for infectious mononucleosis. *Amer J Clin Path* **21**:1101–13, 1951.

361. Efrati, P., and Jonas, W.: Chediak's anomaly of leukocytes in malignant lymphoma associated with leukemic manifestations: case report with necropsy. *Blood* **13**:1063–73, 1958.

362. Efrati, P., and Rozenszajn, L.: The morphology of buffy coat in normal human adults. *Blood* **16**:1012–19, 1960.

363. Erwin, W., Weber, R. W., and Manning, R. T.: Complications of infectious mononucleosis. *Amer J Med Sci* **238**:699–712, 1959.

364. Evans, A. S.: Infectious mononucleosis in University of Wisconsin students. Report of a five-year investigation. *Amer J Hyg* **71**:342–62, 1960.

365. Fredricks, R. E., and Moloney, W. C.: The basophilic granulocyte. *Blood* **14**:571–83, 1959.

366. Futterweit, W.: Serum alkaline phosphatase activity in infectious mononucleosis. A clinical study of fifty-five cases. *Arch Intern Med* (Chicago) **108**:253–68, 1961.

367. Gall, E. A., and Stout, H. A.: The histological lesion in lymph nodes in infectious mononucleosis. *Amer J Path* **16**:433–56, 1940.

368. Gavosto, F., Pileri, A., and Maraini, G.: Incorporation of thymidine labelled with tritium by circulating cells of infectious mononucleosis. *Nature* **183**:1691–92, 1959.

369. Ghaemi, A., and Seaman, A. J.: "Swiss cheese" nuclei—an incubation-induced lesion of infectious mononucleosis lymphocytes. *Amer J Clin Path* **39**:492–95, 1963.

370. Gelb, D., West, M., and Zimmerman, H. J.: Serum enzymes in disease. IX. Analysis of factors responsible for elevated values in infectious mononucleosis. *Amer J Med* **33**:249–61, 1962.

371. Hoagland, R. J.: The clinical manifestations of infectious mononucleosis. A report of two hundred cases. *Amer J Med Sci* **240**:21–29, 1960.

372. Hoagland, R. J.: False-positive serology in mononucleosis. *JAMA* **185**:783–85, 1963.

373. Holman, H. R., Deicher, H. R. G., and Kunkel, H. G.: The L. E. cell and the L. E. serum factors. *Bull NY Acad Med* **35**:409–18, 1959.

374. Houck, G. H.: Involvement of the heart in infectious mononucleosis. *Amer J Med* **14**:261–64, 1953.

375. Hovde, R. F., and Sundberg, R. D.: Granulomatous lesions in the bone marrow in infectious mononucleosis. A comparison of the changes in the bone marrow in infectious mononucleosis with those in brucellosis, tuberculosis, sarcoidosis and lymphatic leukemia. *Blood* **5**:209–32, 1950.

376. Jackson, J. F.: Histochemical identification of megakaryocytes from peripheral blood examined for tumor cells. *Cancer* **15**:259–62, 1962.

377. Kritzler, R. A., Terner, J. Y., Lindenbaum, J., Magidson, J., Williams, R., Preisig, R., and Phillips, G. B.: Chediak-Higashi syndrome. *Amer J Med* **36**:583–94, 1964.

378. Lawrence, J. S.: Leukopenia: its mechanism and therapy. *J Chronic Dis* **6**:351–64, 1957.

379. Leibowitz, S.: *Infectious Mononucleosis.* New York: Grune and Stratton, 1953, 163 p.

380. Litwins, J., and Leibowitz, S.: Abnormal lymphocytes ("virocytes") in virus diseases other than infectious mononucleosis. *Acta Haemat* (Basel) **5**:223–31, 1951.

381. Mason, W. R., Jr., and Adams, E. K.: Infectious mononucleosis. An analysis of 100 cases with particular attention to diagnosis, liver function tests and treatment of selected cases with prednisone. *Amer J Med Sci* **236**:447–59, 1958.

382. Miale, J. B.: *Laboratory Medicine—Hematology.* St. Louis: C. V. Mosby Company, 2nd Ed., 1962, pp. 593–626.

383. Nelson, R. S., and Darragh, J. H.: Infectious mononucleosis hepatitis. A clinicopathologic study. *Amer J Med* **21**:26–33, 1956.

384. Oski, F. A., Naiman, J. L., Allen, D. M., and Diamond, L. K.: Leukocytic inclusions—Döhle bodies—associated with platelet abnormality (the

May-Hegglin anomaly). Report of a family and review of the literature. *Blood* **20**:657–67, 1962.

385. Page, A. R., and Good, R. A.: Studies on cyclic neutropenia. A clinical and experimental investigation. *Amer J Dis Child* **94**:623–61, 1957.

386. Payne, R.: Leukocyte agglutinins in human sera. Correlation between blood transfusions and their development. *Arch Intern Med* (Chicago) **99**:587–606, 1957.

387. Payne, R., and Rolfs, M. R.: Fetomaternal leukocyte incompatibility. *J Clin Invest* **37**:1756–63, 1958.

388. Pisciotta, A. V., Ebbe, S., Lennon, E. J., Metzger, G. O., and Madison, F. W.: Agranulocytosis following administration of phenothiazine derivatives. *Amer J Med* **25**:210–23, 1958.

389. Raftery, M., Schumacher, E. E., Jr., Grain, G. O., and Quinn, E. L.: Infectious mononucleosis and the Guillain-Barré syndrome. Report of three cases. *Arch Intern Med* (Chicago) **93**:246–53, 1954.

390. Riley, H. D., Jr.: Acute infectious lymphocytosis. Report of two cases in the same family. *New Eng J Med* **248**:92–95, 1953.

391. Skendzel, L. P., and Hoffman, G. C.: The Pelger anomaly of leukocytes: forty-one cases in seven families. *Amer J Clin Path* **37**:294–301, 1962.

392. Smith, C. H.: Acute infectious lymphocytosis: a specific infection. *JAMA* **125**:342–49, 1944.

393. Smith, J. N., Jr.: Complications of infectious mononucleosis. *Ann Intern Med* **44**:861–73, 1956.

394. Southam, C. M., Goldsmith, Y., and Burchenal, J. H.: Heterophile antibodies and antigens in neoplastic diseases. *Cancer* **4**:1036–42, 1951.

395. Tanaka, K. R., Valentine, W. N., and Fredricks, R. E.: Diseases or clinical conditions associated with low leukocyte alkaline phosphatase. *New Eng J Med* **262**:912–18, 1960.

396. Tullis, J. L.: The role of leukocyte and platelet antibody tests in management of diverse clinical disorders. *Ann Intern Med* **54**:1165–80, 1961.

397. Walford, R. L.: *Leukocyte Antigens and Antibodies*. New York: Grune and Stratton, 1960, 182 p.

398. Wiseman, B. K.: The treatment of infectious mononucleosis. *J Chronic Dis* **6**:347–50, 1957.

399. Zarafonetis, C. J. D., Oster, H. L., and Colville, V. F.: Cold agglutination of sheep erythrocytes as a factor in false-positive heterophile agglutination tests. *J Lab Clin Med* **41**:906–12, 1953.

400. Zarafonetis, C. J. D., and Kent, J. F.: Serologic tests for syphilis in infectious mononucleosis. *J Lab Clin Med* **43**:253–58, 1954.

Chapter 8. Leukemia

401. Baldini, M., Fudenberg, H. H., Fukutake, K., and Dameshek, W.: The anemia of the Di Guglielmo syndrome. *Blood* **14**:334–63, 1959.

402. Bentley, H. P., Reardon, A. E., Knoedler, J. P., and Krivit, W.: Eosinophilic leukemia. Report of a case with review and classification. *Amer J Med* **30**:310–22, 1961.

403. Bethell, F. H.: The relative frequency of the several types of chronic leukemia and their management. *J Chronic Dis* **6**:403–20, 1957.

404. Block, M., and Jacobson, L. O.: Preleukemic acute human leukemia. *JAMA* **152**:1018-28, 1953.

405. Bluefarb, S. M.: *Leukemia Cutis.* Springfield, Ill.: Charles C Thomas, 1960, 489 p.

406. Boggs, D. R., Wintrobe, M. M., and Cartwright, G. E.: The acute leukemias. Analysis of 322 cases and review of the literature. *Medicine* (Balt) **41**:163–225, 1962.

407. Bouroncle, B. A., Wiseman, B. K., and Doan, C. A.: Leukemic reticuloendotheliosis. *Blood* **13**:609–30, 1958.

408. Brescia, M. A., Santora, E., and Sarnataro, V. F.: Congenital leukemia. *J Pediat* **55**:35–41, 1959.

409. Brill, A. B., Tomonaga, M., and Heyssel, R. M.: Leukemia in man following exposure to ionizing radiation. A summary of the findings in Hiroshima and Nagasaki, and a comparison with other human experience. *Ann Intern Med* **56**:590–609, 1962.

410. Bryan, W. R., Moloney, J. B., O'Connor, T. E., Fink, M. A., and Dalton, A. J.: Viral etiology of leukemia (Combined Clinical Staff Conference at the National Institutes of Health). *Ann Intern Med* **62**:376–99, 1965.

411. Burchenal, J. H., Murphy, M. L., and Tan, C. T. C.: Treatment of acute leukemia. *Pediatrics* **18**:643–60, 1956.

412. Burnet, M.: Leukemia as a problem in preventive medicine. *New Eng J Med* **259**:423–31, 1958.

413. Carbone, P. P., Tjio, J. H., Whang, J., Block, J. B., Kremer, W. B., and Frei, E., III: The effect of treatment in patients with chronic myelogenous leukemia. Hematologic and cytogenetic studies. *Ann Intern Med* **59**:622–28, 1963.

414. Chen, H. P., and Smith, H. S.: Eosinophilic leukemia. *Ann Intern Med* **52**:1343–52, 1960.

415. Chodos, R. B., and Ross, J. F.: The use of radioactive phosphorus in the therapy of leukemia, polycythemia vera and lymphomas: a report of 10 years' experience. *Ann Intern Med* **48**:956–77, 1958.

416. Clark, P. A., Hsia, Y. E., and Huntsman, R. G.: Toxic complications of treatment with 6-mercaptopurine. Two cases with hepatic necrosis and intestinal ulceration. *Brit Med J* **1**:393–95, 1960.

417. Court Brown, W. M., and Abbott, J. D.: The incidence of leukaemia in ankylosing spondylitis treated with x-rays. A preliminary report. *Lancet* **1**:1283–85, 1955.

418. Craddock, C. G., and Nakai, G. S.: Leukemic cell proliferation as determined by *in vitro* deoxyribonucleic acid synthesis. *J Clin Invest* **41**:360–69, 1962.

419. Cronkite, E. P., Moloney, W., and Bond, V. P.: Radiation leukemogenesis. An analysis of the problem. *Amer J Med* **28**:673–82, 1960.

420. Dameshek, W.: The outlook for the eventual control of leukemia. *New Eng J Med* **250**:131–39, 1954.

420a. Dameshek, W., Necheles, T. F., Finkel, H. E., and Allen, D. M.: Therapy of acute leukemia, 1965. *Blood* 26:220–25, 1965.

421. Dameshek, W., and Baldini, M.: The Di Guglielmo syndrome. *Blood* 13:192–94, 1958.

422. Dameshek, W., and Gunz, F.: *Leukemia.* New York: Grune and Stratton, 2nd Ed., 1964, 608 p.

423. Di Guglielmo, G.: Les maladies érythrémiques. *Rev Hemat* (Paris) 1:355–98, 1946.

424. Dittman, W. A., and Ward, J. R.: Demecolcine toxicity. A case report of severe hematopoietic toxicity and a review of the literature. *Amer J Med* 27:519–24, 1959.

425. Ebbe, S., Wittels, B., and Dameshek, W.: Autoimmune thrombocytopenic purpura ("ITP" type) with chronic lymphocytic leukemia. *Blood* 19:23–37, 1962.

426. Ellison, R. R., and Burchenal, J. H.: Therapy of acute leukemia in adults. *J Chronic Dis* 6:421–36, 1957.

427. Evans, T. S.: Monocytic leukemia (general review of the subject). *Medicine* (Balt) 21:421–56, 1942.

428. Fahey, J. L., and Boggs, D. R.: Serum protein changes in malignant diseases. I. The acute leukemias. *Blood* 16:1479–90, 1960.

429. Fernbach, D. J., Sutow, W. W., Thurman, W. G., and Vietti, T. J.: Clinical evaluation of cyclophosphamide. *JAMA* 182:30–37, 1962.

430. Ferrebee, J. W., and Thomas, E. D.: Transplantation of marrow in man. *Arch Intern Med* (Chicago) 106:523–31, 1960.

431. Field, J. B., and Williams, H. E.: Artifactual hypoglycemia associated with leukemia. *New Eng J Med* 265:946–48, 1961.

432. Fitzgerald, P. H., Adams, A., and Gunz, F.: Chronic granulocytic leukemia and the Philadelphia chromosome. *Blood* 21:183–96, 1963.

433. Freeman, J. A.: The ultrastructure and genesis of Auer bodies. *Blood* 15:449–65, 1960.

434. Frei, E., III, Freireich, E. J., Gehan, E., et al. (Acute Leukemia Group B): Studies of sequential and combination antimetabolite therapy in acute leukemia: 6-mercaptopurine and methotrexate. *Blood* 18:431–54, 1961.

435. Frenkel, E. P., and Meyers, M. C.: Acute leukemia and pregnancy. *Ann Intern Med* 53:656–71, 1960.

436. Friedman, B. I., Will, J. J., Freiman, D. G., and Braunstein, H.: Tissue mast cell leukemia. *Blood* 13:70–78, 1958.

437. Friend, C.: Immunological relationships of a filterable agent causing a leukemia in adult mice. I. The neutralization of infectivity by specific antiserum. *J Exp Med* 109:217–28, 1959.

438. Furth, J.: Recent studies on the etiology and nature of leukemia. *Blood* 6:964–75, 1951.

439. Galton, D. A. G., Wiltshaw, E., Szur, L., and Dacie, J. V.: The use of

chlorambucil and steroids in the treatment of chronic lymphocytic leukemia. *Brit J Haemat* **7**:73–98, 1961.

439a. Goh, K., and Swisher, S. N.: Identical twins and chronic myelocytic leukemia. Chromosomal studies of a patient with chronic myelocytic leukemia and his normal identical twin. *Arch Intern Med* (Chicago) **115**:475–78, 1965.

440. Gross, L.: Viral etiology of "spontaneous" mouse leukemia. A review. *Cancer Res* **18**:371–81, 1958.

441. Gunz, F. W., and Atkinson, H. R.: Medical radiations and leukaemia: a retrospective survey. *Brit Med J* **1**:389–93, 1964.

442. Gunz, F. W., and Fitzgerald, P. H.: Chromosomes and leukemia. *Blood* **23**:394–400, 1964.

443. Gunz, F. W., and Hough, R. F.: Acute leukemia over the age of fifty: a study of its incidence and natural history. *Blood* **11**:882–901, 1956.

444. Haurani, F. I., Repplinger, E., and Tocantins, L. M.: Attempts at transplantation of human bone marrow in patients with acute leukemia and other marrow depletion disorders. *Amer J Med* **28**:794–806, 1960.

445. Haut, A., Abbott, W. S., Wintrobe, M. M., and Cartwright, G. E.: Busulfan in the treatment of chronic myelocytic leukemia. The effect of long term intermittent therapy. *Blood* **17**:1–19, 1961.

446. Haut, A., Altman, S. J., Wintrobe, M. M., and Cartwright, G. E.: The influence of chemotherapy on survival in acute leukemia. Comparison of cases treated during 1954 to 1957 with those treated during 1947 to 1954. *Blood* **14**:828–47, 1959.

447. Haut, A., Wintrobe, M. M., and Cartwright, G. E.: The clinical management of leukemia. *Amer J Med* **28**:777–93, 1960.

448. Hayhoe, F. G. J.: *Leukemia. Research and Clinical Practice.* Boston: Little, Brown and Company, 1960, 335 p.

449. Heyssel, R., Brill, A. B., Woodbury, L. A., Nishimura, E. T., Ghose, T., Hoshino, T., and Yamasaki, M.: Leukemia in Hiroshima atomic bomb survivors. *Blood* **15**:313–31, 1960.

450. Hotchkiss, D. J., Jr., and Block, M. H.: Effect of splenic irradiation on systemic hematopoiesis. *Arch Intern Med* (Chicago) **109**:695–711, 1962.

451. Houghie, C.: The early diagnosis and natural history of chronic lymphatic leukemia. *Ann Intern Med* **45**:39–55, 1959.

452. Hunt, W. E., Bouroncle, B. A., and Meagher, J. N.: Neurologic complications of leukemias and lymphomas. *J Neurosurg* **16**:135–51, 1959.

453. Hyman, C. B., Bogle, J. M., Brubaker, C. A., Williams, K., and Hammond, D.: Central nervous system involvement by leukemia in children. I. Relationship to systemic leukemia and description of clinical and laboratory manifestations. *Blood* **25**:1–12, 1965.

454. Johnson, I. S., Armstrong, J. G., Gorman, M., and Burnett, J. P., Jr.: The vinca alkaloids: a new class of oncolytic agents. *Cancer Res* **23**:1390–1427, 1963.

455. Johnston, A. W.: The chromosomes in a child with mongolism and acute leukemia. *New Eng J Med* **264**:591–94, 1961.

456. Kaplan, H. S.: On the etiology and pathogenesis of the leukemias: a review. *Cancer Res* **14**:535–48, 1954.

457. Kiossoglou, K. A., Rosenbaum, E. H., Mitus, W. J., and Dameshek, W.: Multiple chromosomal aberrations in a patient with acute granulocytic leukemia associated with Down's syndrome and twinning. Study of a family with a possible tendency to nondisjunction. *Blood* **24**:134–59, 1964.

458. Klatte, E. C., Yardley, J., Smith, E. B., Rohn, R., and Campbell, J. A.: The pulmonary manifestations and complications of leukemia. *Amer J Roentgen* **89**:598–609, 1963.

459. Krakoff, I. H.: Mechanisms of drug action in leukemia. *Amer J Med* **28**:735–50, 1960.

460. Krakoff, I. H., and Meyer, R. L.: Prevention of hyperuricemia in leukemia and lymphoma. *JAMA* **193**:1–6, 1965.

461. Kritzler, R. A.: Anuria complicating the treatment of leukemia. *Amer J Med* **25**:532–38, 1958.

462. March, H. C.: Leukemia in radiologists, ten years later. *Amer J Med Sci* **242**:137–49, 1961.

463. Martin, W. J., and Bayrd, E. D.: Erythroleukemia, with special emphasis on the acute or incomplete variety. Report of five cases. *Blood* **9**:321–39, 1954.

464. Mathé, G.: Application of hematopoietic cell grafts to the treatment of leukemias and allied diseases. A critical review. *Blood* **16**:1073–88, 1960.

464a. Meyers, M. C., Hines, D. R., and Bishop, R. C.: Acute leukemia in adolescents and adults. Results of treatment over three consecutive 5-year periods. *Ann Intern Med* **63**:411–15, 1965.

465. Miller, D. G.: Patterns of immunological deficiency in lymphoma and leukemias. *Ann Intern Med* **57**:703–16, 1962.

466. Miller, D. G., Diamond, H. D., and Craver, L. F.: The clinical use of chlorambucil. *New Eng J Med* **261**:525–35, 1959.

467. Miller, R. W.: Radiation, chromosomes and viruses in the etiology of leukemia: evidence from epidemiologic research. *New Eng J Med* **271**:30–36, 1964.

468. Moertel, C. G., and Hagedorn, A. B.: Leukemia or lymphoma and coexistent primary malignant lesions: a review of the literature and a study of 120 cases. *Blood* **12**:788–803, 1957.

469. Moore, E. W., Thomas, L. B., Shaw, R. K., and Freireich, E. J.: The central nervous system in acute leukemia. *Arch Intern Med* (Chicago) **105**:451–68, 1960.

470. Nathan, D. G., and Berlin, N. I.: Studies of the rate of production and life span of erythrocytes in acute leukemia. *Blood* **14**:935–49, 1959.

470a. Nies, B. A., Thomas, L. B., and Freireich, E. J.: Meningeal leukemia. A follow-up study. *Cancer* **18**:546–53, 1965.

471. Norris, H. J., and Wiener, J.: The renal lesions in leukemia. *Amer J Med Sci* **241**:512–18, 1961.

472. Oliner, H., Schwartz, R., Rubio, F., and Dameshek, W.: Interstitial pulmonary fibrosis following busulfan therapy. *Amer J Med* **31**:134–39, 1961.

473. Osgood, E. E.: The threshold dose of P^{32} for leukemic cells of the lymphocytic and granulocytic series. *Blood* **16**:1104–21, 1960.

474. Osgood, E. E., and Seaman, A. J.: Treatment of chronic leukemias. Results of therapy by titrated, regularly spaced total body radioactive phosphorus, or roentgen irradiation. *JAMA* **150**:1372–79, 1955.

475. Page, A. R., Hansen, A. E., and Good, R. A.: Occurrence of leukemia and lymphoma in patients with agammaglobulinemia. *Blood* **21**:197–206, 1963.

476. Pearson, H. A., Grello, F. W., and Cone, T. E., Jr.: Leukemia in identical twins. *New Eng J Med* **268**:1151–56, 1963.

477. Pierce, M. I.: The acute leukemias of childhood. *Pediat Clin N Amer* **4**:497–530, 1957.

478. Pierce, M. I.: Leukemia in the newborn infant. *J Pediat* **54**:691–706, 1959.

479. Pisciotta, A. V., and Hirschboeck, J. S.: Therapeutic considerations in chronic lymphocytic leukemia. Special reference to the natural course of the disease. *Arch Intern Med* (Chicago) **99**:334–45, 1957.

480. Pisciotta, A. V., Jermain, L. F., and Hinz, J. E.: Chronic lymphocytic leukemia, hypogammaglobulinemia and autoimmune hemolytic anemia—an experiment of nature. *Blood* **15**:748–57, 1960.

481. Prolla, J. C., and Kirsner, J. B.: The gastrointestinal lesions and complications of the leukemias. *Ann Intern Med* **61**:1084–1103, 1964.

482. Quaglino, D., and Hayhoe, F. G. J.: Periodic-acid-Schiff positivity in erythroblasts with special reference to Di Guglielmo's disease. *Brit J Haemat* **6**:26–33, 1960.

483. Quattrin, N., Dini, E., and Palumbo, E.: Basophile leukämien, *Blut* **5**:166–87, 1959.

484. Raab, S. O., Hoeprich, P. D., Wintrobe, M. M., and Cartwright, G. E.: The clinical significance of fever in acute leukemia. *Blood* **16**:1609–28, 1960.

485. Reinhard, E. H., Neely, C. L., and Samples, D. M.: Radioactive phosphorus in the treatment of chronic leukemias: long-term results over a period of 15 years. *Ann Intern Med* **50**:942–58, 1959.

486. Roath, S., Israels, M. C. G., and Wilkinson, J. F.: The acute leukemias: a study of 580 patients. *Quart J Med* **33**:257–83, 1964.

487. Sandberg, A. A., Cartwright, G. E., and Wintrobe, M. M.: Studies on leukemia. I. Uric acid excretion. *Blood* **11**:154–66, 1956.

488. Sandberg, A. A., Ishihara, T., Crosswhite, L. H., and Hauschka, T. S.: Comparison of chromosome constitution in chronic myelocytic leukemia and other myeloproliferative disorders. *Blood* **20**:393–423, 1962.

489. Schwartz, D. L., Pierre, R. V., Scheerer, P. P., Reed, E. C., Jr., and Linman, J. W.: Lymphosarcoma cell leukemia. *Amer J Med* 38:778–86, 1965.

490. Schwartz, E. E., and Upton, A. C.: Factors influencing the incidence of leukemia: special consideration of the role of ionizing radiation. *Blood* 13:845–64, 1958.

491 Schwartz, S. O., and Critchlow, J.: Erythremic myelosis (Di Guglielmo's disease). Critical review with report of four cases, and comments on erythroleukemia. *Blood* 7:765–93, 1952.

492. Schwartz, S. O., and Schoolman, H. M.: The etiology of leukemia: the status of the virus as causative agent—a review. *Blood* 14:279–94, 1959.

493. Scott, R. B.: Leukaemia. *Lancet* 1:1053–58, 1957.

494. Shanbrom, E., and Miller, S.: Critical evaluation of massive steroid therapy of acute leukemia. *New Eng J Med* 266:1354–58, 1962.

495. Shaw, R. K., Boggs, D. R., Silberman, H. R., and Frei, E., III: A study of prednisone therapy in chronic lymphocytic leukemia. *Blood* 17:182–95, 1961.

496. Sinn, C. M., and Dick, F. W.: Monocytic leukemia. *Amer J Med* 20:588–602, 1956.

497. Smith, C. H.: *Blood Diseases of Infancy and Childhood.* St. Louis: C. V. Mosby Company, 1960, pp. 379–421.

498. Southam, C. M., Craver, L. F., Dargeon, H. W., and Burchenal, J. H.: A study of the natural history of acute leukemia with special reference to the duration of the disease and the occurrence of remissions. *Cancer* 4:39–59, 1951.

499. Steinberg, A. G.: The genetics of acute leukemia in children. *Cancer* 13:985–99, 1960.

500. Syverton, J. T., and Ross, J. D.: The virus theory of leukemia. *Amer J Med* 28:683–98, 1960.

501. Szweda, J. A., Abraham, J. P., Fine, G., Nixon, R. K., and Rupe, C. E.: Systemic mast cell disease. A review and report of three cases. *Amer J Med* 32:227–39, 1962.

502. Talbott, J. H.: Gout and blood dyscrasias. *Medicine* (Balt) 38:173–205, 1959.

503. Tartaglia, A. P., Scharfman, W. B., and Propp, S.: Splenic rupture in leukemia. *New Eng J Med* 267:31–33, 1962.

504. Thomas, E. D., Lochte, H. L., Jr., and Ferrebee, J. W.: Irradiation of the entire body and marrow transplantation: some observations and comments. *Blood* 14:1–23, 1959.

505. Tivey, H.: The prognosis for survival in chronic granulocytic and lymphocytic leukemia. *Amer J Roentgen* 72:68–93, 1954.

506. Tivey, H.: The natural history of untreated acute leukemia. *Ann NY Acad Sci* 60:322–58, 1954.

507. Tough, I. M., Court Brown, W. M., Baikie, A. G., Buckton, K. E., Harnden, D. G., Jacobs, P. A., King, M. J., and McBride, J. A.:

Cytogenetic studies in chronic myeloid leukaemia and acute leukaemia associated with mongolism. *Lancet* 1:411–17, 1961.

508. Troup, S. B., Swisher, S. N., and Young, L. E.: The anemia of leukemia. *Amer J Med* 28:751–63, 1960.

509. Valentine, W. N.: The metabolism of the leukemic leukocyte. *Amer J Med* 28:699–710, 1960.

510. Wasi, P., and Block, M.: The mechanism of anemia in untreated chronic lymphatic leukemia. *Blood* 17:597–609, 1961.

511. Weinstein, A. W., and Weinstein, E. D.: A chromosomal abnormality in acute myeloblastic leukemia. *New Eng J Med* 268:253–55, 1963.

512. Weintraub, L. R., Penner, J. A., and Meyers, M. C.: Acute uric acid nephropathy in leukemia. Report of a case treated with peritoneal dialysis. *Arch Intern Med* (Chicago) 113:111–14, 1964.

513. Wetherley-Mein, G., Epstein, I. S., Foster, W. D., and Grimes, A. J.: Mechanisms of anaemia in leukaemia. *Brit J Haemat* 4:281–91, 1958.

514. Woolley, D. W.: Antimetabolites. *Science* 129:615–21, 1959.

515. Xefteris, E., Mitus, W. J., Mednicoff, I. B., and Dameshek, W.: Leukocytic alkaline phosphatase in busulfan induced remissions of chronic granulocytic leukemia. *Blood* 18:202–6, 1961.

516. Zuelzer, W. W., and Flatz, G.: Acute childhood leukemia: a ten-year study. *Amer J Dis Child* 100:886–907, 1960.

Chapter 9. Lymphoma

517. Aisenberg, A. C.: Studies on delayed hypersensitivity in Hodgkin's disease. *J Clin Invest* 41:1964–70, 1962.

518. Aisenberg, A. C.: Hodgkin's disease—prognosis, treatment and etiologic and immunologic considerations. *New Eng J Med* 270:508–14; 617–22, 1964.

519. Arends, T., Coonrad, E. V., and Rundles, R. W.: Serum proteins in Hodgkin's disease and malignant lymphoma. *Amer J Med* 16:833–53, 1954.

520. Bayrd, E. D., Paulson, G. S., and Hargraves, M. M.: Hodgkin's specific cells in bone marrow aspirations. A brief review and report of two cases. *Blood* 9:46–56, 1954.

521. Berman, L.: Malignant lymphomas. Their classification and relation to leukemia. *Blood* 8:195–210, 1953.

522. Bethell, F. H., Andrews, G. A., Neligh, R. B., and Meyers, M. C.: Treatment of Hodgkin's disease with roentgen irradiation and nitrogen mustards. *Amer J Roentgen* 64:61–74, 1950.

523. Block, J. B., Edgcomb, J., Eisen, A., and Van Scott, E. J.: Mycosis fungoides. Natural history and aspects of its relationship to other malignant lymphomas. *Amer J Med* 34:228–35, 1963.

524. Bostick, W. L.: Evidence for the virus etiology of Hodgkin's disease. *Ann NY Acad Sci* 73:307–34, 1958.

525. Bouroncle, B. A., Old, J. W., Jr., and Vazques, A. G.: Pathogenesis of jaundice in Hodgkin's disease. *Arch Intern Med* (Chicago) **110**:872–83, 1962.

526: Brody, J. I., and Finch, S. C.: Candida-reacting antibody in the serum of patients with lymphomas and related disorders. *Blood* **15**:830–39, 1960.

527. Brody, J. I., and Finch, S. C.: Serum factors of acquired hemolytic anemia in leukemia and lymphoma. *J Clin Invest* **40**:181–87, 1961.

528. Burchenal, J. H., and Diamond, H. D.: Leukemia and lymphoma. *DM* 1958:3–60, Jan.

529. Conn, H. O., and the Medical Resident Staff of the Grace-New Haven Community Hospital (1955–1956): Alcohol-induced pain as a manifestation of Hodgkin's disease. An investigation of its specificity and frequency. *Arch Intern Med* (Chicago) **100**:241–47, 1957.

530. Cook, J. C., Krabbenhoft, K. L., and Leucutia, T.: Lymphosarcoma, reticulum cell sarcoma and giant follicular lymphoma. Long term results following radiation therapy. *Amer J Roentgen* **84**:656–65, 1960.

531. Dameshek, W., Weisfuse, L., and Stein, T.: Nitrogen mustard therapy in Hodgkin's disease. Analysis of fifty consecutive cases. *Blood* **4**:338–79, 1949.

532. Diwani, M., Gabr, M., Essawy, M., and Elwi, A.: Malignant lymphoma in childhood. *Arch Pediat* **77**:406–20, 1960.

533. Evans, T. S., and Doan, C. A.: Giant follicular hyperplasia: a study of its incidence, histopathologic variability, and the frequency of sarcoma and secondary hypersplenic complications. *Ann Intern Med* **40**:851–80, 1954.

534. Finkbeiner, J. A., Craver, L. F., and Diamond, H. D.: Prognostic signs in Hodgkin's disease. *JAMA* **156**:472–77, 1954.

535. Frenkel, R. S.: The history of Hodgkin's disease. *Univ Mich Med Bull* **25**:390–96, 1959.

536. Frost, J. W., Goldwein, M. I., and Bryan, J. A.: Clinical experience with vincaleukoblastine in far-advanced Hodgkin's disease and various malignant states. *Ann Intern Med* **56**:854–59, 1962.

537. Fucilla, I. S., and Hamann, A.: Hodgkin's disease in bone. *Radiology* **77**:53–60, 1961.

538. Goodman, L. S., and Gilman, A.: *The Pharmacological Basis of Therapeutics.* New York: The Macmillan Company, 3rd Ed., 1965, pp. 1345–57.

539. Hall, C. A., and Olson, K. B.: Therapy of the malignant lymphomas. I. A study of 116 cases. II. A review. *Amer J Med* **20**:392–411, 1956.

540. Hennessy, J. P., and Rottino, A.: Hodgkin's disease in pregnancy with a report of twelve cases. *Amer J Obstet Gynec* **63**:756–64, 1952.

541. Hoster, H. A., Dratman, M. B., Craver, L. F., and Rolnick, H. A.: Hodgkin's disease—1832–1947. *Cancer Res* **8**:1–78, 1948.

542. Hunt, W. E., Bouroncle, B. A., and Meagher, J. N.: Neurologic complications of leukemias and lymphomas. *J Neurosurg* **16**:135–51, 1959.

543. Hurst, D. W., and Meyer, O. O.: Giant follicular lymphoblastoma. *Cancer* **14**:753–78, 1961.

544. Jackson, H., Jr., and Parker, F., Jr.: Hodgkin's disease. I. General considerations. II. Pathology. III. Symptoms and course. *New Eng J Med* **230**:1–8, **231**:35–44; 639–46, 1944.

545. Jackson, H., Jr., and Parker, F., Jr.: *Hodgkin's Disease and Allied Disorders.* New York: Oxford University Press, 1947, 177 p.

546. James, A. H.: Hodgkin's disease with and without alcohol-induced pain: a clinical and histological comparison. *Quart J Med* **29**:47–66, 1960.

547. Karnofsky, D. A.: Summary of results obtained with nitrogen mustard in the treatment of neoplastic disease. *Ann NY Acad Sci* **68**:899–914, 1958.

548. Kofman, S., Perlia, C. P., Boesen, E., Eisenstein, R., and Taylor, S. G., III: The role of corticosteroids in the treatment of malignant lymphomas. *Cancer* **15**:338–45, 1962.

549. Kyle, R. A., Kiely, J. M., and Stickney, J. M.: Acquired hemolytic anemia in chronic lymphocytic leukemia and the lymphomas. Survival and response to therapy in twenty-seven cases. *Arch Intern Med* (Chicago) **104**:61–67, 1959.

550. Lacher, M. J.: Role of surgery in Hodgkin's disease. *New Eng J Med* **268**:289–92, 1963.

551. Levinson, B., Walter, B. A., Wintrobe, M. M., and Cartwright, G. E.: A clinical study in Hodgkin's disease. *Arch Intern Med* (Chicago) **99**:519–35, 1957.

552. Levitan, R., Diamond, H. D., and Craver, L. F.: Jaundice in Hodgkin's disease. *Amer J. Med* **30**:99–111, 1961.

553. Limarzi, L. R., and Paul, J. T.: Sternal marrow studies in Hodgkin's disease. A review of the literature and a report of thirty-five cases. *Amer J Clin Path* **19**:929–61, 1949.

554. Littman, M. L., and Zimmerman, L. E.: *Cryptococcosis. Torulosis or European Blastomycosis.* New York: Grune and Stratton, 1956, 205 p.

555. Louis, J.: Management of reticuloendothelial malignancies. *Med Clin N Amer* **46**:171–215, 1962.

556. Lucas, P. F.: Lymph node smears in the diagnosis of lymphadenopathy: a review. *Blood* **10**:1030–54, 1955.

557. Matthias, J. Q., Misiewicz, J. J., and Scott, R. B.: Cyclophosphamide in Hodgkin's disease and related disorders. *Brit Med J* **2**:1837–40, 1960.

558. Miller, D. G., Diamond, H. D., and Craver, L. F.: The clinical use of chlorambucil: a critical study. *New Eng J Med* **261**:525–35, 1959.

559. Moertel, C. G., and Hagedorn, A. B.: Leukemia or lymphoma and coexistent primary malignant lesions: a review of the literature and a study of 120 cases. *Blood* **12**:788–803, 1957.

560. Moore, R. D., Weisberger, A. S., and Bowerfind, E. S., Jr.: An evaluation of lymphadenopathy in systemic disease. *Arch Intern Med* (Chicago) **99**:751–59, 1957.

561. Moss, W. T.: *Therapeutic Radiology.* St. Louis: C. V. Mosby Company, 1959, pp. 325–36.

562. Onat, A., and Cooper, T.: Relation of bone marrow findings to serum protein changes in lymphosarcoma, chronic lymphocytic leukemia and Hodgkin's disease. *Blood* **15**:114–29, 1960.

563. Osgood, E. E.: Methods for analyzing survival data, illustrated by Hodgkin's disease. *Amer J Med* **24**:40–47, 1958.

564. Peters, M. V.: A study of survivals in Hodgkin's disease treated radiologically. *Amer J Roentgen* **63**:299–311, 1950.

565. Primikirios, N., Stutzman, L., and Sandberg, A. A.: Uric acid excretion in patients with malignant lymphomas. *Blood* **17**:701–18, 1961.

566. Razis, D. V., Diamond, H. D., and Craver, L. F.: Familial Hodgkin's disease: its significance and implications. *Ann Intern Med* **51**:933–71, 1959.

567. Razis, D. V., Diamond, H. D., and Craver, L. F.: Hodgkin's disease associated with other malignant tumors and certain non-neoplastic diseases. *Amer J Med Sci* **238**:327–35, 1959.

568. Rebuck, J. W.: The structure of the giant cells in the blood-forming organs. *J Lab Clin Med* **32**:660–99, 1947.

569. Reed, D. M.: On the pathological changes in Hodgkin's disease, with especial reference to its relation to tuberculosis. *Johns Hopkins Hosp Rep* **10**:133–96, 1902.

570. Richmond, J., Sherman, R. S., Diamond, H. D., and Craver, L. F.: Renal lesions associated with malignant lymphomas. *Amer J Med* **32**:184–207, 1962.

571. Rosenberg, S. A., Diamond, H. D., and Craver, L. F.: Lymphosarcoma: survival and the effects of therapy. *Amer J Roentgen* **85**:521–32, 1961.

572. Rosenberg, S. A., Diamond, H. D., Jaslowitz, B., and Craver, L. F.: Lymphosarcoma: a review of 1269 cases. *Medicine* (Balt) **40**:31–84, 1961.

573. Rosenthal, N., Dreskin, O. H., Vural, I. L., and Zak, F. G.: The significance of hematogones in blood, bone marrow and lymph node aspiration in giant follicular lymphoblastoma. *Acta Haemat* (Basel) **8**:368–77, 1952.

574. Rosenthal, M. C., Pisciotta, A. V., Komninos, Z. D., Goldenberg, H., and Dameshek, W.: The auto-immune hemolytic anemia of malignant lymphocytic disease. *Blood* **10**:197–227, 1955.

575. Schier, W. W., Roth, A., Ostroff, G., and Schrift, M. H.: Hodgkin's disease and immunity. *Amer J Med* **20**:94–99, 1956.

576. Shanbrom, E., Miller, S., and Haar, H.: Herpes zoster in hematologic neoplasias: some unusual manifestations. *Ann Intern Med* **53**:523–33, 1960.

577. Shimkin, M. B., Oppermann, K. C., Bostick, W. L., and Low-Beer, B. V. A.: Hodgkin's disease: an analysis of frequency, distribution and mortality at the University of California Hospital, 1914–1951. *Ann Intern Med* **42**:136–53, 1955.

578. Smith, D. F., and Klopp, C. T.: The value of surgical removal of localized lymphomas. *Surgery* **49**:469–76, 1961.

579. Smith, R. B. W., Sheehy, T. W., and Rothberg, H.: Hodgkin's disease and pregnancy. *Arch Intern Med* (Chicago) **102**:777–89, 1958.

580. Sokal, J. E., and Primikirios, N.: The delayed skin test response in Hodgkin's disease and lymphosarcoma. Effect of disease activity. *Cancer* **14**:597–607, 1961.

581. Steiner, P. E.: Hodgkin's disease. The incidence, distribution, nature and possible significance of the lymphogranulomatous lesions in the bone marrow. A review with original data. *Arch Path* (Chicago) **36**:627–37, 1943.

582. Sugarbaker, E. D., and Craver, L. F.: Lymphosarcoma. A study of 196 cases with biopsy. *JAMA* **115**:17–23; 112–17, 1940.

583. Ultmann, J. E., Koprowska, I., and Engle, R. L., Jr.: A cytological study of lymph node imprints. *Cancer* **11**:507–24, 1958.

584. Varadi, S.: Hodgkin's disease: specific findings in sternal puncture material. *Brit J Haemat* **1**:184–88, 1955.

585. Varadi, S.: Reed-Sternberg cells in the peripheral blood and bone-marrow in Hodgkin's disease. *Brit Med J* **1**:1239–43, 1960.

586. Wall, R. L., and Conrad, F. G.: Cyclophosphamide therapy. Its use in leukemia, lymphoma and solid tumors. *Arch Intern Med* (Chicago) **108**:456–82, 1961.

587. Williams, H. M., Diamond, H. D., and Craver, L. F.: The pathogenesis and management of neurological complications in patients with malignant lymphomas and leukemia. *Cancer* **11**:76–82, 1958.

588. Wiseman, B. K.: The blood pictures in the primary diseases of the lymphatic system. Their character and significance. *JAMA* **107**:2016–22, 1936.

Chapter 10. **Plasmacytic Myeloma**

589. Adams, W. S., Alling, E. L., and Lawrence, J. S.: Multiple myeloma. Its clinical and laboratory diagnosis with emphasis on electrophoretic abnormalities. *Amer J Med* **6**:141–61, 1949.

590. Adams, W. S., and Skoog, W. A.: The management of multiple myeloma. *J Chronic Dis* **6**:446–56, 1957.

591. Bantzel, C. J., Carbone, P. P., and Rosenberg, L.: The effect of prednisone on calcium metabolism and Ca^{47} kinetics in patients with multiple myeloma and hypercalcemia. *J Clin Invest* **43**:2132–45, 1964.

592. Bayrd, E. D.: The bone marrow on sternal aspiration in multiple myeloma. *Blood* **3**:987–1018, 1948.

593. Bayrd, E. D., and Heck, F. J.: Multiple myeloma. A review of eighty-three proved cases. *JAMA* **133**:147–57, 1947.

594. Best, W. R., Pisciotta, A. V., Donnelly, W. J., Fowler, W. M., Linman, J. W., Schwartz, S. O., and Louis, J.: Multiple myeloma. General aspects of diagnosis, course, and survival. *JAMA* **188**:741–45, 1964.

595. Braunsteiner, H., and Pakesch, F.: Electron microscopy and the functional significance of a new cellular structure in plasmocytes: a review. *Blood* **10**:650–54, 1955.

596. Brownell, E. G.: Multiple myeloma. Review of sixty-one proved cases. *Arch Intern Med* (Chicago) **95**:699–704, 1955.

597. Carson, C. P., Ackerman, L. V., and Maltby, J. D.: Plasma cell myeloma. A clinical, pathologic and roentgenologic review of 90 cases. *Amer J Clin Path* **25**:849–88, 1955.

598. Christopherson, W. M., and Miller, A. J.: A re-evaluation of solitary plasma-cell myeloma of bone. *Cancer* **3**:240–52, 1950.

599. Clark, H., and Muirhead, E. E.: Plasmacytosis of bone marrow. *Arch Intern Med* (Chicago) **94**:425–32, 1954.

600. Costanza, D. J., and Smoller, M.: Multiple myeloma with the Fanconi syndrome. *Amer J Med* **34**:125–33, 1963.

601. Engle, R. L., Jr., Woods, K. R., Castillo, G. B., and Pert, J. H.: Starch gel electrophoresis of serum proteins and urinary proteins from patients with multiple myeloma, macroglobulinemia, and other forms of dysproteinemia. Demonstration of diversity and complexity of protein alterations in 72 cases. *J Lab Clin Med* **58**:1–22, 1961.

602. Fahey, J. L.: Heterogeneity of myeloma protein. *J Clin Invest* **42**:111–23, 1963.

602a. Fahey, J. L.: Antibodies and immunoglobulins. I. Structure and function. II. Normal development and changes in disease. *JAMA* **194**:71–74; 255–58, 1965.

603. Farmer, R. G., Cooper, T., and Pascuzzi, C. A.: Cryoglobulinemia. Report of twelve cases with bone marrow findings. *Arch Intern Med* (Chicago) **106**:483–95, 1960.

604. Glenchur, H., Zinneman, H. H., and Hall, W. H.: A review of fifty-one cases of multiple myeloma. Emphasis on pneumonia and other infections as complications. *Arch Intern Med* (Chicago) **103**:173–83, 1959.

605. Györkey, F., and Curd, G. W., Jr.: Plasma cell leukemia. *Ann Med Intern Fenn* **50**:137–48, 1961, Fasc. 3.

606. Hayes, D. W., Bennett, W. A., and Heck, F. J.: Extramedullary lesions in multiple myeloma. Review of literature and pathologic studies. *Arch Path* (Chicago) **53**:262–72, 1952.

607. Heremans, J. F., Laurell, A. H. F., Mårtensson, L., Heremans, M. -Th., Laurell, C. -B., Sjöquist, J., and Waldenström, J.: Studies on "abnormal" serum globulins (M-components) in myeloma, macroglobulinemia and related diseases. *Acta Med Scand* **170** (Suppl. **367**):1–126, 1961.

608. Humphrey, J. H., and Fahey, J. L.: The metabolism of normal plasma proteins and gamma-myeloma protein in mice bearing plasma-cell tumors. *J Clin Invest* **40**:1696–1705, 1961.

609. Innes, J., and Newall, J.: Myelomatosis. *Lancet* 1:239–45, 1961.

610. Kenny, J. J., and Moloney, W. C.: Multiple myeloma: diagnosis and management in a series of 57 cases. *Ann Intern Med* 46:1079–91, 1957.

611. Klein, H., and Block, M.: Bone marrow plasmacytosis. A review of sixty cases. *Blood* 8:1034–41, 1953.

612. Korst, D. R., Clifford, G. B., Fowler, W. M., Louis, J., Will, J., and Wilson, H. E.: Multiple myeloma. II. Analysis of cyclophosphamide therapy in 165 patients. *JAMA* 189:758–62, 1964.

613. Korst, D. R., Frenkel, E. P., and Nixon, J. C.: Multiple myeloma. Studies of mouse plasma cell tumor and human myeloma responsiveness to cyclophosphamide (Cytoxan). *Ann Intern Med* 60:217–30, 1964.

614. Kyle, R. A., and Bayrd, E. D.: "Primary" systemic amyloidosis and myeloma. Discussion of relationship and review of 81 cases. *Arch Intern Med* (Chicago) 107:344–53, 1961.

615. Luttgens, W. F., and Bayrd, E. D.: Treatment of multiple myeloma with urethane. Experience with sixty-six cases over a two-and-a-half year period. *JAMA* 147:824–27, 1951.

616. Mackay, J. R., Eriksen, N., Motulsky, A. G., and Volwiler, W.: Cryo- and macroglobulinemia. Electrophoretic, ultracentrifugal and clinical studies. *Amer J Med* 20:564–87, 1956.

617. Martin, W. J., Mathieson, D. R., and Eigler, J. O. C.: Pyroglobulinemia: further observations and review of 20 cases. *Proc Mayo Clin* 34:95–101, 1959.

618. Moseley, J. E.: Patterns of bone change in multiple myeloma. *J Mount Sinai Hosp NY* 28:511–36, 1961.

619. Osserman, E. F.: Plasma-cell myeloma. II. Clinical aspects. *New Eng J Med* 261:952–60; 1006–14, 1959.

620. Osserman, E. F.: The plasmocytic dyscrasias. Plasma cell myeloma and primary macroglobulinemia. *Amer J Med* 31:671–75, 1961.

621. Osserman, E. F., and Lawlor, D.: Immunoelectrophoretic characterization of the serum and urinary proteins in plasma cell myeloma and Waldenström's macroglobulinemia. *Ann NY Acad Sci* 94:93–109, 1961.

622. Osserman, E. F., and Takatsuki, K.: Plasma cell myeloma: gamma globulin synthesis and structure. *Medicine* (Balt) 42:357–84, 1963.

623. Owen, J. A., and Got, C.: The biological significance of the anomalous serum and urinary proteins of myelomatosis, lymphoma, and other conditions. *J Clin Path* 13:58–68, 1960.

624. Perillie, P. E., and Conn, H. O.: Acute renal failure after intravenous pyelography in plasma cell myeloma. *JAMA* 167:2186–89, 1958.

625. Potter, M.: Plasma cell neoplasia in a single host: a mosaic of different protein-producing cell types. *J Exp Med* 115:339–56, 1962.

626. Potter, M., Fahey, J. L., and Pilgrim, H. I.: Abnormal serum protein and bone destruction in transmissible mouse plasma cell neoplasm (multiple myeloma). *Proc Soc Exp Biol Med* 94:327–33, 1957.

627. Putnam, F. W.: Aberrations of protein metabolism in multiple myeloma. Interrelationships of abnormal serum globulins and Bence-Jones proteins. *Physiol Rev* **37**:512–38, 1957.

628. Putnam, F. W.: Plasma-cell myeloma and macroglobulinemia. I. Physicochemical, immunochemical and isotopic turnover studies of the abnormal serum and urinary proteins. *New Eng J Med* **261**:902–8, 1959.

629. Rundles, R. W., Dillon, M. L., and Dillon, E. S.: Multiple myeloma. III. Effect of urethane therapy on plasma cell growth, abnormal serum protein components and Bence Jones proteinuria. *J Clin Invest* **29**:1243–60, 1950.

630. Snapper, I., Turner, L. B., and Moscovitz, H. L.: *Multiple Myeloma.* New York: Grune and Stratton, 1953, 168 p.

631. Solomon, A., and Fahey, J. L.: Bence Jones proteinemia. *Amer J Med* **37**:206–22, 1964.

632. Tomasi, T. B., Jr.: Human gamma globulin. *Blood* **25**:382–403, 1965.

633. Victor, M., Banker, B. Q., and Adams, R. D.: The neuropathy of multiple myeloma. *J Neurol Neurosurg Psychiat* **21**:73–88, 1958.

634. Waldenström, J.: Melphalan therapy in myelomatosis. *Brit Med J* **1**:859–65, 1964.

635. Weiss, D. L., and De Los Santos, R.: Urethane-induced hepatic failure in man. *Amer J Med* **28**:476–81, 1960.

636. Yentis, I.: Radiological aspects of myelomatosis. *Clin Radiol* **12**:1–7, 1961.

637. Zinneman, H. H.: Dysproteinemia. *Postgrad Med* **23**:550–60, 1958.

638. Zinneman, H. H., and Hall, W. H.: Recurrent pneumonia in multiple myeloma and some observations on immunologic response. *Ann Intern Med* **41**:1152–63, 1954.

Chapter 11. Other Myeloproliferative and Lymphoproliferative Disorders

Agnogenic Myeloid Metaplasia

639. Block, M., and Jacobson, L. O.: Myeloid metaplasia. *JAMA* **143**:1390–96, 1950.

640. Bouroncle, B. A., and Doan, C. A.: Myelofibrosis. Clinical, hematologic and pathologic study of 110 patients. *Amer J Med Sci* **243**:697–715, 1962.

641. Dameshek, W., and Gunz, F.: *Leukemia.* New York: Grune and Stratton, 2nd Ed., 1964, pp. 356–402.

642. Erf, L. A., and Herbut, P. A.: Primary and secondary myelofibrosis (a clinical and pathological study of thirteen cases of fibrosis of the bone marrow). *Ann Intern Med* **21**:863–89, 1944.

643. Green, T. W., Conley, C. L., Ashburn, L. L., and Peters, H. R.: Splenectomy for myeloid metaplasia of the spleen. *New Eng J Med* **248**:211–19, 1953.

644. Hill, J. M., and Duncan, C. N.: Leukemoid reactions. *Amer J Med Sci* **201**:847–57, 1941.

645. Korst, D. R., Clatanoff, D. V., and Schilling, R. F.: On myelofibrosis. *Arch Intern Med* (Chicago) **97**:169–83, 1956.

646. Leigh, T. F., Corley, C. C., Jr., Huguley, C. M., Jr., and Rogers, J. V., Jr.: Myelofibrosis. The general and radiologic findings in 25 proved cases. *Amer J Roentgen* **82**:183–93, 1959.

647. Linman, J. W.: Differential diagnosis of massive splenomegaly. Agnogenic myeloid metaplasia versus chronic granulocytic leukemia. *Med Clin N Amer* **46**:49–62, 1962.

648. Linman, J. W., and Bethell, F. H.: Agnogenic myeloid metaplasia. Its natural history and present day management. *Amer J Med* **22**:107–22, 1957.

649. Meilleur, P. A., and Meyers, M. C.: Thrombocytosis: a postsplenectomy complication in agnogenic myeloid metaplasia. *Amer J Med Sci* **241**:68–82, 1961.

650. Mitus, W. J., Bergna, L. J., Mednicoff, I. B., and Dameshek, W.: Alkaline phosphatase of mature neutrophils in chronic forms of the myeloproliferative syndrome. *Amer J Clin Path* **30**:285–94, 1958.

651. Nakai, G. S., Craddock, C. G., and Figueroa, W. G.: Agnogenic myeloid metaplasia: a survey of twenty-nine cases and a review of the literature. *Ann Intern Med* **57**:419–40, 1962.

652. Szur, L., and Smith, M. D.: Red-cell production and destruction in myelosclerosis. *Brit J Haemat* **7**:147–68, 1961.

653. Zucker, M. B., and Woodward, H. Q.: Elevation of serum acid glycerophosphatase activity in thrombocytosis. *J Lab Clin Med* **59**:760–70, 1962.

PRIMARY THROMBOCYTHEMIA

654. Fanger, H., Cella, L. J., Jr., and Litchman, H.: Thrombocythemia. Report of three cases and review of literature. *New Eng J Med* **250**:456–61, 1954.

655. Gunz, F. W.: Hemorrhagic thrombocythemia: a critical review. *Blood* **15**:706–23, 1960.

656. Levinson, B., Jones, R. S., Wintrobe, M. M., and Cartwright, G. E.: Thrombocythemia and pulmonary intra-alveolar coagulum in a young woman. *Blood* **13**:959–71, 1958.

657. Ozer, F. L., Truax, W. E., Miesch, D. C., and Levin, W. C.: Primary hemorrhagic thrombocythemia. *Amer J Med* **28**:807–23, 1960.

PRIMARY MACROGLOBULINEMIA

658. Adner, P. L., Wallenius, G., and Werner, I.: Macroglobulinemia and myelomatosis. *Acta Med Scand* **168**:431–37, 1960.

659. Bayrd, E. D.: Continuous chlorambucil therapy in primary macroglobulinemia of Waldenström: report of four cases. *Proc Mayo Clin* **36**:135–47, 1961.

660. Bloch, H. S., Prasad, A., Anastasi, A., and Briggs, D. R.: Serum protein changes in Waldenström's macroglobulinemia during administration of a low molecular weight thiol (Penicillamine). *J Lab Clin Med* **56**:212–17, 1960.

661. Bouroncle, B. A., Datta, P., and Frajola, W. J.: Waldenström's macroglobulinemia. Report of three patients treated with cyclophosphamide. *JAMA* **189**:729–32, 1964.

662. Butler, E. A., Flynn, F. V., Harris, H., and Robson, E. B.: The laboratory diagnosis of macroglobulinaemia with special reference to starch-gel electrophoresis. *Lancet* **2**:289–93, 1961.

663. Clatanoff, D. V., and Meyer, O. O.: Response to chlorambucil in macroglobulinemia. *JAMA* **183**:40–44, 1963.

664. Clausen, J., Rask-Nielsen, R., Christensen, H. E., Lontie, R., and Heremans, J.: Macroglobulinemia in a transplantable mouse leukemia. *Proc Soc Exp Biol Med* **103**:802–4, 1960.

665. Dutcher, T. F., and Fahey, J. L.: The histopathology of the macroglobulinemia of Waldenström. *J Nat Cancer Inst* **22**:887–918, 1959.

666. Kunkel, H. G.: Macroglobulins and high molecular weight antibodies. In *The Plasma Proteins*, Vol. 1, Putnam, F. W., Ed., New York: Academic Press, 1961, pp. 279–307.

667. Logothetis, J., Silverstein, P., and Coe, J.: Neurologic aspects of Waldenström's macroglobulinemia. Report of a case. *Arch Neurol* (Chicago) **3**:564–73, 1960.

668. Mackay, I. R.: Macroglobulins and macroglobulinaemia. *Aust Ann Med* **8**:158–70, 1959.

669. Mackay, I. R., Eriksen, N., Motulsky, A. G., and Volwiler, W.: Cryo- and macroglobulinemia. Electrophoretic, ultracentrifugal and clinical studies. *Amer J Med* **20**:564–87, 1956.

670. Osserman, E. F., and Lawlor, D.: Immunoelectrophoretic characterization of the serum and urinary proteins in plasma cell myeloma and Waldenström's macroglobulinemia. *Ann NY Acad Sci* **94**:93–109, 1961.

671. Pachter, M. R., Johnson, S. A., Neblett, T. R., and Truant, J. P.: Bleeding, platelets, and macroglobulinemia. *Amer J Clin Path* **31**:467–82, 1959.

672. Ritzmann, S. E., Thurm, R. H., Truax, W. E., and Levin, W. C.: The syndrome of macroglobulinemia. Review of the literature and a report of two cases of macrocryogelglobulinemia. *Arch Intern Med* (Chicago) **105**:939–65, 1960.

673. Rosen, F. S.: The macroglobulins. *New Eng J Med* **267**:491–97; 546–50, 1962.

674. Solomon, A., and Fahey, J.: Plasmapheresis therapy in macroglobulinemia. *Ann Intern Med* **58**:789–800, 1963.

675. Strisower, E. H., and Galleto, A. T.: Waldenström's macroglobulinemia. Differential diagnosis, lipoprotein study, and case report. *Amer J Med* **32**:304–12, 1962.

676. Waldenström, J.: Die makroglobulinämie. *Ergebn Inn Med Kinderheilk* 9:586–621, 1958.

Chapter 12. Hypersplenism

677. Aster, R. H., and Jandl, J. H.: Platelet sequestration in man. II. Immunological and clinical studies. *J Clin Invest* **43**:856–69, 1964.

678. Clough, P. W.: Auto-immunization and auto-antibodies. *Ann Intern Med* **52**:930–39, 1960.

679. Crosby, W. H.: Normal functions of the spleen relative to red blood cells: a review. *Blood* **14**:399–408, 1959.

680. Crosby, W. H.: Hypersplenism. *Ann Rev Med* **13**:127–46, 1962.

681. Dameshek, W.: Hypersplenism. *Bull NY Acad Med* **31**:113–36, 1955.

682. Dameshek, W., Schwartz, R., and Oliner, H.: Current concepts of auto-immunization: an interpretive review. *Blood* **17**:775–83, 1961.

683. Doan, C. A.: Hypersplenism. *Bull NY Acad Med* **25**:625–50, 1949.

684. Evans, R. S., Takahashi, K., Duane, R. T., Payne, R., and Liu, C.: Primary thrombocytopenic purpura and acquired hemolytic anemia. Evidence for a common etiology. *Arch Intern Med* (Chicago) **87**:48–65, 1951.

685. Giblett, E. R., Motulsky, A. G., Casserd, F., Houghton, B. and Finch, C. A.: Studies on the pathogenesis of splenic anemia. *Blood* **11**:1118–31, 1956.

686. Hayhoe, F. G. J., and Whitby, L.: Splenic function. A study of the rationale and results of splenectomy in blood disorders. *Quart J Med* **24**:365–91, 1955.

687. Jandl, J. H., Greenberg, M. S., Yonemoto, R. H., and Castle, W. B.: Clinical determination of the sites of red cell sequestration in hemolytic anemias. *J Clin Invest* **35**:842–67, 1956.

688. Jandl, J. H., Jacob, H. S., and Daland, G. A.: Hypersplenism due to infection. A study of five cases manifesting hemolytic anemia. *New Eng J Med* **264**:1063–71, 1961.

689. Knisely, M. H.: Spleen studies. I. Microscopic observations of the circulatory system of living unstimulated mammalian spleens. *Anat Rec* **65**:23–50, 1936.

690. Lipson, R. L., Bayrd, E. D., and Watkins, C. H.: The postsplenectomy blood picture. *Amer J Clin Path* **32**:526–32, 1959.

691. Mason, D. T., and Morris, J. J.: The variable features of Felty's syndrome. *Amer J Med* **36**:463–69, 1964.

692. Medoff, A. S., and Bayrd, E. D.: Gaucher's disease in 29 cases: hematologic complications and effect of splenectomy. *Ann Intern Med* **40**:481–92, 1954.

693. Motulsky, A. G., Casserd, F., Giblett, E. R., Broun, G. O., Jr., and Finch, C. A.: Anemia and the spleen. *New Eng J Med* **259**:1164–69; 1215–19, 1958.

694. Palmer, J. G., Eichwald, E. J., Cartwright, G. E., and Wintrobe, M. M.: The experimental production of splenomegaly, anemia and leukopenia in albino rats. *Blood* **8**:72–80, 1953.

695. Reich, C., Seife, M., and Kessler, B. J.: Gaucher's disease: a review, and discussion of twenty cases. *Medicine* (Balt) **30**:1–20, 1951.

696. Robinson, T. W., and Sturgeon, P.: Post-splenectomy infection in infants and children. *Pediatrics* **25**:941–51, 1960.

697. Shulman, N. R.: A mechanism of cell destruction in individuals sensitized to foreign antigens and its implications in auto-immunity. *Ann Intern Med* **60**:506–21, 1964.

698. Smith, C. H., Erlandson, M. E., Stern, G., and Hilgartner, M. W.: Postsplenectomy infection in Cooley's anemia. An appraisal of the problem in this and other blood disorders, with a consideration of prophylaxis. *New Eng J Med* **266**:737–43, 1962.

699. Sturgis, C. C.: *Hypersplenism. A Clinical Evaluation.* Springfield, Ill.: Charles C Thomas, 1953, 97 p.

700. Von Hamm, E., and Awny, A. J.: The pathology of hypersplenism. *Amer J Clin Path* **18**:313–22, 1948.

700a. Weiss, L., Ruhenstroth-Bauer, G., and Amorosi, E. L.: Hypersplenism. *Seminars in Hematology* **2**:205–85, 1965.

Chapter 13. Hemorrhagic Disorders

701. Aggeler, P. M., Hoag, M. S., Wallerstein, R. O., and Whissell, D.: The mild hemophilias. Occult deficiencies of AHF, PTC and PTA frequently responsible for unexpected surgical bleeding. *Amer J Med* **30**:84–94, 1961.

702. Alexander, B.: Anticoagulant therapy with coumarin congeners. *Amer J Med* **33**:679–91, 1962.

703. Barnhart, M. I., and Riddle, J. M.: Cellular localization of profibrinolysin (plasminogen). *Blood* **21**:306–21, 1963.

704. Bean, W. B.: *Vascular Spiders and Related Lesions of the Skin.* Springfield, Ill.: Charles C Thomas, 1958, pp. 132–57.

705. Biggs, R., and MacFarlane, R. G.: *Human Blood Coagulation and Its Disorders.* Philadelphia: F. A. Davis Company, 3rd Ed., 1962, 474 p.

706. Bithell, T. C., Didisheim, P., Cartwright, G. E., and Wintrobe, M. M.: Thrombocytopenia inherited as an autosomal dominant trait. *Blood* **25**:231–40, 1965.

707. Blombäck, M., Jorpes, J. E., and Nilsson, I. M.: von Willebrand's disease. *Amer J Med* **34**:236–41, 1963.

708. Bowie, E. J. W., Thompson, J. H., Jr., and Owen, C. A., Jr.: The blood platelet (including a discussion of the qualitative platelet diseases). *Proc Mayo Clin* **40**:625–53, 1965.

709. Breckenridge, R. T., and Ratnoff, O. D.: Studies on the nature of the circulating anticoagulant directed against antihemophilic factor: with notes on an assay for antihemophilic factor. *Blood* **20**:137–49, 1962.

710. Breckenridge, R. T., and Ratnoff, O. D.: Studies on the site of action of a circulating anticoagulant in disseminated lupus erythematosus. Evidence that this anticoagulant inhibits the reaction between activated Stuart factor (factor X) and proaccelerin (factor V). *Amer J Med* **35**:813–19, 1963.

711. Brinkhous, K. M.: Hemophilia—pathophysiologic studies and the evolution of transfusion therapy. *Amer J Clin Path* **41**:342–51, 1964.

712. Bunting, W. L., Kiely, J. M., and Campbell, D. C.: Idiopathic thrombocytopenic purpura. *Arch Intern Med* (Chicago) **108**:733–38, 1961.

713. Castaldi, P. A., Firkin, B. G., Blackwell, P. M., and Clifford, K. I.: An electron microscopic study of the changes in platelets during viscous metamorphosis. *Blood* **20**:566–80, 1962.

714. Cohen, P., Gardner, F. H., and Barnett, G. O.: Reclassification of the thrombocytopenias by the Cr^{51}-labeling method for measuring platelet life span. *New Eng J Med* **264**:1294–99; 1350–55, 1961.

715. Cohen, S. I., and Warren, R.: Fibrinolysis. *New Eng J Med* **264**:79–84; 128–34, 1961.

716. Conley, C. L.: Blood platelets and platelet transfusions. *Arch Intern Med* (Chicago) **107**:635–38, 1961.

717. Didisheim, P.: Hageman factor deficiency (Hageman trait). *Arch Intern Med* (Chicago) **110**:170–77, 1962.

718. Doan, C. A., Bouroncle, B. A., and Wiseman, B. K.: Idiopathic and secondary thrombocytopenic purpura: clinical study and evaluation of 381 cases over a period of 28 years. *Ann Intern Med* **53**:861–76, 1960.

719. Fletcher, A. P., Alkjaersig, N., and Sherry, S.: Fibrinolytic mechanisms and the development of thrombolytic therapy. *Amer J Med* **33**:738–52, 1962.

720. Gaston, L. W.: The blood-clotting factors. *New Eng J Med* **270**:236–42; 290–98, 1964.

721. Glynn, M. F., Movat, H. Z., Murphy, E. A., and Mustard, J. F.: Study of platelet adhesiveness and aggregation, with latex particles. *J Lab Clin Med* **65**:179–201, 1965.

722. Hampton, J. W., Bird, R. M., and Hammarsten, D. M.: Defective fibrinase activity in two brothers. *J Lab Clin Med* **65**:469–74, 1965.

723. Horowitz, H. F., and Fujimoto, M. M.: Acquired hemophilia due to a circulating anticoagulant. Report of two cases, with review of the literature. *Amer J Med* **33**:501–9, 1962.

724. Howell, M.: Acquired factor X deficiency associated with systematized amyloidosis—a report of a case. *Blood* **21**:739–44, 1963.

725. Jorpes, J. E.: Heparin, its chemistry, pharmacology and clinical use. *Amer J Med* **33**:692–701, 1962.

726. Koller, F.: Intravascular clotting and spontaneous fibrinolysis. *Acta Haemat* (Basel) **31**:239–46, 1964.

727. Lechler, E., Webster, W. P., Roberts, H. R., and Penick, G. D.: The

inheritance of Stuart disease. Investigation of a family with factor X deficiency. *Amer J Med Sci* **249**:291–94, 1965.

728. Levine, S., and Searn, M. A.: Thrombotic thrombocytopenic purpura and systemic lupus erythematosus. *Arch Intern Med* (Chicago) **113**:826–36, 1964.

729. Little, A. S., and Bell, H. E.: Painful subcutaneous hemorrhages of the extremities with unusual reaction to injected deoxyribonucleic acid. *Ann Intern Med* **60**:886–91, 1964.

730. MacWhinney, J. B., Jr., Packer, J. T., Miller, G., and Greendyke, R. M.: Thrombotic thrombocytopenic purpura in childhood. *Blood* **19**:181–99, 1962.

731. Marcus, A. J., and Zucker, M. B.: *The Physiology of Blood Platelets. Recent Biochemical, Morphologic and Clinical Research.* New York: Grune and Stratton, 1965, 162 p.

732. Marder, V. J., and Shulman, N. R.: Clinical aspects of congenital factor VII deficiency. *Amer J Med* **37**:182–205, 1964.

733. McElfresh, A. E.: Coagulation during the neonatal period. *Amer J Med Sci* **242**:771–79, 1961.

734. McMillan, C. W., Diamond, L. K., and Surgenor, D. M.: Treatment of classic hemophilia: the use of fibrinogen rich in factor VIII for hemorrhage and for surgery. *New Eng J Med* **265**:224–30; 277–82, 1961.

735. Merskey, C., Johnson, A. J., Pert, J. H., Wohl, H.: Pathogenesis of fibrinolysis in defibrination syndrome: effect of heparin administration. *Blood* **24**:701–15, 1964.

736. Meyers, M. C.: Results of treatment in 71 patients with idiopathic thrombocytopenic purpura. *Amer J Med Sci* **242**:295–302, 1961.

737. Mustard, J. F., Murphy, E. A., Rowsell, H. C., and Downie, H. G.: Factors influencing thrombus formation *in vivo. Amer J Med* **33**:621–47, 1962.

738. Najean, Y., Ardaillou, N., Caen, J., Larrieu, M. and Bernard, J.: Survival of radiochromium-labeled platelets in thrombocytopenias. *Blood* **22**:718–32, 1963.

739. Nussbaum, M., and Morse, B. S.: Plasma fibrin stabilizing factor activity in various diseases. *Blood* **23**:669–78, 1964.

740. Oski, F. A., Naiman, J. L., and Diamond, L. K.: Use of the plasma acid phosphatase value in the differentiation of thrombocytopenic states. *New Eng J Med* **268**:1423–31, 1963.

741. Owen, C. A., Jr., Amundsen, M. A., Thompson, J. H., Jr., Spittell, J. A., Jr., Bowie, E. J. W., Stilwell, G. G., Hewlett, J. S., Mills, S. D., Sauer, W. G., and Gage, R. P.: Congenital deficiency of factor VII (hypoconvertinemia). Critical review of literature and report of three cases, with extensive pedigree study and effect of transfusions. *Amer J Med* **37**:71–91, 1964.

742. Pearson, H. A., Shulman, N. R., Marder, V. J., and Cone, T. E., Jr.: Isoimmune neonatal thrombocytopenic purpura. Clinical and therapeutic considerations. *Blood* **23**:154–77, 1964.

742a. Pechet, L.: Fibrinolysis. *New Eng J Med* **273**:966–73; 1024–34, 1965.

743. Quick, A. J.: *Hemorrhagic Diseases.* Philadelphia: Lea & Febiger, 1957, 451 p.

744. Quick, A. J.: The diagnosis of common hereditary hemorrhagic diseases. *Ann Intern Med* **55**:201–9, 1961.

745. Rabinowitz, Y., and Dameshek, W.: Systemic lupus erythematosus after "idiopathic" thrombocytopenic purpura: a review. A study of systemic lupus erythematosus occurring after 78 splenectomies for "idiopathic" thrombocytopenic purpura, with a review of the pertinent literature. *Ann Intern Med* **52**:1–28, 1960.

746. Ratnoff, O. D.: The therapy of hereditary disorders of blood coagulation. *Arch Intern Med* (Chicago) **112**:92–111, 1963.

747. Ratnoff, O. D.: *Bleeding Syndromes.* Springfield, Ill.: Charles C Thomas, 1960, 287 p.

748. Ruffolo, E. H., Pease, G. L., and Cooper, T.: Thrombotic thrombocytopenic purpura. *Arch Intern Med* (Chicago) **110**:78–82, 1962.

749. Schwartz, R. S., Lewis, F. B., and Dameshek, W.: Hemorrhagic cutaneous anaphylaxis due to autosensitization to desoxyribonucleic acid. *New Eng J Med* **267**:1105–11, 1962.

750. Sharp, A. A.: Present status of platelet aggregation. *New Eng J Med* **272**:89–92, 1965.

751. Simpson, N., and Biggs, R.: The inheritance of Christmas factor. *Brit J Haemat* **8**:191–203, 1962.

752. Sise, H. S., Moschos, C. B., and Becker, R.: On the nature of hypercoagulability. *Amer J Med* **33**:667–78, 1962.

753. Stafford, J. L.: The fibrinolytic mechanism in haemostasis: a review. *J Clin Path* **17**:520–30, 1964.

754. Stefanini, M., and Dameshek, W.: *The Hemorrhagic Disorders.* New York: Grune and Stratton, 2nd Ed., 1962, 614 p.

755. Stefanini, M.: Studies on the hemostatic breakdown during massive replacement transfusions. *Amer J Med Sci* **244**:298–305, 1962.

755a. Strauss, H. S., and Bloom, G. E.: von Willebrand's disease. Use of a platelet-adhesiveness test in diagnosis and family investigation. *New Eng J Med* **273**:171–81, 1965.

756. Sutherland, D. A., and Clark, H.: Hemangioma associated with thrombocytopenia. Report of a case and review of the literature. *Amer J Med* **33**:150–57, 1962.

757. Tocantins, L. M., and Kazal, L. A.: *Blood Coagulation, Hemorrhage and Thrombosis.* New York: Grune and Stratton, 2nd Ed., 1964, 560 p.

758. Troup, S. B., and Lüscher, E. F.: Hemostasis and platelet metabolism. *Amer J Med* **33**:161–65, 1962.

759. Weiss, H. J., and Eichelberger, J. W.: The detection of platelet defects in patients with mild bleeding disorders. Use of a quantitative assay for platelet factor 3. *Amer J Med* **32**:872–83, 1962.

760. Weiss, H. J., and Eichelberger, J. W.: Secondary thrombocytopathia. Platelet factor 3 in various disease states. *Arch Intern Med* (Chicago) **112**:827–34, 1963.

761. Whissell, D. Y., Hoag, M. S., Aggeler, P. M., Kropatkin, M., and Garner, E.: Hemophilia in a woman. *Amer J Med* **38**:119–29, 1965.

762. Wurzel, H. A.: Incidence of various coagulation defects and their association with different diseases. *Amer J Med Sci* **241**:625–31, 1961.

Chapter 14. Blood Groups and Transfusions

763. Allen, J. G., and Sayman, W. A.: Serum hepatitis from transfusions of blood. *JAMA* **180**:1079–85, 1962.

764. Anderson, R. E., and Walford, R. L.: Direct demonstration of A, B, and Rh₀ (D) blood group antigens on human leukocytes. *Amer J Clin Path* **40**:239–45, 1963.

765. Barlas, G. M., and Kolff, W. J.: Transfusion reactions and their treatment, especially with the artificial kidney. *JAMA* **169**:1969–75, 1959.

766. Braude, A. I.: Transfusion reactions from contaminated blood. Their recognition and treatment. *New Eng J Med* **258**:1289–93, 1958.

767. Brittingham, T. E., and Chaplin, H., Jr.: The antigenicity of normal and leukemic human leukocytes. *Blood* **17**:139–65, 1961.

768. Davidsohn, I., and Stern, K.: Blood transfusion reactions: their causes and identification. *Med Clin N Amer* **44**:281–92, 1960.

769. DeGowin, E. L., Greenwalt, T. J., and Merrill, J. P. (Dameshek, W. moderator): Management of an incompatible hemolytic transfusion reaction. *Blood* **10**:1164–72, 1955.

770. Djerassi, I., Farber, S., and Evans, A. E.: Transfusions of fresh platelet concentrates to patients with secondary thrombocytopenia. *New Eng J Med* **268**:221–26, 1963.

771. Freireich, E. J., Kliman, A., Gaydos, L. A., Mantel, N., and Frei, E., III: Response to repeated platelet transfusion from the same donor. *Ann Intern Med* **59**:277–87, 1963.

772. Grove-Rasmussen, M., Lesses, M. F., and Anstall, H. B.: Transfusion therapy. *New Eng J Med* **264**:1034–44, 1961.

773. Jones, A. R., Diamond, L. K., and Allen, F. H., Jr.: A decade of progress in the Rh blood-group system. *New Eng J Med* **250**:283–88, 324–30, 1954.

774. Krevans, J. R., Jackson, D. P., Conley, C. L., and Hartmann, R. C.: The nature of the hemorrhagic disorder accompanying hemolytic transfusion reactions in man. *Blood* **12**:834–43, 1957.

775. Krugman, S.: The clinical use of gamma globulin. *New Eng J Med* **269**:195–201, 1963.

776. Ludbrook, J., and Wynn, V.: Citrate intoxication. A clinical and experimental study. *Brit Med J* **2**:523–28, 1958.

777. Meyers, M. C.: Blood groups and red cells antibodies. In Miller, S. E.:

A Textbook of Clinical Pathology. Baltimore: The Williams and Wilkins Company, 6th Ed., 1960, pp. 226–35.

778. Mollison, P. L.: *Blood Transfusion in Clinical Medicine.* Oxford: Blackwell Scientific Publications, 3rd Ed., 1961, 773 p.

779. Morgan, W. T. J., and Watkins, W. M.: Some aspects of the biochemistry of the human blood-group substances. *Brit Med Bull* **15**:109–13, 1959.

780. Payne, R., and Rolfs, M. R.: Further observations on leukoagglutinin transfusion reactions with special reference to leukoagglutinin transfusion reactions in women. *Amer J Med* **29**:449–58, 1960.

781. Race, R. R., and Sanger, R.: The inheritance of blood groups. *Brit Med Bull* **15**:99–108, 1959.

782. Race, R. R., and Sanger, R.: *Blood Groups in Man.* Oxford: Blackwell Scientific Publications, 4th Ed., 1962, 456 p.

783. Ramgren, O., Skold, E., and Tengberg, J.: Immediate, non-haemolytic reactions to blood transfusion. Analysis of a series of transfusions. *Acta Med Scand* **162**:211–23, 1958.

784. Ruesch, M., Miyatake, S., and Ballinger, C. M.: Continuing hazard of air embolism during pressure transfusions. *JAMA* **172**:1476–82, 1960.

785. Stern, K.: Unusual blood types as a cause of disease. *Med Clin N Amer* **46**:277–94, 1962.

786. Strumia, M. M.: The preservation of blood for transfusion. *Blood* **9**:1105–19, 1954.

787. Strumia, M. M., Crosby, W. H., Gibson, J. G., II, Greenwalt, T. J., Krevans, J. R., and Gannon, H. T.: General principles of blood transfusion. *Transfusion* **3**:301–46, 1963.

788. Trobaugh, F. E., Jr., and De Cataldo, F.: Management of transfusion reactions. *Med Clin N Amer* **43**:1537–51, 1959.

789. Wiener, A. S.: *Advances in Blood Grouping.* New York: Grune and Stratton, 1961, 549 p.

790. Wiener, A. S., and Wexler, I. B.: *Heredity of the Blood Groups.* New York: Grune and Stratton, 1958, 150 p.

Index

Bibliographic numbers are indicated in **boldface** type.

A

ABO blood group system, 521–23
  "Bombay" blood, 521
  genotypes, 522
  H substance, 521
  hemolytic transfusion reactions due to, 532
  inheritance, 521–22, **781, 782, 790**
  phenotypes, relative frequency, 522
  secretors, 521
Acanthocytes, 62
ACD solution, 527
Acetazolamide, in hyperuricemic obstructive uropathy, 361
Acetylcholinesterase, erythrocytic, in paroxysmal nocturnal hemoglobinuria, 151
Achlorhydria, in iron deficiency anemia, 175
  in normal subjects, 215
  in pernicious anemia, 199, 211
Achylia gastrica, in pernicious anemia, 199
Acid hemolysis test, 151
Acid phosphatase, serum, in agnogenic myeloid metaplasia, 435, **653**
  in immunothrombocytopenias, 493, **740**
Acid-citrate-dextrose solution, 527
Addisonian pernicious anemia, 204–11. *See also* Pernicious anemia
Addison's disease, anemia in, 155–56
  erythropoiesis in, 16
Adenosine diphosphate. *See* ADP
Adenosine triphosphate, 75–77
Adolescence, iron requirements, 160, 171

ADP, in erythrocytes, 75–77
  in platelet aggregation, 465
Adrenals, erythropoietic effects, 16
Agammaglobulinemia, leukemia and lymphoma in, 335, **475**
Agnogenic myeloid metaplasia, 430–40. *See also* Myeloid metaplasia, agnogenic
Agranulocytosis, 330–31
AHF. *See* Factor VIII
Alcohol, effect in Hodgkin's disease, 390, **529, 546**
Alder's anomaly, 311
Alkaline phosphatase, granulocyte, in agnogenic myeloid metaplasia, 434
  in chronic granulocytic leukemia, 363, **395, 515**
  in leukemoid reactions, 333
  in paroxysmal nocturnal hemoglobinuria, 151
  in polycythemia vera, 302–303, **330, 341**
  serum, in infectious mononucleosis, 322, **366**
  in plasmacytic myeloma, 421
Alkeran, 426
Alkylating agents, in agnogenic myeloid metaplasia, 439
  in autoimmune hemolytic anemias, 145
  biologic effects, 403, **538**
  in leukemia, 357, 367, 373, **429, 439, 445, 466**
  in lymphoma, 402–406, **531, 538, 547, 557, 558, 586**
  in plasmacytic myeloma, 425–27, **612, 613, 634**